Perspectives In Exercise Science and Sports Medicine
Volume I: Prolonged Exercise

Edited by

David R. Lamb, Ph.D.
Ohio State University

Robert Murray, Ph.D.
The Quaker Oats Company

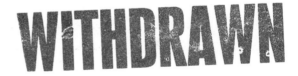

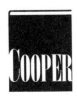

Library of Congress Cataloging in Publication Data:

LAMB, DAVID R., 1939 -

Perspectives In Exercise Science and Sports Medicine
Volume 1: Prolonged Exercise

Cover Design: Gary Schmitt

Library of Congress Catalog Card number: 88-70343

ISBN: 1-884125-34-4

Printed in the United States of America

10 9 8 7 6 5 4 3 2

The Publisher and Author disclaim responsibility for any adverse effects or consequences from the misapplication or injudicious use of the information contained within this text.

Contributors

Elizabeth Aaron, MS
University of Wisconsin
Madison, WI

Steven N. Blair, P.E.D.
Aerobics Institute
Dallas, TX

George A. Brooks, Ph.D.
Department of Physical Education
University of California-Berkeley
Berkeley, CA

Edmund R. Burke, Ph.D.
Spenco Medical Corporation
Waco, TX

John Cantwell, M.D.
Preventive Medicine Institute
Atlanta, GA

Carl J. Casperson, Ph.D.
Center for Health Promotion &
  Education
Center for Disease Control
Atlanta, GA

Edward F. Coyle, Ph.D.
Department of Physical Education
University of Texas
Austin, TX

J. Mark Davis, Ph.D.
Department of Physical Education
University of South Carolina
Columbia, SC

Jerome A. Dempsey, Ph.D.
Department of Preventive Medicine
University of Wisconsin Health Science
  Center
Madison, WI

Rod K. Dishman, Ph.D.
Department of Physical Education
University of Georgia
Athens, GA

Edward R. Eichner, M.D.
Department of Medicine
University of Oklahoma
Oklahoma City, OK

Peter A. Farrell, Ph.D.
Laboratory for Human Performance
  Research
Pennsylvania State University
University Park, PA

Carl V. Gisolfi, Ph.D.
Department of Exercise Science and
  Physical Education
University of Iowa
Iowa City, IA

Philip D. Gollnick, Ph.D.
Department of Veterinary Physiology/
  Pharmacology
Washington State University
Pullman, WA

James Hagberg, Ph.D.
Center for Exercise Science
University of Florida
Gainesville, FL

George A. Halaby, Ph.D.
The Quaker Oats Company
Barrington, IL

David R. Lamb, Ph.D.
School of Health, Physical Education,
  and Recreation
The Ohio State University
Columbus, OH

Daniel M. Landers, Ph.D.
Department of Health, Physical
  Education, and Recreation
Arizona State University
Tempe, AZ

Frank Landy, Ph.D.
Applied Psychology Institute
Pennsylvania State University
University Park, PA

Bruce J. Martin, Ph.D.
Indiana University
Department of Physiology
Bloomington, IN

Lyle J. Micheli, M.D.
Children's Hospital Medical Center
Boston, MA

Robert Murray, Ph.D.
The Quaker Oats Company
Barrington, IL

Ethan R. Nadel, Ph.D.
John B. Pierce Foundation Laboratory
New Haven, CT

Russell R. Pate, Ph.D.
Department of Physical Education
University of South Carolina
Columbia, SC

Peter B. Raven, Ph.D.
Department of Physiology
Texas College of Osteopathic Medicine
Fort Worth, TX

W. Michael Sherman, Ph.D.
School of Health, Physical Education &
    Recreation
The Ohio State University
Columbus, OH

Roy J. Shephard, M.D., Ph.D.
School of Health and Physical
    Education
University of Toronto
Toronto, Ontario
Canada

Glen H. J. Stevens, M.Sc.
Department of Physiology
Texas College of Osteopathic Medicine
Fort Worth, TX

Richard H. Strauss, M.D.
The Ohio State University
Columbus, OH

John R. Sutton, M.D.
McMaster University Medical Center
Hamilton, Ontario
Canada

Ronald L. Terjung, Ph.D.
St. University of New York
Department of Physiology
Upstate Medical Center
Syracuse, NY

Charles M. Tipton, Ph.D.
Department of Exercise and Sport
    Sciences
University of Arizona
Tucson, AZ

Garron Weiker, M.D.
Cleveland Clinic Foundation
Cleveland, OH

Christine L. Wells, Ph.D.
Department of Health and Physical
    Education
Arizona State University
Tempe, AZ

Acknowledgement

The Quaker Oats Company and Gatorade Thirst Quencher are proud to have facilitated this publication which resulted from collective deliberations and contributions during the 1987 Bermuda Conference on Prolonged Exercise. It represents the highest quality of scientific endeavor.

We at The Quaker Oats Company will continue our support of education and research in exercise science and sports medicine. By working together, we hope to make a significant contribution to the science and medicine of exercise.

Philip A. Marineau
Executive Vice President
The Quaker Oats Company

George A. Halaby
Vice President
Research and Development

Foreword

In the past few years The Quaker Oats Company has provided significant support to the area of Exercise Science and Sports Medicine. Internally, Quaker has developed a Sports Science Institute dedicated to the generation and dissemination of knowledge concerning sports science. The company has provided grant-in-aid for many American College of Sports Medicine projects including a Science Writers Conference series, program support to the Annual Meeting, and to the development of an annual Bermuda Conference on topics of concern and interest to the sports medicine specialist.

This represents the initial volume in the Quaker Bermuda Conference series and is the compilation of the efforts of more than forty leading scientists in exercise science and sports medicine. The conference consisted of closed door presentations and discussions of manuscripts concerning "Prolonged Exercise." In my opinion, this volume represents a significant step in the relationship between the scientist/educator and the corporate world, a relationship that will prove mutually beneficial to both worlds. I was happy and honored to be a part of the inaugural conference and wish continued success to all involved in future conferences.

> Peter B. Raven, Ph.D.
> President
> American College of Sports Medicine

Preface

Where does one find authoritative, comprehensive, up-to-date reviews of the scientific and medical aspects of prolonged exercise? We hope this book will provide a unique answer to that question. There are excellent books available about specific types of prolonged exercise, e.g., distance running or cycling, but these books are written by one or two authors who obviously cannot be expert in all aspects of the topic. More general books on exercise physiology or sports medicine obviously do not concentrate on prolonged exercise, and unwarranted extrapolations are often drawn from research done on brief exercise. Furthermore, because there is usually a long time between the initiation and completion of such books, they tend to be somewhat obsolete by the time they are published. In *Prolonged Exercise*, on the other hand, each chapter is written by an internationally acclaimed expert in the field, and a relatively brief 10 months passed between final drafts and publication. Our charge to the authors was to provide scientifically accurate, comprehensive, and readable reviews of the information available on their topics, to focus on evidence obtained from exercise of one to six hours duration, to avoid unwarranted extrapolations from research on less prolonged activity, and to emphasize areas that require further research before reasonable conclusions can be drawn. We are proud of the way the authors have met these objectives, and we believe this book will be a valuable addition to the libraries of those who teach, perform research, or engage in clinical practice related to exercise science, sports medicine, athletic training, and athletic coaching.

The chapters for this book were reviewed by the contributors at a conference held in Bermuda in June of 1987. After each author presented the salient arguments contained in the chapter, an assigned reactor and the other participants engaged in a spirited discussion of the points made and recommended numerous revisions in the text. The multidisciplinary nature of the discussion raised new perspectives for the authors, and the revised chapters reflect many of those viewpoints. The discussion points are presented at the end of each chapter. In some cases, most of the recommendations raised during the discussion were included in the revised chapter, the reactor was included as a coauthor, and the published discussion is thus quite brief. All participants expressed an appreciation for the high quality of the discussion. The only problem that arose was that time constraints meant that contributors sometimes were unable to get their oars deep enough in the debate waters to make their points adequately.

This book and conference in Bermuda would not have been possible without the support of the Quaker Oats Company and Gatorade Thirst Quencher. Quaker has made a major commitment to support high quality research and education in exercise science and sports medicine, and this book is the first in a series of volumes to be part of the commitment. We gratefully acknowledge Quaker's support of this endeavor and the high ethical standards they have established in providing that support.

Finally, we would like to express our appreciation to Leslie Walczak and the folks at McCord Travel and to Pam Schaffter and Mary Coolman, who diligently helped prepare this manuscript.

D. R. Lamb
R. Murray

Contents

Contributors iii
Acknowledgement v
Foreword vii
Preface ix

Chapter 1. Energy Metabolism and Prolonged Exercise 1
P. D. Gollnick
   I. Muscle Energy Reserves 2
   II. Energy Sources External to Muscle 5
   III. Fuel Use During Exercise 7
   IV. Carbohydrate Availability During Exercise 20
   V. Fat Utilization During Exercise 26
   VI. Amino Acid Oxidation During Exercise 30
   Summary 31
   Bibliography 31
   Discussion 37

Chapter 2. Cardiovascular Function and Prolonged Exercise . . 43
P. B. Raven and G. H. J. Stevens
   I. Cardiovascular Adjustments to Prolonged Exercise 44
   II. Cardiovascular Drift 46
   III. Myocardial Fatigue 57
   Summary 65
   Bibliography 67
   Discussion 71

Chapter 3. Pulmonary Function and Prolonged Exercise 75
J. A. Dempsey, E. Aaron and B. J. Martin
   I. Essential Elements of the Normal Response 76
   II. Failure of Pulmonary Gas Exchange 82
   III. Ventilatory Responses During Long-Term Work 85
   IV. Ventilatory Responses and Gas Exchange
      During Competitive Endurance Running 98
   V. Regulation of Breathing in Prolonged Exercise 100
   VI. Do Respiratory Muscles Fatigue During
      Prolonged Exercise? 103
   VII. Training Effects 107

VIII. Aging Effects 111
 IX. Hypoxic Effects 112
  X. Does the Lung Limit Prolonged Exercise
     Performance? 114
Bibliography 116
Discussion 119

Chapter 4. Temperature Regulation and Prolonged
              Exercise 125
E. R. Nadel
   I. Heat Transfer in the Body 127
  II. Heat Transfer from the Body 129
 III. Physiological Control of Heat Transfer Rates 131
  IV. Temperature Regulation During Prolonged Exercise ... 133
   V. Body Water Shifts During Exercise 135
  VI. Effects of Improved Fitness and Heat Acclimation 142
Summary 144
Bibliography 146
Discussion 147

Chapter 5. Endocrine Responses to Prolonged Exercise 153
J. R. Sutton and P. Farrell
    I. Endocrine Responses During Prolonged Exercise 156
   II. Endocrine Responses Associated with the Provision
       of Fuels for Prolonged Exercise 156
  III. Glucose Transport into Muscle: Insulin Receptors ... 158
   IV. Plasma Glucose and Prolonged Exercise 159
    V. Hormonal Changes Relevant to Glucose
       Homeostasis 162
   VI. Cortisol 170
  VII. Growth Hormone 174
 VIII. Reproductive Hormones 179
   IX. Endorphins and Enkephalins 187
    X. Fluid and Electrolyte Balance 191
   XI. What are the Implications of the Hormonal
       Response to Prolonged Exercise for the Physician, the
       Coach, and the Athlete? 194
Summary 197
Bibliography 198
Discussion 208

Chapter 6. Nutrition and Prolonged Exercise 213
W. M. Sherman and D. R. Lamb
    I. Energy Expenditure of Exercise 215

II. Dietary Practices of Athletes in Training 218
III. Fuel Reserves of the Body 221
IV. Nutrition During Training 229
V. Nutrition During the Week Before an Important
Performance 239
VI. The Preexercise Meal 244
VII. Water as a Primary Nutrient for Prolonged
Exercise 253
VIII. Gastric Emptying of Solutions Consumed
During Prolonged Exercise 261
IX. Carbohydrate Feedings During Prolonged Exercise . . .264
Summary 270
Bibliography 270
Discussion 277

Chapter 7. Psychological Factors and Prolonged Exercise 281
R. K. Dishman and F. J. Landy
I. Responses to Training in Top Athletes 283
II. Acute and Chronic Responses to Exercise in
Non-Athletes 294
III. Correlates of Performance During Acute Exercise 311
IV. Adherence to Prolonged Exercise in Preventive
Medicine 320
V. Motivation Models for the Study of Prolonged
Exercise 330
VI. Limitations of Research Design and Methodology 338
VII. Implications for Applied Research and Practice 341
Bibliography 343
Discussion 354

Chapter 8. Training for Performance of Prolonged Exercise . .357
C. L. Wells and R. R. Pate
I. Principles of Training for Prolonged Exercise 359
II. Current Training Regimens 368
III. Special Training Problems 378
Summary 383
Bibliography 386
Discussion 389

Chapter 9. Injuries and Prolonged Exercise 393
L. J. Micheli
I. Types of Overuse Injuries 394
II. Running Injuries 396
III. Risk Factors: Running 397

    IV. Assessing Risk Factors 398
     V. Sites of Running Injuries 400
    VI. Lower Leg Overuse Injuries 401
   VII. Swimming Injuries 403
  VIII. Cycling Injuries 403
    IX. Triathlon Injuries 404
  Summary...404
  Bibliography 405
  Discussion..407

Chapter 10. Other Medical Considerations in
               Prolonged Exercise **415**
  E. R. Eichner
     I. Sports Hematology 428
    II. Prolonged Exercise and the Urinary Tract 429
  III. Prolonged Exercise and the Gastrointestinal Tract 434
  Bibliography 437
  Discussion..440

Chapter 11. Exercise, Health, and Longevity.................**443**
  S. N. Blair
     I. Epidemiology of Physical Activity 446
    II. Participation in Physical Activity 448
  III. Prolonged Physical Activity and Health..............452
  IV. Treatment and Rehabilitation 466
    V. Risks of Exercise and Physical Activity...............468
  VI. Prolonged Physical Activity and Longevity 472
  VII. Recommendations 474
 VIII. Public Health Approach to Physical Activity
      and Exercise......................................475
  Summary...479
  Bibliography 480
  Discussion..484
  Index 489

1

Energy Metabolism and Prolonged Exercise

PHILIP D. GOLLNICK, PH.D.

INTRODUCTION
  I. MUSCLE ENERGY RESERVES
    A.   Adenosine Triphosphate (ATP)
    B.   Creatine Phosphate (CP)
    C.   Carbohydrates
    D.   Muscle Glycogen Stores
    E.   Fats
    F.   Fat Storage In Muscle
  II. ENERGY SOURCES EXTERNAL TO MUSCLE
    A.   Carbohydrates
    B.   Lipid Storage in Adipose Tissue
    C.   Total Body Fat Stores
  III. FUEL USE DURING EXERCISE
    A.   ATP
    B.   Creatine Phosphate
    C.   Carbohydrates
    D.   Muscle Glycogen Use
    E.   Control of Glycogenolysis at the Onset of Exercise
    F.   Glycogenolysis During Short, Heavy Exercise
    G.   Glycogenolysis During Prolonged Exercise
    H.   Energy Production From Carbohydrate
    I.   Energy Production from Lactate Formation
    J.   Energy Production from Carbohydrate Oxidation
    K.   Training and Carbohydrate Use
    L.   Patterns of Glycogen Depletion
    M.   Identification of Fuel Use During Exercise
    N.   Influence of Training on Fuel Use During Exercise
    O.   Disadvantages of Carbohydrate as Fuel
  IV. CARBOHYDRATE AVAILABILITY DURING EXERCISE
    A.   Carbohydrate Availability and Work Capacity
    B.   Consequence of Glycogen Depletion in Muscle
    C.   Gluconeogenesis
    D.   Repletion of Muscle Glycogen Following Exercise

V. FAT UTILIZATION DURING EXERCISE
   A.   Contribution of Plasma FFA
   B.   Intramuscular Lipids as Fuel
   C.   Effect of Training on Fat Metabolism
   D.   Repletion of Body Fat Stores After Exercise
VI. AMINO ACID OXIDATION DURING EXERCISE
SUMMARY
BIBLIOGRAPHY
DISCUSSION

INTRODUCTION

Muscular exercise is accomplished by the transformation of chemical energy to mechanical energy within skeletal muscle. The primary source of fuel for this energy conversion is provided by the oxidation of carbohydrates and fats. The relative contribution that each fuel makes to the overall energy consumption during exercise depends on:

1. Exercise intensity.
2. Exercise duration.
3. Athlete's fitness.
4. Athlete's diet and nutritional status.
5. Presence of metabolic diseases and genetic errors in metabolism.

I. MUSCLE ENERGY RESERVES

A. Adenosine Triphosphate (ATP)

ATP is the metabolic intermediary in the energy flow from stored energy compounds (primarily carbohydrates and fats) and muscular contraction. ATP is formed during the oxidation of carbohydrates and fats and is eventually hydrolyzed by contracting muscle to adenosine diphosphate (ADP) and inorganic phosphate. The amount of ATP present in skeletal muscle can only power intense exercise for a few seconds. There are differences in the ATP concentrations between the major fiber types of animals (Fig. 1-1), particularly in the rat (88). Attempts to establish the existence of differences in the ATP concentrations to the different fiber types in human skeletal muscle (121) have produced less definitive results.

B. Creatine Phosphate (CP)

The role of CP is to rephosphorylate ADP to ATP. The concentration of CP in muscle is three to four times greater than that of ATP (Fig. 1-1). There are differences in the concentration of CP be-

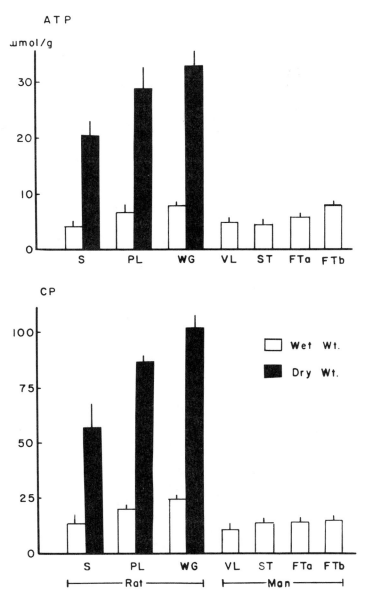

FIGURE 1-1. *ATP (top panel) and CP (bottom panel) concentrations in the different muscle and fiber types of rat and human skeletal muscle. Data are adopted from Kelso et al. (88) and Saltin and Gollnick (121). Values are presented both as wet and dry weight concentrations. Kelso et al. (88) have also presented these values on the basis of protein and total creatine.*

tween the major fiber types of muscle, CP concentration being highest in fast twitch (low oxidative) muscle fibers.

C. Carbohydrates

Carbohydrates are compounds having a ratio of one carbon atom to water ($C:H_2O$). Glucose, fructose, and galactose, all $C_6H_{12}O_6$, are common dietary carbohydrates. Of these monosaccharides, glucose is the most important in metabolism. Glucose is stored in plant and animal cells in polymer form. In plants, the storage form of glucose is called starch, a straight chain polymer ranging widely in molecular weight from 50,000 to several million. In animals, glucose is stored in cells as glycogen and the polymerization process includes branchings that result in a tree-like formation.

The branched structure of glycogen increases the number of terminal glucose units. This is advantageous during periods of high intensity exercise because rapid degradation is needed to provide energy. The many terminal sites that are available to the glycogen phosphorylase enzyme enhance the rapidity of glycogen breakdown (glycogenolysis). Conversely, the many end points on the glycogen molecule provide multiple sites for the addition of glucose units during glycogen synthesis (glycogenesis).

The branch points in glycogen complicate its degradation by requiring the action of debranching and transferase enzymes, in addition to phosphorylase. These enzymes are necessary since phosphorylase can degrade the straight chain part of the glycogen molecule only when it is longer than 4 glucosyl units. When the straight chains are reduced to 4 glucosyl units, the so-called "limit dextran," the transfer process, catalyzed by the transferase enzyme, produces another straight chain. Free glucose is formed within muscle as a result of the debranching process. Since about 8% of the glucosyl units in glycogen are at branch points, significant amounts of free glucose are produced in muscle when the rate of glycogenolysis is high. The glucose produced during glycogenolysis can be released from muscle cells or phosphorylated to glucose-6 phosphate (G-6-P) via the hexokinase reaction.

Glycogen is stored in tissue with 2.7 g of water per g glycogen (106). This reduces the effective caloric value of glycogen (i.e., the energy to wet weight ratio) as an energy reserve.

D. Muscle Glycogen Stores

The glycogen concentration of skeletal muscle of individuals consuming a mixed diet is approximately 80 mmol of glucose units $\cdot$ kg wet muscle^{-1} or about 15 g glycogen $\cdot$ kg muscle^{-1}. With skeletal muscle representing about 40% of body weight, an 80 kg person would store 480 g of glycogen in skeletal muscle, or about 2000 kcal. This assumes, probably incorrectly, that all skeletal muscles have similar glycogen concentrations. The glycogen concentration in skeletal muscle at rest depends upon the athlete's immediate past history relative to diet, exercise, and state of training (48). Thus, values of twice normal or more, as well as below normal, exist in human skeletal muscle. There are differences in the concentrations of glycogen within the different types of skeletal muscle in the rat (88) but there is less variation for human muscle (121) (Fig. 1-2). As indicated in Fig. 1-2, human skeletal muscle also appears to contain more stored fat than does rat limb muscle.

E. Fats

Fats, like carbohydrates, are also composed of carbon, hydrogen, and oxygen. Fats differ from carbohydrates in that about 90% of the molecule is carbon and hydrogen. The most important types of fat, from the standpoint of fuel use by muscle, are the fatty acids. Fatty acids have the general formula $CH_3(CH_2)_nCOOH$, where n represents the number of repeating CH_2 groups. Most fatty acids that are important for mammalian energy metabolism during exercise have from 12 to 18 total carbons. The turnover of palmitic acid, $CH_3(CH_2)_{14}COOH$, is a good indicator of the use of all free fatty acids (FFA) in the plasma (67).

F. Fat Storage in Muscle Fibers

The amount of energy stored in the muscle fibers, as triglycerides, is rather small as compared to glycogen, ranging from 7 to 25 umol·g wet muscle^{-1}. There is considerable variation in the amount of fat stored within regions of fibers and between the different fiber types for both man and animals (Fig. 1-2). Highly oxidative fibers possess more stored lipid than the low oxidative fibers, and lipid storage may increase with training (114).

II. ENERGY SOURCES EXTERNAL TO MUSCLE

A.   Carbohydrates

The major source of carbohydrate located outside of the muscle fiber, and yet available to it, is found in liver (103,104,105). The liver, with an average weight of 1.2 kg, contains about 100 g of glycogen (85 g·kg wet weight^{-1}). However, this ranges widely, from nearly zero to 110 g·kg^{-1}, depending on the athlete's nutritional state, fitness, and exercise history. In a fed state, the average caloric value of liver glycogen is about 400 kcal. Liver glycogenolysis and the subsequent release of glucose into the bloodstream is an essential mech-

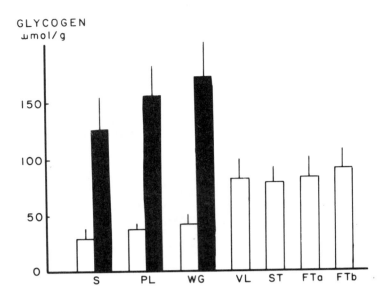

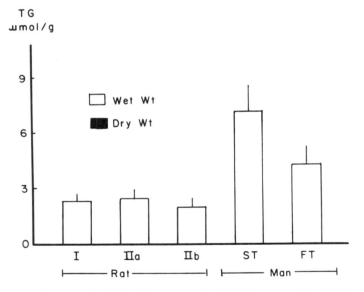

FIGURE 1-2. *Glycogen and triglyceride concentration in different muscles and fibers found in rat and human skeletal muscle. Data are adapted from Saltin and Gollnick (121). Values for glycogen are in umoles of glucose units.*

anism for maintaining normal blood glucose levels during exercise and between meals.

The concentration of glucose in blood and other extracellular fluids is 1 $g \cdot L^{-1}$ or 5.55 $mmol \cdot L^{-1}$. This amounts to approximately 10 g for the 10 to 15 liters of extracellular fluid. Although the glucose in blood supports the metabolism of erythrocytes and leukocytes, it is also important for other peripheral tissues, notably the nervous system. The glucose in blood and extracellular fluid can be thought of as carbohydrate in transport, and is relatively unimportant as an energy reserve, unless it is continually replenished by the liver. The importance of the liver in providing a continual supply of glucose is illustrated by the fact that the average oxygen consumption of the brain is approximately 50 $mL \cdot min^{-1}$, which is equal to a consumption of approximately 4 grams of glucose $\cdot h^{-1}$. Therefore, unless the blood glucose content is constantly replenished by the liver, hypoglycemia will quickly occur.

B. Lipid Storage in Adipose Tissue

Lipids are stored primarily in adipose tissue, where fatty acids are complexed to glycerol to form neutral fats, also commonly referred to either as triglycerides or triacylglycerols (TG). These TGs within the fat cell (adipocytes) are a relatively undiluted store of energy. Thus, the ratio of energy to wet weight is high. The chemical characteristics of the lipids stored in and used by the body are influenced by diet.

C. Total Body Fat Stores

The total amount of fat energy stored in the human body varies widely. The minimum fat content compatible with normal health is approximately 5% of the body weight. This fat is contained in such tissues as skin, nerves and brain, and bone marrow. It is perhaps impossible to establish the upper limit for total fat storage. However, fat storage is known to exceed 50% of the total body weight in severely obese individuals. On average, males are between 15% to 25% fat, whereas, in females, the range is between 25% and 35%, with women having more essential fat than men. The fat weight of male and female athletes is comparably less but also varies widely. Based on the body weight of 60 kg, this fat store amounts to an energy reserve in excess of 150,000 kcal.

III. FUEL USE DURING EXERCISE

A. ATP

It may seem inappropriate to consider ATP as a metabolic fuel since it appears to always be in a state of turnover. The end result of ATP turnover is that, for most exercise conditions, the ATP content of muscle remains constant. However, since the demand for ATP by the contractile elements establishes the metabolism of the muscle, it is appropriate to begin any discussion of fuels for muscular contraction with a short examination of the dynamics that surround the status of ATP within the muscle.

In one of the first reports of a decline of ATP during exercise in man, ATP was observed to have been reduced by approximately 20% following heavy exercise (76). Saltin and co-workers (85,86,89) observed reductions in ATP ranging from 10% to 45% in response to exercise ranging in intensity from 20% to 114% of the $\dot{V}O_2$max (Fig. 1-3). These estimates of the decline in ATP following exercise were made from samples obtained with the needle biopsy method. Since some time can elapse between termination of the exercise and collection of the sample (during which time a restoration of ATP can occur), the magnitude of the decline in ATP provoked by the exercise may have been underestimated in these studies. However, similar reductions in the ATP concentration in human skeletal muscle have been observed with ^{31}P nuclear magnetic resonance (127), where, presumably there is no time delay. It should be pointed out that a decline in ATP is not always observed at the point of exhaustion (127).

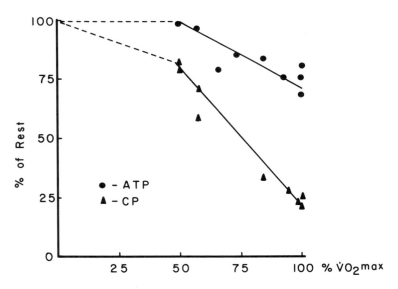

FIGURE 1-3. *Effect of different intensities of exercise on the ATP and CP concentrations in human skeletal muscle. Data are adopted from Karlsson et al. (86).*

Tetanic stimulation of rat muscle can reduce the ATP concentration (129) to approximately 50% of that at rest, a value similar to that observed in human muscle after voluntary exercise. These reductions are similar for both high and low oxidative type muscle.

Although the ATP concentration in muscle declines with exercise, the change is small when related to the total turnover of ATP within the active muscle cell. Thus, an oxygen uptake of 150 $mL \cdot kg^{-1} \cdot min^{-1}$ of muscle is equivalent to more than a 40-fold turnover of ATP every minute. It should be noted that an oxygen uptake of 150 $mL \cdot kg^{-1} \cdot min^{-1}$ is less than 50% of the maximal capacity of muscle (4) and far below the capacity of muscle to use ATP. Training reduces the magnitude of the decline in ATP that occurs during various intensities of exercise (86).

The small amount of ATP within muscle is not quantitatively an important energy store. Nonetheless, a significant change in its content within skeletal muscle during exercise could have important implications for the cells' ability to continue contracting. The advantage of using ATP as an immediate energy source is that it is contained in muscle at the contractile site, and there is no metabolism required to produce it at the onset of activity. It is, thus, a true anaerobic energy source. The major disadvantage of ATP as an energy source is its limited availability in muscle. Although the ATP content of muscle may decline during exercise, the magnitude of this decrease varies widely and cannot be used as an indicator of fatigue (127).

B. Creatine Phosphate

The concentration of CP in skeletal muscle is only three or four times that of ATP. The CP content in muscle can be nearly depleted (64,76,86), depending upon the duration and intensity of exercise (Fig. 1-3). If there were no resynthesis of CP during exercise, CP depletion would occur after only a few seconds of maximal contractile activity. Although the CP concentration of muscle can decline to nearly zero, there is no evidence that its depletion per se is responsible for fatigue. The decline in CP during exercise is less after, as compared to before, training (86).

A long-held view has been that the role of CP is to donate high energy phosphate and thereby prevent a fall in ATP during exercise. An alternative view is that CP is part of a system for translocating ATP from its site of synthesis within the mitochondria to the site of its hydrolysis at the interaction of the actin and myosin filaments. This has been referred to as the "creatine-creatine phosphate shuttle". The evidence for the existence of this shuttle system has been summarized by Bessman and Carpenter (13). The shuttle system is envisaged as delivering high energy phosphate directly to the site of its use during contraction without requiring intracellular transport of the relatively large ATP molecule. Currently, no evidence exists that the translocation of ATP generated from the Embden-Meyerhof pathway to the site of use in muscle contraction is via a CP shuttle system. However, the demonstration that the enzymes of this system are bound in an ordered manner to cellular components makes this an attractive possibility. The high concentration of CP found in low oxidative muscle should create a favorable environment for the operation of such a system. Although the relative importance of CP in energy production and as a high energy phosphate carrier within the cell is being debated, the fact remains that the concentration of CP in skeletal muscle declines during exercise.

The advantages and disadvantages of CP as energy sources during exercise are the same as those for ATP. Thus, ATP and CP are important energy sources during high intensity exercise lasting only a few seconds. In such cases, ATP and CP may be the only energy sources utilized.

C. Carbohydrates

Glucose is the principal currency for carbohydrate metabolism by active skeletal muscle. Glucose can originate either from muscle glycogen or from glucose taken up from the blood. Glucosyl units are cleaved from the glycogen molecule by action of phosphorylase, which produces glucose⁻1-PO$_4$ (G-1-P), as described above. The glucose that enters the cell from the blood is phosphorylated to G-6-P by hexokinase at the expense of ATP. Neither G-1-P nor G-6-P can diffuse out of the cell, and, therefore, glucose is captured either for the immediate energy needs of the muscle cell or for storage.

Liver cells can dephosphorylate G-6-P via the action of the enzyme glucose-6-phosphatase and by this mechanism, the liver releases glucose into the blood. In this manner, the liver can function as a glucose reservoir for maintaining a relatively constant blood glucose concentration. Though lacking glucose-6-phosphatase, muscle can release carbohydrate either as free glucose, produced by cleavage at the glycogen branch points, or as a glucose precursor, lactate. Both free glucose and lactate can diffuse out of the cell and can be taken up by other cells.

D. Muscle Glycogen Use

Muscle glycogen use varies as a function of the time and duration of the exercise (Fig. 1-4). There also appears to be an order in the manner that glycogen is depleted from the different fibers of

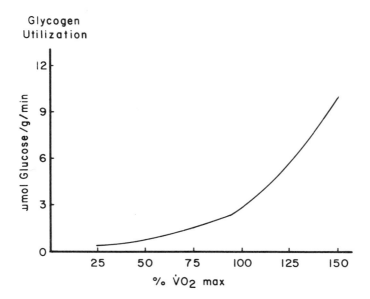

FIGURE 1-4. *The relationship between the rate of glycogen utilization and exercise intensity expressed as a percent of the maximal oxygen uptake.*

muscle (Fig. 1-5). Of special importance is the observation that during moderately intense exercise, requiring between 60% to 80% of the $\dot{V}O_2$max, fatigue occurs when muscle glycogen stores are depleted. The relative contribution that glycogen makes to the total metabolism during exercise depends upon the factors listed above.

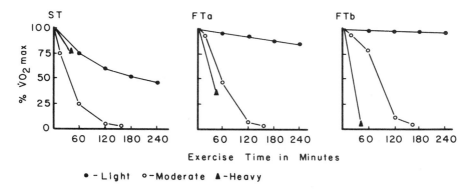

FIGURE 1-5. *Rate of glycogen disappearance from the different fiber types of human skeletal muscle during exercise of varying intensities expressed as percentages of the maximal oxygen uptake. Light, moderate, and heavy exercise are at 30%–40%, 60%–70%, and about 90% of the maximal oxygen uptake, respectively.*

ENERGY METABOLISM AND PROLONGED EXERCISE **11**

The role of glycogen as a fuel during exercise can be summarized by the following points:

1. Glycogen storage in muscle can range from 10 to 50 $g \cdot kg$ wet muscle^{-1}.
2. Glycogen has a high energy yield per liter of oxygen uptake (approximately 5.1 $kcal \cdot L \ O_2^{-1}$).
3. Glycogen can be metabolized both aerobically and anaerobically.
4. There is a rapid activation of the metabolic pathways for glycogen metabolism at the onset of exercise.
5. Glycogen concentration can be greatly increased by training and diet.
6. Glycogen can be the sole source of energy during heavy exercise.

E. Control of Glycogenolysis at the Onset of Exercise

Glycogen is broken down under the influence of the enzyme phosphorylase (PHOS) (69). Glycogenolysis is a regulated process, since PHOS, at times of low metabolism (e.g., at rest), exists in a form (PHOS b) that is inactive except in the presence of AMP. At the onset of muscular contraction there is a rapid conversion of PHOS b to PHOS a, the enzyme form that is most active. This conversion results in a rapid phosphorylysis of glycogen with the formation of glucose-1-phosphate (G-1-P) units (22,26,37,92,93,110). Activation of PHOS occurs by activation of the enzyme phosphorylase b kinase, which is also inactive in resting muscle when the free calcium concentration is low and muscle pH is around 7.0 (92,93). At the onset of contraction, a rapid elevation in free calcium and alkalization occurs in muscle (96). These events trigger activation of phosphorylase b kinase, which converts PHOS b to PHOS a. Thus, activation of glycogenolysis is linked to the contractile activity of the muscle fibers.

Activation of another key regulator enzyme, phosphofructokinase, occurs in concert with that of PHOS (131). This coordinates the further degradation of the glucosyl units through the Embden-Meyerhof pathway to generate pyruvate for both the anaerobic and aerobic production of ATP. In addition to the activation of PHOS by calcium and the initial rise in pH, there are many other factors that control the breakdown of glycogen to pyruvate. Included are increases in adenosine monophosphate (AMP), inorganic phosphate, ammonium, and fructose-1,6-bisphosphate, all of which modulate the activity of phosphofructokinase (131). It is unclear how all these factors operate to regulate the total amount of glycogen breakdown and flux through the Embden-Meyerhof pathway.

F.   Glycogenolysis During Short, Heavy Exercise

During short, heavy exercise there is a rapid breakdown of gly-cogen and a large production of lactate. The rate of lactate produc-tion in human skeletal muscle under such exercise conditions may be as high as 40 mmol $\cdot$ kg^{-1} $\cdot$ min^{-1} (23). This increase in lactate pro-duction is linearly related to the lowering of muscle pH (117). It is commonly claimed that this decline in pH depresses the flux of glu-cosyl units through the Embden-Meyerhof pathway. This is thought to occur by an inhibition of the key enzyme phosphofructokinase (PFK). The most frequently cited evidence for this inhibition is the study of Trevidi and Danforth (131), in which it was reported that the PFK activity in homogenates of frog muscle was almost abol-ished at a pH of about 6.9. When considered from the standpoint of events that are known to occur both in intact mammalian and in isolated frog muscle, the near complete inhibition of PFK at such a high pH seems unlikely. The conclusion that the Embden-Meyerhof pathway is not as sensitive to relatively small changes in pH is based on the following line of reasoning:

1. There are numerous reports of skeletal muscle pH in the 6.2 to 6.4 range after exercise. In fact, a muscle pH of 5.9 was reported using NMR.
2. The major cause for the decline in pH of muscle during ex-ercise is the free protons released into the cytosol during lac-tate production.
3. For the pH of skeletal muscle to decline below 6.8, there must be a continued production and accumulation of lactate in muscle.
4. Lactate production continues well beyond the concentration that results in a skeletal muscle pH of 6.8.
5. A close examination of the properties of PFK, under condi-tions where other modulators were adjusted to mimic those within the cell, suggests that PFK is not as pH labile as orig-inally thought (36).

G.   Glycogenolysis During Prolonged Exercise

As exercise becomes prolonged, there is a decline in the per-centage of PHOS in the *a* form, and yet glycogenolysis continues (22,26). This may be linked to the fact that, as exercise continues, the initial alkalization is replaced either by a return to a normal pH with light exercise or to a reduced pH with heavy exercise (73,117). The reduction in pH is closely coupled to the concentration of lac-tate within the muscle. Glycogenolysis can also be initiated by the action of hormones, particularly epinephrine and norepinephrine, from the sympathetic nervous system and adrenal medulla (37,69,110). Although some (46) have suggested that glycogenolysis is tightly coupled with a release of catecholamines from the adrenal medulla, it is hard to understand the role these hormones play in the control of glycogenolysis, since there is a decline in PHOS *a* with prolonged exercise while glycogen breakdown continues. Moreover, there is ample evidence demonstrating that glycogenolysis can be initiated and sustained in skeletal muscle and liver in the absence of these hormones (21,22,37,49,65,110,122). With very prolonged exercise, the contribution of glycogen metabolism declines as the oxidation of fatty acids increases (38). Thus, with prolonged exercise, there are shifts in the manner in which glycogenolysis is regulated.

H. Energy Production From Carbohydrate

Energy can be released both from lactate production (an anaerobic process), and from the terminal oxidation of glucose to CO_2 and H_2O (an aerobic process). The efficiency of the energy captured as ATP by each of these processes is actually fairly similar when related to the fall in free energy within the system. There is a fall in total free energy of 47 kcal when 1 mol of glucose is oxidized to 2 mol of pyruvate (or lactate). The energy conserved in the net synthesis of 3 mol of ATP (21 kcal) during pyruvate or lactate formation indicates that 45% (21/47) of the available energy is transferred to ADP. When glucose oxidation proceeds to CO_2 and H_2O the total fall in free energy is 686 kcal with 252 kcal of energy conserved as ATP (36 mol ATP at 7 $kcal \cdot mol^{-1}$), an efficiency of 37% (252/686). The difference in the anaerobic and aerobic energy production from carbohydrate is not in the biochemical conservation of energy but in the fall in free energy within the muscle cell in relation to the amount retained as ATP. There is still a large amount of energy in the lactate that diffuses from the muscle fiber, and the escape of lactate from the muscle cell is equivalent to "throwing it away." Since this energy is subsequently recovered by the oxidation of lactate either within active muscle or other tissues, or with resynthesis of lactate to glucose or glycogen, this energy is surely not lost to the body, but is lost only (and perhaps only temporarily) from the muscle from which lactate escapes. In this sense, any method that the muscle can use to produce energy without the release of lactate is beneficial to the overall energy status of the cell.

I. Energy Production from Lactate Formation

Lactate production can make a significant contribution to the overall energy production of muscle. The energy added to the total energy pool by lactate formation varies between muscle fiber types as a function of the concentration of enzymes for the Emdben-Meyerhof (glycolytic) pathway. (For a discussion of fiber type classification, fiber metabolic potentials, and blood supply, see Saltin and Gollnick (121), Gollnick and Hodgson (58), and Armstrong and Laughlin (5).) For the rat, the maximal rate of lactate production by fibers with high concentrations of glycolytic enzymes (Type II fibers) is about 0.5 umol $\cdot$ g^{-1} wet weight $\cdot$ s^{-1}, whereas fibers with low concentrations of these enzymes (Type I fibers) have a maximal rate of about half this (128). Lactate has been observed to accumulate in human muscle at a rate of about 0.9 umol $\cdot$ g^{-1} wet weight $\cdot$ s^{-1}. With an ATP production of 1.5 umol ATP $\cdot$ umol^{-1} lactate, maximal lactate production in human muscle would result in an ATP production of approximately 1.35 umol $\cdot$ g wet weight$^{-1} \cdot$ s^{-1}. The maximal rate of ATP utilization is approximately 3.0 umol $\cdot$ g wet weight$^{-1} \cdot$ s^{-1}. This energy production can therefore cover nearly half of the energy requiried for maximal contractile activity of human skeletal muscle during brief exercise. Thus, ATP production from lactate formation is important to the total energy consumption of muscle under some circumstances.

J. Energy Produced from Carbohydrate Oxidation

The energy oxidation equivalent for the terminal oxidation of glucose to CO_2 and H_2O is about 5.1 kcal $\cdot$ L^{-1} of oxygen. The number of kcal liberated from the terminal oxidative process can then be calculated from the oxygen consumption and will simply be a function of the $\dot{V}O_2$ multiplied by 5.1 when carbohydrate is the only substrate being oxidized.

K. Training and Carbohydrate Use

There is extensive evidence demonstrating a decreased use of carbohydrate during submaximal exercise after training (9,24,25,8). The respiratory exchange ratio is lower and increases in blood lactate are minimized during exercise following endurance training. These data have been verified by studies in which direct measurements of muscle glycogen and respiratory quotients (RQ) across the muscles were recorded and from evaluation of muscle and blood lactate dynamics (55,70,87).

L. Patterns of Glycogen Depletion

With exercise there is an ordered recruitment of motor units in skeletal muscle (Fig. 1-4). (For a more detailed description of motor units and their control during exercise see Saltin and Gollnick (121).) The essential element of this recruitment order is that the slow-twitch motor units (Type I) are the most easily activated and are consequently the first to be activated during exercise. With prolonged exercise, these fibers may be the first to fatigue with subsequent recruitment of high oxidative fast-twitch units (Type IIa). With continued activity low oxidative fast-twitch (Type IIb) motor units can be recruited. With high intensity exercise, all motor units can be engaged at the onset of exercise. The pattern of motor unit recruitment can be determined by the pattern of glycogen depleted from the different fiber types (See Armstrong et al. (6) and Gollnick et al. (51–55).)

M.   Identification of Fuel Use During Exercise

Several methods are available to evaluate the contribution of different fuels to metabolism during exercise. The simplest method employs the respiratory exchange ratio RER (R-value), which is the ratio of carbon dioxide production to oxygen uptake ($\dot{V}CO_2/\dot{V}O_2$). An RER value of 1.0 is indicative that carbohydrate metabolism is predominating. This conclusion is based on the stoichiometry for the oxidation of carbohydrates, which is $C_6H_{12}O_6 + 6\ O_2 \rightarrow 6\ CO_2 + 6\ H_2O$. This can be contrasted to the oxidation of the fat molecule (e.g., palmitate, $C_{16}H_{32}O_2$), where the RER is about 0.7 ($C_{16}H_{32}O_2 + 23\ O_2 \rightarrow 16C_2 + H_2O$). The volume of O_2 for fat oxidation is determined by using this equation:

$$\text{Oxygen for Fat} = \text{Total } O_2 \text{ uptake} \times (1 - \text{RER}) / 0.3$$

Intermediate RER values (between .70 and 1.0) indicate a mixed contribution of fat and carbohydrate to energy metabolism. The contribution of fat and carbohydrate to energy production is best estimated during steady state conditions where the respiratory exchange over the lungs accurately reflects tissue metabolism.

The influence of exercise duration on fuel metabolism during exercise was originally based on RER values. Such studies revealed shifts in the source of energy during the course of prolonged exercise. An example of this is the study of Edwards, Margaria, and Dill (38), in which the metabolism of subjects was followed during the course of six h of moderate exercise. Initially, approximately 90% of the energy was derived from carbohydrate oxidation. With the passage of time, there was a progressive shift toward a reliance on fat oxidation, such that fat provided approximately 90% of the energy in the latter stages of exercise. During the six h of exercise, approximately 1700 kcal was derived from carbohydrate oxidation. This is equivalent to 425 g of glucose. A similar caloric contribution from fat during this period of time was equal to a combustion of only 183 g of fat.

Direct analysis of glycogen stores in liver and skeletal muscle has also been used for estimating the contribution of carbohydrate to energy production at rest and during exercise. As indicated above, the rate of glycogen degradation during exercise depends on exercise intensity (119), increasing exponentially as a function of the relative exercise intensity (% of the maximal oxygen uptake [$\dot{V}O_2$max]) (Fig. 1-5). Thus, the rate of carbohydrate use is low at a low percentage of the $\dot{V}O_2$max. When exercise requires a $\dot{V}O_2$ near or above the $\dot{V}O_2$max, there is nearly a complete dependency upon carbohydrate as a fuel, with most derived from the muscle glycogen stores (48,119). Considerable intersubject variation exists in the contribution of fat and carbohydrate to metabolism during submaximal exercise. This is related in part to the subject's state of training (see below).

Fuel use during heavy exercise cannot be estimated from the RER value, due to hyperventilation and/or acidification of the blood. Under these conditions, the volume of CO_2 expired does not reflect its production from metabolism in the working muscle. Therefore, it is impossible to state that fats are not oxidized during such exercise. However, if fats are used, the total amount consumed is likely small. Moreover, the glycogen depletion from muscle under such conditions correlates closely with estimates of its oxidation and conversion to lactate. The almost exclusive reliance on muscle glycogen under these conditions may be related to transport limitations for fatty acids and glucose.

The analysis of muscle tissue samples can be used to assess the rate of glycogen depletion during exercise. Initially, muscle samples for such studies were collected from anesthetized or sacrificed animals. However, development of the percutaneous needle biopsy method (10) greatly expanded the potential for studying metabolism in human and animal muscle. As a result, many studies have confirmed the estimates made by earlier workers on the basis of RER values.

As previously mentioned, one advantage of carbohydrate as a fuel is that it can be degraded both aerobically and anaerobically. Thus, in the absence of O_2, glycogen can be broken down to pyruvate with the formation of 3 mol of ATP per 2 mol of pyruvate formed. In the absence of oxygen, the pyruvate can be converted to lactate by the action of the enzyme lactate dehydrogenase. However, except in very short, heavy exercise, where blood flow is impaired, it is rare that muscles are devoid of O_2. Moreover, lactate production can occur in the presence of O_2. Lactate production occurs whenever pyruvate production exceeds that needed to fuel the oxidative process in mitochondria. The reduction of pyruvate to lactate is often incorrectly assumed to indicate that the muscle cell is anoxic. Ample evidence exists to demonstrate that lactate production can occur in fully oxygenated muscle cells (27). Lactate production occurs as the result of excess pyruvate being reduced to lactate by the mass action effect of the enzyme lactate dehydrogenase. However, anaerobic lactate production does represent an inefficient use of muscle glycogen.

N.   Influence of Training on Fuel Use During Exercise

Training, particularly endurance training, reduces the amount of glycogen used by muscle during submaximal exercise, while fat oxidation increases. This phenomenon was observed in early studies (9,24,25) in which the RER was the indicator of fuel use (38,87). The training-induced shift to increased fat metabolism was subsequently confirmed in studies using the muscle biopsy technique (87) and in studies in which the energy consumption of working muscle was measured from the O_2 and CO_2 contents of arterial and venous blood, in combination with blood flow measures. Thus during a standard submaximal exercise test, RER is lower, muscle glycogenolysis is less, lactate accumulation is less, and fatty acid oxidation is greater after, as compared to before, training (55,87,120). Similar responses were also observed with subjects who trained only one leg, and where subsequent measurements were performed with either one or both legs (55,70,120).

The shift to a greater fat use during exercise after endurance training is related to the increased oxidative capacity of muscle, resulting from an increased concentration of mitochondrial protein per unit tissue. This increases the potential of the citric acid cycle, beta-oxidation, ketone body oxidation, and the electron transfer system (34,121). A theoretical basis for the shift in substrate choice, based on enzyme regulation, has been discussed elsewhere (56,57).

The greater fat oxidation during submaximal exercise after endurance training is not due to the increases in stroke volume and maximal cardiac output which endurance training also produces (15). Cardiac output, arteriovenous O_2 difference, and blood flow through muscle are similar in the non-trained and trained conditions during the same submaximal exercise load (5,15). The observation of a similar cardiac output and blood flow through active muscle before and after endurance training does not preclude the possibility of an adjustment in the regional perfusion within contracting muscle with a greater delivery of O_2 to contracting motor units. If this occurs, and there is a greater $\dot{V}O_2$ by active motor units, this would widen the arteriovenous O_2 difference across the muscle. These questions are currently unsettled.

In addition to an elevated fat use during submaximal exercise after training, there is a decreased lactate accumulation in muscle and blood. This effect of endurance training is an old (9) and often replicated observation (86,87,118). Based on the general cardiovascular adjustment described above, altered response in muscle and blood lactate cannot be attributed to differences in the delivery and uptake of O_2 after endurance training. As stated above, considerable evidence supports the concept that the lactate accumulation in blood and muscle is not always indicative of anaerobiosis in muscle (27). The delay in lactate accumulation produced by training is related to the increased mitochondrial protein concentration within muscle and an improved ability to more closely balance pyruvate production and its oxidation within mitochondria (34,56,57).

The decreased lactate production and enhanced fat utilization are important from two standpoints. First, lactate production and accumulation in muscle lowers intracellular pH. This can adversely affect such processes as the speed of contraction and relaxation, function of the sarcoplasmic reticulum, mitochondrial oxidation, and activity of enzymes. Secondly, lactate production is an inefficient use of glycogen for ATP production, yielding only three mol of ATP for each mol of glucose converted to lactate. Conversely, oxidation of one mol of glucose to CO_2 and H_2O yields 12 times more ATP than from lactate production.

The differential energy production from lactate formation, as opposed to terminal oxidation of glucose, though important, is also not the prime consideration. Of paramount importance in the shift to fat oxidation is the conservation of intramuscular glycogen stores. During moderately intense exercise, depletion of muscle glycogen stores requires either that the exercise be terminated or its intensity be reduced. Since carbohydrates are used continually during submaximal exercise, the ability to conserve this energy reserve and to forestall its depletion are important physiological adaptations resulting from endurance training.

The delayed onset of lactate accumulation in muscle and blood does not mean that the skeletal muscle of trained individuals cannot produce large amounts of lactate, but only that the relative work load (% $\dot{V}O_2$max) for lactate accumulation is higher after training. During maximal efforts, the lactate concentration in blood and muscle may actually be higher for trained than for non-trained individuals (71). During such efforts, the production of lactate may be important in providing ATP to the contractile elements of muscle.

O. Disadvantages of Carbohydrate as a Fuel

There are disadvantages in the use of carbohydrate as fuels.

1. Glycogen is stored with a large amount of water, 2.7 g $H_2O \cdot g$

glycogen^{-1}. This reduces the caloric value of the storage form to 1.11 kcal · g glycogen^{-1} (wet weight).
2. The total amount of glycogen available to the body is, even in the trained state, relatively small.
3. Although glycogen can be used both aerobically and anaerobically, anaerobic use results in an accumulation of lactate that lowers intramuscular pH, a response that may interfere with a number of cellular processes, including continued energy production.
4. Muscle cells appear to have a dependence upon their internal glycogen stores, and, when these stores are depleted, moderately heavy exercise cannot be continued.

IV. CARBOHYDRATE AVAILABILITY DURING EXERCISE

The contribution of glycogen to metabolism during exercise depends upon its availability. The foundation for the role of glycogen availability during exercise was laid by the early work of Frentzel and Reach (41), Marsh and Murlin (99) and Christensen and Hansen (25), who demonstrated that alterations in diet either increased or decreased carbohydrate use during exercise. These results were confirmed by studies with man in which small muscle samples were collected before, during and after exercise in subjects who had consumed different diets (11,12,72). These studies demonstrated that the glycogen stores of muscle were altered by diet and a combination of previous exercise and diet. Additionally, it was found that the rate of glycogen use and depletion from muscle was positively related to its initial concentration in the skeletal muscle. Further investigation into these relationships involved the selective altering of the glycogen content of the muscle of only one leg (55,107). These studies demonstrated that local concentrations of glycogen, rather than the availability for blood glucose or liver glycogen, are crucial in regulating fuel choice. A greater rate of glycogen depletion also occurs during electrical stimulation in rat muscle with a high glycogen content (116).

A. Carbohydrate Availability and Work Capacity

Attempts to prolong work capacity by providing the body with carbohydrate during prolonged exercise are among the early efforts concerning metabolism during exercise. Dill and colleagues (35) observed that an unfed dog ran for 4.5 h on a treadmill, whereas it ran for 17 h when given sugar during the run. Similarly, Christensen and Hansen (25) reported that subjects who ingested 200 g of glucose at the point of exhaustion were able to exercise for another h. The lack of an increase in the RER value following glucose ingestion in many of these studies suggests that, rather than providing fuel for the working skeletal muscles, exogenous glucose may affect central nervous function. The ingestion and infusion of glucose into the blood of both man and animals can retard the rate of glycogen depletion of skeletal muscle and liver during exercise and can delay the onset of fatigue (8,14,32,63,77,81,83,84,95).

Ingestion of glucose prior to exercise can have a detrimental effect on the maintenance of normal blood glucose concentration. This is the result of glucose absorption producing a substantial rise in the insulin concentration in the blood (17,30,31,47,90,91,111). When such an insulinemic response occurs prior to exercise, there is a facilitation of glucose uptake during exercise, which can produce a pronounced decline in blood glucose. Such glucose ingestion can also inhibit fatty acid mobilization. These effects can be avoided by not starting the glucose ingestion until close to or after the onset of exercise, when the increased activity of the sympathetic nervous system depresses the release of insulin from the pancreas, resulting in a decline in insulin concentration in blood. Since insulin receptors are sensitive to concentration, rather than total availability (expressed as insulin concentration times blood flow), this reduced insulin concentration in blood will obviate any rapid intake of glucose by the muscle.

It has been known for some time that the ingestion of glucose can extend work tolerance during exercise. The ingestion of glucose during such exercise results in 1) a rise in blood glucose concentration, 2) a fall in plasma FFA levels, 3) an increased use of glucose by the working muscle, 4) an increased splanchnic release of glucose, 5) a decreased uptake of gluconeogenic percursors by the liver, and 6) a decline in hepatic oxygen uptake (133).

Animal studies suggest that glucose infusion can partially substitute for muscle glycogen. In one study (135), it was noted that, in comparison to ingestion of a water placebo, there was a greater total carbohydrate use associated with ingestion of a carbohydrate drink during exercise. The similar rates of muscle glycogen use suggested a greater use of blood borne carbohydrate with ingestion of the carbohydrate solution; this theory is supported by higher RER values and higher blood glucose and lower low plasma free fatty acid concentrations in the late stages of the exercise when subjects consumed the carbohydrate beverage. Interestingly, when fed carbohydrate, the subjects exercised an additional hour, even though the concentration of muscle glycogen was reduced to the level that existed in the control condition when fatigue occurred. This might be interpreted as indicating that muscle glycogen is not as important an indicator of fatigue as has been previously suggested (137). Here, it should be noted that in the study of Coyle et al. (135), the concentration of glycogen in the exercising muscle at the point of fatigue was about 40 mmol·kg^{-1}. This value can be contrasted to the value reported in the studies of Hermansen et al. (137) in which fatigue occurred when glycogen content reached 5 mmol·kg^{-1}. Thus, these recent data cannot be used to support or refute the concept that depletion of muscle glycogen occurs in concert with the onset of fatigue in man.

Recently there has been interest regarding the form of carbohydrate to be ingested before, during, or following exercise. One sugar that has received some attention as a potential aid for extending work capacity is fructose. For human subjects, the ingestion of fructose prior to exercise has produced disparate results. In some cases, there has been no difference in exercise capacity or the rate of glycogen utilization (91) with or without fructose ingestion, whereas, in other studies, it has been claimed that fructose exerted a glycogen sparing effect (95). Part of this disparity may be due to differences in the exercise intensities employed, since low intensity, prolonged exercise (approximately 55% VO$_2$max) after fructose ingestion had no effect on muscle glycogen, whereas glycogen depletion was delayed during moderately heavy (approximately 75% VO$_2$max) exercise.

When fructose was given to rats, there was a sparing of the glycogen stores of both liver and muscle observed in one study (123), but in another study, in which the feedings included glucose, fructose, or sucrose prior to exercise, no such sparing was noted (1).

The biochemical basis for suspecting that fructose would produce a glycogen sparing effect on muscle and liver is obscure. Fructose is a normal part of the diet and is ingested with fruits or in sucrose; it is taken up by the liver and converted to glucose by the action of fructokinase, which phosphorylates fructose to fructose-1-phosphate. The fructose-1-phosphate is then split into glyceraldehyde and dehydroxyacetone phosphate by a specific fructose-1-phosphate aldolase. The glyceraldehyde is phosphorylated to glyceraldehyde-3-phosphate by triose kinase, which allows it to enter glycolysis. Skeletal muscle hexokinase can phosphorylate fructose to fructose-6-phosphate, enabling it to enter the glycolytic pathway. There are a number of factors to be considered when evaluating the suitability of fructose as a source of carbohydrate. Although the hexokinase of muscle can phosphorylate fructose to fructose-6-phosphate, the affinity of this enzyme in muscle is only about one-tenth that for glucose (33) and hexokinase may actually be inhibited by fructose (60). Therefore, for fructose to compete on an equal basis with glucose for entry into muscle glycolysis, its concentration in blood would have to be 10 times higher than that of glucose. This would produce a considerable diuresis. Thus, not only would fructose not compete well at the level of entry into the metabolism of muscle, but it may actually inhibit glucose uptake from the blood. Second, fructose absorption from the gut is slower than that of glucose (28,29). The oral ingestion of large amounts of fructose can cause gastric distress. Third, it appears that there is a much more rapid removal of fructose by the liver than by muscle, with synthesis of glycogen being more rapid when fructose is infused into the blood of man, as compared to an isocaloric infusion of glucose (105). The principal advantage of fructose ingestion, as compared to glucose, is that fructose produces a much smaller increase in plasma insulin concentration (17,90,91). This could be important in that fructose provides some carbohydrate without concomitantly raising plasma insulin levels or depressing fatty acid mobilization. From a biochemical point of view, however, there are considerations to suggest that it is not likely that fructose is better than glucose as a carbohydrate supplement during exercise or for replenishing carbohydrate after exercise.

B. Consequence of Glycogen Depletion in Muscle

During prolonged exercise of moderate intensity (65% to 75% $\dot{V}O_2$max), the depletion of muscle glycogen is often associated with the onset of exhaustion. This exhaustion is typified by an inability to continue the exercise at the desired intensity; exercise can only continue if the intensity of the exercise is reduced. This fatigue can occur in spite of the existence of fairly high levels of glucose and FFA in the blood. These data suggest that there is an absolute glucose requirement within the contracting fibers that, at some exercise intensities, cannot be met by the uptake of glucose from the blood.

Muscle glycogen is important for short, heavy work, as well as for prolonged exercise, as demonstrated by the reduction in $\dot{V}O_2$max after glycogen depletion (7,68). This raises the question of why skeletal muscle is so dependent upon glycogen for all but the mildest of exercise. The answer to this question appears to be that the uptake of substrate by muscle from the blood cannot occur rapidly enough to support heavy exercise. An example in nature that supports this contention comes from human subjects with McArdle's disease. These individuals lack myophosphorylase and, therefore, cannot use the glycogen stored in the muscles, but rely upon the uptake of glucose and fatty acids from the blood to support the exercise metabolism. Affected persons have a low exercise tolerance and $\dot{V}O_2$max, but the intravenous infusion of glucose can increase the relative contribution of carbohydrate to metabolism (62). Thus, immediate access to the glucose stored in glycogen appears to be essential for maintaining muscle metabolism during moderate to heavy exercise. The relative work load that can be sustained if muscle were to rely solely upon the exclusive oxidation of FFA is unknown.

C. Gluconeogenesis

The importance of gluconeogenesis stems from the fact that, with exercise, a major decline in the body's total carbohydrate stores can occur. Since the brain consumes about 120 g of glucose per day, it is imperative that the body's reserve of glucose be maintained. During exercise, this is accomplished by the generation of glucose from lactate (141), a reaction occuring principally in the liver. Ahlborg et al. (134) reported that gluconeogenesis was responsible for approximately 25% of the total splanchnic glucose output in resting subjects. This contribution fell to 16% after moderate exercise lasting 40 min and to 6% with short, heavy exercise. However, with light, prolonged exercise, hepatic gluconeogenesis contributed as much as 45% of the total glucose released from the liver. This glucose production was associated with an increased uptake of lactate, pyruvate, alanine, and glycerol by the liver (134). It should be remembered that the production of glucose via gluconeogenesis is not without cost to the body, since the production of 1 mol of glucose from pyruvate requires the use of 6 mol of ATP. In conclusion, it can be stated that, during prolonged exercise, gluconeogenesis is a major source of glucose production.

D. Repletion of Muscle Glycogen Following Exercise

The ability to replenish the glycogen stores of muscle following depletion has been examined in man and animals. In an early study by Bergström and Hultman (11), it was observed that glycogen concentration had returned to near normal within 24 h after being depleted by exercise. However, the maximal concentration, a supercompensation of glycogen stores, was not reached until three days postexercise. This supercompensation occurred during a high carbohydrate intake. Since then, a number of reports have appeared which demonstrated that a significant carbohydrate intake is needed for the replenishment of glycogen in both the liver and skeletal muscle (31,53,77,97,98,101,108,128). Piehl (108,109) observed that 46 h were required for the muscle glycogen to return to the preexercise concentration. McDougall and associates (101) found the glycogen concentration of muscle to be normal 24 h following depletion to approximately 20% of preexercise values. Further, there was no difference in the glycogen replenishment rate between subjects fed a diet containing about 50% carbohydrate and those given a supplemental feeding of 2500 kcal of carbohydrate.

Numerous reports exist concerning the rate of glycogen replenishment in the muscles of animals following exercise-induced depletion. Lamb et al. (94) observed that the glycogen content of guinea pig muscle was about 30% greater than normal 24 h after its depletion. However, the time course of the return to normal and supercompensation was not followed. Terjung and co-workers (128) followed the time course of the return of liver and muscle glycogen of the rat and observed a normal value for muscle 4 h after its depletion. The greatest glycogen synthesis rate occurred between 30 and 60 min after termination of the exercise. A similar finding has been reported for fasted rats (45). In these experiments, liver glycogen was normal only at 24 h after exercise. Studies with the horse revealed a time course for glycogen repletion similar to that of man (75).

Since there is an ordered pattern of glycogen depletion during exercise based on recruitment of motor units, there might also be a consistent sequence for its replenishment to prepare the fibers for subsequent activation. Factors involved in such a differential glycogen repletion would be the relative concentration of the key enzymes for glycogen synthesis (glycogen synthase) within the fibers, regulation of the enzymes, and the delivery of glucose to the enzyme. The concentration of glycogen synthase has been examined in the different types of fibers for a number of animal species. The general observation has been that the more oxidative fibers, identified either as red or intermediate or as Type I and Type II, have higher concentrations of glycogen synthase than do the low oxidative fibers (16,74,82,109,124). Differential rates of glycogen repletion have been observed in rats, with the order being heart > red part of the vastus muscle > soleus muscle > white part of the vastus muscle (128). The rate of glycogen replenishment in the red portion of the vastus lateralis muscle was three times that of the white part of this muscle. The order of glycogen repletion in the horse was in reverse order of its depletion with low oxidative Type II fibers > high oxidative Type II fibers > Type I fibers. No information is available concerning the relative concentration of glycogen synthase in the different types of fibers in equine muscle. Examination of the relative rate of glycogen repletion in human muscle (109) did not reveal any consistent differences among fiber types.

Since the rate of glycogen repletion may be controlled by the concentration of glycogen synthase in a muscle, the effect of training on this property of muscle has been studied. There is general agreement that the glycogen synthase concentration in muscle increases with endurance training (82,94,109,125). Taylor et al. (126) observed a nearly two-fold higher activity of the glycogen debranching enzyme in the muscle of trained, as compared to sedentary, subjects. This may explain the higher concentration of muscle glycogen in trained as compared to non-trained individuals.

The regulation of glycogen synthase is important in the glycogen repletion process. Part of this regulation is due to the existence of two interconvertible forms of glycogen synthase. One form is active only in the presence of glucose-6-phosphate and is designated as synthase-D (D-form), whereas the other form, whose activity is independent of glucose-6-phosphate, is identified as synthase-I (I-form) (2). Of these, synthase-I is the most active. Following exercise, there is an increased percentage of synthase-I, which progressively returns to normal with time (109). However, since there can also be a high glucose-6-phosphate concentration in muscle after exercise, both forms of the enzymes are probably involved in the early glycogen restoration in skeletal muscle. However, with time, the D-form predominates in the control of glycogen synthesis.

Another factor involved in glycogen synthesis in muscle after exercise is the availability of glucose, the prime source of which is the blood. In the rat, regional blood flow differs, with the highly oxidative portions of muscle having greater blood flow at rest and during exercise than the low oxidative regions (5). This blood flow pattern would result in the delivery of larger amounts of glucose to the highly oxidative fibers, a scenario that is consistent with the more rapid return of glycogen to the resting concentration in these fibers after exercise. The heterogeneity in the fiber distribution of human skeletal muscle, compared to the rat and guinea pig, is such that differences in blood flow to the different fiber types at rest or during exercise have not been established.

A more rapid replenishment of glycogen in the oxidative fibers would be a reasonable response, since these fibers are the first to be used in normal activity, and this would ready them for additional contractile activity.

V. FAT UTILIZATION DURING EXERCISE

As indicated earlier, fat is a very concentrated energy form, with about 90% of the molecule comprised of carbon and hydrogen. Thus, fat offers some distinct advantages as an energy store and metabolic fuel.

1. Fat has the highest energy value of any fuel, $9.3 \text{ kcal} \cdot \text{g}^{-1}$.

2. Fat can be stored in large amounts in various sites throughout the body.
3. Fat is a stable energy source, yet it can be mobilized for use during exercise.

Conversely, there are some disadvantages to fat as a metabolic fuel for muscular exercise. These can be summarized as follows:

1. Compared to glycogen, the total caloric value of intramuscle fiber lipid stores is small.
2. Energy release from fat occurs only with an uptake of oxygen.
3. The oxidation of fat yields less energy per liter of oxygen taken up (4.62 kcal $\cdot$ L^{-1}) than does carbohydrate.
4. Since the storage of fat is mainly outside the muscle fiber and since fats are not soluble in water, there is a delayed transport of FFA to the muscle, and consequently FFAs are not readily available at the onset of exercise.
5. Fats cannot serve as the sole source of energy for anything except mild exercise.

At rest, the RER of man is usually around 0.80. This signifies that about 65% of the energy consumption of the body is derived from the oxidation of fat. During prolonged exercise, with an RER value of 0.85, 50% of the energy production is derived from fat oxidation. The relative contribution that fat can make to the exercise metabolism depends upon the intensity and duration of the exercise and the athlete's fitness.

As the intensity of exercise increases, the relative contribution that fat makes to metabolism becomes less. In all cases, the longer the exercise is sustained, the greater is the contribution of fat to the metabolism. This was observed by Edwards and co-workers (38); at the end of a 6 h period of exercise, approximately 90% of the energy could be attributed to the oxidation of fat. This was exercise that was supported by an oxygen uptake of about 2.3 L $\cdot$ min^{-1}, equivalent to the oxidation of about 62 g of fat (574 kcal). Over the same time span, the oxidation of 18.6 g of carbohydrate occurred (75 kcal). These rather old data illustrate the important role that the oxidation of fat can play during prolonged exercise.

B. Contribution of Plasma FFA

As was illustrated in the work of Edwards et al. (38), there is a considerable time lag between the onset of exercise and the point at which fat becomes a major contributor to metabolism. There is very little lipid stored within skeletal muscle, and there is a considerable time lag between the between the onset of exercise, lipolysis of TG in adipose tissue, and the release of FFA into the plasma. The sluggishness of the rise in plasma FFA is related to the fact that lipolysis in adipose tissue is accelerated primarily by the sympathetic nervous system and that diffusion barriers exist at several sites in the system. This is illustrated in Fig. 1-6. The rise in plasma FFA is essential, since there is a close relationship between the concentration of FFA in plasma and FFA contribution to metabolism (66). Under normal conditions, the time between the onset of exercise and the existence of a significant rise in plasma FFA is between 20 and 30 min (19,20,50,59,66,107,112).

An acceleration of the mobilization of lipolysis (as is thought to occur with caffeine ingestion), promotes an early elevation in plasma FFA, and has been suggested to result in an increased use of fat and a sparing of muscle glycogen (30,81,115). Although there are claims that such a response results in increased work capacity, this claim has been contested (113,132).

During short, heavy exercise, there may actually be an inhibition of FFA mobilization, and there is a reduction in the concentration of FFA in plasma (8,18,40,59,79). This has been demonstrated to be closely associated with the lactate concentration in the blood, which may have an inhibitory effect on lipolysis in fat cells.

B. Intramuscular Lipids as Fuel

There is currently considerable uncertainty and debate as to the role that intra-fiber TG stores contribute to the total fuel utilization of exercise. The inability of early investigators to account for all of the fat oxidized as coming from fat delivered by the blood prompted these researchers to conclude that there was an oxidation of lipids stored within the muscle fibers. Attempts to quantify the magnitude of the contribution of such lipids have been difficult and have brought disparate results. For example, Masoro et al. (100) were unable to demonstrate a major role for intramuscular TG in the muscles of monkeys, following prolonged electrical stimulation. In contrast, Issekutz and co-workers (78,80) concluded, on the basis of energy balance studies, that there had to be a major use of intramuscular lipid stores. A number of studies, in which the lipid content of muscle was measured either before and after exercise or in which comparisons between muscles were obtained from exercised and non-exercised animals, have supported the theory regarding a major decline in this energy source (42,43,44,114). In studies with man, there are reports of declines in the TG concentrations of muscle after exercise lasting from 1 to 12 h (39,120). In direct contrast are reports of no changes in intramuscular TG (54,100).

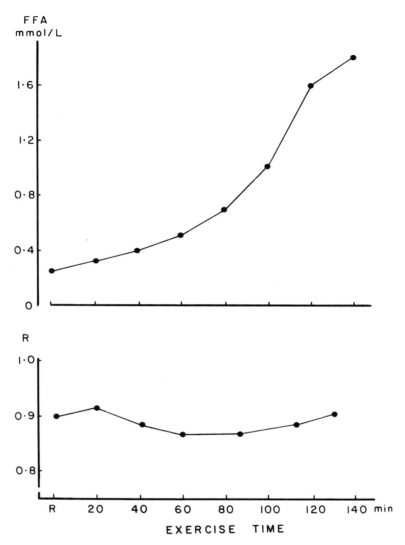

FIGURE 1-6. *Plasma free fatty acid (FFA) concentrations and R value during the course of exhaustive exercise performed at 75% to 80% of the maximal oxygen uptake. Note the delayed increase in plasma FFA and that the R value increased as exhaustion approached. Adopted from Gollnick et al. (58).*

The regional variation in TG deposits that exist both within and around the fibers presents a major problem in evaluating the contribution of intramuscular lipids during exercise. Moreover, extrafiber lipid must also be accounted for to ensure that the lipid being measured is only that found within the fibers. Attempts to circum-

ENERGY METABOLISM AND PROLONGED EXERCISE **29**

vent the regional variation of muscle lipid stores have included the assaying of relatively large pieces of muscle. When this has been done (44), reduction in muscle TG of from 2.6 to 15.8 umol $\cdot$ g^{-1} have been observed after exercise requiring a total caloric expenditure of 6000 or more kcal. Under these conditions, the total contribution of intramuscular TG would have been only about 5% of the total kcal consumed. The limited ability of intramuscular TG to contribute to the total energy demands of the muscle can be illustrated by the fact that the complete depletion of all of the TG in muscle would have been equivalent to only 10% of the total caloric expenditure.

C. Effect of Training on Fat Metabolism

There is a greater utilization of fat during submaximal exercise after endurance training. This is not produced by a greater or more rapid mobilization of FFA from adipose tissue (61,87). It is related to the enhanced oxidative capacity and capillarization of trained muscle (121). The increase in capillarization does not increase the supply or uptake of oxygen by the muscle at a standard submaximal exercise intensity. But capillarization does result in a greater transit time for blood through the capillary bed, thereby allowing a longer time for the exchange of materials between the blood and the muscle fiber. The elevation in mitochondrial enzymes includes increases in enzymes for beta-oxidation. The theoretical basis for this has been discussed elsewhere (56,57).

D. Repletion of Body Fat Stores after Exercise

In the normal, well-nourished person, the total amount of fat stores are so large that the amount used during most exercise does not require a special dietary regimen to return them to an acceptable level. Moreover, any excess carbohydrate or protein that is consumed can be converted to fat. Thus, it is not necessary to institute any special measures to replete the fat stores following exercise.

Miller et al. (102) observed that prolonged high fat feeding of rats enhanced fat oxidation during work. In these studies there were increases in the enzymes for muscle beta-oxidation, exercise endurance was greater, and glycogen depletion and increases in blood lactate were less. These data suggest that with prolonged exposure to a high fat diet there can be adaptations in the muscle that enhance the capacity for fatty acid oxidation.

VI. AMINO ACID OXIDATION DURING EXERCISE

The role of amino acids as fuels during exercise metabolism has been estimated from the oxidation of radiolabeled amino acids infused into man and animals, the oxidation of amino acids in electrically stimulated perfused animal muscle, and from nitrogen excretion. The possible benefits of the oxidation of protein include a) conversion of amino acids to citric acid cycle intermediates to support the oxidation of fat and carbohydrate derived acetyl-CoA, b) generation of carbon skeletons for gluconeogenesis, and c) the direct oxidation of amino acids within muscle to produce ATP. This topic has been reviewed by Dohm et al. (136). On the basis of changes in serum urea and excretion of urea in sweat, Lemon and Mullin (140) estimated that protein oxidation accounted for 4% and 10% of the caloric cost of one h of exercise that required about 60% $\dot{V}O_2$max under conditions of low and high glycogen, respectively. Lefebvre (139), using nitrogen excretion, estimated that about 3% of a total of 2200 to 2400 kcal expended during 4 hours of treadmill exercise could be accounted for by protein oxidation.

The oxidation of amino acids has been reported to increase during exercise (138,142). The major conclusion from such studies is that although the total amount of amino acids oxidized increases during exercise, contribution of amino acids to the total carbon flux declines. These data suggested that, under normal conditions, the contribution of amino acids to the total oxidative process of muscle is small and does not increase in proportion to that of fat and carbohydrate during exercise.

SUMMARY

Although both fats and carbohydrates are used as fuels by muscle during exercise, the greatest concern for the endurance athlete for in maintaining carbohydrate stores. This conclusion is based on the fact that, during moderately intense exercise, exhaustion coincides with the depletion of glycogen from the active skeletal muscles. Depletion of liver glycogen can also occur during exercise. Although the glucose released into the blood from the liver can be used by muscle as an energy source, this glucose is also important for maintaining the function of the central nervous system. Thus, depletion of liver glycogen can lead to hypoglycemia, which will also result in impaired exercise capacity. Based on this information, it is essential that the endurance athlete use both dietary manipulation and training-induced shifts in metabolism to conserve glycogen and improve performance capacity.

BIBLIOGRAPHY

1. Addington, E.E., and K.K. Gurenwald. Preexercise feedings of glucose, fructose or sucrose effects on fuel homeostasis in rats. *Fed Proc.* 45:972, 1986.
2. Adolfsson, S. Regulation of glycogen synthesis in muscle. Thesis, Department of Physiology, University of Göteborg, Sweden, 1972.

3. Anderson, P., and J. Henriksson. Capillary supply of the quadriceps femoris muscle of man: adaptive response to exercise. *J Physiol* (London) 270:677–690, 1977.
4. Anderson, P., and B. Saltin. Maximal perfusion of skeletal muscle in man. *J Physiol.* (London) 366:233–249, 1985.
5. Armstrong, R.B., and M.H. Laughlin. Metabolic indicators of fiber recruitment in mammalian muscle during locomotion. *J Exp Biol.* 115:201–213, 1985.
6. Armstrong, R.B., C.W. Saubert, IV, W.L. Sembrowich, R.E. Shepherd, and P.D. Gollnick. Glycogen depletion in rat skeletal muscle fibers at different intensities and durations of exercise. *Pflügers Arch.* 352:243–256, 1974.
7. Åstrand, P.O., I. Hallback, R. Hedman, and B. Saltin. Blood lactates after prolonged severe exercise. *J Appl Physiol.* 18:619–622, 1963.
8. Bagby, G.J., H.J. Green, S. Katsuta, and P.D. Gollnick. Glycogen depletion in exercising rats infused with glucose, lactate, or pyruvate. *J Appl Physiol.* 45:425–429, 1978.
9. Bang, O. The lactate content of blood during and after exercise in man. *Skand Arch Physiol.* 74:51–82, 1936.
10. Bergström, J. Muscle electrolytes in man. *Scand J Clin Lab Invest Suppl.* 68, 1962.
11. Bergström, J., and E. Hultman. Muscle glycogen syntheses after exercise: an enhancing factor localized to the muscle cells in man. *Nature.* 210:309–310, 1966.
12. Bergström, J., L. Hermansen, E. Hultman, and B. Saltin. Diet, muscle glycogen and physical performance. *Acta Physiol Scand.* 71:140–150, 1967.
13. Bessman, S.P., and C.L. Carpenter. The creatine-phosphate energy shuttle. *Ann Rev Biochem.* 54:831–862, 1985.
14. Bjorkman, O., K. Sahlin, L. Hagenfeldt, and J. Wahren. Influence of glucose and fructose ingestion on the capacity for long-term exercise in well trained men. *Clin Physiol Oxf.* 4:483–494, 1984.
15. Blomqvist, C.G., and B. Saltin. Cardiovascular adaptations to physical training. *Ann Rev. Physiol.* 45:169–189, 1983.
16. Bocek, R., and C.H. Beatty. Glycogen synthetase and phosphorylase in red and white muscle of rat and rhesus monkey. *J Histochem Cytochem.* 14:549–559, 1966.
17. Bohannon, V.V., J.H. Haram, and P.H. Forsham. Endocrine response to sugar ingestion in man. *J Am Diet Assoc.* 76:555–560, 1980.
18. Boyd, A.E., S.R. Giamber, M. Mager, and H.E. Lebovitez. Lactate inhibition of lypolysis in exercising man. *Metabolism.* 23:531–542, 1974.
19. Carlson, L.A., and B. Pernow. Studies on blood lipids during exercise. I. Arterial and venous plasma concentration of unesterified fatty acids. *J Lab Clin Med.* 58:833–841, 1959.
20. Carlson, L.A., L. Ekelund, and S.O. Fröberg. Concentration of triglycerides, phospholipids, and glycogen in skeletal muscle and of free fatty acids and beta-hydroxbutyric acid in blood in man in response to exercise. *Europ J Clin Invest.* 1:248–254, 1971.
21. Carlson, K.I., J.C. Marker, D.A. Arnall, M.L. Terry, H.T. Yang, L.G. Lindsay, M.E. Bracken, and W.W. Winder. Epinephrine is unessential for stimulation of liver glycogenolysis during exercise. *J Appl Physiol.* 58:544–548, 1985.
22. Cartier, L.J., and P.D. Gollnick. Sympathoadrenal system and activation of glycogenolysis during muscular exercise. *J Appl Physiol.* 58:1122–1127, 1985.
23. Cheetham, M.E., L.H. Boobis, S. Brooks, and C. Williams. Human muscle metabolism during spring running. *J Appl Physiol.* 61:54–60, 1986.
24. Christensen, E.H., Der Stoffweschsel und de respiratorischen Funktionen bei schwerer köperliche Arbeit. *Arbeitsphysiologie* 5:463–478, 1932.
25. Christensen, E.H., and O. Hansen. Arbeitsfähigkeit und Ehrnährung. *Skand Ark Physiol.* 81:160–175, 1939.
26. Conlee, R.K., J.A. McLane, M.J. Rennie, W.W. Winder, and J.O. Holloszy. Reversal of phosphorylase activation in muscle despite continued contractile activity. *Am J Physiol.* 237:R291–R296, 1979.
27. Connett, R.J., T.E. Gayeski, and C.R. Honig. Lactate accumulation in fully aerobic, working dog gracilis muscle. *Am J Physiol.* 246:H120–H128, 1984.
28. Cori, C.F. The fate of sugar in the animal body. I. The rate of absorption of hexoses and pentoses from the intestinal tract. *J Biol Chem.* 66:691–715, 1925.
29. Cori, C.F. The fate of sugar in the animal body. III. The rate of glycogen formation in the liver of normal and insulinized rats during the absorption of glucose, fructose, and galactose. *J Biol Chem.* 70:477–585, 1926.
30. Costill, D.L., E. Coyle, G. Dalsky, W. Evans, W. Fink, and D. Hoopes. Effects of elevated plasma FFA and insulin on muscle glycogen usage during exercise. *J Appl Physiol.* 43:695–699, 1977.
31. Costill, D.L., W.M. Sherman, W.J. Fink, C. Maresh, M. Witten, and J.M. Miller. The role of dietary carbohydrates in muscle glycogen synthesis after strenuous running. *Am J Clin Nutr.* 34:1831–1836, 1981.

32. Coyle, E.F., J.M. Hagberg, B.F. Hurley, W.H. Martin, A.A. Ehsani, and J.O. Holloszy. Carbohydrate feeding during prolonged strenuous exercise can delay fatigue. *J Appl Physiol.* 55:230–235, 1983.

33. Crane, R.K., and A. Sols. The non-competitive inhibition of brain hexokinase by glucose-6-phosphate and related compounds. *J Biol Chem.* 210:597–606, 1954.

34. Davies, K.J.A., L. Packer, and G.A. Brooks. Biochemical adaptations of mitochondria, muscle, and whole-animal respiration to endurance training. *Arch Biochem Biophys.* 209:539–554, 1981.

35. Dill, D.B., H.T. Edwards, and J.H. Talbott. Studies in muscular activity. VII. Factors limiting the capacity for work. *J Physiol.* 77:49–62, 1932.

36. Dobson, G.P., E. Yamamoto, and P.W. Hochachka. Phosphofructokinase control in muscle: nature and reversal of pH-dependent ATP inhibition. *Am J Physiol.* 250:R71–R76, 1986.

37. Drummond, G.I., J.P. Harwood, and C.A. Powell. Studies on the activation of phosphorylase in skeletal muscle by contraction and by epinephrine. *J Biol Chem.* 244:4235–4240, 1969.

38. Edwards, H.T., R. Margaria, and D.B. Dill. Metabolic rate, blood sugar and the utilization of carbohydrate. *Am J Physiol.* 108:203–209, 1934.

39. Essén, B. Intramuscular substrate utilization during prolonged exercise. *Ann NY Acad Sci.* 301:30–44, 1977.

40. Fredholm, B.B. Inhibition of fatty acid release from adipose tissue by high arterial blood lactate concentrations. *Acta Physiol Scand.* 77:Suppl. 330, 1969.

41. Frentzel, J., and F. Reach. Untersuchungen zur Frage nach der Quelle der Muskeldraft. *Pflügers Arch.* 83:477–508, 1901.

42. Fröberg, S.O. Effect of acute exercise on tissue lipids in rats. *Metabolism.* 20:714–720, 1971.

43. Fröberg, S.O. Effect of training and of acute exercise in trained rats. *Metabolism.* 20:1044–1051, 1971.

44. Fröberg, S.O., and F. Mossfeldt. Effect of prolonged strenuous exercise on the concentrations of triglycerides, phospholipids, and glycogen in muscle of man. *Acta Physiol Scand.* 82:167–171, 1971.

45. Gaesser, G.A., and G.A. Brooks. Glycogen repletion following continuous and intermittent exercise to exhaustion. *J Appl Physiol.* 49:722–728, 1980.

46. Galbo, H., N.J. Christensen, and J.J. Holst. Catecholamines and pancreatic hormones during autonomic blockade in exercise. *Acta Physiol Scand.* 101:428–437, 1977.

47. Ganda, O.P., J.S. Soeldner, R.W. Gleason, I.H.M. Cleator, and C. Reynolds. Metabolic effects of glucose, mannose, galactose, and fructose in man. *J Clin Endocrinol Met.* 49:616–622, 1979.

48. Gollnick, P.D. Metabolism of substrates: energy substrate metabolism during exercise and as modified by training. *Fed Proc.* 44:353–357, 1985.

49. Gollnick, P.D., R.G. Soule, A.W. Taylor, C. Williams, and C.D. Ianuzzo. Exercise-induced glycogenolysis and lipolysis in the rat: hormonal influence. *Am J Physiol.* 239:729–733, 1970.

50. Gollnick, P.D., C.D. Ianuzzo, C. Williams, and T.R. Hill. Effect of prolonged, severe exercise on the ultrastructure of human skeletal muscle. *Int Z Angew Physiol.* 27:257–265, 1969.

51. Gollnick P.D., R.B. Armstrong, W.L. Sembrowich, R.E. Shepherd, and B. Saltin. Glycogen depletion pattern in human skeletal muscle fibers after heavy exercise. *J Appl Physiol.* 34:615–618, 1973.

52. Gollnick, P.D., R.B. Armstrong, C.W. Saubert, IV, W.L. Sembrowich, R.E. Shepherd, and B. Saltin. Glycogen depletion patterns in human skeletal muscle fibers during prolonged work. *Pflügers Arch.* 344:1–12, 1973.

53. Gollnick, P.D., K. Piehl, C.W. Saubert, IV, R.B. Armstrong, and B. Saltin. Diet, exercise and glycogen depletion in different fiber types. *J. Appl Physiol.* 33:421–425, 1972.

54. Gollnick, P.D., K. Piehl, and B. Saltin. Selective glycogen depletion pattern in human muscle fibers after exercise of varying intensity and at varying pedaling rates. *J Physiol.* (London) 241:45–57, 1974.

55. Gollnick, P.D., B. Pernow, B. Essén, E. Jansson, and B. Saltin. Availability of glycogen and plasma FFA for substrate utilization in leg muscle of man during exercise. *Clin Physiol.* 1:27–42, 1981.

56. Gollnick, P.D., B. Pernow, B. Essén, E. Jansson, and B. Saltin. Availability of glycogen and plasma FFA for substrate utilization in leg muscle of man during exercise. *Clin Physiol.* 1:27–42, 1981.

57. Gollnick, P.D., M. Riedy, J.J. Quintinskie, and L.A. Bertocci. Differences in metabolic potential of skeletal muscle fibers and their significance for metabolic control. *J Exp Biol.* 115:191–199, 1985.

58. Gollnick, P.D., and D.R. Hodgson. The identification of fiber types in skeletal muscle: a

continual dilemma. *Exer Sports Sci Rev.* 14:81–104, 1986.

59. Green, H.J., M.E. Huston, J.A. Thomson, J.R. Sutton, and P.D. Gollnick. Metabolic consequences of supramaximal arm work performed during prolonged submaximal leg work. *J Appl Physiol.* 46:249–255, 1976.
60. Grossbard, L., and R.T. Schimke. Multiple hexokinases of rat tissue purification and comparison of soluble forms. *J Biol Chem.* 241:3546–3560, 1966.
61. Gyntelberg, F., M.J. Rennie, R.C. Hickson, and J.O. Holloszy. Effect of training on the response of plasma glucagon to exercise. *J Appl Physiol.* 43:302–308, 1977.
62. Haller, R.G., S.F. Lewis, J.D. Cook, and C.G. Blomqvist. Myophosphorylase deficiency impairs muscle oxidative metabolism. *Ann Neurol.* 17:196–199, 1985.
63. Hargreaves, M., D.L. Costill, A. Coggan, W.J. Fink, and I. Nishibata. Effect of carbohydrate feedings on muscle glycogen utilization and exercise performance. *Med Sci Sports Exer.* 16:219–222, 1984.
64. Harris, R.C., R.H.T. Edwards, E. Hultman, L.O. Nordesjö, B. Nylind, and K. Sahlin. The time course of phosphorylcreatine resynthesis during recovery of the quadriceps muscle in man. *Pflügers Arch.* 367:137–142, 1976.
65. Hashimoto, I., M.B. Knudson, E.G. Noble, G.A. Klug, and P.D. Gollnick. Exercise-induced glycogenolysis in sympathectomized rats. *Jap J Physiol.* 32:153–160, 1982.
66. Havel, R.J., A. Naimark, C.R. Borchgrevink. Turnover rate and oxidation of free fatty acids of blood plasma in man during exercise: studies during continuous infusion of palmitate-l-C14. *J Clin Invest.* 42:1054–1063, 1959.
67. Havel, R.J., L.A. Carlson, L.G. Ekelund, and A. Holmgren. Turnover rate and oxidation of different free fatty acids in man during exercise. *J Appl Physiol.* 19:613–618, 1964.
68. Heigenhauser, G.J.F., J.R. Sutton, and N.L. Jones. Effect of glycogen depletion on the ventilatory response to exercise. *J Appl Physiol.* 54:470–474, 1983.
69. Helmreich, E., and C.F. Cori. Regulation of glycolysis in muscle. *Advan in Enzyme Reg.* 3:91–107, 1964.
70. Henriksson, J. Training induced adaptations of skeletal muscle and metabolism during submaximal exercise. *J Physiol.* (London) 270:661–675, 1977.
71. Hermansen, L. Anaerobic energy release. *Med Sci Sports.* 1:32–38, 1969.
72. Hermansen, L., E. Hultman, and B. Saltin. Muscle glycogen and prolonged severe exercise. *Acta Physiol Scand.* 71:129–139, 1967.
73. Hermansen, L., and J.B. Osnes. Blood and muscle pH after maximal exercise in man. *J Appl Physiol.* 32:304–308, 1972.
74. Hess, R., and A.G.E. Pearse. Dissociation of uridine diphosphate glucose-glycogen transglucosylase from phosphorylase activity in individual muscle fibers. *Proc Soc Exp Biol Med.* 107:569–571, 1961.
75. Hodgson, D.R. *Studies on Equine Muscle.* Thesis. 1984. University of Sydney. Sydney, Australia.
76. Hultman, E., J. Bergström, and N. McLennan Anderson. Breakdown and resynthesis of phosphorylcreatine and adenosine triphosphate in connection with muscular work in man. *Scand J Clin Lab Invest.* 19:56–69, 1967.
77. Hultman, E., and L.H. Nilsson. Liver glycogen in man. Effect of different diets and muscular exercise. In: *Muscle Metabolism During Exercise.* Edited by B. Pernow and B. Saltin. Plenum, New York, 1971, 143–152.
78. Issekutz, B., Jr., and P. Paul. Intramuscular energy sources in exercising normal and pancreatomized dogs. *Am J Physiol.* 215:197–204, 1968.
79. Issekutz, B., Jr., W.A. Shaw, and T.B. Issekutz. Effect of lactate on the FFA and glycerol turnover in resting and exercising dogs. *J Appl Physiol.* 39:349–353, 1975.
80. Issekutz, B., Jr., H.I. Miller, P. Paul, and K. Rodahl. Source of fat oxidation in exercising dogs. *Am J Physiol.* 207:583–587, 1964.
81. Ivy, J.L., D.L. Costill, W.J. Fink, and R.W. Lower. Influence of caffeine and carbohydrate feedings on endurance performance. *Med Sci Sports.* 11:6–11, 1979.
82. Jeffress, R.N., J.B. Peter, and D.R. Lamb. Effects of exercise on glycogen synthetase in red and white skeletal muscle. *Life Sci.* 7:957–960, 1968.
83. Jenkins, A.B., S.M. Furler, D.J. Chisholm, and E.W. Kraegen. Regulation of hepatic glucose output during exercise by circulating glucose and insulin in humans. *Am J Physiol.* 250:R411–R417, 1986.
84. Jenkins, A.B., D.J. Chisholm, D.E. James, K.Y. Ho, and E.W. Kraegen. Exercise-induced hepatic glucose input is precisely sensitive to the rate of systemic glucose supply. *Metabolism.* 34:431–436.
85. Karlsson, J., and B. Saltin. Oxygen deficit and muscle metabolites in intermittent exercise. *Acta Physiol Scand.* 82:115–122, 1971.
86. Karlsson, J., L.O. Nordesjö, L. Jorfeldt, and B. Saltin. Muscle lactate, ATP, and CP levels

during exercise after physical training in man. *J Appl Physiol.* 33:199–203, 1972.
87. Karlsson, J., L.O. Nordesjö, and B. Saltin. Muscle glycogen utilization during exercise after physical training. *Acta Physiol Scand.* 90:210–217, 1974.
88. Kelso, T.B., D.R. Hodgson, A.R. Visscher, and P.D. Gollnick. Some properties of different skeletal muscle fiber types: Comparison of reference bases. *J Appl Physiol.* 62:1436–1441, 1987.
89. Knuttgen, H.G., and B. Saltin. Oxygen uptake and high-energy phosphate, and lactate in exercise under acute hypoxic conditions in man. *Acta Physiol Scand.* 76:368–376, 1973.
90. Koivisto, V.A., S.L. Karonen, and E.A. Nikkilä. Carbohydrate ingestion before exercise: comparison of glucose, fructose, and sweet placebo. *J. Appl Physiol.* 51:783–787, 1981.
91. Koivisto, V.A., M. Härkonen, S.L. Karonen, P.H. Groop, R. Elovainio, E. Ferrannini, L. Sacca, and R.A. Defronzo. Glycogen depletion during prolonged exercise: influence of glucose, fructose, or placebo. *J Appl Physiol.* 58:731–737, 1985.
92. Krebs, E.G., D.R. Graves, and E.H. Fischer. Factors affecting the activity of muscle phosphorylase *b* kinase. *J Biol Chem.* 234:2869–2873, 1959.
93. Krebs, E.G., D.S. Lover, G.E. Bartovold, K.A. Tayser, W. Meyer, and E.H. Fischer. Purification and properties of rabbit skeletal muscle phosphorylase *b* kinase. *Biochemistry.* 3:1022–1033, 1964.
94. Lamb, D.R., J.B. Peter, R.N. Jeffress, and H.A. Wallace. Glycogen, hexokinase, and glycogen synthetase adaptations to exercise. *Am J Physiol.* 217:1628–1632, 1969.
95. Levine, L., W.J. Evans, B.S. Cararette, E.C. Fisher, and B.A. Bullen. Fructose and glucose ingestion and muscle glycogen use during submaximal exercise. *J Appl Physiol.* 55:1767–1771, 1983.
96. MacDonald, V.W., and F.F. Jöbsis. Spectrophotometric studies on the pH from skeletal muscle: pH change during and after contractile activity. *J Gen Physiol.* 68:179–195, 1976.
97. Maehlum, S. Muscle glycogen synthesis after glucose infusion during postexercise recovery in diabetic and non-diabetic subjects. *Scand J Clin Lab Invest.* 38:349–354, 1978.
98. Maehlum, S., P. Felig, and J. Wahren. Splanchnic glucose and muscle glycogen metabolism after glucose feeding during postexercise recovery. *Am J Physiol.* 235:E255–E260, 1978.
99. Marsh, M.E., and J.R. Murlin. Muscular efficiency on high carbohydrate and high fat diets. *J Nutr.* 1:105–137, 1928.
100. Masoro, E.J., L.B. Rowell, R.M. McDonald, and B. Steiert. Skeletal muscle lipids. II. Nonutilization of intracellular lipid esters as an energy source for contractile activity. *J Biol Chem.* 241:2626–2634, 1966.
101. McDougall, J.D., G.R. Ward, D.G. Sale, and J.R. Sutton. Muscle glycogen repletion after high-intensity intermittent exercise. *J Appl Physiol.* 42:129–132, 1977.
102. Miller, W.C., G.R. Bryce, and R.K. Conlee. Adaptations to a high-fat diet that increases exercise endurance in male rats. *J Appl Physiol.* 56:78–83, 1984.
103. Nilsson, L.H., and E. Hultman. Liver glycogen in man—the effect of total starvation or a carbohydrate-poor diet followed by carbohydrate refeeding. *Scand J Clin Lab Invest.* 32:325–330, 1973.
104. Nilsson, L.H., P. Fürst, and E. Hultman. Carbohydrate metabolism of the liver in normal man under varying dietary conditions. *Scand J Clin Lab Invest.* 32:331–337, 1974.
105. Nilsson, L.H., and E. Hultman. Liver and muscle glycogen in man after glucose and fructose infusion. *Scand J Clin Lab Invest.* 33:5–10, 1974.
106. Olsson, K.E., and B. Saltin. Variations in total body water with muscle glycogen changes in man. *Acta Physiol Scand.* 80:11–18, 1970.
107. Pernow, B., and B. Saltin. Availability of substrates and capacity for prolonged exercise in man. *J Appl Physiol.* 31:416–422, 1971.
108. Piehl, K. Time course for refilling the glycogen stores in human muscle following exercise-induced glycogen depletion. *Acta Physiol Scand.* 90:297–302, 1974.
109. Piehl, K., S. Adolfsson, and K. Nazar. Glycogen storage and glycogen synthetase activity in trained and untrained muscle of man. *Acta Physiol Scand.* 90:779–788, 1974.
110. Posner, J.B., R. Stern, and E.G. Krebs. Effect of electrical stimulation and epinephrine on muscle phosphorylase, phosphorylase *b* kinase, and adenosine 3', 5' phosphate. *J Biol Chem.* 240:682–685, 1965.
111. Pruett, E.D.R. Glucose and insulin during prolonged work stress in men living on different diets. *J Appl Physiol.* 28:199–208, 1970.
112. Pruett, E.D.R. FFA mobilization during and after prolonged severe muscular work in man. *J Appl Physiol.* 29:809–815, 1970.
113. Ravussin, E., C. Bogardus, K. Scheidegger, B. LaGrange, E.D. Horton, and E.S. Horton. Effect of elevated FFA on carbohydrate and lipid oxidation during prolonged exercise in humans. *J Appl Physiol.* 60:1986.

ENERGY METABOLISM AND PROLONGED EXERCISE **35**

114. Reitman, J., K.M. Baldwin, and J.O. Holloszy. Intramuscular triglyceride utilization by red, white, and intermediate skeletal muscle and heart during exhaustive exercise. *Proc. Soc Expt Biol Med.* 142:628–631, 1973.
115. Rennie, M., W.W. Winder, and J.O. Holloszy. A sparing effect of increased free fatty acids on muscle glycogen content in exercising rats. *Biochem J.* 156:647–655, 1976.
116. Richter, E.A., and H. Galbo. High glycogen levels enhance glycogen breakdown in isolated contracting skeletal muscle. *J Appl Physiol.* 61:827–831, 1986.
117. Sahlin, K. Intracellular pH and energy metabolism in skeletal muscle. *Acta Physiol Scand.* Suppl. 455, 1978.
118. Saltin, B., L.H. Hartley, Å. Kilbom, and I. Åstrand. Physical training in sedentary middle-aged and older men. II. Oxygen uptake, heart rate and blood lactate concentration at submaximal and maximal exercise. *Scand J Clin Lab Invest.* 24:323–334, 1969.
119. Saltin, B., and J. Karlsson. Muscle glycogen utilization during work of different intensities. In: *Muscle metabolism during exercise.* Edited by B. Pernow and B. Saltin, Plenum, New York, 1971, 289–299.
120. Saltin, B., K. Nazar, D.L. Costill, E. Stein, E. Jansson, B. Essen, and P.D. Gollnick. The nature of the training response: peripheral and central adaptations to one-legged exercise. *Acta Physiol Scand.* 96:289–305, 1978.
121. Saltin, B., and P.D. Gollnick. Skeletal muscle adaptability: significance for metabolism and performance. In: *Handbook of Physiology—Skeletal Muscle.* Edited by L.D. Peachy, R.H. Adrian, and S.R. Geiger, Williams & Wilkins, Baltimore, 1983, 555–631.
122. Sembrowich, W.L., C.D. Ianuzzo, C.W. Saubert, IV, R.E. Shepherd, and P.D. Gollnick. Substrate mobilization during prolonged exercise in 6-hydroxydopamine treated rats. *Pflügers Arch.* 349:57–62, 1974.
123. Sonne, B., and H. Galbo. Carbohydrate metabolism in fructose-fed and food-restricted running rats. *J Appl Physiol.* 61:1457–1466, 1986.
124. St. George Stubbs, S., and M.C. Blanchaer. Glycogen phosphorylase and glycogen synthetase activity in red and white skeletal muscle of the guinea pig. *Can J Biochem.* 43:463–468, 1965.
125. Taylor, A.W., R. Thayer, and S. Rao. Human skeletal muscle glycogen synthetase activities with exercise and training. *Can J Physiol Pharmacol.* 50:411–415, 1972.
126. Taylor, A.W., J. Stothart, M.W. Booth, R. Thayer, and S. Rao. Human skeletal muscle glycogen branching enzyme activities with exercise and training. *Can J Physiol Pharmacol.* 52:119–122, 1974.
127. Taylor, D.G., P. Styles, P.M. Matthews, D.A. Arnold, D.G. Gadian, P. Bore and G.K. Radda. Energetics of human muscle: exercise-induced ATP depletion. *Magn Res Med.* 3:44–54, 1986.
128. Terjung, R.L., K.M. Baldwin, W.W. Winder, and J.O. Holloszy. Glycogen repletion in different types of muscle and in liver after exhausting exercise. *Am J Physiol.* 226:1387–1391, 1974.
129. Terjung, R.L., G.A. Dudley, and R.A. Meyer. Metabolic and circulatory limitation to muscular performance at the organ level. *J Exp Biol.* 115:307–318, 1985.
130. Thronheim, K., and J.M. Lowenstein. Control of phosphofructokinase from rat skeletal muscle. *J Biol Chem.* 251:7322–7328, 1976.
131. Trivedi, B., and W.H. Danforth. Effects of pH on the kinetics of frog muscle phosphofructokinase. *J Biol Chem.* 2421:310–322, 1966.
132. Winder, W.W. Effect of intravenous caffeine on liver glycogenolysis during prolonged exercise. *Med Sci Sports Exer.* 18:192–196, 1986.
133. Ahlborg, G., and P. Felig. Influence of glucose ingestion on fuel-hormone response during prolonged exercise. *J Appl Physiol.* 41:683–688, 1976.
134. Ahlborg, G., P. Felig, L. Hagenfeldt, R. Hendler, and J. Wahren. Substrate turnover during prolonged exercise in man: splanchnic and leg metabolism of glucose, free fatty acids, and amino acids. *J Clin Invest.* 53:1080–1090, 1974.
135. Coyle, E.F., A.R. Coggan, M.K. Hemmert, and J.L. Ivy. Muscle glycogen utilization during prolonged strenuous exercise when fed carbohydrate. *J Appl Physiol.* 61:165–172, 1986.
136. Dohm, G.L., G.J. Kasperek, E.B. Tapscott, and H.A. Barakat. Protein metabolism during endurance exercise. *Fed Proc.* 44:348–352, 1985.
137. Hermansen, L., E. Hultman, and B. Saltin. Muscle glycogen during prolonged severe exercise. *Acta Physiol. Scand* 71:129–139, 1967.
138. Hood, D.A., and R.L. Terjung. Leucine metabolism in perfused rat skeletal muscle during contraction. *Am J Physiol.* 253:E636–E647, 1987.
139. Lefebvre, P.J. Availability of sugars ingested before or during prolonged-duration moderate-intensity exercise in man. *Biochemical Aspects of Physical Exercise.* edited by G. Benzi, L. Packer, and N. Siliprandi, Elsevier, Amsterdam, 1986, 295–298.
140. Lemon, P.W.R., and J.P. Mullin. Effect of initial muscle glycogen levels on protein ca-

tabolism during exercise. *J Appl Physiol.* 48:624–629, 1980.

141. Wahren, J. Glucose turnover during exercise in man. *N.Y. Acad Sci.* 301:45–55, 1977.

142. White, T.P., and G.A. Brooks. [U-14C]-glucose, alanine, and levcine oxidation in rats at rest and at two intensities of running. *Am J Physiol.* 240:E155–E165, 1981.

DISCUSSION

BROOKS: If you look at subjects exercising for one to two hours, you see that the respiratory exchange ratios (RER) are really pretty high and that glycogen utilization is also pretty high. That really emphasizes the importance of carbohydrates. Some have reported that the better the marathon runner, the higher the RER, with an average RER of about .93 to .95, for well-prepared marathon runners. In fact, slower guys were around three hours, and their RERs were a lot lower.

GOLLNICK: I think we should not lose sight of the fact that carbohydrates are important for so many types of exercise.

FARRELL: You made the point that as the muscles become depleted of glycogen, there may be an increased central drive. That occurs even where you have euglycemia. What do you make of that?

GOLLNICK: Well, that's an interesting point. It appears to me that you cannot take glucose up fast enough to support the total muscular activity that some people have. The data that I used to support that is data from the Dallas group. They used MacArdle patients, who, of course, can't break down their muscle glycogen. One interesting experiment that they did in Dallas was to infuse glucose and elevated blood glucose level. When they did that, work capacity and oxygen consumption went up. That suggests to me that if you get enough glucose into the muscle, then you can sustain contraction. Why can you do that when you raise the blood glucose? Well, that's because of the transport mechanism of the glucose molecule. This is facilitated transport that obeys standard saturation kinetics, and if you raise blood glucose, then you change the saturation point. So blood glucose uptake is more concentration than flow dependent.

DEMPSEY: In short-term exercise, do you see any changes in muscle glycogen?

GOLLNICK: If you go to 150 percent of the $\dot{V}O_2$max, you can see a decline in glycogen after one minute. We published that in 1970.

DEMPSEY: Is it significant?

GOLLNICK: Yes, it is.

SHEPHARD: And you saw what fractional decrease, roughly?

GOLLNICK: Oh, it's about 10% or 15%.

BROOKS: You don't know from those data where the 10% to 15% are coming from.

GOLLNICK: You can't see it yet, because the glycogen depletion at that point is not big enough to allow you to note differences among fiber types.

GISOLFI: How low does muscle glycogen have to be in order to affect exercise performance?

GOLLNICK: I don't know. It has not been studied in a systematic way.

DEMPSEY: But that is a topic of controversy, isn't it? How good a marker of fatigue is glycogen depletion? How much depletion do you need before performance suffers?

BROOKS: In the short-term, I don't know. It shouldn't make much of a difference, because I don't think the Vmax of phosphorylase is affected too much by the glycogen content. So, I mean if you have lots of glycogen in muscle, it can be half depleted without affecting the Vmax of phosphorylase.

COYLE: I think 40 or 50 mmols per kilogram wet weight is when depletion begins to affect animals with high intensity exercise performance.

GOLLNICK: Well, Eric Hultman thinks that since the glycogen is bound to the phosphorylase complex, that if you start to deplete it, then you won't have enough glycogen immediately available for the phosphorylase enzyme. So that could be an issue. But he has no data to support that: he's just suggesting it.

BROOKS: Carl's first question was how much glycogen can be depleted before you affect the rate of glycogenolysis.

GOLLNICK: Actually, the rate of glycogenolysis falls rather sharply. It's usually an initial burst, and then it starts to fall, and that is the same pattern that you see in phosphorylase a. After the initial burst of phosphorylase a formation, it starts to decline.

RAVEN: What affect does intracellular dehydration have on that?

GOLLNICK: I have no way to know.

LAMB: Would it be your prediction that if you infused glucose into somebody and kept them at high glucose levels that they ought to be able to work at higher rates for longer periods of time?

GOLLNICK: Of course, those studies have been done. They've been done on animals. We did them on rats. We infused glucose some years ago in rats, and they were able to run an extra hour. And they've also been done on man. There's an Australian group who recently infused glucose into human subjects and prolonged their work. From a fuel standpoint, it appears that if you can give enough fuel, the muscle can take it up and then prolong the work.

LAMB: Do you care to speculate on what the limits of the intensity of exercise may be? Do you think infused subjects could work for six hours at say, 75% of $\dot{V}O_2$max, rather than 60% of $\dot{V}O_2$max?

GOLLNICK: I don't know for certain that it's possible.

COYLE: We've got some data now. We've been infusing glucose in glycogen-depleted subjects to see how long exercise can be continued. And they go on for 45 minutes to an hour while being infused. We've done some other studies looking at the work rate limitations. We find they can't exercise any more intensely than 75% of $\dot{V}O_2$max for more than a few minutes, while muscle glycogen is low, and we assume that blood glucose is a primary source of carbohydrate. So there's a work rate limitation which is just about equal to their lactate threshold. With glucose infusion, they can go 45 minutes, and they fatigue, with no indication that they're lacking carbohydrate. In other words, their RER values are still in the range that was acceptable to them before. We don't know if fatigue is due to some other factors besides carbohydrate depletion at that point.

DAVIS: Was this glucose infusion done after prolonged exercise?

COYLE: Yes. These subjects used glucose at over 1.1 grams per minute but we're not sure if that's because of their having low glycogens or having exercised three hours.

GOLLNICK: We did our studies with constant infusion. But I don't think there's any question that if you infuse glucose, you can prolong endurance.

NADEL: What are the kinetics of lactate under these circumstances?

GOLLNICK: It's very difficult to know.

BLAIR: As an epidemiologist who doesn't know much about this, what are we supposed to call this phenomenon of lactate accumulation?

GOLLNICK: Well, why not call it "the point of lactate accumulation." Or do you want to call it "lactate threshold"? The Scandanavians use what they call "OBLA" onset of blood lactate accumulation. But generally, "threshold" has a certain connotation that the muscles are hypoxic and the tissue oxygen content is below what you need to drive the aerobic process, so you're forced into lactate production. There's much evidence to suggest that that's not so.

BROOKS: We've been talking about glycogen utilization from specific depots, for instance, glycogen in the quadriceps during cycling. Two recent papers suggest that glycogenolysis can proceed on a global scale and provide substrates. One muscle can fuel another. Subjects did arm training, while researchers looked at exchanges across the legs. They did leg training, and the investigators looked at exchange across the arms. Their first report, I think, was with leg cycling. What they found is that after awhile in leg cycling, the legs weren't losing any lactate. But blood lactate was still elevated. They estimated that much of the lactate was being produced by the arms and was being taken up by the liver to make glucose. This glucose was then delivered to the legs during leg cycling. More recently they did the reverse. They saw that the rested legs were releasing lactate in a fairly large amount, and that was perfusing the liver. The liver was producing glucose, and the glucose was going back to make glycogen in the arms.

GOLLNICK: There's no reason, of course, that the lactate itself can't serve as a fuel to the working muscle. It's essentially a carbohydrate, and there's no reason that it has to go back to the liver to generate glucose, as far as I can see, because it's fairly diffusible across the muscle membrane. Once dehydrogenated, lactate is a nice fuel for the aerobic pathway. I don't see why we have to worry so much about whether it goes back to the liver.

BROOKS: Nobody's arguing with that particular point. I think the point is how significant a fuel it is.

GOLLNICK: I don't have any problem there. There's no reason that lactate can't, in fact, come across from one fiber to another.

BROOKS: Well, that's one of our current ideas. One fiber can interact with an adjacent fiber, by way of the capillary. Once it reaches the capillary, it could go to any of the fibers anywhere. There are two other things I did want to mention. One is the use of amino acids. Classically, it's been believed that amino acids don't constitute much of a fuel, but there's a growing mass of evidence that they do. And this is based on a variety of stable isotope work in humans and radiotracer work in animals. For instance, leucine could supply about 1% of the energy in exercise. Now scaling up from leucine being one amino acid, you just can't multiply that by 20, because leucine is probably one of the most important amino acids. It's purely ketogenic, and it is a fuel. But it might be that a small percent of the energy in prolonged work could be provided by amino acids. And, especially in the longer work, then, it might be more than a small percent. It might be 5% to 10%.

Now the question is how important is 5% to 10%? It could be that 5% to 10% is not that important. But in competition, seldom are first and last places separated by more than 1%. Also when you think about amino acids, you have to think about all the diverse ways in which they can enter into metabolic pathways and support the whole metabolism. They really sustain, allow the metabolism to go, even though other fuels provide the majority of the substrates. So I think there's some evidence that amino acids are involved. And as you increase the metabolism in exercise, then all the substrates become involved. And, finally, I want to say something about the glucose paradox.

The glucose paradox is based on mostly animal experimentation. If you feed glucose after fasting, most of the carbohydrate enters the portal circulation and bypasses the liver. So the liver apparently does not make glycogen from an immediate precursor such as glucose, which escapes and goes systemically. Some believe that glucose goes systemically and gets made mainly into lactate which reperfuses the liver. The liver then actually prefers to make glycogen from gluconeogenic precursers. Fructose appears better than glucose in recovery from exercise in terms of liver glycogen restitution. Apparently, what the liver does is clear the fructose, whereas the glucose largely escapes. So that's the glucose paradox.

NADEL: As you suggest, an increase in leucine oxidation may occur, but some have showed no change in blood urea nitrogen. So it implies that some of the amino acids may be oxidized, and others not.

BROOKS: We exhausted rats and then didn't feed them. We found that the heart will replenish its glycogen reserves in a few hours, even if the animal is starved. When you look at the total amount of lactate and glucose in the animal, it can't account for the glycogen repletion. So there's something else: this leaves the door open for some other kind of precursor, perhaps amino acids, to supply glycogen.

SHEPHARD: You could get a minimum estimate of the protein metabolism from the increment in blood urea content, and that was about five or six percent.

NADEL: We don't think there's any major contribution of protein metabolism. There's no question that there is oxidation of some of the amino acids. Animal studies and human studies have shown this.

FARRELL: How efficient is it to use amino acids? It seems to me from basic chemistry that it is a very inefficient way to make ATP.

GOLLNICK: It depends upon which amino acid you're looking at. Some of them are more efficient than others. But I personally feel that if I had a choice, I would take carbohydrates.

I think fructose is rather unimportant as an energy source for the muscle during exercise, and my reason is simple: the affinity of hexokinase in muscle is only one-tenth for fructose that it is for glucose. This means that you have to have a concentration of fructose at least ten times that of glucose in blood to compete effectively to enter the metabolism. You just don't see those kinds of fructose levels. If you look at all the fructose studies that are in the literature, almost nobody measured blood fructose. They give fructose, but they don't measure it. And why? It's very difficult to measure. So there's no indication in any of those studies that there's really a big enough elevation in fructose to make it interesting.

I think fructose is probably more interesting in the postexercise phase than it might be in the exercise phase. Fructose has a good ability to replenish liver glycogen. Liver handles fructose differently than how the muscle handles fructose. Fructokinase is a very active enzyme in the liver, and that's why you probably don't see much fructose appearing in the blood; as the fructose enters the blood it's rapidly cleared by the liver.

There is another problem that you might want to concern yourself with if you're thinking about giving fructose to athletes. If you give a large bolus, you are bound to have intestinal problems. Some people are actually allergic to it.

Fructose may ultimately come back out of the liver as glucose and provide some fuel. One of the advantages of that is fructose doesn't seem to produce the insulin surge that glucose does. So that's one reason that people try to use it. But I think the biochemical basis for using fructose directly is very, very weak.

HAGBERG: With training you use more fat. Where does it come from?

GOLLNICK: Well, I think, primarily fatty acids come from the stores that we have as adipose tissue, and probably to some degree from fat contained in the muscle itself. In order to really analyze how much fat is being used, you have to isolate the fiber. You have to be very careful with fibers, because the fat is not distributed as nicely as glycogen is with the fiber. There's also a lot of fat in between fibers. It's a difficult problem.

TIPTON: Don't intramuscular triglycerides really increase with training?

GOLLNICK: I'm saying it's very, very difficult to be absolutely certain they increase because you have regional variation. There's quite a lot of variability between samples.

2

Cardiovascular Function and Prolonged Exercise

PETER B. RAVEN, PH.D.

GLEN H.J. STEVENS, M.SC.

INTRODUCTION
  I. CARDIOVASCULAR ADJUSTMENTS TO PROLONGED EXERCISE
 II. CARDIOVASCULAR DRIFT
    A. Cardiovascular Drift and Body Temperature
    B. Cardiovascular Drift and Cutaneous Blood Flow
    C. Cardiovascular Drift and Blood Flow in Splanchnic, Hepatic, and Renal
       Circulation
    D. Cardiovascular Drift and Blood Volume Changes
    E. Cardiovascular Drift and Alterations in Central Command
III. MYOCARDIAL FATIGUE
SUMMARY
BIBLIOGRAPHY
DISCUSSION

INTRODUCTION

Despite accumulating evidence that increased physical activity contributes to the prevention of cardiovascular disease and to an increase in longevity (55,73,74,75,79,82,83,118), many questions have been raised with respect to the benefits and safety of prolonged exercise. One of these questions is whether or not strenuous exercise increases the risk of sudden cardiac death, both in healthy persons and in those with coronary artery disease (22,35,36,61). For example, Noakes et al. (80) documented six cases of myocardial infarction in highly-trained marathon runners with documented coronary artery disease, and Zoltic et al. (117) have reported that 50% of the sudden deaths recorded for United States Army personnel were associated with exercise.

Earlier reports by Jokl and Melzer (51) suggested that sudden cardiac death could not occur as a result of over-exertion of a healthy heart. Haskell (45), on the other hand, cautioned against optimism and cited the Green et al. (38) case finding, which reported on a 44-year-old male trained marathon runner who collapsed at mile 24 of the Boston Marathon. The runner died from an extensive transmural anterior myocardial infarction, yet on autopsy was found to be free of coronary artery disease.

It is apparent that questions concerning the efficacy and safety of prolonged exercise remain. Also, our understanding of cardiovascular regulation during prolonged exercise of one to six h in duration is incomplète. In this chapter, we describe the circulatory and hemodynamic responses to prolonged exercise. We have approached the issue with the focus that the cardiovascular system works during prolonged exercise to maintain blood pressure to assure adequate perfusion of vital organs and working muscles, despite the ever-increasing competitive demand on the circulating blood volume to dissipate heat (88,90).

I. CARDIOVASCULAR ADJUSTMENTS TO PROLONGED EXERCISE

Cardiovascular responses to an acute bout of prolonged exercise appear similar in both trained and untrained individuals (6,19,29). The differences associated with training appear more related to the onset of skeletal muscle fatigue, intensity of the exercise, and the temperature regulatory capacity, than to cardiovascular function, per se.

Many studies have utilized prolonged exercise protocols ranging from greater than 15 min to a termination time of one to six h (3,4,7,19,28,29,30,31,32,88,89,90,95,96,98,107). In this section, we will define the cardiovascular adjustment to prolonged exercise as that which occurs during constant load exercise for 60 min or longer at a level of intensity greater than 50% of maximal oxygen uptake ($\dot{V}O_2$max). Regardless of the exercise position (upright or supine), the consensus finding is that if the work load is greater than 50% $\dot{V}O_2$max, and maintained longer than 10 min, (in which time the acute hemodynamic response achieves a new steady state), there is a progressive increase in heart rate over time with a corresponding decrease in stroke volume. The degree of change observed in these responses appears related to environmental temperature (76,97,99) and the relative work load (97) (Fig. 2-1). This phenomenon has been termed "cardiovascular drift" (88,90), and the decrease in stroke volume counteracts the increase in heart rate to maintain cardiac output constant over time.

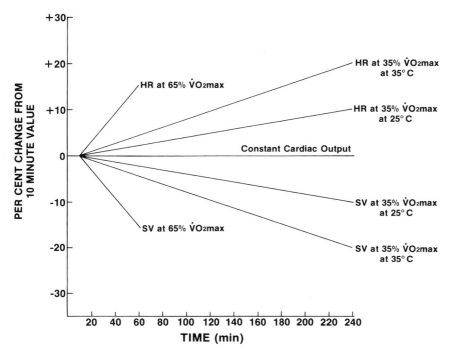

FIGURE 2-1. *A composite of data presented in references #29 and 37 depicting the effect of intensity of work and environmental temperature on the heart rate and stroke volume response to prolonged work.*

During prolonged exercise, the organism is faced with two physiological problems. First, thermal stress invokes cutaneous vasodilation, which displaces the circulating blood volume into cutaneous veins and thereby lowers central blood volume, cardiac filling pressure and, subsequently, stroke volume. Second, the working muscles must receive adequate perfusion for the delivery of oxygen, which if inadequate, will hinder performance or work. If cutaneous blood flow is reduced below the thermoregulatory needs, then hyperthermia will occur, which may prove debilitating in the highly-motivated athlete. The competition between these two physiological processes does not become manifest as "cardiovascular drift" until the workload exceeds 50% of the individual's maximal capacity (>50% $\dot{V}O_2$max).

The cardiovascular response to prolonged exercise begins with the initial phase of adjustment to a new steady state that is related directly to the metabolic demand of the exercise. The initial adjustment is followed by the phase of "cardiovascular drift," which is related to an individual's V̇O₂max, the relative workload, the environmental conditions, and the level of hydration of the individual. Finally, if exercise is of long enough duration and the intensity of work is severe enough, a stage of exhaustion or "myocardial fatigue" may ensue.

As noted previously, the initial phase of cardiovascular adjustment will not be described here. However, the mechanisms associated with "cardiovascular drift" and "myocardial fatigue" will be discussed.

II. CARDIOVASCULAR DRIFT

Clearly the primary event associated with "cardiovascular drift" is the translocation of the circulating blood volume into the cutaneous circulation (90). Johnson and Rowell (50) have suggested that the progressive decrements in central venous pressure, stroke volume, and mean arterial pressure seen during prolonged exercise by Ekelund and Holmgren (31) and Ekelund (29) (Fig. 2-2) were primarily due to progressive increments in cutaneous blood flow.

In an earlier investigation, Kamon and Belding (54) evaluated the changes in "effective" dermal blood flow (BF$_e$) (calculated from

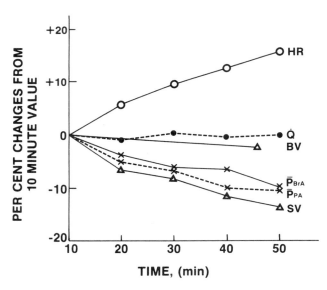

FIGURE 2-2. *Hemodynamic responses during long-term exercise in six subjects. BV = Blood volume, Q = Cardiac output, SV = Stroke volume, $\bar{P}_{BrA}$ = Mean brachial artery pressure, and $\bar{P}_{PA}$ = Mean pulmonary artery pressure. Data are presented as percent change from 10 min value. (Modified from data presented in reference #32.)*

heat uptake) in trained subjects exercising at a $\dot{V}O_2$ of 600 mL $\cdot$ min^{-1} $\cdot$ (m^2)$^{-1}$ for one h. During the first 10 min they found that BF$_e$ to the hand decreased with no change in BF$_e$ to the forearm. Because brachial artery pressure simultaneously increased, they suggested that dermal vasoconstriction had occurred. However, after 10 min, BF$_e$ in the hand and forearm increased 20% to 50% above control. This suggested a secondary release of vasoconstriction during more prolonged exercise to assist in thermal balance. However, it was unclear whether the increase was due to increases in blood flow to the skin or muscle. During prolonged exercise, the blood supply to active skeletal muscle increases, while, at the same time, the body attempts to maintain thermal balance. Johnson and Rowell (50) found a sustained fall in forearm muscle blood flow during exercise indicating regional muscular vasoconstriction. This confirmed that the increase in forearm blood flow they found was confined to the cutaneous beds, presumably to promote heat dissipation. Rowell et al. (91) and Zitnik et al. (116) have found a continuous decrease in venous tone during exercise or with local heating, following an initial vasoconstriction. These findings further support the contention that blood translocation to the skin is a primary response during prolonged exercise.

In the studies of Ekelund (29), heart rate increased continuously throughout a constant prolonged workload, regardless of exercise position. However, the rate of increase in heart rate was greater during the first 30 min of exercise, as compared to the final 30 min. The increased heart rate was positively correlated to the increase in core temperature (r = 0.72) and, as has been reported previously (19,20,21,32,98), the decrease in stroke volume matched the increase in heart rate (Fig. 2-3). Subjects that were at a greater relative work load showed greater increases in heart rate and greater decreases in stroke volume, once again confirming that fitness plays only a relative part in the cardiovascular response. A significant correlation was found between the decrease in stroke volume from 10 minutes to the end of the exercise and the corresponding change in heart rate during the same time period. Other measurements included right ventricular pressure, pulmonary artery pressure, and brachial artery pressure (Fig. 2-3). From rest to 10 min of exercise, a continuous increase in all pressures was seen, but from the 10th minute to the end of exercise the pressures continuously decreased. The mean brachial artery pressure decreased by 6-10 Torr from the 10th min to the end of exercise, with the greatest decrease seen in those subjects exercising at the highest relative load. The decrease in brachial pressure was a combination of decreases in both systolic and diastolic pressures, suggestive of progressive vasodilation and de-

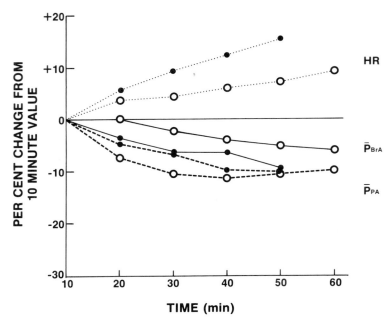

FIGURE 2-3. *Responses of heart rate, HR (dotted line), mean brachial artery pressure* P_{BrA} *(continuous line), and mean pulmonary artery pressure* P_{PA} *(dashed line) during prolonged exercise. Data are presented as percent change from 10 min value (modified from data presented in reference #29.) Exercise was performed in the sitting position at two intensities: solid circles represent higher intensity work (77% W_{170}) than open circles.*

creasing total peripheral resistance. Right ventricular end-diastolic pressure decreased some 2.2 to 2.6 Torr from minute 10 until the end of exercise in all studies.

A. Cardiovascular Drift and Body Temperature

Presumably cardiovascular drift is related to the thermoregulatory need to increase skin blood flow. Ekelund (29) reported that increases in heart rate were positively correlated to increases in body temperature. In addition, Jose et al. (52) found that intrinsic heart rate increased 7 beats $\cdot$ min$^{-1} \cdot °$ C^{-1} rise in core temperature. Similar results have been shown in the dog heart-lung preparation (59). The relation between intrinsic heart rate and core temperature explains some 88% of the variance, whereas the correlation between functional heart rate and core temperature accounts only for 55% of the variance. Therefore, it is doubtful that the change in heart rate observed in experiments involving cardiovascular drift can be totally attributable to absolute changes in core temperature. Furthermore, Christensen (15) has shown that with prolonged exercise at a given steady state heart rate, body temperature increases; in experiments where body temperature was maintained constant, heart rate increased. Saltin and Hermansen (97) clearly demonstrated that core temperature was directly related to relative work loads and was independent of absolute load. Given that increases in intrinsic heart rate were more strongly correlated with increases in core temperature, we submit that a thermally mediated redistribution of blood volume plays an important part in the phenomenon of cardiovascular drift. However, increases in core temperature can only partially explain the redistribution of blood volume and increasing heart rate.

B. Cardiovascular Drift and Cutaneous Blood Flow

After an initial increase, cardiac output has been shown to remain constant during prolonged exercise (29,98). After the first few minutes of exercise, blood flow to visceral organs decreases and then shows only minor changes with prolonged exercise (39,92). If both blood flow to active skeletal muscle and venous return remain constant, then blood flow to skin must suffer, and thermal balance may become compromised (49). But this scenario does not occur in prolonged exercise. At the beginning of leg exercise, vasoconstriction is seen in the forearm and hand, but this constriction is succeeded by a steady vasodilation as exercise continues (8,10).

Rowell (88,89,93) suggested that the progressively decreasing stroke volume during prolonged exercise was due to an increased core temperature that results in a relative vasoconstriction of active skeletal muscle and peripheral displacement of blood volume to the cutaneous blood vessels (Fig. 2-4). Subsequently, Johnson and Rowell (50) demonstrated that after one h of continuous leg exercise at 100 to 125 W, there was a continuous increase in forearm blood flow (FBF) and heart rate (Fig. 2-5). The FBF increased an average 8.26 $ml \cdot dL^{-1} \cdot min^{-1}$ over 60 min of exercise, while muscle blood flow decreased. This indicated that the increased FBF must have been directed to the cutaneous beds. This concept is supported by Ekelund's data (28,31) on six male subjects who exercised in the upright position at a constant workload. The mean stroke volume in Ekelund's subjects decreased from 123 mL after 10 min to 106 mL, i.e., 13.8% of the 10 min value. Heart rate increased an average of 30 $beats \cdot min^{-1}$, whereas mean arterial pressure decreased, and cardiac output did not change. Although oxygen uptake increased over time, it was attributed to a decrease in work efficiency because, as time passed the subjects' gross motor movements increased.

The ventilation/perfusion ratio also increased, which, along with an increased dead space ventilation, indicated a decrease in perfu-

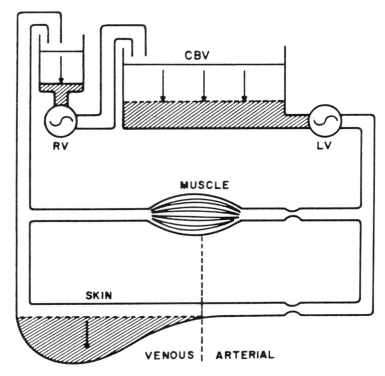

FIGURE 2-4. *Schematic illustration of the effects of cutaneous vasodilation and the pre-loads of the right (RV) and left ventricles (LV). The increasing cutaneous volume produces a decreasing venous return. Central or thoracic blood volume is represented by CBV. (Reprinted with permission from L.R. Rowell and the American Physiological Society reference #89).*

sion of the upper parts of the lung (28,31). In the supine position, where hydrostatic forces imposed by gravity were obviated, the cardiovascular responses were similar to those found in the upright position. The pulmonary artery pressure decreased 20% from the 10th to the 20th min of exercise, indicating an increase in the capacitance of the pulmonary bed. In addition, a reduction in central venous pressure and a change in the distribution of the circulating blood volume were observed (28,31). The decreased central venous pressure, coupled with a decrease in pulmonary artery pressure, clearly indicated that the shift in blood volume was a result of a progressive translocation of blood from the central capacitance vessels to the periphery. Therefore, measurements reflecting decreases in filling pressures and pulmonary artery pressure with cardiac output maintained at a constant level are clearly a part of the cardiovascular drift.

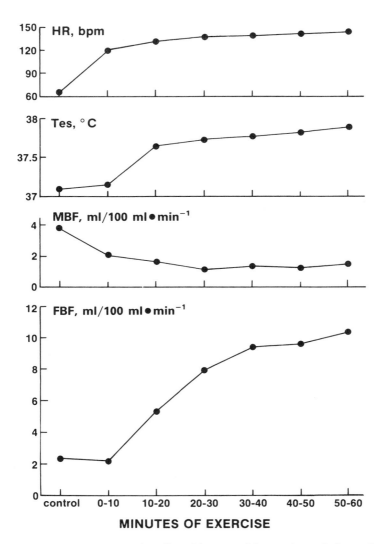

FIGURE 2-5. *Average responses from five subjects exercising continuously for one h at 100 to 125 W. Heart rate, (HR) esophageal temperature (T_{es}), muscle blood (MBF), forearm blood flow (FBF). (Replotted from data presented in reference #50.)*

Hartley (42,43) and Johnson (49) have both described the competition that exists between the cutaneous vessels and the circulatory beds. Indirect evidence of this competition was obtained by Sawka et al. (99) who had subjects exercise at 70% of $\dot{V}O_2$max for 80 min followed by a 90 min rest. Following the work/rest session, each subject repeated the 70% $\dot{V}O_2$max exercise bout for 80 min.

CARDIOVASCULAR FUNCTION **51**

Although fluid replacement was allowed *ad libitum,* body weight decreased by 2%. The second bout of exercise exacerbated the cardiovascular drift in that the heart rate was higher and stroke volume lower than during the first exercise bout. Also, it was noted that cardiac output tended to decrease near the end of the second bout of exercise. In addition, the rectal temperature was higher during the second run. The investigators suggested that the decreasing cardiac output was due to the competition for circulation between the dilated skeletal muscle beds and the cutaneous vessels and that as oxygen uptake was maintained during the repeat exercise bout, increases in oxygen extraction at the working muscles must have occurred.

In summary, during prolonged exercise, vasodilation of vessels within the active skeletal muscle occurs along with vasoconstriction in the non-active muscle beds and organs. These alterations are temporally related to oxygen delivery to the working muscles, whereas vasodilation of the cutaneous beds is directly and temporally related to the need to dissipate heat.

C. Cardiovascular Drift and Blood Flow In Splanchnic, Hepatic, and Renal Circulation

Diminished circulation during prolonged exercise has been reported in non-active tissues, such as the splanchnic-hepatic and renal vascular beds (39,88). At the start of exercise, Clausen and Trap-Jensen (18) showed that for a given steady-state exercise that resulted in constant oxygen uptake or cardiac output, the increase in heart rate and the proportionate increase in vasoconstriction of the splanchnic-hepatic vascular beds had a common time course. These findings confirm Rowell's (88,90) statement that "increased sympathetic nervous outflow to the heart to increase its rate is accompanied by a proportionate increase in sympathetic vasomotor outflow to the visceral organs."

Vasoconstriction to splanchnic organs occurs rapidly during the first few minutes of exercise (9,18). When exercise at a constant yet moderate oxygen uptake was prolonged, heart rate and norepinephrine concentrations increased in concert with increases in splanchnic and renal vascular resistance (17). Both Christensen (17) and Hartley et al. (43) have clearly documented the activation of the sympathetic nervous system during prolonged exercise. Despite this increase in sympathetic stimulation leading to reduced flow in splanchnic, hepatic, and renal circulation and presumably leading to increased inotropy, stroke volume continues to decrease during the phenomenon of cardiovascular drift. Therefore, it is apparent that neither vasodilation in visceral organs nor decreased sympathetic discharge to the heart can account for cardiovascular drift.

Despite the suggestion that cardiovascular drift appears directly related to the increasing cutaneous circulation, two other phenomena may contribute to the overall degree of response. These are (1) a progressively decreasing blood volume due to dehydration and (2) an increasing "central command."

D. Cardiovascular Drift and Blood Volume Changes

Progressive reductions in blood volume occur during the first 10 min of prolonged exercise that are attributable to the initial osmotic and hydrostratic changes within the exercising muscle. Subsequently, in Rowell's many investigations into cardiovascular drift, blood volume due to dehydration was maintained constant by infusion of isotonic saline during the exercise (90).

However, earlier work had shown that alterations in body position and the hemodynamic change associated with the initiation of exercise from rest produces an alteration in the amount of circulating blood volume (40,101). This change in volume is primarily related to changes in plasma volume (40,101). Because of this phenomenon, it was postulated that, during prolonged exercise, the progressively increasing need for sweating to dissipate internally generated heat would further reduce the plasma volume such that circulating blood volume and stroke volume would be similarly decreased. The reduced stroke volume would require a compensatory increase in heart rate to maintain cardiac output, thereby providing a plausible explanation for cardiovascular drift.

Initially, Thompson et al. (106) demonstrated that plasma volume (PV) decreased on changing from the supine to the standing position or from supine or sitting rest to exercise. These findings have been confirmed by Hagan et al. (40), and Senay et al.(101). More recently, Wells et al. (112) reported that after a marathon plasma volume decreased 8% in females and 13% in males. The plasma volume returned to normal in 8 hours. However, in laboratory studies, Kozlowski and Saltin (60) found very small decreases in extracellular fluid after exercise dehydration that suggested a greater loss of water from intracellular stores. Subsequently, Saltin (95) used a sauna to dehydrate subjects and then perform exercise in a supine and sitting position for an hour at 45% VO_2max. The subjects exhibited a 25% decrease in plasma volume after the dehydration. However, when the decreased stroke volume and increased heart rate and cardiac output were compared with the same exercise load without prior dehydration in the sitting position, no differences were observed. The same comparison in the supine position also showed no car-

TABLE 2-1. *Hemodynamic Changes Associated with Dehydration and Body Position**

BWD, %	Work Position	$\dot{V}O_2$ (L · min^{-1})		Heart Rate (beats · min^{-1})		O^2 Pulse	
		PRE	POST	PRE	POST	PRE	POST
3.93	Supine	3.10	2.98	148	147	21.1	20.5
	Sitting	3.14	3.06	154	163	20.7	19.0

Mean data from three subjects at a submaximal work load before (PRE) and after (POST) thermal dehydration (BWD = body weight decrease).
*From data in Reference 95.

diovascular differences (Table 2-1). In addition, no change was seen in maximal oxygen uptake, cardiac output or stroke volume between exercise with and without dehydration. However, work time was decreased with dehydration, and the levels of blood lactate at the end of exercise were less. A significant correlation was found between the relative decrease in plasma volume and change in stroke volume for submaximal work. Saltin (95) suggested that the shorter maximal work time represented a decreased ability to perform muscular work and implied an intra-cellular limitation of the skeletal muscle.

In contrast to Wells et al. (112), Astrand and Saltin (5,6) found that total water loss after an 85 km race was 5.9 L, but that plasma volume increased 11% and red blood cells volume decreased 3.2%, hence, total blood volume increased 3.5%. They also found a decreased work capacity after the race. Since the subjects exercised in a cold environment, the thermal load was not regarded as significant. The increase in plasma volume was thought to be partially mediated by water released from combusted glycogen. A later study by Harrison et al. (41) examined the concept of thermally mediated plasma volume shifts in six men exercising for 50 min at either 25% $\dot{V}O_2$max at 42° C or 30° C, and 50% $\dot{V}O_2$max at both temperatures at different times. During exercise at 25% $\dot{V}O_2$max in the cooler environment (30° C), they saw little change in plasma volume after the initial hemoconcentration but did see a decreased plasma volume with exercise at 42° C. These changes were increased at the 50% $\dot{V}O_2$max workload. Therefore, it was thought that plasma volume decreased in the subjects due to the fluid volume shifts brought about by exercising in a hot environment. It was theorized that a rapid secretion of hypotonic sweat occurred in the hot environment, thereby establishing a greater concentration gradient between extravascular and intravascular compartments than in cooler environments. Presumably, the difference in gradient subsequently drew water from the intravascular compartment. During the prolonged exercise in the cool environment, it was thought that the proteins in the intravascular compartment acted to maintain oncotic pressure and thus favor water retention within the intravascular compartment.

Ekelund (29,32) examined different work intensities and body positions during prolonged exercise. During the first 10 min of sitting exercise, blood volume measured using I^{131} labeled albumin, was decreased 9.3%, and plasma volume was decreased 14.3% from rest to the end of exercise. Between the 10th and 60th min of exercise, there was no change in plasma volume or blood volume. During sitting exercise at a lower work intensity, blood volume decreased 7.5% between rest and exercise, and plasma volume decreased 10%. Again, no change between 10 and 60 minutes of exercise was observed. In the supine position, blood volume decreased 5% and plasma volume decreased 7.4% after 10 min of exercise with no further change in plasma volume. In all three exercise states, no significant change in cardiac output was seen after 10 min of exercise, during which time heart rate continued to increase as stroke volume decreased.

In 1972, Costill (20) provided a case study report in which a well trained marathon runner exercised to exhaustion during a 20 mile treadmill run. The typical cardiovascular drift was observed, with heart rate increasing from 159 beats $\cdot$ min^{-1} at 6 min to 175 beats $\cdot$ min^{-1} at 101 min; stroke volume decreased 13 mL $\cdot$ beat^{-1} during the same time interval. Body weight loss was greater than 8%, yet plasma volume was only slightly decreased, suggesting that intracellular dehydration occurred in order to maintain plasma volume. In a later study, Costill and Saltin (21) demonstrated that fluid loss occurred equally from both intracellular and extracellular compartments, thereby raising questions as to the influence of environmental temperature, workload, body position, and exercise duration on fluid volume shifts.

In summary, progressive dehydration does not usually produce a progressive loss in plasma volume or total blood volume (1,6,20,28,29,30,31,32,41,98), and loss of plasma volume does not make a major contribution to cardiovascular drift. However, fluid shifts producing intracellular dehydration during prolonged exercise may well be a component of the complex phenomenon known as muscular fatigue.

E. Cardiovascular Drift and Alterations in Central Command

Another possible factor contributing to the degree of cardiovascular drift is an increased "central command." In many of the studies of prolonged submaximal exercise at levels of >50% $\dot{V}O_2$max, a progressive increase in oxygen uptake (metabolic drift) occurs despite a constant work load and constant cardiac output (30,31,43,98). Ekelund and Holmgren (31) attributed this decrease in efficiency to an increasing recruitment of motor units (increasing central command) to accomplish the same work task. Hartley (42) suggested that metabolic drift alone could explain the cardiovascular drift.

In a more recent investigation, Davies and Thompson (23) demonstrated an average 9.1% increase in $\dot{V}O_2$ (metabolic drift) for well-trained marathon runners performing four h of work at 60% to 70% $\dot{V}O_2$max. Although rehydration fluids were available *ad libitum* body weight decreased 5.5%. However, plasma volume was not altered, confirming the work of Kozlowski and Saltin (60) and others (6,21,29,32,95). The classic cardiovascular drift was present with a 17% increase in heart rate and a 17% decrease in stroke volume over the four h. The fact that the metabolic drift was only half as great as the cardiovascular drift speaks against a "cause and effect" association between the two. Heart rate was increased in parallel to the increasing rectal temperature ($r = 0.99$), suggesting once again that a major component of the cardiovascular drift is the translocation of blood to the periphery to assist in temperature regulation. Alterations in body weight or fuel source could not explain the increasing oxygen uptake observed.

In a recent investigation in our laboratory (115), in which 38 subjects walked to exhaustion at a constant work load of 70% $\dot{V}O_2$max, we observed an average 4% increase in oxygen uptake and a 13% increase in heart rate. It would appear, therefore, that in light of a constant cardiac output (23) the metabolic drift is accomplished by an increasing oxygen extraction at the tissue level. Furthermore, as in other studies (23,31), the increase in heart rate was substantially in excess of the increase in metabolic rate, and, therefore, the increasing metabolic demand can explain only a portion of the increasing heart rate.

The concept of a centrally mediated descending neural stimulus that reflexly adjusts skeletal muscle force generation to accomplish a fatiguing work task was initially described by McCloskey and Mitchell (68) and is a modification of Krogh and Lindhard's (62) concepts of an increasing spread of neural activity, i.e., central command. Thus, in the central command model, the finding of an increasing oxygen uptake links the increase in neural drive to maintain muscle force output by fiber recruitment (71) with an increased sympathetic stimulus (43,44,109) that increases heart rate (16). The functional pathways for this feedback detection and subsequent increased central drive have been clearly described during static exercise (Fig. 2-6). However, the stimulus and the signal detecting organ re-

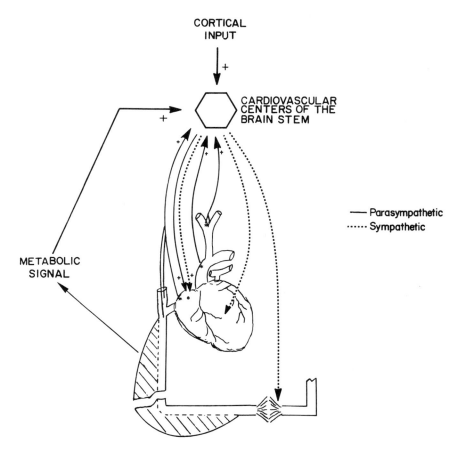

CORTICAL
INPUT

CARDIOVASCULAR
CENTERS OF THE
BRAIN STEM

——— Parasympathetic
······· Sympathetic

METABOLIC
SIGNAL

FIGURE 2-6. *A schematic depiction of the integration of input from central command (cortical input) to cardiovascular centers of the brain stem with metabolic signals from the muscle (Type III and Type IV afferents), information from aortic and carotid baroreceptors via the Hering-Bruer nerve, and with information from direct vagal afferents or C-fiber input from cardiac volumes. Subsequent sympathetic afferent traffic (dashed line) governing heart rate, myocardial contractility and peripheral vasomotion depicted along with vagal withdrawal (continuous line) at the S-A node.*

quire further elucidation, and the functionality of this mechanism during dynamic exercise has yet to be described.

III. MYOCARDIAL FATIGUE

With the advent of the modern marathon, concern has been raised that the combination of severe exercise intensity and prolonged duration might produce catastrophic sequelae of cardiovascular events that would induce failure of cardiac muscle function similar to that observed when skeletal muscle is severely exercised and hyperthermically stressed. Despite Rowell's (90) contention "that no direct evidence exists to suggest that the inherent mechanical properties of the myocardium are reduced during prolonged exercise," sufficient data are available to support the possibility of damage to the heart and its performance.

As early as 1899, Williams and Arnold (114) reported that following the Boston Marathon, run at a pace of 7 min·mile^{-1}, the postrace pulse rates were weak in all subjects and weight loss ranged from 1.1% to 4.9% of initial body weight. Furthermore, in 10 runners evaluated, seven showed a relative increase and two a decrease in the area of the left ventricle. It was also noted after the race that the majority of the runners had mitral valve murmurs, which was thought to indicate muscular incompetence (or fatigue) of the mitral valve. This was the first suggestion that exercise performance was limited because of the heart, especially when it was noted that the first and second place finishers in the race had no murmurs.

Most studies suggest an increase in heart size as an effect of training (56,64,72,84,114). The findings with respect to postrace heart size have been much more variable, with groups reporting decreases (7), increases (11) or variable changes (29,30,114). Interestingly, Maron and Horvath (67) in their review note that Hug (48) had earlier reported that early marathon finishers had smaller hearts after the race, whereas the slower runners had dilated hearts. As will be noted later, an enlarging heart for a given venous return accompanied by an increasing heart rate is thought to be clear evidence of adverse myocardial functional changes. Previous reviews of cardiac adaptation to training exist in the literature, and this topic will not be discussed further here. For a comprehensive analysis, see the reviews by Schaible and Scheuer (100), Dowell (26), and Peronnet et al. (84).

Ekelund et al. (23,32) determined heart volumes during upright and supine prolonged exercise. The roentgenological heart volume was measured at end-diastole. During prolonged exercise at a constant work load, there was a decrease in heart volume, which was accompanied by an increased heart rate. An average 37.5 mL decrease in heart volume for each 10 beats·min^{-1} increase in heart rate was found when the subjects exercised at 71% and 67% of working capacity at a heart rate of 170 beats·min^{-1} in the upright and supine position, respectively. However, as exhaustion approached, six of the 10 subjects in the sitting position showed an average 52 mL increase in heart volume (Fig. 2-7). A negative slope relating heart rate to heart volume was observed. This fits well with the concept that

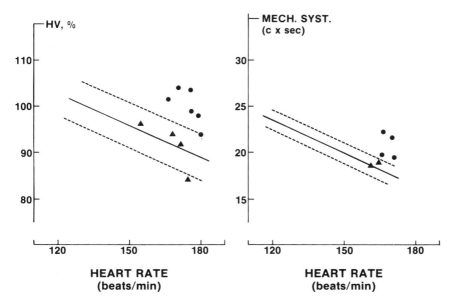

HEART VOLUME

MECHANICAL SYSTOLE

FIGURE 2-7. *Regression line ±1 SD for heart volume (HV), in percent of first exercise heart volume, and mechanical systole at specific heart rates during exercise in the sitting position (c × sec = 1/100 second). Solid circles represent final values for individual subjects during exercise that are equal to or greater than ±1 SD above the predicted values. The triangles represent volumes that were either below or less than ±1 SD above the regression line. (This figure was replotted from data presented in references #29 and 32.)*

if both venous return and cardiac output remain constant, then an increase in heart rate will accompany a smaller heart size and a smaller stroke volume. However, the increase in heart volume that occurred in six of the 10 subjects at the end of the upright exercise was thought to be evidence of myocardial dysfunction.

Ekelund (29) further evaluated the concept of myocardial dysfunction by determining the relationship between mechanical systole and heart rate. In the sitting position, the subjects exercised at either a relatively high or low intensity. After six min at the higher intensity, the average heart rate was 139 beats · min^{-1}; it increased to 171 beats · min^{-1} after 56.5 min. As noted, the heart volume showed a continuous decline during prolonged exercise, decreasing an average 81.1 mL (or 10.4%) of the 3rd to 9th min value. When the relationship between mechanical systole and heart rate was plotted for the high intensity work loads, the mechanical systole was longer than predicted in five of the six subjects (Fig. 2-7). If the regression of the mechanical systole on heart rate was plotted for the lower intensity exercise, all points were near the regression line. This indirect evidence of a longer ejection time at the end of 60 min of exercise in the more exhausted group again suggests the possibility of myocardial dysfunction (29,98,107). It appears that the increase in heart size at the end of exhaustive prolonged exercise (29,98,107) and in the presence of a maintained central filling pressure (28,31) coupled with the documented increase in mechanical systole, are suggestive of myocardial dysfunction. This myocardial dysfunction, if confirmed, may be related to myocardial fatigue or damage.

The concept of myocardial fatigue has intrigued many investigators. It has been reasoned that if fatigued or damaged myocardium were a factor in myocardial dysfunction, then, as with damaged skeletal muscle (12,46) and other organs (12,34,46), one should be able to detect release into the blood of specific cardiac isoenzymes for creatine phosphokinase (CPK) and lactate dehydrogenase (LDH) (2,13,24,87,108). Indeed, experiments indicate greater levels of the CPK isoenzyme specific to the heart (CPK-MB) and the LDH enzyme pattern of LDHI>LDHII following exercise (13,53,57,81,86,103,104). In fact, in many instances (53,57,81) postrace enzyme patterns were similar to those observed following myocardial infarction (104,108) (Fig. 2-8). However, the temporal relationships of the LDHI>LDHII patterns and peaks in CPK, as well as the absolute levels of total enzymes (CPK and LDH), were different for the postexercise pattern compared to the postmyocardial infarction pattern. Changes in total LDH and CPK activities have been shown by many to be more related to changes in skeletal muscle than to exercise effects on cardiac muscle (53,111).

Two studies that suggested myocardial fatigue used similar protocols but different measurement techniques to determine the cardiovascular response to prolonged exercise at 70% to 75% $\dot{V}O_2$max (98,107). Maximal exercise tests were conducted before and after prolonged submaximal exercise. Saltin and Stenberg (98) reported the classical cardiovascular drift during prolonged exercise, i.e., a 14% increase in heart rate and an 8% decrease in stroke volume (Fig. 2-9). Cardiac output was maintained constant, yet mean arterial pressure and total peripheral resistance declined, probably as a result of cutaneous vasodilation to facilitate dissipation of metabolic heat. After 90 min of rest following the submaximal exercise a further 15 min 75% submaximal bout was accompanied by a further decrease in stroke volume and increase in heart rate. This occurred in both upright and supine exercise and suggested central cardiovascular (myocardial) fatigue. Subsequently, when compared with a baseline maximal test, a maximal exercise test after prolonged ex-

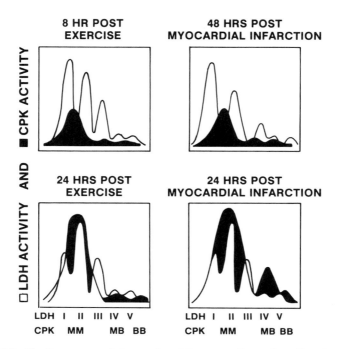

FIGURE 2-8. *The time course of changes in relative proportions of creatine phosphokinase (CPK) and lactate dehydrogenase (LDH) isoenzymes following 48 and 24 h after myocardial infarction and 8 and 24 h after acute exercise. (Modified from data presented in reference #53.)*

ercise elicited a 10% decrease in $\dot{V}O_2$max, a 5% increase in stroke volume and cardiac output, and a 3% to 10% reduction in mean arterial pressure with a marked decrease in work time and postexercise lactate.

In contrast, Upton et al. (107) using MUGA studies to evaluate circulatory hemodynamics, report an average $2\ L \cdot min^{-1}$ increase in cardiac output, a $9\ beats \cdot min^{-1}$ increase in heart rate, and a stable stroke volume over 110 min of work at 70% maximal work (Fig. 2-10 and Table 2-2). During the final minutes of work, cardiac output increased further as a result of an increasing heart rate (Table 2-2). Finally, at the end of the prolonged work, during a 10 min maximal exercise test values for cardiac output, stroke volume, $\dot{V}O_2$max, work time, and lactate level were all reduced compared to a control day maximal exercise test (Table 2-2). Significantly, three subjects were found to have reduced ejection fractions during the prolonged work. Because of the uncertainties involved in determining cardiac volumes from MUGA scans, one must question the discrepancies in findings concerning cardiac output and stroke volume between the

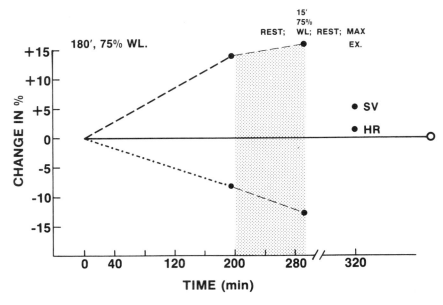

FIGURE 2-9. *Values are plotted as percent change from 10 min exercise value. Subjects exercised at 75% $VO_2max[=WL]$ for 180 min with a 15 min rest period for a total time of 195 min. The subjects then rested for 90 min, exercised again at 75% $VO_2max[=WL]$ for 15 min, rested again for 30 min, and then performed a maximal effort. The dashed lines represent change in heart rate (HR) and dotted and dashed lines represent change in stroke volume (SV). The maximal exercise values at 320 min are given as change from a maximal exercise test carried out on a separate day without prior prolonged exercise. (Modified from data presented in reference #98.)*

studies of Saltin and Stenberg (98) and Upton et al. (107). More recently, Niemela et al. (77) performed an echocardiographic evaluation of 13 athletes involved in a 24 h running race. Resting diastolic dimensions of the athletes confirmed the often reported increase in heart volume due to training (63). After the 24 h race, a 4.2% decrease in body weight was seen, but hemoglobin, hematocrit, and serum electrolytes were unchanged thus it was doubtful that circulating blood volume was reduced. The postrace echocardiographic data indicated a decrease in fractional shortening and mean velocity of circumferential fiber shortening of 16% and 9%, respectively. However, it is well known that alterations in preload and afterload influence these indices of contractility (85). A poor correlation was found between change in end-diastolic dimension and change in fractional shortening (r = 0.22). Also, the relationship of the change in end-diastolic dimension to the change in end-systolic dimension was negative (r = −0.66), suggesting a decrease in contractile function. Furthermore, end-systolic diameter increased after

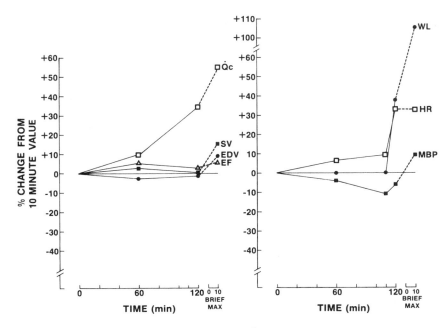

FIGURE 2-10. *Subjects exercised at 60–70% of $\dot{V}O_2$max for the initial 110 min and then workload (WL) was gradually increased over the next 10 min to maximum tolerated. Values are presented as percent change from 10 min value. The dotted lines represent the difference between a max effort after prolonged exercise vs an acute max test. Q_c = cardiac output, EDV = end-diastolic volume, EF = ejection fraction, HR = heart rate, SV = stroke volume, MBP = mean blood pressure (Redrawn from data presented in reference #107.)*

the race, despite a significant decrease in the afterload as indicated by a decrease in blood pressure from a prerace mean value of 136/80 Torr to postrace values of 109/65 Torr. As end-systolic fiber length in a normally functioning heart is directly proportional to afterload (94), the negative relationship found after exercise between end-sys-

TABLE 2-2. *Hemodynamic Measurements During Brief and Prolonged Exercise*

	Prolonged Exercise[1]		10 min Exercise
	Submaximal	Maximal	Maximal
HR (beats · min^{-1})	135 ± 12	180 ± 10	180 ± 9
Mean BP (mmHg)	102 ± 9	96 ± 9	112 ± 10
SV (mL)	129 ± 19	130 ± 19	150 ± 19
EF (%)	79 ± 6	81 ± 5	84 ± 5
EDV (mL)	164 ± 23	162 ± 24	179 ± 22
CO (L · min^{-1})	17.4 ± 2.9	23.4 ± 3.7	26.9 ± 3.1

BP = blood pressure; SV = stroke volume; EF = ejection fraction; EDV = end-diastolic volume; CO = cardiac output.
[1]Prolonged exercise was performed without maintaining euhydration.

tolic diameter and blood pressure further indicated a decrease in contractility or a failing heart. This depressed contractile state was reversed after two to three days of recovery.

As with other studies (78,81) of prolonged exercise, total creatine kinase activity was elevated following the race in the report by Niemala et al. (77). The CPK-MB fraction was also increased, but the percentage of the total (<4%) was not changed from the prerace levels. Because no electrocardiographic evidence of myocardial injury was seen after the race, it was felt that injury to the heart had not occurred and that the increase in CPK-MB fraction was not of cardiac origin. However, functional indices of depressed contractile function were evident and may explain the decreasing stroke volume that existed during the prolonged exercise. In addition, free fatty acids (FFA) were found to be elevated after the race, i.e., 0.15 ± 0.1 mM to 0.62 ± 0.16 mM after the race. Although it has been suggested that elevated FFA together with reduced cardiac glycogen subsequent to prolonged exercise results in reduced myocardial performance (63,70), it is doubtful that the 4-fold increase in FFA in Niemala's study (77) was enough to account for the change in left ventricular function.

During the 90 km Comrades Marathon in Johannesburg, two highly trained marathon runners developed hemoptysis and left ventricular failure (69,70), which was clinically reversible within 36 h after the race. These findings were suggestive of pulmonary edema of cardiac origin. However, the postexercise examination using electrocardiography, echocardiography, phonocardiography or coronary angiography provided no evidence of cardiac disease. A postulated mechanism was that with prolonged exercise, an increase in circulating free fatty acids, along with a decrease in cardiac glyogen stores and circulating insulin, produced a decreased level of cardiac energy production from glycogenolysis (70). This might result in a decreased rate of myocardial relaxation that would effectively decrease compliance of the myocardium. This decreased compliance, along with shorter filling time in the presence of tachycardia, could precipitate left ventricular failure (or fatigue).

Maher et al. (66) evaluated isolated ventricular trabecular muscles from sedentary controls and exercised exhausted rats and found that the resting length-tension (L-T) curve was unchanged with exhaustion, but that the active tension of the exhausted rats was depressed to 44% of that at rest. The force-velocity curve for the exhausted group was shifted downward and to the left. Furthermore, the exhausted rat myocardium displayed a diminished response to exogenous catecholamines. No structural changes were seen. However, King and Gollnick (58) have reported myofibrillar distortion and mitochondrial damage in the rat heart following exhaustive exercise.

In contrast to the proposed myocardial fatigue, Chan et al.(14) reported no cardiac symptoms during a 3000-km, 55-day Beijing to Hong Kong Marathon. Sugimoto et al.(105) found that the rat heart can be pumped maximally in excess of two h without measurable tissue damage.

Obviously, the evaluation of the concept of cardiac muscle fatigue has suffered from the problems associated with field investigations, individual susceptibility, and differences in exercise intensity and duration. Consistently, in all laboratory investigations, cardiovascular drift is progressive over the duration of the exercise. Also, in those studies in which a careful evaluation of myocardial function has been performed, significant decreases in cardiac function, analogous to that observed in skeletal muscle during long-term exercise, have been reported. However, whether these changes are progressive and causally related to the decrease in stroke volume remains to be elucidated. Despite later ideas disputing the concept of myocardial fatigue, exercise-induced changes in heart size and function and their relation to cardiac fatigue remain a significant phenomena to be evaluated by more sophisticated measurement techniques.

SUMMARY

It is apparent from the above discussion that the competition for the circulating blood volume between the working muscles and the skin is closely linked to cardiovascular drift. Increasing core temperature explains only a portion of the early increase in heart rate, and further increases in heart rate may be directly linked to increases in central command. The heightened sympathetic stimulation associated with the increased central command results in increased tachycardia and inotropy. Nevertheless, a continuous fall in stroke volume occurs, which may be a result of decreasing central filling pressure or a decrease in beta receptor responsiveness. In some investigations, despite the maintenance of cardiac output, systemic arterial pressures also decline (21,31). This suggests a possible fatigue of alpha receptor responsiveness in resistance vessels and/or a decreased baroreceptor sensitivity. Perhaps the entire sympathetic mechanism suffers from a decreasing responsiveness at the receptor level.

It would appear that reductions in the circulating blood volume do not ordinarily contribute to cardiovascular drift. However, dehydration exacerbates the drift during prolonged exercise, suggesting that the maintenance of circulating volume is a primary need (95,99). Consequently, cardiovascular drift associated with dehydration compromises temperature regulation and cellular function such that the muscular fatigue is heightened and performance decreased (27,65).

Finally, the concept of myocardial fatigue was presented because of its historical importance in the field of prolonged exercise. There are recently documented instances of catastrophic hemoptysis and myocardial infarction (38,45,70) which suggests that perhaps the heart, unlike skeletal muscle, has a nonprogressive point of breakdown which results in a significant dysfunction. Historical evidence of an increase in heart size and time of mechanical systole (32) and subsequent indices of a failing pump function remain to be explained. However, without convincing evidence concerning alterations in myocardial compliance, contractility, or substrate utilization, one must conclude that the progressive nature of the cardiovascular drift cannot be adequately explained by myocardial fatigue.

Practical considerations lead us to ask whether cardiovascular drift affects work performance. Irma Astrand (4) had subjects walk on a treadmill at 50% $\dot{V}O_2$max for one h. From the 10th min until the end of the exercise, oxygen uptake decreased from 1.04 to 0.98 $L \cdot min^{-1}$, heart rate decreased 4 beats $\cdot min^{-1}$ and ventilation volumes decreased 2 to 8 $L \cdot min^{-1}$. All subjects performed the work without subjective fatigue. In a later study, Irma Astrand (3) had two males and two females alternate walking on a treadmill or riding a cycle ergometer for 50 min followed by ten min rest and repeated until seven h. Each subject exercised at 50% $\dot{V}O_2$max. Food and water were given *ad libitum*. Although all subjects were fatigued after 7 h, it was felt that the exercise at 50% $\dot{V}O_2$max could have been repeated the next day. However, after one h, progressive rises in oxygen uptake (metabolic drift) and heart rate were seen.

Many studies by Costill (20) have shown that well-trained marathon runners can perform for 2 to 2.5 h at 85–95% $\dot{V}O_2$max utilizing 90% of maximum cardiac output and 95% of maximum stroke volume without generating any serum lactate. In Costill's research, cardiovascular drift presumably occurred, as it apparently exists in all exercise periods performed for more than one h, if exercise intensity is greater than 50% $\dot{V}O_2$max, and when ambient temperature allows central temperature to stabilize (4). Accordingly, there is no direct evidence that cardiovascular drift impedes performance. However, this question has also not been directly investigated.

Endurance training may reduce the severity of cardiovascular drift. The more well trained the exercising subject, the less the degree of drift for a given exercise load. However, it is likely that the degree of drift will be similar for exercise at similar *relative* intensities. Because hyperthermia is one of the primary limiting factors in prolonged exercise (1,27,65), it would be appropriate to maintain hydration to reduce functional skeletal muscle fatigue associated with dehydration (6,98). Furthermore, adequate hydration may help sustain heat dissipation by sweating and thereby minimize the thermoregulatory requirement for translocation of blood volume to the skin.

BIBLIOGRAPHY

1. Adams, W.C., R. H. Fox, A.J. Fry, and I.C. MacDonald. Thermoregulation during marathon running in cool, moderate, and hot environments. *J Appl Physiol.* 38:1030–1037, 1975.
2. Anderson, M.G. The effect of exercise on the lactic dehydrogenase and creating kinase isoenzyme composition of horse serum. *Res Vet Sci.* 20:191–196, 1976.
3. Astrand, I. Aerobic work capacity in men and women with special reference to age. *Acta Physiol Scand.* 49 (Suppl 169) p. 69, 1960.
4. Astrand, I., P.O. Astrand, and K. Rodahl. Maximal heart rate during work in older men. *J Appl Physiol.* 14(4):562–566, 1959.
5. Astrand, P.O., I. Hallback, R. Hedman, and B. Saltin. Blood lactate after prolonged severe exercise. *J Appl Physiol.* 18(3):619–622, 1963.
6. Astrand, P.O., and B. Saltin. Plasma and red cell volume after prolonged severe exercise. *J Appl Physiol.* 19(5):829–832, 1964.
7. Beckner, G.L., and T. Winsor. Cardiovascular adaptations to prolonged physical effort. *Circulation.* 9:835–846, 1954.
8. Bevegard, B.S., and J.T. Shepherd. Reaction in man of resistance and capacity vessels in forearm and hand to leg exercise. *J Appl Physiol.* 21(1):123–132, 1966.
9. Bishop, J.M., K.W. Donald, S.H. Taylor, and P.N. Wormald. Changes in arterial-hepaticvenous oxygen content differences during and after supine leg exercise. *J Appl Physiol* (Lond). 137:309–317, 1967.
10. Blair, D.A., W.E. Glover, and I.C. Roddie. Vasomotor responses in the human arm during leg exercise. *Circ Res.* 9:264–274, 1961.
11. Blake, J.B., and R.C. Larrabee (eds.) Observations upon long distance runners. *Boston Med Surg J.* 148:195–206, 1903.
12. Bloor, C.M., and N.M. Papadopoulos. Plasma lactic dehydrogenase activity and myocardial cellular changes after cessation of training. *J. Appl Physiol* 26:371, 1969.
13. Bolter, C.P., and J.B. Critz. Plasma enzyme activities after simulation of cardiovascular responses to exercise. *Am J Physiol.* 220(5):1444–1447, 1971.
14. Chan, K.M., P. Diamond, C.K. Law, P.C. Leung, S.Y. So, R. Wang, and W.Y. Shen. Case study Beijing to Hong Kong super-marathon—sports medicine research. *Brit J Sports Med.* 19(3):145–147, 1985.
15. Christensen, E.H. Beitrage zur physiologic schwerer korperlicher arbeit. *Arbeitsphysiologie* 4:453–469, 1931.
16. Christensen, N.J., and O. Brandsborg. The relationship between plasma catecholamine concentration and pulse rate during exercise and standing. *Eur J Clin Invest.* 3:299–306, 1973.
17. Christensen, N.J., H. Galbo, J.F. Hansen, B. Hesse, E.A. Richter, and J.T. Jensen. Catecholamines and exercise. *Diabetes.* 28 (Suppl. 1): 58–62, 1979.
18. Clausen, J.P., and J. Trap-Jensen. Arteriohepatic venous oxygen difference and heart rate during initial phases of exercise. *J. Appl. Physiol.* 37(5):716–719, 1974.
19. Cobb, L.A., and W.P. Johnson. Hemodynamic relationships of anaerobic metababolism and plasma free fatty acids during prolonged strenuous exercise in trained and untrained subjects. *J Clin Invest.* 42(6):800–810, 1963.
20. Costill, D.L. Physiology of marathon running. *JAMA* 221(9):1024–1029, 1972.
21. Costill, D.L. and B. Saltin. Muscle glycogen and electrolytes following exercise and thermal dehydration. In: *Metabolic Adaptation to Prolonged Physical Exercise*, edited by H. Howald and J.R. Poortmans. Basel: Berkhauser Verlag, 352–360, 1975.
22. Currens, J.H., and P.D. White. Half a century of running: Clinical, physiological and autopsy findings in the case of Clarence DeMar. *N Engl J Med.* 16:988–993, 1961.

23. Davies, C.T.M. and M.W. Thompson. Physiological responses to prolonged exercise in man. *J Appl Physiol* 61:611–617, 1986.
24. Dawson, D. and J. Fine. Creatine kinase in human tissues. *Arch Neurol.* 16:175–179, 1967.
25. Dick, R.W. and P.C. Cavanagh. An explanation of the upward drift in oxygen uptake during prolonged sub-maximal downhill running. *Med Sci Sports Exerc.* 19:310–317, 1987.
26. Dowell, R.T. Cardiac adaptations to exercise. *Exerc Sports Sci Rev.* 11:99–117, 1983.
27. Drinkwater, B.L. Heat as a limiting factor in endurance sports. *Am Acad Phys Ed.* 18:93–100, 1984.
28. Ekelund, L.G. Circulatory and respiratory adaptations during prolonged exercise in the supine position. *Acta Physiol Scand.* 68:382–396, 1966.
29. Ekelund, L.G. Circulatory and respiratory adaptations during prolonged exercise. *Acta Physiol Scand.* (Suppl 292) 70:5–38, 1967.
30. Ekelund, L.G. Circulatory and respiratory adaptations during prolonged exercise of moderate intensity in the sitting position. *Acta Physiol Scand.* 69:327–340, 1967.
31. Ekelund, L.G., and A. Holmgren. Circulatory and respiratory adaptations, during long-term, non-steady state exercise, in the sitting position. *Acta Physiol Scand.* 62:240–255, 1964.
32. Ekelund, L.G., A. Holmgren, and C,O. Ovenfors. Heart volume during prolonged exercise in the supine and sitting position. *Acta Physiol Scand.* 70:88–98, 1967.
33. Forsburg, A., P. Tesch and J. Karlsson. Effect of prolonged exercise on muscle strength performance. In: *Biomechanics* IV-A, edited by E. Asmussen and K. Jorgensen. Baltimore, MD: University Park, 1979, 6:62–67.
34. Fowler, W.M. et al. Changes in serum enzyme levels after exercise in trained and untrained subjects. *J Appl Physiol.* 17:934, 1962.
35. Fox, S.M. III, J.P. Naughton, and W.L. Haskell. Physical activity and prevention of coronary heart disease. *Ann Clin Res.* 3:404–432, 1971.
36. Froericher, V.P., and A. Oberman. Analysis of epidemiological studies in physical inactivity as a risk factor for coronary artery disease. *Prog Cardiovasc Dis.* 15:41–65, 1972.
37. Gliner, J.A., P.B. Raven, S.M. Horvath, B.L. Drinkwater and J.C. Sutton. Mans physiological responses to long-term work during thermal and pollutant stress. *J Appl Physiol.* 39:628–632, 1975.
38. Green, L.H., S.I. Cohn, and G. Kurlan. Fatal myocardial infarction in marathon racing. *Ann Int Med* 84:704–706, 1976.
39. Grimby, G. Renal clearances during prolonged supine exercise at different workloads. *J. Appl Physiol.* 20(6):1294–1298, 1965.
40. Hagan, R.D., F.J. Diaz, R.G. McMurray, and S.M. Horvath. Plasma volume changes related to posture and exercise. *Proc Soc Exp Biol Med.* 165:155–160, 1980.
41. Harrison, M.H., R.J. Edwards, and D.R. Leitch. Effect of exercise and thermal stress on plasma volume. *J Appl Physiol* 39(6):925–931, 1975.
42. Hartley, L.H. Central circulatory function during prolonged exercise. *Annal NY Acad Sci.* 301:189–194, 1977.
43. Hartley, L.H., J.W. Mason, R.P. Hogan, L.G. Jones, T.A. Kotchen, E.H. Mougey, F.E. Wherry, L.L. Pennington, and P.T. Ricketts. Multiple hormonal responses to prolonged exercise in relation to physical training. *J Appl Physiol.* 33(5):607–610, 1972.
44. Hartley, L.H., B. Perow, J. Haggendal, J. Lacour, J. De Lattre and B. Saltin. Central circulation during submaximal work preceded by heavy exercise. *J Appl Physiol.* 29(6):818–823, 1970.
45. Haskell, W.L. Sudden cardiac death during vigorous exercise. *Int J Sports Med.* 3:45–48, 1982.
46. Highman, B., and P.D. Altland. Serum enzyme rise after hypoxia and effect of autonomic blockade. *Am J Physiol.* 199:981, 1960.
47. Horwitz, L.D., and J. Lindenfeld. Effects of enhanced ventricular filling on cardiac pump performance in exercising dogs. *J Appl Physiol.* 59:1886–1890, 1985.
48. Hug, O. Sportarztliche Beobachtugen vom I. Schweizerischen Marathonlauf 1927, unterbesonderer Berucksichtigung des Verhaltens der Kreislauforgane und der Atmung. *Schweiz Med Wochenschr.* 58:453–461, 1928.
49. Johnson, J.M. Regulation of skin circulation during prolonged exercise. *Ann NY Acad Sci.* 301:195–212, 1977.
50. Johnson, J.M., and L.B. Rowell. Forearm skin and muscle vascular responses to prolonged leg exercise in man. *J Appl Physiol.* 39(6):920–924, 1975.
51. Jokl E., and L. Melzer. Acute fatal non-traumatic collapse during work and sport. *S Afr J Med Sci.* 5:4, 1940.
52. Jose, A.D., F. Stitt, and B. Collison. The effects of exercise and changes in body temperature on the intrinsic heart rate in man. *Am Heart J.* 79(4):488–498, 1970.
53. Kaman, R.L., P.B. Raven, R.W. Patton, J. Ayres, and B. Goheen. The effects of near maximum exercise on serum enzymes: The exercise profile vs. the cardiac profile. *Clin Chim Acta.* 81:145–152, 1977.

54. Kamon, E., and H. Belding. Dermal blood flow in the resting arm during prolonged leg exercise. *J Appl Physiol.* 26(3):317–320, 1969.
55. Kannel, W.B. Habitual levels of physical activity and risk of coronary heart disease: the Framingham study. *Can Med Assoc J.* 96:811–812, 1967.
56. Keul, J., H.H. Dickhuth, M. Lehmann, and J. Staiger. The athlete's heart—haemodynamics and structure. *Int J Sports Med.* 3:33–43, 1982.
57. Kielblock, A.J., M. Manjoo, J. Booyens, and I.E. Katzeff. Creatine phosphokinase and lactyate dehydrogenase levels after ultra long-distance running. *S Afr Med J.* 55:1061–1064, 1979.
58. King, D.W., and P.D. Gollnick. Ultrastructure of rat heart and liver after exhaustive exercise. *Am J Physiol* 218(4):1150–1155, 1970.
59. Knowlton, F.P., and E. Starling. The influence of variations in temperature and blood pressure on the performance of the isolated mammalian heart. *J Physiol.* 44:206, 1912.
60. Kozlowski, S., and B. Saltin. Effect of sweat loss on body fluids. *J Appl Physiol.* 19(6):1119–1124, 1964.
61. Kreger, B.E., L.A. Cupples, and W.B. Kannel. The electrocardiogram in prediction of sudden death: Framingham study experience. *Am Heart J.* 113(2):377–382, 1987.
62. Krogh, A., and J. Lindhard. The regulation of respiration and circulation during the initial stages of muscular work. *J Physiol.* 45:112–135, 1913.
63. Longhurst, J.D., A.R. Kelly, W.J. Gonyea, and J.H. Mitchell. Cardiovascular responses to static exercise in distance runners and weight lifters. *J Appl Physiol.* 49:676–683, 1980.
64. Liedtke, A.J., S. Nellis, and J.R. Neely. Effects of excess free fatty acids on mechanical and metabolic function in normal and ischemic myocardium in swine. *Cir Res.* 43:652–661, 1978.
65. MacDougall, J.D., W.G. Reddan, C.R. Layton, and J.A. Dempsey. Effects of metabolic hyperthermia on performance during prolonged exercise. *J Appl Physiol.* 36:538–544, 1974.
66. Maher, J.T., A.L. Goodman, R. Francesconi, W.D. Bowers, L.H. Hartley, and E.T. Angelakos. Responses of rat myocardium to exhaustive exercise. *Am J Physiol.* 222(1):207–212, 1972.
67. Maron, M.B., and S.M. Horvath. The marathon: a history and review of the literature. *Med Sci Sports.* 10(2):137–150, 1978.
68. McCloskey D.I. and J.H. Mitchell. Reflex cardiovascular and respiratory responses originating in exercising muscle. *J Physiol* (Lond). 224:173–186, 1972.
69. McKechnie, J.K., W.P. Leary, and S.M. Joubert. Some electrocardiographic and biochemical changes recorded in marathon runners. *S Afr Med J.* 722–725, 1967.
70. McKechnie, J.K., W.P. Leary, T.D. Noaks, J.C. Kallmeyer, E.T.M. MacSearraigh, and L.R. Oliver. Acute pulmonary oedema in two athletes during a 90 Km running race. *S Afr Med J.* 56:261–265, 1979.
71. Mitchell, J.H., M.P. Kaufman, and G.A. Iwamoto. The exercise pressor reflex: Its cardiovascular effects mechanisms, and central pathways. *Ann Rev Physiol.* 45:229–242, 1983.
72. Morganroth, J., and B.J., Maron. The athlete's heart syndrome: a new perspective. *Ann NY Acad Sci.* 301:931–941, 1977.
73. Morris, J.N., J.A. Heady, and P.A.B. Raffle. Physique of London busmen. *Lancet* 569–570, 1959.
74. Morris, J.N., J.A. Heady, P.A.B. Raffle, C.G. Roberts, and J.W. Parks. Coronary heart-disease and physical activity of work. *Lancet* 1054–1057, 1953.
75. Morris, J.N., J.A. Heady, P.A.B. Raffle, C.G. Roberts, and J.W. Parks. Coronary heart-disease and physical activity of work. *Lancet* 1111–1120, 1953.
76. Nadel, E.R., E. Cafarelli, M.F. Roberts, and B. Wenger. Circulatory regulation during exercise in different ambient temperatures. *J Appl Physiol.* 46(3):430–437, 1979.
77. Niemela, K.O., I.J. Palatsi, M.J. Ikaheimo, J.T. Takkunen, and J.J. Vuori. Evidence of impaired left ventricular performance after an interrupted competitive 24 hour run. *Circulation* 70(3):350–356, 1984.
78. Noakes, T.D., and J.W. Carter. Biochemical parameters in athletes before and after having run 160 kilometres. *S Afr Med J.* 50:1562–1566, 1976.
79. Noakes, T.D., and L.H. Opie. Marathon runners and impending heart-attacks. (letter) *Lancet* May 8, p. 1020, 1976.
80. Noakes, T.D., L. Opie, W. Beck, J. McKechnie, A. Benchimol, and K. Desser. Coronary heart disease in marathon runners. *Ann NY Acad Sci.* 301:593–619, 1977.
81. Oliver, L.R., A De Waal, F.J. Retief, J.D. Marx, J.R. Kriel, G.P. Human, and G.M. Potgieter. Electrocardiographic and biochemical studies on marathon runners. *S Afr Med J.* 53:783–787, 1978.
82. Paffenbarger, R.S. Factors predisposing to fatal stroke in longshoreman. *Prev Med.* 1(4):522–527, 1972.
83. Paffenbarger, R.S., W.E. Hales. Work activity and coronary heart mortality. *N Engl J Med.* 292(11):545–550, 1975.

84. Peronnet, F., R.J. Ferguson, H. Perrault, G. Ricci, and D. Lajoie. Echocardiography and the athlete's heart. *Phys Sports Med* 9(5):102–112, 1981.
85. Quinones, M.A., W.H. Gaasch, J.S. Cole, and J.K. Alexander. Echocardiographic determination of left ventricular stress-velocity relations in man with reference to the effect of loading and contractility. *Circulation* 51:689–700, 1975.
86. Roberts, R., K.S. Gowda, P.A. Ludbrook, and B.E. Sobel. Specificity of elevated serum MB creatine phosphokinase activity in the diagnosis of acute myocardial infarction. *Am J Cardiol.* 36:433–437, 1975.
87. Rosalki, S.B. Creative phosphokinase isoenzymes. *Nature* 207:414–415, 1965.
88. Rowell, L.B. Human cardiovascular adjustments to exercise and thermal stress. *Physiol Rev.* 54(1):75–159, 1974.
89. Rowell, L.B. Cardiovascular adjustments to thermal stress. Chapter 27 in *Handbook of Physiology,* Vol. III. Sect. 2. Edited by J.T. Shephard, F.M. Abboud, S.R. Geiger. Publ. by Amer. Physiol. Soc., Washington, D.C., 967–1023, 1983.
90. Rowell, L.B. *Human Circulation Regulation During Physical Stress.* New York: Oxford Press, 308–322, 356–374, 257–286, 1986.
91. Rowell, L.B., G.L. Brengelmann, J.M.R. Detry, and C. Wyss. Venomotor responses to rapid changes in skin temperature in exercising man. *J Appl Physiol* 30(1):64–71, 1971.
92. Rowell, L.B., K.K. Kraning, T.O. Evans, J.W. Kennedy, J.R. Blackmon, and F. Kusumi. Splanchnic removal of lactate and pyruvate during prolonged exercise in man. *J Appl Physiol* 21(6):1773–1783, 1966.
93. Rowell, L.B., C.R. Wyss, and G.L. Brengelmann. Sustained human skin and muscle vasoconstriction with reduced baroreceptor activity. *J Appl Physiol* 34(5):639–643, 1973.
94. Sagawa, K. The end-systolic pressure-volume relation to left ventride: definition, modifications and clinical use. *Circulation* 65:1223–1227, 1981.
95. Saltin, B. Circulatory responses to submaximal and maximal exercise after thermal dehydration. *J Appl Physiol.* 19(6):1125–1132, 1964.
96. Saltin, B. Aerobic and anaerobic work capacity after dehydration. *J Appl Physiol.* 19(6):1114–1118, 1964.
97. Saltin, B., and L. Hermansen. Esophageal, rectal, and muscle temperature during exercise. *J Appl Physiol* 21(6):1757–1762, 1966.
98. Saltin, B., and J. Stenberg. Circulatory responses to prolonged severe exercise. *J Appl Physiol.* 19(5):833–838, 1964.
99. Sawka, M.N., R.C. Knowlton, and J.B. Critz. Thermal and circulatory responses to repeated bouts of prolonged running. *Med Sci Sports Exerc.* 11(2):177–180, 1979.
100. Schaible, T.F., and J. Scheuer. Cardiac adaptations to chronic exercise. *Prog Cardiov Dis.* 27(5):297–324, 1985.
101. Senay, L.C., and J.M. Pivarnick. Fluid shifts during exercise. *Exerc Sports Sci Rev.* 13:335–387, 1985.
102. Sherman, W.M., L.E. Armstrong, T.M. Murray, F.C. Hagerman, D.L. Costill, C. Staron, and J.L. Ivy. Effect of a 42.2 km footrace and subsequent rest or exercise on muscular strength and work capacity. *J Appl Physiol.* 57:1668–1673, 1984.
103. Smith, O.A., R.F. Rushnaer, and E.P. Lasher. Similarity of cardiovascular responses to exercise and diencephalec stimulation. *Am J Physiol.* 198:1139–1142, 1960.
104. Smith, A.F., D. Radford, C.P. Wong, and M.F. Oliver. Creatine kinase MB isoenzyme studies in diagnosis of myocardial infarction. *Br Heart J.* 38:225–232, 1976.
105. Sugimoto, T., J.L. Allison, and A.C. Guyton. Effect of maximal workload on cardiac function. *J Heart J.* 14:146–153, 1973.
106. Thompson, W.O., P.K. Thompson, and M.E. Daily. The effect of posture upon the composition and volume of the blood in man. *J Clin Invest.* 5:573–604, 1928.
107. Upton, M.T., S.K. Rerych, J.R. Roeback Jr., G.E. Newman, J.M. Douglas Jr., A.G. Wallace, and R.H. Jones. Effect of brief and prolonged exercise on left ventricular function. *Am J Cardiol.* 45:1154–1160, 1980.
108. Van der Veen, K.J. and A.F. Willebrane. Isoenzymes of creatine phosphokinase in tissue extracts and in normal and pathological sera. *Clin Chim Acta* 13:312–317.
109. Victor, R.G., D.R. Seals and A.L. Mark. Differential control of heart rate and sympathetic nerve activity during dynamic exercise: Insight from direct intraneural recordings in humans. *J Clin Invest.* 79:508–516, 1987.
110. Wagner, G.S., C.R. Roe, L.E. Limbird, R.A. Rosati, and A.G. Wallace. The importance of identification of the myocardial specific isoenzyme of creatine phosphokinase (MB form) in the diagnosis of acute myocardial infarction. *Circulation* 47:262–269, 1973.
111. Warren, S.G., G.S. Wagner, C.F. Bethea, C.R. Roe, H.N. Oldham, and Y. Kong. Diagnostic and prognostic significance of electrocardiographic and CPK isoenzyme changes following coronary bypass surgery: correlation with findings at one year. *Am Heart J.* 93(2):189–196, 1977.

70 *PERSPECTIVES IN EXERCISE*

112. Wells, C.L., J.R. Stern, and L.H. Hecht. Hematological changes following a marathon race in male and female runners. *Eur J Appl Physiol.* 48:41–49, 1982.
113. Wilhelm, A.H., and J.K. Todd. Limited diagnostic value of CK-MB (Letter) *Clin Chem.* 23(8):1509–1510, 1977.
114. Williams, H., and H.D. Arnold. The effects of violent and prolonged muscular exercise upon the heart. *Phil Med J.* 1233–1239, 1899.
115. Wilson, J.R., P.B. Raven, S.A. Zinkgraf, W.P. Morgan and A.W. Jackson. Alterations in physiological and perceptual variables during exhaustive endurance work while wearing a "pressure-demand" respirator. *Am Ind Hyg Assoc J.* (Submitted), 1987.
116. Zitnik, R.S., E. Ambrosioni, and J.T. Shepherd. Effect of temperature on cutaneous venomotor reflexes in man. *J Appl Physiol.* 31(4):507–512, 1971.
117. Zoltic, J.M., R. Virmani, J. Kishel, W. Fitzgerald, M. Robinowitz, and J. Bedynek. Cardiovascular screening and autopsy findings in sudden cardiac death in middle aged males. *Med Sci Sports Exerc.* Suppl 19:S91 (abstract), 1987.
118. Zukel, W.J., R.H. Lewis, P.E. Enterline et al. A short-term community study of the epidemiology of coronary heart disease: a preliminary report on the North Dakota study. *Am J Public Health* 49:1630–1639, 1959.

DISCUSSION

TIPTON: Considering cardiovascular drift, the issue, it seems to me is, what is primary and what is secondary? We are seeing a whole host of changes, and consequently, it's difficult to recognize which change is occurring because of a preliminary or preceding change. And even though five components are listed in this chapter it would seem to me that it is conceivable and perhaps defensible that the drift is initiated because of a change in central command. I'm not so sure that central command might not be associated to some extent with respiratory drift, but Dempsey and I can argue this out later. The point is that I think the initiation of many of these changes is probably because of a change in central drive.

Concomitant with that central drive, I think there's probably an alteration of autonomic drive. Now, Peter mentions that it could be questionable that this could occur, but I'm not so sure it couldn't occur, particularly when we have a competition and a shift between the masking effect of many of our receptors. We do not know, for type 3 or 4 receptors, or even in the alpha and beta receptors, whether their responsiveness has changed. I would suggest that perhaps it has. And consequently, the afferent information is going to impinge and have a cascading effect. I also feel that the baroreceptor issue is in need of amplification. If baroreceptor responsiveness is being altered, clearly we could find that those changes could explain, to some extent, the increased amount of circulating catecholamine, even though those catecholamines may not necessarily have the same effect because of a change in the receptor responsiveness.

I would concur that perhaps a very good discriminator of cardiovascular function during prolonged exercise is the change in stroke volume. However, I would not be too much enamored by changes in heart size. I think the emphasis on change in heart size that you alluded to historically is interesting, but I'm not so sure that heart size is a very good discriminator. And the emphasis on heart size changes is more for historical than scientific value. I think the ejection fraction or the stroke volume is a variable that we should focus on. I would define myocardial fatigue as a change in the stroke volume or ejection fraction and let it go at that. A size change to me is not necessarily indicative of fatigue. I also believe that looking at the serum CPK values is interesting, but I think you need to put that with histological data to make a case for myocardial damage. I don't think there is hard evidence, histological evidence in the myocardium, that there is myocardial damage caused by exhaustive exercise. The case can be made that the CPK values are indicative that, indeed, you do have a permeability change in the myocardium in prolonged exercise, and this could potentially be "damage." But I think the inference that it is damage should be a little more subdued.

Substrate utilization by the myocardiam deserves attention, even though it clearly hasn't been explored, even though it has been demonstrated that myocardial glycogen can be changed. So substrate utilization could be a contributing factor here to the drift that is being noticed.

Finally, I agree that the intracellular and extracellular fluid shifts are very important variables and cannot be ignored. I really don't understand the data that suggest or imply that you don't have a change in blood volume with prolonged exercise. I think the majority of the evidence is rather impressive that most people do lose volume and plasma volume.

CANTWELL: What about this question of myocardial fatigue as indexed by systolic and diastolic fatigue?

RAVEN: If the end-systolic index is showing that contractility is going down, and if blood pressure is going down, and if the relationship between volume or pump function and blood pressure is reversing, then something's going on. Something's going wrong with the pump.

TIPTON: That's just a qualitative descriptor. My point is that you should be more quantitative about what you define. Don't just use heart size as a discriminator. There are other data that show changes in compliance in animals. I think that's a very strong argument.

GOLLNICK: There are some points that ought to be brought up here about the structural aspects. In our own work, we saw some ultrastructural damage to the myofibrils and mitochondria in rats we had swim for prolonged durations. We saw what looked like swollen SR tubules, and that was subsequently confirmed by others. There might be some damage going on in muscle, at least focal damage. And then there is evidence of a disturbed sarcoplasmic reticulum that is associated with fatigue. There is an indication there may be some changes occurring in the excitation-contraction process. I was also disturbed when you just dismissed the idea that CPK in plasma during exercise is not coming from the heart. You can't say that. There could very well be myocardial as well as skeletal muscle damage.

CANTWELL: The group from Finland did show myocardial fatigue, and, I think, most of us would accept this. Be reminded that this was after a 24-hour race. I think that maybe exceeds our definition of prolonged exercise.

RAVEN: The data I've seen from the Beijing to Hong Kong race, which took 55 days, show no cardiovascular problems.

MICHELI: Isn't change in electroconductivity of the heart a physiologic response to prolonged exercise? Perhaps there should be some discussion of this because for the medical clinician and the physiological clinician, that's the major tool used to assess the heart.

RAVEN: I did not approach this particular chapter to look at electrocadiographic variations that you see in athletes. There are some major variances in these people that can be tremendous. When you start seeing resting heart rates at 30 and 32, you start wondering. You often don't know what's going on.

NADEL: The cardiovascular drift that's seen in prolonged exercise should be considered further. You're in a pretty dynamic state during prolonged exercise. For one thing, ambient temperature does affect water and volume loss. Another is that water intake will affect those conditions. So I think those ought to be addressed.

RAVEN: Well, in a way I did that. When you're in a cool environment, for example, there's no plasma volume change at 25° C; but when you get over 35° C, there is a change. So I would agree, if one is dehydrated, the drift's going to be worse.

PATE: Peter, I'm wondering if you think that the cardiovascular drift that you described has functional significance for the endurance athlete. Do you think it's a cause or an effect of fatigue? Or both?

RAVEN: As a muscle is fatiguing, you get a fiber recruitment increase, and perhaps peripheral feedback from fatiguing skeletal muscles influences the change in heart rate. I guess it also depends on how you define central command. Is central command purely a cognitive function, or is it a feedback from the muscle and afferents integrating with the central function? I think that's one part of the cause of cardiovascular drift. The other is the temperature regulatory need. I think myocardial fatigue is a crisis in waiting. It can become a crisis. That's why we see these people with pulmonary edema during marathon runs and why we see anterior wall infarcts without any indication that should have had an infarct.

BLAIR: Except there are other possible mechanisms, like spasm, thrombosis, and so forth that could be implicated.

EICHNER: Here, I think, is a good example of the problem we face in determining what is cause and what is effect. On a very hot day in Boston, a runner collapsed at the 24th mile, and it's largely believed by clinicians that he collapsed with heat stroke. He was on a respirator for 40 or 50 days, and then he died. He had an anterior myocardial infarction. It's certainly, at the very least, not a clean case. But he did not die from a heart attack. Most people feel perhaps he collapsed and died from heat stroke. I guess that's just a mini-example of the difference between the physiologic and clinical approach.

SUTTON: Very specifically, when we're actually talking about exercise, we need to specify the duration of exercise, to specify the type of exercise, the intensity of exercise, and the true nature of it. So we really must be absolutely clear about all those conditions, because the responses can be so different. In a publication like this where we tend to lump things together, we can get differences in interpretation. In talking about fatigue, and particularly cardiovascular fatigue, we have to be very clear about definition. Clarification is terribly important.

We see physiologists grabbing a little bit of information and jumping on that. And the clinicians say, "We want to hear much more." For instance, the two cases from South Africa about pulmonary edema reported as a result of prolonged exercise—that was not clear. And I just happened to review another case where a guy actually went into pulmonary edema following the Pittsburgh Marathon last year. In that instance, he also had central filling pressures measured, and the best evidence was that this was noncardiogenic pulmonary edema. So that type of pulmonary edema is not reflective of myocardial dysfunction.

And my final question concerns the importance of the sympathetic system in catecholamine response to exercise in these circumstances. Is there any evidence of changes in sensitivity to autonomic function, particularly during prolonged exercise?

RAVEN: I didn't find any evidence of unloading of the baroreceptors, yet people who are well trained seem to have altered baroreceptor function. The receptor responsiveness may be different. Baroreceptors may be resetting.

3

Pulmonary Function and Prolonged Exercise

JEROME A. DEMPSEY, PH.D.

ELIZABETH AARON, MS

BRUCE J. MARTIN, PH.D.

INTRODUCTION
   I. ESSENTIAL ELEMENTS OF THE NORMAL RESPONSE
     A. Control of Exercise Hyperpnea
     B. Pulmonary Gas Exchange
  II. FAILURE OF PULMONARY GAS EXCHANGE
 III. VENTILATORY RESPONSES DURING LONG-TERM WORK
     A. Long-Term Work in a Controlled Environment
       1. Ventilatory Response
       2. Pulmonary Gas Exchange and Acid-Base Regulation
       3. Composition of Venous Effluent Blood from Working Muscle
       4. Effects of Relative Work Intensity and Exercise Mode
 IV. VENTILATORY RESPONSES AND GAS EXCHANGE DURING
     COMPETITIVE ENDURANCE RUNNING
  V. REGULATION OF BREATHING IN PROLONGED EXERCISE
 VI. DO RESPIRATORY MUSCLES FATIGUE DURING PROLONGED
     EXERCISE?
     A. Metabolic Considerations in Animals
     B. Neuro-Mechanical Evidence in Humans
     C. Central "Inhibition" of Respiratory Muscle Force Development
     D. The "Cost" of Exercise Ventilation
 VII. TRAINING EFFECTS
VIII. AGING EFFECTS
  IX. HYPOXIC EFFECTS
   X. DOES THE LUNG LIMIT PROLONGED EXERCISE PERFORMANCE?
BIBLIOGRAPHY
DISCUSSION

INTRODUCTION

The pulmonary system is primarily concerned with ensuring adequate gas exchange at a minimum of physiologic cost and cognitive effort. In most cases in health, this aim is accomplished; however, there are some notable exceptions. This chapter analyzes the adequacy of the pulmonary system's response to exercise and the regulatory mechanisms underlying this response in a variety of physiologic and environmental states. We will start with a brief synopsis of the "essential elements" in the pulmonary response to exercise, as usually defined during short term exercise in healthy, young adults. Then we will proceed to analyze the special problems presented by prolonged exercise. Finally, we will examine any changes in this response resulting from the chronic effects of physical training, aging and hypoxia.

I. ESSENTIAL ELEMENTS OF THE NORMAL RESPONSE

Table 3-1 lists some of the major demands imposed on the pulmonary system by an increasing tissue O_2 consumption and CO_2 production. This increasing metabolic rate in working skeletal muscle dictates an increasing O_2 desaturation and acidity in the mixed venous blood presented to the lung for gas exchange. Hence, the requirement of the gas exchange system for maintaining iso-capnic and iso-oxic conditions in arterial blood is increased several fold, and yet the reduced time spent by the desaturated hemoglobin molecule in the pulmonary capillary provides less and less time for the lung to meet this requirement. Also noted in Table 3-1 are examples of key "responses", such as alveolar ventilation and pulmonary blood flow. While the magnitude and precision of these responses are essential to adequate gas exchange and acid-base regulation during

TABLE 3-1. *Demands on pulmonary control systems*

	Rest	Mild	Max	"Max"	Units	
$\dot{V}O_2(\dot{V}CO_2)$	0.3	1	3	5	$L \cdot min^{-1}$	Metabolic "demand"
$C\bar{v}O_2$	15	11	6	<2	$mL \cdot 100\ mg^{-1}$	Gas exchange "requirement"
$P\bar{v}CO_2$	46	52	65	>75–80	mmHg	
Alveolar Ventilation	5	25	90	140	$L \cdot min^{-1}$	
Pulmonary blood flow	5	11	20	27	$L \cdot min^{-1}$	"Response"

Maximum refers to work requiring a $\dot{V}O_2$ max in an untrained (Max) and highly trained athlete ("Max").

exercise, it is also crucial that these responses be accomplished with minimal physiologic cost to the lung and chest wall.

At least three tightly interrelated control systems combine forces to ensure that the lung's gas exchange functions are met both adequately and efficiently during exercise—namely, control of exercise hyperpnea, control of mechanical work done by the lung and chest wall, and control of alveolar to arterial gas exchange.

A.   Control of Exercise Hyperpnea

A general scheme of ventilatory control during exercise is shown in Fig. 3-1. We consider this highly complex control system in two interrelated sections that are concerned with the overall regulation of alveolar ventilation and with the mechanical efficiency of each breath.

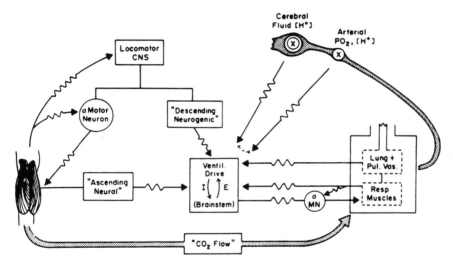

FIGURE 3-1. *Functional pathways for control of exercise hyperpnea. Three primary stimuli are shown, each with input to respiratory center neurons: 1) CO_2 flow ($Q:C\bar{v}Co_2$), sensed in the lung and mediated via the vagus nerves; 2) a descending neurogenic drive linking central commands to locomotor skeletal muscle to respiratory center neurons; and 3) an ascending neurogenic stimulus from contracting skeletal muscle. Three types of error detection or feedback effects are shown: 1) from intercostal muscle spindles to phrenic motor neurons (segmetal reflex) and to the CNS; and 2) from lung and airway receptors to the CNS. These feedbacks from the chest wall and lung are concerned with mechanical events (flow-pressure-volume-tension relationships) and their optimization via control of breathing pattern and lung volume. These feedback pathways may also affect the magnitude of inspiratory neural drive as a compensatory response to mechanical loads imposed on the lung and/or chest wall; and 3) feedback from peripheral (carotid body) chemoreceptors sensitive to arterial blood PO_2 and $[H^+]$ and from central (medullary) chemoreceptors affected by extracellular (and probably intracellular cerebral fluid $[H^+]$. (Neural feedback from working locomotor muscle to higher CNS and to motor neurons for fine control of limb locomotion are also shown.) (From Dempsey, Vidruk & Mitchell, 1985.)*

There are at least three types of documented primary afferent inputs to ensure that the output of medullary inspiratory neurons and magnitude of the neural input to inspiratory muscles is proportional to rising metabolic demands (26,95). The critical primary neural drives include descending influences from the higher CNS proportional to locomotor activity (29), ascending influences from working skeletal muscle, and a humoral input related to increasing metabolic CO_2 production. At the same time, it is likely that a significant amount of "error" exists in the precision of these feed forward primary drives with respect to changing metabolic requirements; thus feedback or error detection is required. First, a mechanoreceptor-type feedback is operative, which adjusts neural drive in response to any mechanical impedance presented by the lung and/or chest wall, to ensure that the final ventilatory output is sufficient to meet metabolic requirements. Second, peripheral and intra-cranial chemoreceptors sensitive to changes in acid-base status and arterial oxygenation may account for a significant portion of the total inspiratory drive, even during mild to moderate exercise. The net effect of these influences is that arterial PCO_2 and pH are controlled fairly close to resting values (although this regulation may not be perfect, as $PaCO_2$ rises a few mmHg in mild bicycle exercise and will tend toward slight hypocapnia if the subject jogs rather than walks (23,45).

As exercise intensity increases beyond 65% to 70% of maximum effort, a cumulative metabolic acidosis presents an additional and substantial homeostatic requirement. This demand is responded to by an increasing alveolar ventilation out of proportion to increasing VCO_2, resulting in a significant hyperventilatory compensation of arterial [H+]. Thus arterial [H+] is maintained at 50% to 60% of the level which would be expected without any compensatory hypocapnia (7.25 − 7.30 arterial pH at $PaCO_2$ 25 to 30 mmHg vs <7.20 at $PaCO_2$ 40 mmHg). This additional neural drive in heavy exercise must be in part mediated by chemoreceptor feedback, but has also been shown to occur in the absence of metabolic acidosis (27,51). One additional feed-forward afferent input may arise in heavy work if the primary neurogenic drive rises alinearly at high work rates coincident with the increase in output from CNS locomotor centers needed to "compensate" for the development of fatigue in limb locomotor muscles (27).

The portion of this control system concerned with minimization of respiratory muscle effort may be especially important during exercise—even in health. Although mechanisms for load compensation and optimization have received little attention and remain poorly understood, several recent observations and some old ones point to the fact that the control system is "aware" of and responds to mechanical needs of the chest wall during exercise:

1. Breathing frequency and tidal volume are controlled by meeting a given overall ventilatory command so as to maintain tidal volume close to the fairly linear portion of the pressure:volume relationship, i.e. V_T rarely exceeds 60% to 65% of vital capacity.

2. Accessory muscles of respiration are activated during even the mildest levels of exercise. These include: a) Activation of the abductor muscles of the larynx which both increases airway diameter at the point of greatest potential resistance and stiffens the airway to accept the large subatmospheric pressures to be generated during exercise. These muscles' activation, together with the relaxation of bronchiolar smooth muscle and the switch from nasal to predominantly oral breathing ensures that airflow resistance during even heavy exercise remains essentially unchanged despite a) A very large increase in flow rate; b) Increasing inspiratory parasternal intercostal muscles and scalene muscle activity to assist the diaphragm and expand the ribcage; c) Expiratory abdominal muscle activation occurs even in very mild exercise (43,86). The advantage of this active expiration is that inspiration can be completed in the shorter time available during exercise— in fact, end-expiratory lung volume actually is reduced during exercise as much as 0.8 to 1.1 liters during heavy exercise. In turn, this reduced lung volume permits tidal volume to be increased over a much wider range of the linear pressure:volume relationship without affecting lung compliance; d) This active expiration also is of substantial assistance to the subsequent inspiration in two ways: (1) It can effectively lengthen the diaphragm, thereby putting it at a more favorable portion of its length-tension relationship during the ensuing inspiration; and (2) Upon sudden relaxation of expiratory muscles, stored energy may be expended by a marked negative swing in abdominal pressure at the onset of inspiration, thus actually creating a significant contribution to the "passive" generation of inspiratory pleural pressure and flow. Of course, there may be limits to this reduction in end-expiratory lung volume (47). While on the one hand, a modest reduction in EELV will permit $\dot{V}_T$ to increase without encroaching on the *upper* stiffer alinear portion of the pressure:volume relationship, an exaggerated reduction in EELV would *cause* a reduced compliance by encroaching on the lower

alinear portion of the pressure:volume relationship. This would require an increased work load on the lung by the chest wall, thereby negating in part the inspiratory assist provided via active expiration. (Additional problems of this type might also arise in the aged individual during exercise, see below).

3. The normal impedance presented by the lung is large enough—especially during exercise—so that it must be compensated for by increasing inspiratory motor output beyond that primary underlying drive to breathe which normally results from the exercise hyperpneic stimulus, per se. This normal compensatory effort was demonstrated during even mild exercise by observing that inspiratory effort—as judged by diaphragmatic EMG (or mouth occlusion pressure) is reduced immediately upon reduction of the lung impedance by breathing a reduced-density gas (52). These contributions of this "load compensating" effort to total inspiratory drive increase in significance as work load increases (22).

4. A final example of mechanical proprioceptive feedback may be seen when comparing ventilatory work during voluntary ventilation versus heavy exercise ventilation at identical flow rates and lung volumes. Voluntary methods always generated excessively high pressures during expiration and, therefore, increased ventilatory work (19)—as if cortical control was overriding (and ignoring) mechanical feed-back control. A practical implication of this comparison is that coaches should not try to change the spontaneously adopted breathing pattern in the endurance athlete. Surely the pattern and level of ventilation achieved by the athlete to serve mechanical efficiency and chemical homeostasis must be far superior to any attempt at voluntary override of this normal physiologic feedback.

B. Pulmonary Gas Exchange

The healthy lung appears to represent the ultimate in ideal design characteristics, ensuring adequate pulmonary gas exchange by preventing an inordinate widening of the alveolar to arterial PO_2 difference in the face of a reduced mixed venous O_2 content and increased pulmonary blood flow. Thus, in healthy subjects working up to approximately 3.5 L·min^{-1} $\dot{V}O_2$, arterial PO_2 is maintained constant, because the alveolar to arterial PO_2 is increased sufficiently so that the arterial PO_2 remains very close to resting levels. Key mechanisms underlying this homeostasis are outlined in Table 3-2 and include the following:

TABLE 3-2. *Determinants of alveolar to end-pulmonary capillary to arterial gas transport and their changes with short-term upright exercise in healthy young men.*

Determinants	Rest	Hard Work	Units
Alveolar-mean capillary PO_2	$100 - 92 = 8$	$120 - 70 = 50$	mmHg
Pulmonary blood flow	5	20–25	L · min
Pulmonary capillary blood volume	70	200–250	mL
Right heart stroke volume	70	150	mL
Mean RBC transit time	0.9	0.5[a]	secs
Pulmonary arterial pressure	15	25[b]–35	mmHg
Pulmonary wedge pressure	5	15–25	mmHg
Pulmonary vascular pressure	1.5–2.0	0.2–0.5	units
Ventilation: Perfusion (V_A:Qc)			
Mean	1	4–6	
Dispersion			
(St. Dev. Distribution)	±0.3	0.4–0.6	
Range	0.5–2.0	1–8	
Arterial PO_2	90	90	mmHg
Alveolar-Arterial PO_2 Diff	10	20–30	mmHg
Arterial PCO_2	40	25–32	mmHg
Arterial pH	7.40	7.20–7.30	

[a]Estimated average RBC transit time in pulmonary capillary would be ~0.2 seconds if pulmonary capillary blood volume remained unchanged from resting levels.

[b]Reports of exercise effects on Ppa are variable and may show little or no change from resting values, depending upon the exercise posture, duration, or recent exercise history. In general, in the upright position, mean Ppa increases about 1 mmHg for every L · min increase in cardiac output.

a) The architectural "reserve" of the alveolar-capillary surface area in terms of maximum available alveolar (140 m^2) and capillary (125 m^2) total surface areas and an air-blood barrier which is 1/50th the thickness of a sheet of air-mail stationery—both of which aid equilibrium of alveolar and end-capillary blood for O_2 (93).

b) A low resistance pulmonary vasculature which is capable of expanding its capillary blood volume about three fold above the resting volume during heavy exercise. Capillary recruitment during exercise occurs primarily from apical lung regions which were markedly underperfused at rest. This expansion in the pulmonary capillary bed is a purely passive phenomenon, as both pulmonary artery and wedge pressures increase with increasing blood flow and vascular resistance falls. This expansion in the pulmonary bed is critical to maintaining adequate transit time for equilibration of alveolar gas with deoxygenated mixed venous blood in the pulmonary capillary (see Table 3-2).

c) Increases in overall ventilation to perfusion ratio ($\dot{V}_A$:Qc) reach 4 to 5 times the resting level in heavy work (so that P_AO_2 is maintained high). This ensures that low $\dot{V}_A$:Qc areas of the lung (which are the main causes of hypoxemia, especially at low $C\bar{v}O_2$) do not occur, because even the lowest $\dot{V}_A$:Qc areas during exercise exceed the highest $\dot{V}_A$:Qc regions in the resting lung (38). In heavy exercise this excessive ventilation is important not only to compensate for metabolic acidosis but also to maintain arterial oxygenation in the face of a rising alveolar to arterial PO_2 difference.

d) The lung is protected from extra-vascular fluid accumulation when blood flow increases during exercise by minimizing increases in pulmonary vascular pressures and because of the extensive capacity for lymphatic drainage from the lung (87). Thus, as Q increases, lung lymph flow increases from 4 to 5 mL·h^{-1} at rest to 15 to 20 mL·h^{-1} during moderate exercise, as shown in the sheep (14). This increased lymph flow is not attributable to significant changes in either transvascular or oncotic hydrostatic pressures or to increased permeability of exchange vessels; but rather to the increase in exchange surface area secondary to capillary recruitment, together with perhaps some increase in filtration pressure with small increases in left atrial pressure (14). Despite these increases in lymph flow, given the large capacity for lymphatic drainage from the lung, it seems doubtful that extravascular lung water would actually accumulate in the lung interstitium during exercise, at least during exercise requiring less than 20 to 25 L·min^{-1} in pulmonary blood flow (see below). Indeed, "heavy" exercise in the dog was shown to cause no change in the wet weight:dry weight ratio of the lung (69).

e) The uniformity of VA:Qc distribution *does* change during exercise, becoming more uniform topographically (among lung regions)—but less uniform *within* lung regions. The net result is a less uniform $\dot{V}_A$:Qc distribution (see Table 3-2), which contributes significantly to the underlying alveolar to arterial PO_2 difference (38).

II. FAILURE OF PULMONARY GAS EXCHANGE

There are limits to homeostasis of gas exchange in healthy persons, and these are frequently exceeded when highly trained athletes are capable of achieving very high work rates and metabolic demands for a period of two to six minutes, primarily because of the very large capacities of their cardiovascular and neuromuscular systems (22). The result may often be arterial hypoxemia as shown by contrasting responses in athletes and nonathletes at maximum exercise (see Table 3-3). Note that the arterial hypoxemia in the athlete is attributable to two general causes. First, alveolar PO_2 is lower in the trained *vs.* untrained, for reasons that are not totally clear but certainly related to the much higher alveolar ventilation required at the athlete's higher max $\dot{V}O_2$ and $\dot{V}CO_2$. For example, in order for the trained runner at 5 L·min^{-1} $\dot{V}O_2$ to achieve the same high alveolar PO_2 and low PCO_2 as in the untrained exercising at 3 L·min^{-1} $\dot{V}O_2$, he would have to sustain a ventilation in excess of 200 L·min^{-1} whereas the untrained individual would only need to achieve about 120 L·min^{-1} (see Table 3-3) (19).

An excessive widening of the alveolar to arterial PO_2 difference is the other major reason for the hypoxemia. The causes are speculative. Any contribution from a pulmonary shunt is ruled out since slight elevations in inspired O_2 during heavy exercise raise alveolar and arterial PO_2 equally (22). A worsening of $\dot{V}_A$:Qc distribution with increasing workload does occur and would be expected to contribute more to the increasing alveolar to arterial O_2 difference as $P\bar{v}O_2$ falls. So, just as in the untrained, in trained athletes, the imperfections in $\dot{V}_A$:Qc distribution and the small anatomical shunt in the face of a falling mixed venous O_2 content cause most of the widening of the alveolar to arterial O_2 difference. We think the additional factor brought out by the high work load in the trained is a significant contribution from the inability of mixed venous blood to equilibrate with alveolar gas by the time the desaturated blood reaches the end of the pulmonary capillary, i.e. diffusion limitation.

The high metabolic demand of the athlete creates a susceptibility to diffusion limitation by exerting negative effects on several determinants of diffusion (see Table 3-3): a) the transit time in the pulmonary capillary is greatly shortened because blood flow continues to increase as pulmonary capillary blood volume reaches its maximum morphologic capacity; (see fig. 3-1); and b) the rate of equilibration is also slowed—or the time required to reach equilibration of mixed venous blood with alveolar PO_2 is prolonged—because of the relatively low alveolar PO_2 and driving pressure for diffusion (90). Thus, for the trained runner at max $\dot{V}O_2$ with alveolar PO_2 equal to 100 mmHg and $P\bar{v}O_2$ approximating 20 mmHg, the estimated mean transit time *available* (0.45 seconds) is significantly shorter than the estimated average time *required* (0.60 seconds) for completeness of equilibration of mixed venous blood with alveolar gas by the end of the pulmonary capillary. Since there must be significant variation around this mean transit time, diffusion disequilibrium probably exists in a significant fraction of the end-pulmonary capillary blood leaving the trained runner's lung.

A *potential* cause of the widened alveolar to arterial O_2 difference might be found in an increased extra-vascular lung water at high

TABLE 3-3. *Untrained vs. trained* young adults—effects on pulmonary transport at max (short-term) exercise*

	$\dot{V}O_2$ L·min⁻¹	a-$\dot{V}O_2\Delta$ (mLO$_2$ ·100 mL⁻¹)	Blood Flow (L·min⁻¹)	Blood Volume (mL)	Transit** Time Available (secs)	Time "Required"⁺*** (secs)	$\dot{V}E$ (L·min⁻¹)	Alveolar PO$_2$ (mmHg)	Arterial PO$_2$ (mmHg)	Alv-art. PO$_2$ (mmHg)	Arterial PCO$_2$ (mmHg)
					Pulmonary Capillary						
Untrained	3–4	16–17	19–24	175–210	.53–.55	0.4	110–120	120	90	20–30	25–32
Trained	5–6	18–19	28–33	210	.38–.45	0.6	160–180	100	55–75	34–45	35–40

*Not all highly trained athletes show hypoxemia at max work (see Dempsey, et al. 1984).

**Transit time "*available*" = capillary blood vol. + blood flow.

⁺***Refers to the time in the pulmonary capillary *required* to bring capillary PO$_2$ into equilibrium with alveolar PO$_2$. This was estimated (Dempsey, 1987) from the rate of the diffusion equilibration calculations as determined by Wagner (1982). Note that in the highly trained, the time *required* for equilibration is longer than that in the untrained and exceeds the time *available* for equilibration.

exercise loads. To date, findings are inconclusive. As discussed above, at lower work levels requiring 4-fold increases in pulmonary blood flow, lung lymph flow increases but extra-vascular lung water probably does not accumulate. However, Younes et al.(98) have recently shown that the *in situ* dog lung lobe accumulates weight as blood flow increases in excess of four times the resting level and pulmonary atrial pressure (Ppa) increases greater than 25–30 mmHg—even though left atrial pressure was held constant. In humans, during very heavy exercise Ppa can approach the 30–40 mmHg range (Table 3-2), so the potential for excessive leakage into the interstitial fluid space from the plasma does exist. On the other hand, indications of extra-vascular lung water accumulation in the human are indirect and inconsistent. Thus, immediately following short-term, heavy exercise, a relative tachypnea may occur (99), presumably secondary to fluid accumulation in the lung. Unfortunately, these effects are inconsistent. Sufficiently sensitive techniques for the *in vivo* measurement of extra-vascular lung water are sorely needed.

Finally, we note, that even if extra-vascular lung water did accumulate in heavy work, it is not clear that alveolar to arterial gas exchange would be affected. The water will accumulate first in interstitial fluid "cuffs" around larger extra-alveolar vessels and airways—this would probably not affect alveolar capillary diffusion distance, because the intra-alveolar septal diameter apparently does not change in these initial stages of fluid accumulation (87). $\dot{V}_A:\dot{Q}c$ distribution might be affected if cuffing causes increased resistance to blood or airflow in these bronchioles or arterioles—but there is doubt if vascular or bronchiolar resistance is affected by cuffing in these regions (76). If the accumulated extra-vascular lung water proceeds to the state of alveolar flooding, then, of course, the stability of the alveolus is lost, and gas exchange will clearly be severely impaired. It is unlikely that this extreme would ever be reached in the healthy lung during the most severe short-term exercise.

III. VENTILATORY RESPONSE DURING LONG-TERM WORK

Clearly the essential elements of the pulmonary system response during short-term exercise apply in principal to long-term exercise. On the other hand, there are special requirements placed on the pulmonary control system peculiar to very long-term, heavy exercise, which affect facets of ventilatory regulation, chest wall mechanics, pulmonary gas exchange, and acid-base regulation.

Various responses of the pulmonary system to long-term exercise are shown in Figures 3-2 through Figure 3-6 (45,89). Subjects

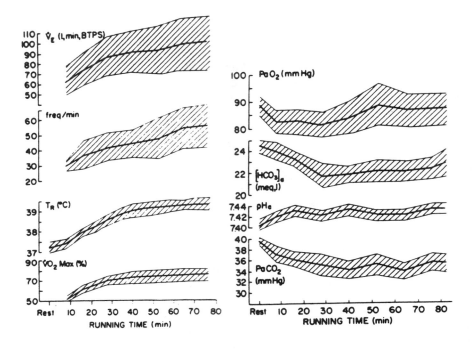

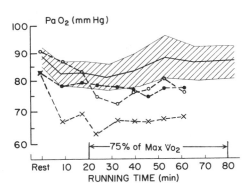

FIGURE 3-2A (Upper Left). *Minute ventilation ($\dot{V}_E$), breathing frequency (f) and rectal temperature (T_R) during continuous treadmill running at 3 work intensities: 55% (8 min), 65% (8 min) and 70% to 75% $\dot{V}O_2max$ (60 min). (N = 13, age 31 ± 4 years) ($\dot{V}O_2max$ = 68 ± 4 mL · kg · $^{-1}min^{-1}$, Max $\dot{V}_E$ = 163 ± 14 L · min^{-1}, & Max fb · min^{-1} = 61 ± 8). (From short-term progressive max test.) (From Hanson et al., 1982.)*

FIGURE 3-2B (Upper Right). *Arterial blood gases & acid-base status during prolonged treadmill running (see Fig. 3-2A).*

FIGURE 3-2C (Lower). *Group mean arterial PO_2 and individual exceptions to the trend of a constant PaO_2 during prolonged treadmill running (see Figure 3-2A). (From Dempsey, 1987.)*

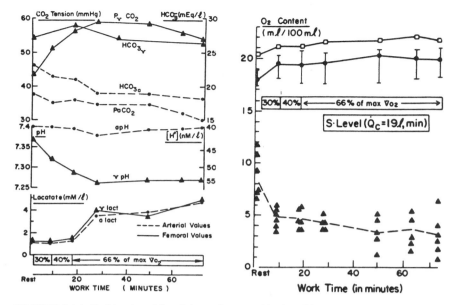

FIGURE 3-3A (Left). *Arterial and femoral venous blood acid-base status during prolonged treadmill walking (N = 6); $\dot{V}O_2max = 51 \pm 3 \; mL \cdot kg^{-1} \cdot min^{-1}$; age 33 $\pm$ 2 years). (From Thompson et al. 1974.)*

FIGURE 3-3B (Right). *Mean arterial O_2 carrying capacity ($\square$); arterial O_2 content ($\bullet$) and individual subject values for femoral venous O_2 content ($\blacktriangle$) during prolonged heavy exercise (see 3-3A legend).*

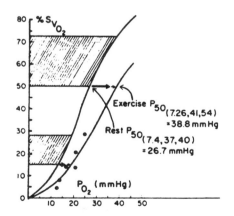

FIGURE 3-4. *Effect of prolonged walking exercise to exhaustion on HbO_2 dissociation in femoral venous blood at 50% Svo_2 [i.e., P_{50} (in vivo) mean value] and at the observed in vivo Svo_2 (mean and individual values). Shifts in the curve are partitioned according to the temperature effect (long arrow) and pH effect (short arrow). Hatched areas indicate potential HbO_2 desaturation (22.7% at P_{50} and 13% at in vivo [Svo_2]) attributed to the observed rightward shift in the curve. (From Thomson et al., 1974.)*

PULMONARY FUNCTION AND PROLONGED EXERCISE   **87**

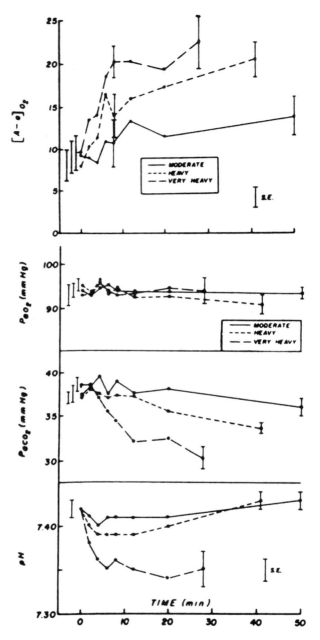

FIGURE 3-5A. *Changes in arterial blood gases and acid-base status and in the alveolar to arterial PO_2 difference during prolonged bicycle exercise to exhaustion at $\dot{V}O_2$ 1.2 $L \cdot min^{-1}$ (419 kgm $\cdot$ min^{-1}), 1.9 $L \cdot min^{-1}$ (737 kpm) and 2.7 $L \cdot min^{-1}$ (1018 kpm). (N = 10, untrained adult males, ages 23–30 yrs.) (From Wasserman et. al., 1967.)*

88   *PERSPECTIVES IN EXERCISE*

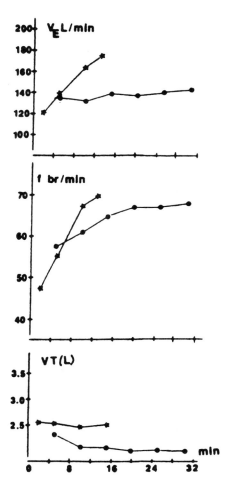

FIGURE 3-5B. *Time-dependent effects on breathing pattern in a highly trained 21-year-old oarsman bicycling at 85% (●) and 95% (*) of $\dot{V}O_2max$ to exhaustion. ($\dot{V}O_2max$ = 63 mL·kg^{-1}min, 5.41 L·min^{-1}; 2600 kpm, max $\dot{V}_E$ = 169 L·min^{-1}; V_T = 2.6 L and fb = 69; Vit. Cap. = 6.8 L.) (From Aaron, E., et al., unpublished findings.) In three of six subjects $\dot{V}_E$ reached at the end of 95% $\dot{V}O_2max$ exercise load to exhaustion was > $\dot{V}_E$ at (short-term) $\dot{V}O_2max$ and in all subjects fb was > fb at $\dot{V}O_2max$.*

shown here were all young male adults and were habitual exercisers, but the level of physical training varied greatly. Max $\dot{V}O_2$ ranged from a mean of 51 ± 2 mL·kg^{-1}·min^{-1}, for the subjects in Figure 3-3, to 68 ± 5 for subjects in Figures 3-2 and 3-6. Training effects on the responses reported here are discussed later, as are the effects of aging, changing environments and varying exercise intensities.

PULMONARY FUNCTION AND PROLONGED EXERCISE **89**

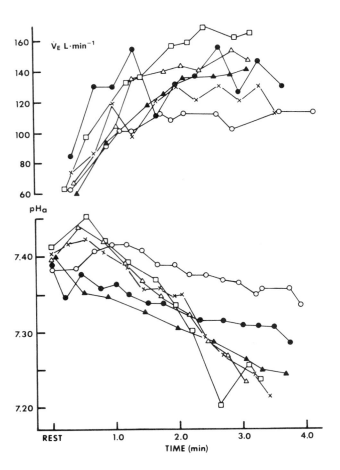

FIGURE 3-5C. *Time-dependent changes in $\dot{V}_E$ and arterial pH in extremely heavy exercise could be maintained for four to six mins. ($\dot{V}O_2max = 74\ mL \cdot kg^{-1}$, % $\dot{V}O_2max = 82\%$ to 97%). Note the variable, but progressive, metabolic acidosis over time in all subjects; while $\dot{V}_E$ rose progressively up to 1.5 to 2 min of exercise but then tended to level off in most cases. (From Dempsey et al., 1984.)*

A. Long Term Work in a Controlled Environment

1. Ventilatory Response. Several time-dependent phases of the ventilatory response to exercise have been described, beginning with the immediate hyperpnea in the initial seconds of exercise, followed by a slow, further rise over one to two minutes to steady state. Thereafter, if the relative work intensity is less than 40% to 50% $\dot{V}O_2max$, a time dependent ventilatory drift occurs with prolongation of exercise, as shown in Figures 3-2 and 3-3 (45,70,89). This is characterized by a 15 to 40% increase in breathing frequency over time, due to reductions in expiratory and inspiratory times. Tidal volume usually falls 10% to 15%. These changes in pattern are accompanied by a coincident rise in $\dot{V}_E$. The increase in $\dot{V}_E$ is out of proportion to a small (5% to 10%) time-dependent increase in $\dot{V}CO_2$ and $\dot{V}O_2$.

Dead space ventilation as a fraction of total ventilation falls in the initial few minutes of exercise ($V_D{:}V_T = .35$ at rest to $.15$–$.20$ during exercise), but then tends to increase as breathing frequency rises over time. Given that the aim of the ventilatory response is to deliver sufficient alveolar ventilation to maintain alveolar PCO_2, this tachypneic response is clearly an inefficient one. The consequences of a change in breathing pattern on alveolar ventilation and gas exchange may be seen in the following relationships:

$$\dot{V}_A = \dot{V}_E - \dot{V}_D$$
$$\dot{V}_A = (V_T - \dot{V}_D) \cdot f_b$$
$$\dot{V}_A = \frac{\dot{V}CO_2 \cdot k}{P_A CO_2}$$

where $\dot{V}_E$ = total ventilation
$\dot{V}_A$ = alveolar ventilation
$\dot{V}_D$ = dead space ventilation volume
V_T = tidal volume
f_b = breathing frequency
$P_A CO_2$ = alveolar PCO_2
k = a constant

Thus, at any given metabolic rate ($\dot{V}CO_2$) during exercise and for a given $\dot{V}_E$ as frequency increases and V_T is reduced, alveolar ventilation will be reduced and $PaCO_2$ will rise; thus, overall $\dot{V}_E$ must increase to preserve gas exchange as breathing frequency increases from the beginning to end of long-term exercise. With very few exceptions, subjects "chose" either to maintain $PaCO_2$ or to further reduce it, and either option must occur at the expense of a 10% to 30% increase in a $\dot{V}_E$, which would not have been necessary had tidal volume been preserved throughout long-term exercise (see Table 3-4).

Based on data from much shorter time periods of 15 minutes of heavy work (86), we would presume that the increase in tidal volume during prolonged exercise—like that during short-term exercise—is obtained from an encroachment on both the inspiratory and expiratory reserve lung volumes. Thus, inspiratory muscles would enjoy the advantages of reduced end-expiratory lung volume, as they

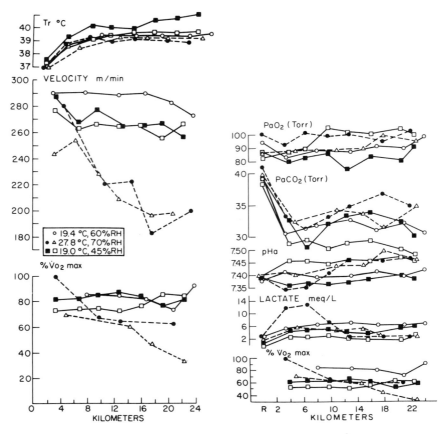

FIGURE 3-6A (Left). *Running velocity, relative work intensity (%$\dot{V}O_2$max) and rectal temperature during road racing. Values are shown for each of five individual subjects. Environmental temperature and relative humidity (RH) are listed for each of the road races. For each subject, $\dot{V}O_2$max $\dot{V}_E$max fb (on short-term progressive max test) and total race times were, respectively; (open circles) 72 ml · kg^{-1}min^{-1}; 147 L · min^{-1}; 54/min and 86 min; (closed circles) 64, 146, 54, and 132 min; (triangles) 58, 216, 92 and 132 min; (closed squares) 60, 157, 46 and 90 min; (closed squares) 59, 146, 63 and 89 min. (From Hanson et al, 1982.)*

FIGURE 3-6B (right). *Blood gases and acid-base status during a 24 km road race. (See Fig. 3-6A legend.)*

did in short-term exercise (see previous section). On the other hand, in cases where extreme tachypnea and shortening of (TE) occurred, perhaps a reduced end-expiratory lung volume could not have been maintained or perhaps may even have risen over 60+ minutes of long-term exercise. Given the potential importance of this occurrence to inspiratory muscle tension development, this possibility deserves further study.

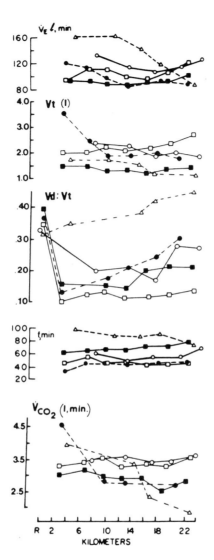

FIGURE 3-6C. *Breathing pattern and dead space ventilation during 24 km road race. (See Fig. 3-6A legend and Table 3-4).*

2. Pulmonary Gas Exchange and Acid Base Regulation. Arterial pH usually remains alkaline throughout prolonged exercise, with changes in resting levels varying from no change to as high as 7.49 to 7.52. These changes reflect the changing influences of lactic acid concentration in arterial blood *vs.* the degree of alveolar hy-

TABLE 3-4. *Ventilating inefficiency due to the tachypneic response to prolonged exercise.*

Group Mean (n = 8)	6 min	60 min with observed increased fb	60 min with no increased fb
fb (per min)	40	54	40
V_T (L)	2.2	1.8	2.3
V_D/V_T	0.18	0.23	0.18
$\dot{V}_E$ (L·min^{-1})	86	98	92
$\dot{V}_A$ (L·min^{-1})	71	75	75
$\dot{V}CO_2$ (L·min^{-1})	3.1	3.1	3.1
Extreme Case (n = 1)			
fb (per min)	48	93	48
V_T (L)	2.4	1.7	2.5
V_D/V_T	0.23	0.36	0.23
$\dot{V}_E$ (L·min^{-1})	116	153	120
$\dot{V}_A$ (L·min^{-1})	90	98	98
$\dot{V}CO_2$ (L·min^{-1})	3.5	3.5	3.5

perventilation and hypocapnia. Plasma lactate usually rises 2 to 4 mEq·L^{-1} (and bicarbonate falls about the same), and $PaCO_2$ falls 5 to 10 mmHg at the initiation of exercise requiring 65% to 75% $\dot{V}O_2$max. Thereafter, arterial lactate (and [HCO_3^-]) either stayed constant or fell toward resting levels, as the level of hypocapnia either remained steady or was further reduced with time.

Arterial blood PaO_2 usually stayed within 5 mmHg of resting levels during most of the exercise and occasionally increased as hyperventilation occurred later in the exercise. The alveolar to arterial PO_2 difference rose to 20 to 25 mmHg (or about 2 to 2.5 times resting levels) and remained constant throughout. This implies that $\dot{V}_A$:$\dot{Q}c$ distribution probably did not worsen with exercise time, nor was the exchange surface area diminished; although there is some evidence that some important determinants of gas exchange have not remained constant thoughout prolonged work. First, pulmonary arterial pressure and pulmonary vascular resistance were shown to fall substantially (back toward resting values) between 10 and 60 minutes of upright exercise (28); and significant pulmonary vasodilation in a resting subject was noted for a considerable time following prolonged exercise (96). The reason for these changes in the pulmonary vasculature with prolonged exercise are not clear; they are suggestive of some exercise-induced vasodilation of medial smooth muscle (as occurs in skeletal muscle), but available evidence points to a purely passive regulation of pulmonary vasculature. As in short-term exercise, pulmonary lymph flow would be expected to increase as gas exchange surface area increased, but again there is no evidence of *accumulation* of interstitial lung water (also see below).

We note that not all subjects maintain homeostasis of arterial blood PO_2 during prolonged, heavy exercise. Note in Figure 3-2C that 3 of 26 subjects studied during prolonged work at 65% to 85% $\dot{V}O_2$max did show a reduction in arterial PO_2 to less than 75 mmHg, a reduction evident during most of the exercise. Two of these cases of hypoxemia were due to excessive widening of the alveolar to arterial PO_2 difference (to > 35 mmHg) and the third subject showed inadequate hyperventilation (38 mmHg $PaCO_2$) with a normal widening of A-aDO_2.

3. **Composition of Venous Effluent Blood from Working Muscle (Fig. 3-3A, B).** The arterial to femoral venous differences for PO_2 and O_2 content widen with increasing work load; PCO_2 and pH differences also widen with increasing work load but stay relatively constant or fall slightly with further exercise duration. This reflects the fairly well maintained ratio of perfusion to metabolism in working skeletal muscle (Fig. 3-3A and B). PO_2 in femoral venous blood did fall as low as 10 mmHg and HbO_2 saturation to less than 10% toward the termination of exercise.

Hydrogen ion buffering in femoral venous blood is enhanced during prolonged work because of the marked HbO_2 desaturation in venous blood. This makes Hb a weaker acid and a more effective hydrogen ion acceptor, i.e., the Haldane effect. Note the increasing or constant femoral venous [HCO_3] during prolonged exercise, despite the 4-fold increase in venous lactate concentration. Another effective regulator of femoral venous [H+] is P_vCO_2, which is reduced 5 to 8 mmHg during prolonged exercise coincident with alveolar hyperventilation and arterial hypocapnia.

Unfortunately, the fact that hypocapnia is readily reflected across metabolizing organs also means that the brain's cerebral fluid PCO_2 is reduced during prolonged exercise. In turn, brain ECF pH is increased substantially because: a) CSF is a protein-free and, therefore, very poorly buffered fluid; and b) a high lactic-acid concentration in the systemic circulation is not readily transported across the tight junctions of the blood-brain barrier into the cerebral interstitial fluid. Cerebral arterioles constrict in an attempt to protect against alkalinization of brain pH by preventing CO_2 removal via the cerebral venous effluent. This effect of hypocapnia overrides the normal autoregulation during exercise, whereby total cerebral blood flow is maintained constant at a time when flow to systemic vascular beds is undergoing marked changes. Thus, when sufficient hyperventilation accompanies exercise ($P_aCO_2 < 30$mm Hg) a 30% to 40% reduction in cerebral blood flow and in cerebral O_2 transport will occur, which is maintained for up to one hour of constant exercise (25). The repercussions of this reduced flow to cerebral neurotransmitter metabolism or neuronal function are unknown. However, one could imagine some deterioration of mental acuity and judgment with such sustained and substantial reductions in cerebral O_2 transport. This problem may become manifest during or following exhaustive, prolonged exercise in the heat (see below), especially if dehydration is excessive and systemic blood pressure is reduced. Combining this reduced perfusion pressure to the brain with acute hypocapnic-induced vasoconstriction of cerebral arterioles may cause dramatic reductions in cerebral flow.

Just as deoxygenation assisted pH regulation in femoral venous blood during prolonged exercise (Fig. 3-3B), acid-base changes along with large increases in vascular temperature provide at least a theoretical advantage to O_2 off-loading at the muscle. Note, in Fig. 3-4, that a substantial rightward shift of the HbO_2 dissociation curve occurs with exhaustive exercise secondary to the femoral venous acidity and the substantial rise in venous blood temperature in excess of 41° C. Accordingly, this shift should preserve off-loading of O_2 to the muscle during prolonged exercise by minimizing the reduction in muscle capillary PO_2—and thereby protecting the diffusion gradient—as HbO_2 is reduced during its transit through the muscle. In arterial blood, PO_2 is maintained high, and the temperature changes are less than one-half those in venous blood; thus, the curve shift is very small, and arterial HbO_2 saturation and O_2 content are preserved very close to resting values. Thus, O_2 delivery is optimized here by affecting a rightward shift in the HbO_2 dissociation curve at the level of working muscle, while O_2 "on loading" at the level of the pulmonary capillary is preserved.

4. **Effects of Relative Work Intensity and Exercise Mode.** The relative intensity of the prolonged exercise is an important determinant of response. A steady-state for ventilatory response and acid-base status is probably achieved during exercise at less than 40% to 50% of max $\dot{V}O_2$ in most healthy individuals. These work loads can be sustained indefinitely. At higher work levels, in the 60% to 75% to 80% $\dot{V}O_2$max range, the major effect of exercise duration is the "drift" of ventilation and breathing frequency with fairly stable regulation of acid-base status and O_2 exchange. Metabolic acid concentrations in arterial blood are stable at mildly elevated levels or dedcrease with time. Vascular and core temperatures increase but usually plateau at some duration of the exercise. Reasonably fit subjects can tolerate these loads for at least one to three hours, and marathons may be completed by the highly fit under these reasonably steady-state conditions (67,17).

Of course, all subjects must eventually achieve a work load in which they are unable to maintain even a quasi-steady state (see Fig. 3-5A and C). One hallmark of having reached this critical intensity is that metabolic acidosis occurs early in the work task and keeps increasing to a plateau after approximately 20 minutes (see Fig. 3-5A); with the next increase in work intensity, no plateau in acidosis ever occurs (Fig. 3-5C) so that the work load is tolerable for only 5 to 10-15 minutes. $\dot{V}O_2$ and $\dot{V}CO_2$ also show a significant upward "creep" over time at these exercise intensities, as do core temperature and probably circulating catecholamines. An unrelenting time-dependent tachypnea and hyperventilation occur at these very high intensities, and dyspnea is progressive. Note that the highly fit subject shown in Fig. 3-5B is capable of maintaining a near-steady state at 85% $\dot{V}O_2$max but not at 95% $\dot{V}O_2$max. The relative intensity at which these various responses occur must vary among healthy subjects and are undoubtedly dependent on fitness level (17). Work loads requiring 90 to 95% $\dot{V}O_2$max probably represent the peak load at which a tolerable and reasonably steady state response of the pulmonary system could be maintained for as long as 30 minutes, even in the most highly fit.

In our consideration of the pulmonary system's response to prolonged exercise, we have dealt almost exclusively with running or, to a lesser extent, stationary bicycle ergometry. Certainly, many of the principles discussed apply to any form of exercise, because an increased metabolic demand is clearly a major instigator of pulmonary system response (see Table 3-1). On the other hand, the *mode* of exercise is probably also crucial, although little work has been done on this topic. Running or jogging is different in many respects from walking or stationary bicycling. For example, at any given $\dot{V}CO_2$, jogging causes a higher breathing frequency and more hyperventilation and respiratory alkalosis than does walking (45). Running also produces increases in intra-abdominal pressure commensurate with each footplant. This reflects a stiffening of the abdominal wall, which presumably assists in shock absorption from the footplant but must also have an effect on the role diaphragm descent and abdominal wall displacement contribute to increasing tidal volume with exercise (47). Stationary bicycling for a longer period causes ventilatory drift and tachypneic drift, much like that observed in the runner or walker (see example in Figure 3-5B). However, actual competitive bicycling requires an almost prone posture for the trunk, which will probably influence the way lung volume and respiratory muscle length changes during exercise. Furthermore, with increased air convection during cycling, temperature regulation becomes more precise and is, therefore, probably less of a contributing factor in the regulation of breathing. Similar considerations of posture and temperature would occur during endurance crawl swimming. Additional constraints of the ventilatory response in this mode of exercise include the added pressure exerted on the abdominal contents by the water environment and the importance of stroke frequency as a determinant of breathing pattern.

IV. VENTILATORY RESPONSES AND GAS EXCHANGE DURING COMPETITIVE ENDURANCE RUNNING

Unlike the constancy of conditions protected by the laboratory environment, competitive road races include variable terrain, temperature, humidity, motivational forces provided by competitors, etc. Measurements of physiologic responses during races are rare (45,67). They have been obtained in a few highly trained runners over durations of 24 to 36 kilometers and over times of 1.5 to 2.6 hours of exercise (see Fig. 3-6A-C). Usually, running velocity and $\dot{V}O_2$ were maintained remarkably constant between 75% and 85% $\dot{V}O_2$max—with some notable exceptions due to changes in terrain or race "tactics" and with changing environment (see below). Under these conditions of fairly constant metabolic demand, many responses are qualitatively similar to those in the laboratory; as tachypneic hyperventilation persisted with $\dot{V}_E$ maintained in the range of 85 to 130 $L \cdot min^{-1}$, $PaCO_2$ was maintained between 28 and 33 mmHg, in the range of lactate 2 to 6 $mEq \cdot L^{-1}$ throughout, and arterial pH was usually equal or slightly alkaline to resting values. A-aDO$_2$ is maintained at two to three times the resting level and PaO_2 within 10 mmHg of resting levels.

Two competitors ran in hot, humid conditions and progressively fatigued, so that running velocity and metabolic rate fell throughout most of the race (Fig. 3-6A-C). As $\dot{V}O_2$ and $\dot{V}CO_2$ fell, lactate concentration also fell, and arterial pH rose; but $\dot{V}_E$ fell only slightly, breathing frequency remained high, and $\dot{V}_D:V_T$ rose throughout exercise. $PaCO_2$ tended to be slightly elevated in these two subjects toward the termination of the race. This ventilatory response and, especially, the frequency response seem to bear little relationship to metabolic demand or chemical stimulation, as exercise was prolonged under these demanding environmental conditions.

Some measurements made *immediately following* long distance races (including marathons) would suggest that these stresses may somehow cause small airway closure or at least narrowing. Initial observations of highly significant but variable reductions in vital capacity (−0.2 to 2 liters) were first made following the 1923 Boston

Marathon by Gordon (39). Maron et al. (68) confirmed and extended these findings to an analysis of lung volume subdivisions and flow:volume relationships following a marathon (see Fig. 3-7). They found TLC to remain unchanged, but residual lung volume increased consistently in all 10 subjects. Flow rate was not affected during inspiration or during expiratory flow at high lung volumes, i.e., where flow rate is effort-dependent, but expiratory flow rate was reduced at low lung volumes where it is effort-independent. Subjects returned to normal by 24 hours following the marathon.

PULMONARY FUNCTION AFTER MARATHON RUNNING

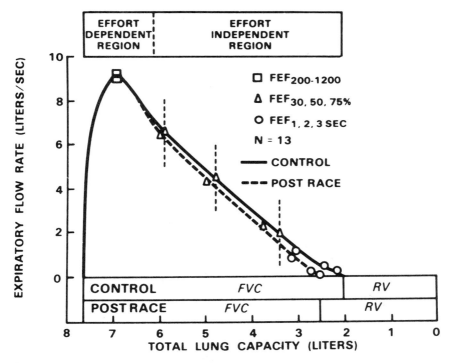

FIGURE 3-7. *Control and post-marathon max. expiratory flow:volume curves reconstructed from average data. Squares (□) refer to average values for $FEF_{200-1200}$, while circles (○) denote (reading from TLC to RV) average values for FEF_1, FEF_2, and FEF_3. Triangles (△) denote expiratory flows at 30%, 50% and 75% FVC. Note that these percentages of FVC fall at higher flow rate. The points of intersection between the post-race curve and the perpendicular dashed lines refer to post-race flow rates at lung volumes corresponding to pre-race absolute lung volumes of 30%, 50% and 75% FVC. While an average flow reduction was observed at higher lung volumes, the differences did not become statistically significant until FEV_1 was reached. The figure shows that flow was unaffected in the effort-dependent region and only became significantly reduced within the effort-independent region. (From Maron, et al., 1979.)*

Similar increases in residual lung volume and in the lung volume at which airways "close," or at least narrow substantially, have been reported following shorter runs of five miles or less (77).

These data are clearly suggestive that prolonged exhaustive exercise may cause increased airway closure at higher lung volumes. Two possibilities appear that are worth exploring. First, similar changes in airway closure may occur secondary to peribronchiolar edema and are produced in resting, normal humans, following rapid infusion of saline (15). Isolated cases of haemoptysis, with clinical signs of left ventricular failure, have been reported in highly trained runners during exhaustive runs of 90 kilometers (74). On the other hand, as we discussed earlier, clear evidence is lacking to document either: a) increases in extravascular lung water as a result of exercise; or b) that any changes in peribronchiolar edema actually cause airway closure. Contraction of bronchiolar smooth muscle in the peripheral airway is another less likely explanation for expiratory flow limitation. If this occurs, it is most likely restricted to the postexercise period, as bronchodilation usually occurs *during* most types of exercise.

Prolonged competitive exercise in the out-of-doors may be complicated and potentially compromised by environmental pollutants. The bulk of the available literature deals with the influence of ozone, a major constituent of photochemical smog. Ozone has two influences on the lung relevant to an acute exposure during prolonged exercise: it increases airway resistance, while simultaneously provoking rapid, shallow breathing (3). These effects are dosage dependent, in terms of both ozone concentration and the minute ventilation maintained during exercise (61). Since prolonging and intensifying work increases exposure, athletes in endurance competition may most seriously be affected. Both the consequences and mechanisms of the ozone effect are fairly well understood. Symptoms of dyspnea can, in some individuals, shorten long-term work performance (3,61); short-term exercise tolerance may not be affected (33,85). Intrapulmonary vagal receptors are responsible for the rapid, shallow breathing induced by ozone in conscious dogs (62). Airway resistance increases after O_3 exposure in two phases, the first dependent upon parasympathetic control and the second upon histamine release (44).

V. REGULATION OF BREATHING IN PROLONGED EXERCISE

A number of factors may be identified as potential contributors to the progressive hyperventilation and tachypnea in prolonged, heavy exercise. We view these as disturbing influences that override the usual precise association of $\dot{V}_A$ to $\dot{V}CO_2$. Several candidates for these disturbing influences have been put forward.

A compensatory response of ventilation to metabolic acidosis is well documented and may have contributed in a minor way to the hyperventilation observed at least at the initiation of prolonged exercise. However, the predominant trend was toward alkalinity during all phases of exercise and/or increasing alkalinity with time, as plasma lactate fell, and hypocapnia persisted. The level of arterial [H+] is apparently determined by, rather than a determinant of, the hyperventilatory response. This contrasts with heavier short-term or sustained work loads (Fig. 3-5A), where metabolic acidosis is progressive. In these cases, increasing arterial [H+] is a potentially major contributor to hyperventilation—but as previously discussed, for short-term, heavy exercise conditions, elevated levels of arterial [H+] may not be *obligatory* to *any* type of exercise hyperventilation.

Elevations in body temperature in excess of 1 to 1.5° C caused by external heating (at rest or exercise) cause hyperventilation (65,82). Furthermore, skin cooling, which prevents at least some of the normal rise in body temperature during prolonged exercise, reduces hyperventilatory response (25,65). During prolonged, heavy work (Figs. 3-2 and 3-3) a significant ventilatory stimulus, linked to accumulation of metabolic heat production, is implicated by the magnitude of the observed increases in core and blood temperatures and by the dominant tachypneic breathing pattern. This almost "panting-like" tachypnea, with increasing dead-space ventilation, is a unique response to ventilatory stimuli in humans, in whom the major mode of response to chemoreceptor stimuli and to exercise, per se, is a rising tidal volume. On the other hand, ventilatory drift in some types of prolonged exercise has also been observed when the increase in core temperature is <1.0° C and insufficient (as tested in the resting subject) to cause a hyperventilatory response (70).

Long-term exercise and, especially, road-racing cause marked increases in circulating norepinephrine, which are fairly well correlated over time with the ventilatory drift (45,70). However, the relative effectiveness of these humoral changes as ventilatory stimuli remains unclear. Adrenergic blockade was shown to have no effect on the hyperventilation accompanying heavy, short-term exercise, during which levels of circulating adrenergic amines coexisted with metabolic acidosis. There is also disagreement concerning the effectiveness of exogenous norepinephrine as a ventilatory stimulus in the absence of a hypoxic background (45).

The tachypneic response and drift during prolonged exercise is a response which is unique among most physiologic ventilatory stimuli applied to humans. When this occurs in heavy, short-term exercise, one usually invokes a mechanical feedback reflex related to lung inflation; but this is not apparently applicable in long-term work, where tidal volume is usually less than 45% of vital capacity, at a time when frequency is increasing and tidal volume falling. We have previously emphasized the importance and uniqueness of temperature changes as a cause of increased breathing frequency (see above); but there are also other possibilities related to mechanical changes in the lung or thorax. First, pulmonary congestion and increased pulmonary venous or lung interstitial fluid pressure is known to produce a tachypneic response—presumably via the activation of C fiber endings in the lung parenchyma and vagal afferent activity (80). Secondly, respiratory muscle fatigue or impending fatigue has been associated with the adoption of a tachypneic breathing pattern (84). Of course, these possibilities are highly theoretical, because neither the accumulation of extravascular lung water nor respiratory muscle fatigue has been established during exercise of any type of duration.

Related to these influences is the possibility that the pattern of breathing adopted during exercise by healthy subjects may be largely "behaviorally" selected, in response to sensory information (56). Indeed, given that the internal mechanical "load" on the inspiratory muscles is augmented with the hyperpnea of exercise, then this load must be "sensed" to some extent to minimize the magnitude of the pleural pressure generated and to optimize the breathing pattern. The immediacy and magnitude of mechano-receptor feedback from the lung and/or chest wall is markedly dependent on the wakeful state, as shown by the absence of response to internal or external resistive or elastic loads during quiet sleep (55). Killian and associates (56,59) claim that it is the actual "perception" of respiratory effort that may be important for compensation of the breathing pattern so that sensory magnitude as well as mechanical force development might be minimized. Certainly, cortical manifestation of loads—when it is present—must be important to load compensation; and this purely "behavioral response" probably does occur in some instances during the tachypnea of heavy, prolonged work. On the other hand, the rapidity of response to partially unloading the normal respiratory system (for example, with low density gas (52)) suggests that sensory information may not require processing by the higher CNS to provide appropriate compensatory responses. So, while the conscious state does seem crucial to providing sufficient gain for most types of mechanical load compensation, a truly cortical "perception" of the load is not obligatory.

As in most other questions involving organ system regulation in the whole animal, regulation of time-dependent tachypneic hyperventilation of the human during prolonged, heavy exercise is multifaceted and obviously unresolved. It would be most helpful in this regard to know the importance of vagal feedback—in the *human*—to the regulation of the breathing pattern (80).

VI. DO RESPIRATORY MUSCLES FATIGUE DURING PROLONGED EXERCISE?

This question remains unanswered, although it has received considerable attention in recent years because of evidence that diaphragm muscle in healthy subjects can be made to fatigue by breathing heavily against resistive loads and the ensuing speculation that diaphragm fatigue occurs in many patients with varying forms of lung and airway disease (84). We very briefly summarize some of the key considerations of this question here and refer the reader to recent specific reviews on the subject (12,20,56). This question is reasonable, given the magnitude of ventilatory response to heavy exercise and the ability of athletes to sustain ventilations in excess of 120 liters per minute throughout one to two hours or more of competition. Nonetheless, in the authors' opinion, respiratory muscle fatigue, per se, does not occur in healthy humans during physiologic exercise.

A. Metabolic Considerations in Animals

The fiber type of the diaphragm is similar to predominantly fast-twitch limb muscle, such as the plantaris, (60% fast twitch, 40% slow twitch). However, the diaphragm has a very high oxidative capacity, similar to a red oxidative muscle like the soleus and less than that in the heart. During exercise in the dog and rat, blood flow increases substantially to the diaphragm similar to that in other exercising skeletal muscles (31). In the pony, at heavy, short-term exercise, there is some evidence that maximum vasodilation has actually occurred in the diaphragm's vascular bed (66). In fact, the amount of vasodilator reserve for the diaphragm at max. exercise was significantly less than that in heart or limb locomotor muscle. So, as discussed above, even though the control system is geared to "spare" the work of the diaphragm by the use of accessory inspiratory and expiratory muscles and the control of the breathing pattern, clearly, its metabolic demand is increased substantially by heavy exercise.

Is this increased demand able to be met by blood-borne substrates, or does anaerobic glycolysis occur in the diaphragm? If so, is it predictive of fatigue? These questions have been studied to date only in the rat, which shows a brisk ventilatory and tachypneic response to prolonged, heavy exercise, maintained arterial oxygenation, high lactate production, but fairly precise [H+] regulation, with high blood flow delivered to the respiratory and locomotor muscles (34). All studies of sustained, heavy exercise to exhaustion (38 minutes to 5 hours) show some glycogen usage by the diaphragm and most show less glycogen loss in diaphragm than in locomotor muscle of similar fiber type. The results are highly variable: a) Moore and Gollnick (79) showed a 90% depletion in diaphragm muscle after a one hour run to exhaustion; b) Iannuzzo et al. (54) and Gorski et al. (40) showed 43 and 50% reduction after 48 minutes of running and 5 hours of swimming, respectively, in the diaphragm vs. 75% depletion in the plantaris; c) Fregosi and Dempsey (35) reported an average reduction of 25% in diaphragm glycogen, which was inconsistent and statistically insignificant, vs. a 75% reduction in plantaris after 38 minutes of exercise at 84% $\dot{V}O_2$max to exhaustion. They also found virtually no measurable change in diaphragm glycogen vs. 55% reduction in plantaris muscle following 54 minutes of exhaustive exercise at a lighter load (68% $\dot{V}O_2$max) (35). All of the above studies showed a significant although highly variable, reduction in intercostal muscle glycogen content following prolonged, heavy exercise to exhaustion. A consensus of these data is that respiratory muscles in the rat do utilize their glycogen stores to some extent during some, but not all types, of prolonged, exhaustive exercise; however, this usage is substantially less than that shown by locomotor muscles of similar fiber type, but of different enzyme profile. Furthermore, since most data show that at least 50% of the diaphragm's glycogen is still remaining, even at the termination of exhaustive exercise, it doesn't seem reasonable to conclude that glycogen "depletion" is limiting diaphragmatic function (or pulmonary ventilation) during prolonged exhaustive exercise. To the contrary, this evidence by itself would support the notion that the diaphragm was not fatigued at a time when locomotor muscles had reached a critical level of substrate depletion. Finally, we note that like locomotor muscle, diaphragm lactic acid concentrations do increase substantially during heavy exercise to exhaustion. This may mean that respiratory muscles, like the heart, may take up circulating lactate for use as a substrate during prolonged exercise (35). This situation changed when exhaustive exercise was carried out in a hypoxic environment; under these conditions of increased hyperventilation, increased circulating catecholamines and reduced oxygen transport, the diaphragm mimicked the plantaris, showing substantial glycogen depletion and an apparent increase in lactate production.

B. Neuro-Mechanical Evidence in Humans

Several approaches have been devised to determine indices to measure or predict respiratory muscle fatigue or capacity and apply them to exercise. One common method is to use a voluntary test of ventilatory muscle "capacity", such as MVV or maximal sustainable ventilation or maximum "isometric" pressure development against a closed airway. Then, these indices are compared to the actual spontaneous ventilation *or* to the esophageal pressure or trans-diaphragmatic pressure (P_{di}) or to such indices as the "tension-time index" of the diaphragm, which include parameters of breath-timing and P_{di}, as developed during exhaustive exercise. These comparisons are intended to provide an estimate of the fraction of the ventilatory or of the respiratory muscle "capacity" used in the exercise. These are probably unrealistic comparisons because: a) the voluntary-type maximum ventilation tests are not controlled for end-expiratory lung volume (i.e., respiratory muscle length) or pressure development (particularly during forced expiration), which differ markedly from those obtained during spontaneous breathing in heavy exercise (48,19); and b) tests of maximum pressure development during airway occlusion do not consider the pressure lost due to muscle shortening and, therefore, greatly overestimate the maximum pressure *available* for spontaneous breathing in exercise.

Other approaches are to perform voluntary maximum ventilation tests or occlusion pressure tests before and after exhaustive exercise supposedly to determine if respiratory muscles fatigue. In almost all cases, these tests show reduced performances following exhaustive exercise of minutes-to-hours duration (10,64). There are serious problems associated with these tests. Variables such as lung volume and/or rate of muscle shortening during the tests are not carefully controlled or accounted for in the pre vs. postexercise test. For example, we discussed earlier the significant increases in lung volume following marathon running which, by itself, would decrease max trans-diaphragmatic pressure (P_{di}). Further, the tests are purely volitional, and it is questionable whether one can distinguish between a true reduction in respiratory muscle function and reductions in all volitional efforts due to "general" body fatigue. A new test using supermaximal phrenic nerve stimulation removes a volitional portion of the test but remains especially sensitive to change in muscle length either at the initiation or during the stimulation (8). In short, truly quantitative, validated tests of respiratory muscle fatigue are desperately needed; but a good starting point here should be to discard the maximum voluntary ventilatory output tests from any serious consideration as mimikers of physiology.

During exercise, it has been virtually impossible to determine whether respiratory muscles are failing. For example, reductions in P_{di} might simply mean accessory muscle recruitment; a changing power spectrum frequency in the diaphragmatic EMG during exercise is extremely difficult to measure accurately and has not been convincingly shown to change coincidentally with mechanical failure. Changes in output variables, such as breathing pattern or even gas exchange and arterial PCO_2 are not valid markers of respiratory muscle fatigue, as they are influenced by many factors which have little to do with respiratory muscle function, per se.

C. Central "Inhibition" of Respiratory Muscle Force Development

Exhaustive exercise may cause respiratory muscle "limitation," but perhaps this is a preventative neural feedback mechanism to *avoid* impending muscle fatigue. One example here may be found in the highly trained athlete working at very high metabolic demand (see Table 3-3), who apparently "permits" often rather severe hypoxemia and acidosis to occur rather than produce the huge ventilatory volumes required for adequate alveolar oxygenation and gas exchange. A more appropriate compensatory hyperventilation was only provided when pulmonary impedance and, therefore, respiratory muscle "load" was reduced via inhalation of a low density gas (22). Similar "protection" has been invoked to spare fatigue and damage of limb skeletal muscles during exhaustive exercise. Appropriate proprioceptors exist in the chest wall and afferent pathways are available in the vagus nerves, spinal cord and phrenic nerves to provide this inhibitory feedback. As with the regulation of the breathing pattern (see above), the cortical perception of impending "hard times" in the respiratory muscles may form an important (behavioral) contribution to this proposed inhibition of respiratory muscle force development. This proposed inhibition might be viewed as a form of central "fatigue." We do not know if it is actually operative in an exercising human.

In *summary*, the jury is clearly not in on this highly complex question of exercise-induced respiratory muscle fatigue. This is really not a surprising or unique dilemma, given the similar controversies and technical problems concerning even locomotor muscle fatigue during exercise or the problem of whether respiratory muscle fatigue actually exists even in the presence of the chronic loads presented by lung disease. Most currently-used methods are seriously limited in usefulness, especially as they have been applied to assessing the relative load represented by exercise ventilation. The cautious and precise use of phrenic nerve supra-maximal stimulation may offer a promising objective definition of exercise-induced changes in diaphragmatic force development.

D. The "Cost" of Exercise Ventilation

A closely related question concerns the energy and blood flow "stolen" by the respiratory muscles. As stated above, animal studies clearly indicate extremely high metabolic demand, as shown by the marked increases in blood flow to the diaphragm. However, the ventilatory response to exercise in quadrupeds is substantially different than that in humans, in terms of the breathing pattern and probably also respiratory muscle recruitment, given the prone posture of the animal and the complex interplay of locomotor and respiratory muscles in the chest wall during exercise and the greater use of ventilation for heat dissipation. In the human, we can only conclude with certainty that respiratory muscles will always require a significant amount of $\dot{V}O_2$ and blood flow, which, of course, reduces that available to working skeletal muscle. The problem here is that this required quantity has really not been measured under experimental conditions which truly mimic the ventilatory work and muscle recruitment which occurs during maximum exercise. The efficiency of breathing and mechanical work required is critically dependent on a number of factors, including muscle length, velocity of shortening, duty cycle of contractions and the use of accessory muscles. Commonly used procedures which voluntarily imitate exercise ventilation or the use of CO_2 to stimulate ventilation do not mimic the true energy cost of the respiratory muscles that are used during physiologic exercises. Current estimates range anywhere from 5% to 25% max of total exercise $\dot{V}O_2$ (78,81).

VII. TRAINING EFFECTS

Two types of training effects might influence the pulmonary system's response to prolonged, heavy exercise: 1) direct training effects on the lung and/or chest wall, per se; and 2) those effects which influence the capacity of "extra-pulmonary" structures in the cardiovascular or neuromuscular systems.

Does physical training or "athleticism" change the structural capacities of the lung? An extreme test of this question may be found in those studies dealing with phylogenetic adaptation. Weibel, Taylor and associates have proposed and tested the concept of "symmorphosis," whereby the structural design of organ systems is commensurate with functional needs (88,93). Their most recent findings show athletic animals (i.e., dog and horse) with $\dot{V}O_2$max which averaged 2.5 times that of more sedentary animals of similar body mass (goat and calf). Proportional adaptations occurred in the volume density of skeletal muscle mitochondria and convective transport capacity of the circulation (16,50,57). The diffusion surface area of the lung was also larger in the athletic species, but by a substantially smaller factor (1.5x) (94). In human athletes, especially swimmers, total lung capacity and vital capacity and FRC are commonly increased approx. 5% to 15% at any given height (6,100); however maximum diffusion capacity of the lung and pulmonary capillary blood volume are similar in athletes and nonathletes (19,21,83). Furthermore, training commonly shows no significant effect on the dimensions of alveolar capillary diffusion in rats (7), and humans show increased max $\dot{V}O_2$ with training which is not accompanied by changes in rest or exercise diffusion capacity (83), even when the training is carried out at high altitudes (21). A consensus of these data seems to favor some very limited degree of adaptability in lung morphology to increasing metabolic demands. These limited changes contrast sharply with those accompanying truly chronic stressors, such as hypoxia or pneumonectomy, which have been shown to exert marked effects on gas exchange surface morphology (11).

Are respiratory muscles adaptable to increased metabolic demands? In the athletic *vs.* nonathletic animal groups mentioned above, it was shown that muscle mass, volume density of mitochondria and capillary density (16,50) increased in the diaphragm of the athletic animal in proportion to that found in limb locomotor skeletal muscles. (One complication here is that the dog, in addition to his higher aerobic capacity, *vs.* the goat also tends to hyperventilate substantially more during exercise for temperature regulation). Human athletes also show some apparent differences in respiratory muscle capacity, as inferred from some volitional performance tests. Thus, maximum pressure development against an occluded airway, or the MVV test, was not found to be different between athletic and nonathletic groups; but the endurance athlete could achieve and sustain a significantly higher percent of his MVV (75%) than could the nonathlete (68%) (72,81). The $\dot{V}O_2$ of this voluntary ventilation was not different in athlete versus nonathlete (72). Most relevant to current consideration is the finding that the athlete could complete exhaustive endurance exercise and yet maintain his MVV performance in the postexercise period; whereas, the nonathlete markedly reduced his MVV following exhaustive endurance exercise (10). Many of these maximum ventilatory performances may be enhanced by specific respiratory muscle training (63). These data are, of course, all concerned with volitional performance tasks. More objective evidence attesting to the chronic adaptability of respiratory muscles may be found when certain lung disease states are simulated in animal models. Thus, aerobic capacity of the diaphragm was markedly increased in surviving animals by chronic marked increases in airway resistance (58), and the length:tension relationship of the hamster diaphragm was significantly changed under conditions of chronic hyperinflation induced via pharmacologically induced reductions in elastic recoil (30). Most impressive is a recent report that chronic stimulation (via phrenic nerve pacing) of the dog diaphragm at 1 to 2 Hz caused this muscle to acquire a histochemical, immunohistochemical and biochemical profile similar to that of slow-twitch muscle—suggesting the suitability of the diaphragm as a contractile autogenous substitute for damaged myocardium (2).

Whether total body physical training can change aerobic capacity of the diaphragm is debatable. Studies in rats show a continuum of findings claiming less than 10% to 15% change in various indices of aerobic capacity with physical training (36,50,75), to 20 to 30% changes (54). However, when comparisons were made among muscles, the training induced changes in diaphragm were consistently less than 25% of those observed in locomotor muscle enzymatic activity (36,50,75). So, while total body physical training will cause significant adaptive changes in respiratory muscle oxidative capacity, this adaptation need not always accompany the acquisition of a highly-trained state. Species specificity is, of course, a major question in extrapolating any of these data to humans. In animals, like the dog and rat, whose diaphragm is so highly oxidative, less redundancy is available for major adaptive shifts in metabolic capacity, except under the most demanding of truly chronic and intense stimulation.

The major non-pulmonary or "indirect" effect of physical training on the pulmonary system's response to exercise is in the training-induced reductions in the ventilatory response to heavy, submaximal short term exercise (21,78). These differences occur at exercise intensities *above* those associated with metabolic acidosis. The most obvious explanation for this reduction in the ventilatory response to heavy exercise is that a ventilatory stimulus has been reduced. In turn, the logical contender here is lactic acidosis, although other potential contributors include training-induced reductions in circulating catecholamines and (for long-term exercise) the enhanced heat dissipation and, therefore, lower core temperatures in endurance-trained athletes. Added to this is the belief by some (but not all) that endurance athletes may have "an inherently suppressed" ventilatory chemosensitivity, which makes them less responsive to any humoral stimulus. However, we have not established which, if any, humoral stimulus during heavy exercise is responsible for the observed hyperventilation. Indeed, less hyperventilation after training may also reflect less neural-induced recruitment (from the CNS) of locomotor and respiratory muscles, as skeletal muscle fatigue is delayed in the trained until a higher work load is reached.

So, what are the implications of these training effects or their absence to the response of the pulmonary system to prolonged, heavy exercise in the trained human?

First, concerning pulmonary O_2 transport, training appears to have little significant effect on the lung's maximum diffusion surface; and we know of no data which suggest that $\dot{V}_A:\dot{Q}c$ distribution is altered or that pulmonary vascular resistance is reduced via physical training. Accordingly, the trained athlete working at 80% $\dot{V}O_2$max will—like the untrained—increases his alveolar to arterial PO_2 difference 2.5 to 3.5 times >, resting levels; thus, to avoid arterial hypoxemia, he must maintain a high overall $\dot{V}_A:\dot{Q}c$ and, therefore, a high alveolar PO_2. These responses do, in fact, occur in the most highly trained roadrunner, and hypoxemia is rare (see Fig. 3-2C). At high pulmonary blood flows, the athlete will probably also achieve a maximally expanded alveolar-capillary surface area, which is maintained for a substantial time period during exercise. Both of these factors point to increased turnover of extravascular lung water. To avoid accumulation of fluid in the lung, lymphatic drainage capacity may require adaptation in the trained endurance athlete.

Second, certain changes with physical training may permit the endurance athlete to sustain very high levels of ventilatory effort for prolonged periods. Most important here would be that for a given metabolic demand, the trained runner will ventilate less and maybe even have less time-dependent ventilatory drift because of reduced stimuli. We do note that even the highly trained do show a hyperventilatory drift and tachypneic response (see Fig. 3-6C), but, presumably, this would be less than in the untrained. Even though ventilatory efficiency, i.e., respiratory muscle work and $\dot{V}O_2$ (per $L \cdot min^{-1} \dot{V}_E$) is similar in the trained and untrained, a reduced $\dot{V}_E$ will also mean a low metabolic "steal" by respiratory muscles, therefore leaving a larger fraction of total blood flow to locomotor muscles. If, in turn, training has provided at least some relatively small enhancement of enzyme profile in the diaphragm and other inspiratory muscles, then respiratory muscles would either not fatigue *or* would be able to achieve and sustain higher ventilatory volumes before a negative feedback inhibition (to avoid fatigue) would constrain the ventilatory response. More firm evidence beyond that achieved in volitional, functional tests is needed in humans to clarify the extent of respiratory muscle adaptation to physical training.

Do respiratory muscles with improved strength and endurance

have any bearing on the ability to achieve and sustain greater alveolar ventilation during heavy exercise? If so, this capability might ensure better acid-base regulation and maintenance of arterial O_2 content; perhaps even exercise performance might be enhanced. One approach to this question might be to use very specific overload of the inspiratory muscles as a part of the endurance athlete's daily training regimen. This training process would simply require that the athlete breathe through an inspiratory resistor sufficient to produce about 70% to 80% of his maximum mouth pressure achieved with maximum voluntary inspiration against an occluded airway. As with any training program, the resistive load would be gradually increased day by day, as the maximum achievable pressure changed, and the duration of the training regimen would be lengthened, as respiratory muscle endurance increased. While limited evidence does exist (using only volitional tests to measure change) that the strength and endurance of healthy respiratory muscles are indeed trainable using these specific techniques, we have no idea that this has any application to the exercise response or to performance. It is of interest here that these training techniques have been tried in patients with chronic, obstructive lung disease, in an attempt to strengthen their apparently fatigued and undernourished chestwall. Only mixed success was achieved with these techniques in this patient population, and in fact, more recently, the emphasis has been on intermittent "rest" for the respiratory muscles of these patients, using mechanical ventilation. Certainly the outcome of specific respiratory muscle training might be quite different with the healthy endurance athlete.

VIII. AGING EFFECTS

Despite the improving fitness level and work capacity of older, healthy persons and the attention given recently to their exercise pathophysiology, few studies have been devoted to detailing the aging effects on the response of the pulmonary system during exercise. Our knowledge of the normal aging process suggests that the pulmonary system response to heavy or prolonged exercise may hamper the older, well-trained athlete.

As with most aging effects, especially those reported in cross-sectional data, the changes in the lung with age are highly variable, but a few important trends do exist, as exemplified in the 70 year-old, non-smoker. A critical change is the loss of lung recoil, as observed mostly at higher lung volumes. This change, in turn, leads to: a) high FRC; and b) closure of airways at higher lung volumes. So, while the airways do not close in young persons until lung volume approaches residual volume, in the aged, airways commonly close—or least become very narrow—at lung volumes very close to and sometimes within their FRC. Expiratory airflow rates are reduced as dynamic compression occurs at higher lung volumes (5,49,60). A second important aging effect is the increasing stiffness of the pulmonary vasculature secondary to changes in either the compliance of the large pulmonary arteries or in the ventricular wall (41,42). Similarly, chest wall compliance is reduced.

At rest, these aging effects may have little effect on pulmonary gas exchange or mechanical efficiency of breathing. However, theoretically at least, in the aged athlete capable of performing prolonged exercise at high demands for gas exchange, these changes may present the following problems to homeostatic regulation. First, if, as in the young, the aged athlete experiences sufficient active expiration during exercise, FRC will be reduced below resting levels. This means that airways may close or narrow during even tidal breathing during exercise, thereby causing underventilation of some lung regions. Even at rest, aging reduces arterial PO_2 and widens alveolar to arterial PO_2 difference. During exercise, when mixed venous O_2 desaturation occurs (see Table 3-1), low $\dot{V}_A:\dot{Q}c$ regions may cause excessive widening of the alveolar to arterial PO_2 difference and even may cause hypoxemia if airways narrow and ventilation is not distributed uniformly.

Secondly, the increased stiffness of the pulmonary vasculature implies that pulmonary vascular resistance may not be so readily reduced as pulmonary blood flow increases with exercise. Indeed, limited data in some healthy, older subjects (mid 60s) even at moderate work loads show pulmonary arterial pressures of greater than 40 mmHg (41,42).

Thirdly, the reduced compliance of the chest wall and shortened inspiratory muscles secondary to hyperinflation may place significant limitations on the ability of inspiratory muscles to sustain a high ventilatory response during prolonged, heavy exercise.

These suggestions as to how heavy, sustained exercise might compromise the adequacy and efficiency of gas exchange, given the normal aging effects in the lung and chest wall, remain untested.

IX. HYPOXIC EFFECTS

Prolonged exercise at high altitudes presents significant problems to regulation in the pulmonary system. The magnitude of the problems presented depends on the length of hypoxic exposure, the degree of hypoxia and the magnitude of the work intensity. The key adaptive mechanism here is hyperventilation, which, along with increasing red cell production after a few days of hypoxic exposure, offers the only significant adaptations in the gas transport system available to the sojourner at high altitude.

Upon acute (less than one hour) hypoxia, the hyperventilatory response is insufficient, and arterial PO_2 and O_2 content are reduced during heavy and maximum exercise (24). This is especially true in the highly trained, who at their very high, metabolic demand, experience significant arterial hypoxemia, even upon acute exposures to high altitudes equivalent to Denver or Mexico City (less than 7500 feet) (22). Ventilatory acclimatization is nearly complete after about one week of sojourn at most high altitudes, and the hyperventilatory response to even mild exercise is substantial. The result is that even at as high as 10 to 12,000 feet, arterial PO_2, during prolonged heavy exercise, is maintained within 10 mmHg of resting levels in the acclimitized sojourner, and arterial pH is also well maintained. Thus, the upper portion of the HbO_2 dissociation curve is slightly shifted left, so as to maintain arterial O_2 saturation greater than 90%. These conditions are maintained during exhaustive exercise of greater than one hour (21). However, this homoestasis is maintained at very high cost, as the tachypnea and hyperventilatory drift during prolonged work exceeds that at sea level, $\dot{V}_E$ exceeds 120 to 140 liters per minute even in the untrained, breathing frequency is commonly in the 60 to 80 per minute range, and $PaCO_2$ is in the 20 to 25 mmHg range. Ventilatory work during heavy exercise at these altitudes is more than twice that of higher work loads at sea level. At higher altitudes (14,000 feet), neither oxygen transport homeostasis *nor* ventilatory efficiency is obtainable even in the acclimatized sojourner. For example, during long-term exercise at 14,000 to 15,000 feet, arterial PO_2 is reduced below 40 mmHg, and arterial HbO_2% saturation is reduced to 70%, even at the outset of exercise and a progressive tachypneic hyperventilaion ensues, never achieving a steady state throughout long-term work. Arterial PCO_2 are reduced below 20 mmHg. Dyspnea is severe and progressive in long-term exercise at these altitudes above 10,000 feet, and perceived dyspnea always occurs prior to perceived leg "fatigue" during prolonged exercise. A special problem with runners attempting to train is that entrainment of locomotion and respiration in any pattern is nearly impossible, and attempts to do so are highly disruptive to performance, as hypoxic ventilatory demands override any conscious attempts at coordination. Only after many years of acclimatization is this highly costly dependence on hyperventilation during exercise in hypoxia supplanted by the truly adaptive, structural changes in the lung's gas exchange surface, enhanced alveolar to arterial gas exchange and a reduced ventilatory response. Of course, this true adaptation occurs only in those "survivors," who choose to live for sufficiently long periods in hypoxia.

X. DOES THE LUNG LIMIT PROLONGED EXERCISE PERFORMANCE?

It is highly unlikely that even maximum metabolic demands in the *untrained*, young, healthy human exceed the ventilatory, diffusion or blood:gas matching capabilities of the healthy lung. Thus, while the exchange is not perfect, arterial PO_2 and HbO_2 saturation are maintained at close to resting levels.

Physical training is the major means through which pulmonary gas exchange, ventilatory cost, and ventilation sustainability may become significant determinants to performance (19). The lung and the chest wall are not as trainable as other links in the chain of gas transport and utilization. Thus, arterial hypoxemia may develop at maximum exercise, and work capacity will be affected. This effect approximates to about a 1% fall in max $\dot{V}O_2$ for every 1% decrement in arterial HbO_2 saturation. Precisely *why* this reduction in arterial O_2 content *causes* a reduced $\dot{V}O_2$max remains unresolved. Long-term exercise must be carried out at sub-maximal levels; thus, arterial hypoxemia, even in the highly trained, is rare (Fig. 3–2C), so long as the hyperventilatory response is substantial and sustained throughout. Pulmonary and blood CO_2 transport and acid-base control are usually adequate in long-term exercise, although when tachypnea is extreme, CO_2 elimination becomes inefficient. Inadequate alveolar ventilation, in terms of $[H+]$ regulation or maintenance of a high alveolar PO_2, may present a problem for the highly trained at maximum work or very high, short-term work loads but is not a problem with long-term submaximal exercise.

Clearly, the physiologic *cost* of hyperventilation during long-term, heavy work presents a significant effect on some determinants of locomotor muscle perfusion and metabolism and perhaps on exercise performance. Endurance performance (running) time is significantly enhanced if the respiratory load is reduced by breathing a low density gas mixture. Wilson & Welch (97) demonstrated this for very short exercise periods of five or six min duration. Aaron et al. (1) studied highly trained athletes (see Fig. 3–5B) who showed highly reproducible performance times to exhaustion. They all showed improvements in performance time while breathing $He:O_2$ of 7% to 58% at both 85% $\dot{V}O_2$max (where times were in the 30 to 51 min range) and at 95% $\dot{V}O_2$max (where performance times were in the 7–20 min range).

What factors might contribute to a significant role for respiratory muscle function as a potential limitation of endurance performance?

(a) Most significant here is the metabolism and perfusion requirement of all respiratory muscles during exercise. Unfortunately, this demand is not yet known precisely (for exercise conditions), but it is assuredly a significant fraction of the total metabolic rate and total cardiac output, and, therefore, must "steal" significantly from locomotor muscles. The metabolic cost of ventilation will become more of a limiting factor the higher the fitness level permits one to work at higher relative work intensity, and, therefore, at a higher ventilatory output.

(b) A second ill-defined contribution is the significant role that dyspnea must make to one's total perception of effort during prolonged exercise, especially as relatively foreign sensations, such as those secondary to progressive tachypnea, are experienced. In the helium breathing study, with enhanced performance times mentioned above (1), at equal exercise times, the subject's perception of both the magnitude of breathlessness and of "total body" effort were substantially reduced while breathing the low density gas.

(c) A third, and we think unlikely, possibility is that of respiratory muscle fatigue during prolonged exercise.

(d) Finally, some environmental factors will push pulmonary limitations to the forefront. Indeed, the panting-like tachypneic hyperventilatory response to prolonged heavy exercise in the heat *or* in some highly polluted environments *or* at even moderately high altitudes must provide a significant curtailment of performance capability in the highly trained competitor.

Finally, we wish to mention briefly a little publicized, poorly understood phenomenon which may link pulmonary reflexes to inhibition of skeletal muscle activity. Paintal (80) and Ginzel and Eldred (37) suggested that vagally-mediated lung reflexes could inhibit skeletal muscle contractility. Indeed, in anesthetized dogs, deep breaths inhibited hind limb EMG and knee-jerk reflexes as much as 30% to 50% (37,13). These inhibitory reflexes are also initiated by lung C fiber stimulation and may also be secondary to distension of the heart and great vessels (13). These inhibitory reflexes are all blocked by vagotomy. While it may seem somewhat farfetched that lung stretch or increased lung interstitial fluid or pulmonary vascular pressures may initiate a significant contribution to locomotor muscle fatigue in the human long-distance runner, given the complexity of fatigue in the whole organism, this idea deserves further attention.

ACKNOWLEDGEMENTS

The original work reported here was supported by Grants from NIH and the American Lung Association. I am indebted to Mary Westervelt for manuscript preparation.

BIBLIOGRAPHY

1. Aaron, E.A., K.G. Henke, D.F. Pegelow, and J.D. Dempsey. "Effects of mechanical unloading of the respiratory system on exercise and respiratory muscle endurance." *Medicine and Science in Sports and Exercise.* 17:290, 1985 (abstract).
2. Acker, M., J. Mannion, W. Brown, S. Salmons, J. Henriksson, T. Bitto, D. Gale, R. Hammond, and W. Stephenson. Canine diaphragm muscle after 1 year of continuous electrical stimulation: its potential as a myocardial substitute. *J Appl Physiol.* 62:1264–1270, 1987.
3. Adams, W.C., W.M. Savin, and A.E. Christo. Detection of ozone toxicity during continuous exercise via the effective dose concept. *J Appl Physiol.* 51:415–422, 1981.
4. Adams, W.C., and E.S. Schelegle. Ozone and high ventilation effects on pulmonary function and endurance performance. *J Appl Physiol.* 55:805–812, 1983.
5. Anthonisen, N.R., J. Danson, P.C. Roberton, and W.R.D. Ross. Airway closure as a function of age. *Resp Physiol.* 8:58–65, 1970.
6. Astrand, P.O., L. Engstrom, B.O. Eriksson, P. Karlberg, I. Nylander, B. Saltin, and S. Thren. Girl swimmers with special references to respiratory and circulatory adaptation and gynecological and psychiatric aspects. *Acta Paediat Scand. Suppl.* 147:43–75, 1963.
7. Bartlett, D. and J.G. Areson. Quantitative lung morphology in Japanese waltzing mice. *J Appl Physiol.* 44:446–449, 1978.
8. Bellemare, F., B. Biglund-Ritchie. Assessment of human diaphragm strength and activation using phrenic nerve stimulation. *Resp Physiol.* 58:263–277, 1987.
9. Bellemare, F. and A. Grassino. Evaluation of human diaphragm fatigue. *J Appl Physiol.* 53:1196–1206, 1982.
10. Bender, P.R. and B.J. Martin. Maximal ventilation after exhausting exercise. *Med Sci Sports Exer.* 17:164–167, 1985.
11. Brody, J.S., S. Lahiri, M. Simpser, E.K. Motoyama and T. Velasquez. Lung elasticity and airway dynamics in Peruvian natives to altitude. *J Appl Physiol.* 42:245–251, 1977.
12. Bye, P.T.P., G.A. Farkas and C. Roussos. Respiratory factors limiting exercise. *Ann. Rev. Physiol.* 45:439–451, 1983.
13. Coast, J.R., E.S. Thompson, S.S. Cassidy. Inhibition of skeletal muscle activity by lung expansion in the dog. *J Appl Physiol.* 62:2058–2065, 1987.
14. Coates, G.H., O'Bradovich, A.L. Jerreries and G.H. Gray. Effects of exercise on lung lymph flow in sheep and goats during normoxia and hypoxia. *J. Clin. Invest.* 74:131–133, 1984.
15. Coates, G., A.C.P. Powles, S.C. Morrison, J.R. Sutton, C.E. Webber and C.J. Zylak. The effects of intravenous infusion of saline on lung volumes, nitrogen washout; computed tomographic scans & chest radiographs in humans. *Am. Rev. Resp. Dis.* 127:91–96, 1983.
16. Conley, K.E., S.R. Kayar, K. Rosler, H. Hoppeler, E.R. Weibel and C.R. Taylor. Capillaries and their relationship to oxidative capacity. *Resp. Physiol.* (In press).
17. Costill, D. Metabolic responses during distance running. *J. Appl. Physiol.* 28:251–255, 1970.
18. Dempsey, J.A. Some exercise-induced imperfections in pulmonary gas exchange. *Can J Sports Sci.* 12:Supp, 66–71, 1987.
19. Dempsey, J.A. Is the lung built for exercise? *Medicine and Science in Sports and Exercise.* 18:2;143–155, 1986.
20. Dempsey, J.A. and R.F. Fregosi. Adaptability of the pulmonary system to changing metabolic requirements. *Am. J. Cardiol.* 55:59D–67D, 1985.
21. Dempsey, J.A., N. Gledhill, W.G. Reddan, H.V. Forster, P.G. Hanson and A.D. Claremont. Pulmonary adaptation to exercise:effects of exercise type and duration, chronic hypoxia and physical training. *Ann. NY Acad. Sci.* 301:243–261, 1977.
22. Dempsey, J.A., P. Hanson and K. Henderson. Exercise-induced arterial hypoxemia in healthy human subjects at sea level. *J. Physiol.* (Lond.) 355:161–175, 1984.
23. Dempsey, J.A., G.S. Mitchell and C.A. Smith. Exercise and Chemoreception. *Am. Rev. Resp. Dis.* 129 (Suppl):S31–S34, 1984.
24. Dempsey, J.A., W.G. Reddan, J. Rankin, M.L. Birnbaum, H.V. Forster, J.S. Thoden and

R.F. Grover. Effects of acute through life-long hypoxic exposure on exercise pulmonary gas exchange. *Resp. Physiol.* 13:62–89, 1971.

25. Dempsey, J.A., J.M. Thomson, S.C. Alexander, H.V. Forster and L.W. Chosy. Respiratory influences on acid-base status and their effects on O_2 transport during prolonged muscular work. In: *Metabolic Adaptation to Prolonged Physical Exercise.* Proceeding of the 2nd International Symposium on Biochemistry of Exercise. H. Howald and J.R. Poortmans (Eds.). Magglingen, Switzerland, Number 7, pp. 56–64, 1975.

26. Dempsey, J.A., E.H. Vidruk, S.M. Mastenbrook. Pulmonary control systems in exercise. *Fed. Proc.* 39:1498–1505, 1980.

27. Dempsey, J.A., E.H. Vidruk, and G.S. Mitchell. Pulmonary control systems in exercise: update. *Fed. Proc.* 44:2260–2270, 1985.

28. Ekelund, L.G. Circulatory and respiratory adaptation during prolonged exercise of moderate intensity in the sitting position. *Acta Physiol. Scand.* 69:327–340, 1967.

29. Eldridge, F.L., D.E. Milhorn, T.G. Waldrop. Exercise hyperpnea and locomotion:parallel activation from the hypothalamus. *Science.* 211-844-846, 1981.

30. Farkas, G.A., C. Roussos. Adaptability of the hamster diaphragm to exercise and/or emphysema. *J. Appl. Physiol.* 53:1263–1272, 1982.

31. Fixler, D.E., J.M. Atkins, J.G. Mitchell and L.D. Horwitz. Blood flow to respiratory cardiac, and limb muscles in dogs during graded exercise. *Am. J. Physiol.* 231:1515–1519, 1976.

32. Folinsbee, L.J., J.F. Bedi and S.M. Horvath. Pulmonary function changes after 1 hour continuous heavy exercise in 0.21 ppm ozone. *J. Appl. Physiol.* 57:984–988, 1984.

33. Folinsbee, L.J., F. Silverman and R.J. Shephard. Decrease of maximum work performance following ozone exposure. *J. Appl. Physiol.* 42:531–536, 1977.

34. Fregosi, R.F. and J.A. Dempsey, Arterial blood acid-base regulation during exercise in rats. *J. Appl. Physiol.* 57:396–402, 1984.

35. Fregosi, R. and J.A. Dempsey. Effects of exercise in normoxia & acute hypoxia on respiratory muscle metabolites. *J. Appl. Physiol.* 60:1274–1283, 1986.

36. Fregosi, R.F., M. Sanjak and D.J. Paulson. "Endurance training does not affect diaphragm mitochondrial respiration." *Resp. Physiol.* 67:225–237, 1987.

37. Ginzel, K. and E. Elched. A Possible physiological role for the depression of somatic motor function by reflexes from the cardiopulomnary region. *Proc. West Pharmacol. Soc.* 13:188–191, 1970.

38. Gledhill, N., A.B. Froese, F.J. Buick and A.C. Bryan. Va:Qc inhomogeneity and $AaDO_2$ in man during exercise:effect of SF_6 breathing. *J. Appl. Physiol.* 45:512–515, 1978.

39. Gordon, B., S.A. Levine and A. Wilmaers. Observations on a group of marathon runners with special reference to the circulation. *Arch. Intern. Med.* 33:425–434, 1924.

40. Gorski, J., Z. Namiot and J. Giedrojc. Effect of exercise on metabolism of glycogen and triglycerides in the respiratory muscles. *Pflugers Arch.* 377-251-254, 1978.

41. Granath, A., B. Jonsson and T. Strandell. Circulation in healthy old men, studied by right heart catheterization at rest and during exercise in supine and sitting position. *Acta Med. Scand.*: 1–22, 1964.

42. Granath, A. and T. Strandell, Relationships between cardiac output, stroke volume, and intracardiac pressures at rest and during exercise in supine position and some anthropometric data in healthy old men. *Acta Med. Scand.* 176:447–466, 1964.

43. Grimby, G., M. Goldman and J. Mead. Respiratory muscle actions inferred from rib cage and abdominal V-P partitioning. *J. Appl. Physiol.* 41:739–751, 1976.

44. Gutner, A., B. Brombeyer-barnea, A.N. Dannenberg, Jr, R. Traystman and H. Menkes. Responses of the lung periphery to ozone and histamine. *J. Appl. Physiol.* 54:640–646, 1983.

45. Hanson, P., A. Claremont, J.A. Dempsey and W. Reddan. Determinants and consequences of ventilatory responses to competitive endurance running. *J. Appl. Physiol.* 52:615–623, 1982.

46. Heistad, D.D., R.C. Wheeler, A.L. Mark, P.G. Schmid and F.M. Abboud. Effects of adrenergic stimulation on ventilation in man. *J. Clin. Invest.* 51:1469–1475, 1972.

47. Henke, K.G., M. Sharratt, D. Pegelow and J. Dempsey. Regulation of end-expiratory lung volume during exercise. *J. Appl. Physiol.* 64:135–146, 1988.

48. Hesser, C.M., D. Linnarsson and L. Fagraeus. Pulmonary mechanics and work of breathing at maximal ventilation and raised air pressure. *J. Appl. Physiol.* 50:747–753, 1981.

49. Holland, J., J. Milic-Emili, P.J. Macklem and D.V. Bates. Regional distribution of pulmonary ventilation & perfusion in elderly subjects. *J. Clin. Inst.* 47:81–92, 1968.

50. Hoppeler, H., S.R. Kayar, H. Claassen, E. Uhlmann and R.H. Karas. Skeletal muscles:setting the demand for oxygen. *Resp. Physiol.* (In press).

51. Hughes, E.F., S.C. Turner and G.A. Brooks. Effects of glycogen depletion and pedaling speed on "anaerobic threshold." *J. App. Physiol.* 52:1598–1607, 1982.

52. Hussain, S.N., R.L. Pardy and J.A. Dempsey. Mechanical impedance as a determinant of

hyperpnea and inspiratory effort during exercise. *J. Appl. Physiol.* 59(2):365–375, 1985.

53. Ianuzzo, C.D., E.G. Noble, N. Hamilton and Dabrowski. Effects of streptozotocin diabetes, insulin treatment, and training on the diaphragm. *J. Appl. Physiol.* 52:1471–1475, 1982.

54. Iannuzzo, C.D., M. J. Spalding and H. Williams. Exercise-induced glycogen utilization by the respiratory muscles. *J. Appl. Physiol.* 62:1405–1409, 1987.

55. Iber, C., A. Berssenbrugge, J.B. Skatrud and J.A. Dempsey. Ventilatory adaptations to resistive loading during wakefulness and non-REM sleep. *J. Appl Physiol.* 52:607–614, 1982.

56. Jones, N.L., K. Killian and D. Stubbing. "The thorax in exercise." In:*The Thorax*, vol. 2, (Ed C. Rousos and P. Macklem. Marcel Dekker, pp. 3–37, 1986.

57. Karas, R.H., C.R. Taylor, J.J. Jones, R.B. Reeves and E.R. Weibel. Flow of oxygen across the pulmonary gas exchanger. *Resp. Physiol.* (In press).

58. Keens, T.G., V. Chen, P. Patel, P. O'Brien, H. Levison and C.D. Ianuzzo. Cellular adaptations of the ventilatory muscles to a chronic increased respiratory load. *J. Appl Physiol.* 44:905–908, 1978.

59. Killian, K.H. and E.J. Campbell. Dyspnea and exercise. *Ann. Rev. Physiol.* 45:465–479, 1983.

60. Krumpe, P.E., R.G. Knudson, G. Parsons and K. Reiser. The aging respiratory system. *Clinics in Geriatric Medicine.* 1:143–175, 1985.

61. Lauritzen, S.K. and W.C. Adams. Ozone inhalation effects consequent to continuous exercise in females: comparison to males. *J. Appl. Physiol.* 59:1601–1606, 1985.

62. Lee, L.Y., T.D. Djokie, C. Dumont, P.D. Graf and J.A. Nadel. Mechanism of ozone-induces tachypneic response to hypoxia and hypercapnia in conscious dogs. *J. Appl. Physiol.* 48:163–168, 1980.

63. Leith, D.E. and M. Bradley. Ventilatory muscle strength and endurance training. *J. Appl. Physiol.* 41(4):508, 1976.

64. Loke, J., D. Mahler and A. Virgulto. Respiratory muscle fatigue after marathon running. *J. Appl. Physiol.* 52:821–824, 1982.

65. MacDougall, J.D., W.G. Reddan, C.R. Layton and J.A., Dempsey. Effects of metabolic hyperthermia on performance during heavy prolonged exercise. *J. Appl. Physiol.* 36:538–544, 1974.

66. Manohar, Murli. Vasodilator reserve in respiratory muscles during maximal exertion in ponies. *J. Appl. Physiol.* 60:1571–1577, 1986.

67. Maron, M., S.M. Horvath, J.E. Wilkerson and J.A. Glimer. Oxygen uptake measurements during competitive marathon running. *J. Appl. Physiol.* 40:836–838, 1976.

68. Maron, M.B., L.H. Hamilton and M.G. Maksud. Alterations in pulmonary function consequent to competitive marathon running. *Med. Sci. Sports.* II(3):244–249, 1979.

69. Marshall, B.E., L.R. Soma and G.R. Neufeld. Lung water volume at rest and exercise in dogs. *J. Appl. Physiol.* 39:7–8, 1975.

70. Martin, B.J., E.J. Morgan, C.W. Zwillich and J.V. Weil. Control of breathing during prolonged exercise. *J. Appl. Physiol.: Respir. Environ. Exercise. Physiol.* 50:27–31, 1981.

71. Martin, B.J., F.E. Sparks, C.W. Zwillich and J.V. Weil. Low exercise ventilation in endurance athletes. *Medical Science Sports.* 11:181–185, 1979.

72. Martin, B.J. and J.M. Stager. Ventilatory endurance in athletes and non-athletes. *Med. Sci. in Sports & Exercise.* 13:21–26, 1981.

73. Martin, B.J., E.J. Morgan, C.W. Zwillich and J.V. Weil. Control of breathing during prolonged exercise. *J. Appl. Physiol.* 50:27–31, 1981.

74. McKechnie, J.K., W.P. Leary, T.D. Noakes, J.C. Kallmeyer, E.T. MacSearraigh, and L.R. Olivier. Acute pulmonary edema in two athletes during a 90-km running race. *S. African Med. Journal.* 56:261–265, 1979.

75. Metzger, J.M. and Fitts. Contractile and biochemical properties of the diaphragm:Effects of exercise training and fatigue. *J. Appl. Physiol.* 60:1752–1758, 1986.

76. Michel, R.P., L. Zocchi, A. Rossi, G.A. Cardinal, Y. Ploy-Sand, R.S. Paulsen, J. Milic-Emili and N.C. Staub. Does interstitial lung edema compress airways and arteries? A morphometric study. *J. Appl. Physiol.* 62:108–115, 1987.

77. Miles, D.S., A.D. Enoch and S.C. Grevey. Interpretation of changes in DLCO & pulmonary function after running five miles. *Resp. Physiol.* 66:135–145, 1986.

78. Milic-Emili, J., J. Petit and R. Deroanne. Mechanical work of breathing during exercise intrained and untrained subjects. *J. Appl. Physiol.* 17:43–46, 1962.

79. Moore, R.L. and P.D. Gollnick. Response of ventilatory muscles of the rat to endurance training. *Pflugers Arch.* 392:268–271, 1982.

80. Paintal, A.S. Vagal sensory receptors and their reflex effects. *Physiol. Rev.* 53:159–227, 1973.

81. Pardy, R.L., S.N. Hussain and P.T. Macklem. The ventilatory pump in exercise. In: Clinics in Chest Medicine. J. Loke (Ed) 5:35–49, 1984.

82. Peterson, E.S. and H. Vejby-Christiansen. Effect of body temperature on steady state ventilation and metabolism in exercise. *Acta. Physiol. Scand.* 38:342–351, 1973.
83. Reuschlein, P.L., W.G. Reddan, J.F. Burpee, J.B.L. Gee and J. Rankin. The effect of physical training on the pulmonary diffusing capacity during submaximal work. *J. Appl. Physiol.* 24:152–158, 1968.
84. Roussos, C.H. and J. Moxham. Respiratory muscle fatigue. In: C.H. Roussos & P. Macklem (Eds.), *The Thorax* (pp. 829–870). New York, Marcel Dekker, 1986.
85. Savin, W.M. and W.C. Adams. Effects of ozone inhalation on work performance and $\dot{V}O_2max$. *J. Appl. Physiol.* 46:309–314, 1979.
86. Sharratt, M., K.G. Henke, E.A. Aaron, D. Pegelow and J.D. Dempsey. Exercise-induced changes in functional residual capacity. *Resp. Physiol.* 70:313–326, 1987.
87. Staub, N.C., H. Nagano and M.L. Pearce. Pulmonay edema in dogs, especially the sequence of fluid accumulation in lungs. *J. Appl. Physiol.* 22:227–240, 1967.
88. Taylor, C.R. E.R. Weibel, R.H. Karas and H. Hoppeler. Structural and functional design principles determining the limits to oxidative metabolism. *Resp. Physiol.* (In press).
89. Thompson, J.M., J.A. Dempsey, L.W. Chosy, N.T. Shahidi and W.G. Reddan. Oxygen transport and oxyhemoglobin dissociation during prolonged muscular work. *J. Appl. Physiol.* 37:658–664, 1974.
90. Wagner, P.D. Influence of mixed venous PO_2 on diffusion of O_2 across the pulmonary blood:gas barrier. *Clin. Physiol.* 2:105–115, 1982.
91. Wasserman, K., A.L. Van Kessel and E.E. Burton. Interaction of physiological mechanisms during exercise. *J. Appl. Physiol.* 22:71–85, 1967.
92. Weibel, E.R. Is the lung built reasonably? *Am. Rev. Resp. Dis.* 128:752–760, 1983.
93. Weibel, E.R. Oxygen demand and the size of respiratory structures in mammals. In: *Evaluation of respiratory processes*, S.C. Wood and C. Lenfant (Eds.). New York:Marcel Dekker, pp. 289–346, 1979.
94. Weibel, E.R., L.B. Marques, M. Constantinopol, F. Doffey, P. Gehr and C.R. Taylor. The pulmonary gas exchanger, *Resp. Physiol.* (In press).
95. Whipp, B.J., K. Wasserman, R. Casaburi, C.E. Juratsch, M.L. Weissman, R.W. Stremel. Ventilatory control characteristics of conditions resulting in isocapnic hyperpnea. In:Fitzgerald R, Lahiri S, Gautier H, (Eds.). *Control of Respiration During Sleep and Anesthesia*. New York:Plenum, 355–365, 1978.
96. Widimski, J., E. Berglund and R. Malmberg. Effect of repeated exercise on the lesser circulation. *J. Appl. Physiol.* 18:983–986, 1963.
97. Wilson, G.D. and H.G. Welch. Effects of varying concentrations of N_2/O_2 and He/O_2 on exercise tolerance in man. *Medicine and Science in Sports and Exercise.* 12(5):380–384, 1980.
98. Younes, M., Z. Bshouty and J. Ali. Longitudinal distribution of pulmonary vascular resistance with very high pulmonary blood flow. *J. Appl. Physiol.* 62:344–358, 1987.
99. Younes, M. and G. Kivinen. Respiratory mechanics and breathing pattern during and following maximal exercise. *J. Appl. Physiol.* 57:1773–1782, 1984.
100. Zinman, R. and C. Gaultier. Maximal static pressures & lung volumes in young female swimmers. *Resp. Physiol.* 64:229–239, 1986.

DISCUSSION

FARRELL: What's wrong with the weighing techniques that are used to look at water accumulation in the lungs?

DEMPSEY: You can imagine trying to get all the fluid out of the lungs. You never can drain them completely. You can never get them out of the animal in time. It's fairly insensitive. There's some excellent work recently published from Winnipeg in an isolated dog lung showing increases of blood flow through the lung by 4- to 6-fold. The lungs were observed starting to gain weight. Now, it's an isolated lobe. So, in that kind of preparation, I think the technique's very useful. In the whole animal, it probably isn't sensitive enough.

RAVEN: That water accumulation in the lung is found in race horses, correct?

DEMPSEY: Some red cells accumulate in the horse's airway following heavy exercise.

RAVEN: So the human parallel may be there.

DEMPSEY: It's found in over 80% of race horses. But that's not been established to the same extent in the human. And, of course, as far as I know, pulmonary vascular pressures in the lung of race horses, at least pulmonary arterial pressures, can exceed 90 mmHg. And we don't get to that extent in a human. Also, I'm not sure that high pulmonary arterial pressure explains why the horse lung bleeds in heavy work. It may be a deterioration of the parenchymal structure of the lung because of the tremendous negative pressure it is exposed to in certain parts of the lung. Plus, the horse almost doubles its hematocrit from rest to very heavy work. So, you have very high viscosity and high pressures there. So, I'm not sure the parallel with humans is there.

MICHELI: Is there significant water loss through the lung in an endurance event?

DEMPSEY: Well, I don't think so. Even though ventilations of 130 $L \cdot min^{-1}$ can be maintained for over 1.5 h of prolonged running in the heat, and, even though panting-like responses occur in some cases, as I understand it, a very small fraction of the total water loss during exercise comes from the lungs.

NADEL: About 15 years ago, we found such water loss to be only 1–2 $g \cdot min^{-1}$, which is trivial in comparison to the fluid lost as sweat.

SHEPHARD: It's more in cold than in the heat.

NADEL: It's related to pulmonary ventilation.

SHEPHARD: Yes, the combination of temperature and ventilation water loss from the lungs can be up to 300 $mL \cdot h^{-1}$ in the cold.

DEMPSEY: I didn't know that. That high, eh?

SHEPHARD: Yes.

NADEL: Oh, that isn't trivial.

GISOLFI: How much of the tachypnea in long-term exercise is associated with the elevation of core body temperature?

DEMPSEY: I think there are several reasons for tachypnea. At one time, I thought it was entirely caused by increased temperature. (One reason I liked that hypothesis was that people didn't believe you, so you know, you put it out just so you could get on people's nerves). Seriously, if you sit people down and heat them, the increased ventilation is primarily a tachypneic response. An that's unique in humans. If you give people CO_2 to breath, make them hypoxic, infuse norepinephrine, any number of things, the response is primarily one of tidal volume (not true of animals, but true in humans). But heating the body seems to produce a unique kind of response, that is, an increased frequency, a tachypneic response. So since hyperpnea in prolonged exercise is roughly correlated with an increase in arterial blood temperature, femoral venous blood temperature, and rectal temperature, I thought it was probably related to the heating. Then we tried an experiment in which we cooled the skin, preventing some, but not all, of the rise in core body temperature, and that prevented a lot of the hyperventilation. I thought, for sure, it was the temperature effect. I don't think that's as good an experiment now as I did then, because I think cooling the skin can have an independent effect on its own of inhibiting breathing. What I did when I cooled the skin was not as pure an experiment as I would have liked. But I think heat has something to do with hyperventilation. Another candidate for causing the hyperventilation is circulating norepinephrine. Another candidate for the tachypneic response is a change in small airway mechanics which stimulates stretch receptors in the lung. This is an excellent possibility. So I think heat has something to do with it, but I don't think it's the whole answer.

Breathing frequencies in the 70s are very common. Just one last note on that: if you do this at high altitude, this is tremendously accentuated. The mean breathing frequency we measured was $80 \cdot \text{min}^{-1}$ in long-term work at even 10,000 and 14,000 feet. So it can be quite a strain.

RAVEN: I wanted to go back to the tachypnea. What's happening to your blood gases when you reach that situation?

DEMPSEY: The control system is maintaining alveolar ventilation over time. So arterial PCO_2 stays fairly normal under conditions where the tachypnea has increased. There is a big increase in minute ventilation and dead space, and alveolar ventilation stays relatively constant. On occasion, you can see $\dot{V}CO_2$ start to creep up a little bit when a guy's ventilating $140 \text{ L} \cdot \text{min}^{-1}$, which is really quite amazing; he pants like a dog.

SUTTON: You see it in a dog as one of the things that occurs in exercise. Dogs can have alveolar ventilations four times normal, in addition to their panting responses, as part of their pulmonary regulation.

DEMPSEY: Indeed, they can achieve very high total (not alveolar) ventilation in panting and so can a human; but I don't think the human does it as efficiently. That's what I'm really saying about the human. Their alveolar ventilation is extremely high. PCO_2 reaches 30 Torr, and this is maintained fairly well. Now somebody can say, "Wouldn't it better if PCO_2 was 25?" Well, I don't think so. PO_2 is regulated very well. Arterial pH is either normal or slightly alkaline. The slight alkalinity in pH may be surprising. It varies from individual to individual, but I rarely see acid pH unless you get to a very heavy prolonged workload, 75% to 95% of max, depending on the individual. If $PaCO_2$ was driven any lower, cerebral vasoconstriction would be extreme and cerebral blood flow greatly compromised.

NADEL: The thing you're talking about is a very inefficient way to dissipate heat. The lung is a poor evaporator. If respiratory water loss is, say 2 $g \cdot min^{-1}$, when you have a potential for losing 30 $g \cdot min^{-1}$ from the skin surface, and you compare the relatively large water loss, that's not a good way to go. And most species don't do well in the heat. They don't have the capacity to get rid of enough heat via the respiratory tract.

RAVEN: But could the panting be a vestigial response to aid brain cooling?

DEMPSEY: It might be, except humans don't have a carotid rete in their brain. We don't have that nice vascular exchange network. In humans, carotid and brain temperature probably are going to change together. But a dog can have an increase of 4 or 5° C in carotid arterial temperature with a normal brain temperature.

GOLLNICK: Do you think that diaphragm blood flow is maximal during exercise, or that the maximal ability to pump blood is reached and you can't perfuse the muscle anymore? You may have a limiting factor of how much blood can be pumped to the diaphragm.

DEMPSEY: Except that it has been shown during max exercise in the pony that limb muscle can still increase blood flow in the presence of a vasodilator, whereas the diaphragm can not.

DEMPSEY: I don't know how else to interpret it.

SHEPARD: The diaphragm could be contracting so forceably that this compresses blood vessels and limits blood flow.

GOLLNICK: I don't think that necessarily means that flow to the diaphragm is maximum.

DEMPSEY: That happens of course, with every inspiration, especially prolonged inspiration, just as it does with every contraction of every limb muscle. But I'm talking about total steady state flow.

GOLLNICK: It depends upon how hard those ponies that were studied were exercising and what their ventilatory frequency was.

DEMPSEY: I don't think so.

GOLLNICK: If they're exercising naturally and are responding with a frequency of $140 \cdot min^{-1}$, then there is not a lot of time to get much of the blood flow through there. I'm not so sure that those studies have really demonstrated that maximum blood flow through that muscle was achieved.

COYLE: Is there any evidence that the referred body pains sometimes experienced toward the end of long exercise, i.e., stitches or whatever, are due to respiratory muscle fatigue?

DEMPSEY: No. There's no evidence of respiratory muscle fatigue at all. The evidence in humans is very poor. You can measure pressure developed across the diaphragm during heavy work with a balloon in the esophagus and one in the stomach. We've done this, and we saw a diaphragmatic pressure change. The problem is that doesn't mean that you've got less contribution from the diaphragm to that inspiration, if you happen to be looking at it then, and more from intercostal muscles. It doesn't say anything about fatigue.

RAVEN: When you do a maximal voluntary ventilation test, don't you do it at two-thirds of vital capacity? And isn't that exactly what they do in long-term exercise? Your tidal volume is two-thirds of your vital capacity.

DEMPSEY: Right. But here's what happens. You might do the test at tidal volume at two-thirds of lung capacity. But the crucial point here is that when you're exercising, you go to a lower lung volume. We found that end expiratory lung volume (FRC) drops about a liter, a liter out of three in heavy work. If you do that, you lengthen the diaphragm. Your diaphragm is operating much more closely to its optimal length:tension relationship. Now, when you do the MVV test, the lung volume just keeps going up: you're breathing at a very high lung volume. So you have similar tidal volumes in the two situations. But one's starting from a large lung volume—that's the voluntary test and the exerciser starts at a smaller end-expiratory volume. That's a big and important difference. The other very important difference is that, for some reason, when we exercise very hard, we know enough that when we get to flow limitation, that is, when we've reached a point where flow is limited on expiration, we don't "push" more with our expiratory muscles. But when we do the voluntary maximal breathing test, for some reason this proprioception is overridden, and we go ahead and push more. We develop these huge expiratory pressures.

RAVEN: That brings me now to my respirator work. People on respirators do push more.

DEMPSEY: When you put an expiratory load on them.

RAVEN: Right. And they're doing endurance work. And their reduction of work under load is significant, e.g., about 40 min out of a 2 h run. You can see that they're uncomfortable. They're not at their voluntary max of ventilation. They're only about 55% of their MVV, and yet they're saying, "We don't want to do it anymore." They're not muscularly fatigued. I say their lungs or their respiratory work is so hard that they won't do it.

DEMPSEY: Of course. I agree. But I don't see what relevance that has to *physiologic* exercise. If you have an expiratory load on these people, the flow resistive work and the end expiratory lung volume are going to be quite high. That's why the breathing apparatus is so important during laboratory exercise tests, because with the slightest expiratory load in heavy work, you're going to change lung volume.

RAVEN: I believe that perhaps respiratory muscle fatigue in long-term work is a factor. Let's say older marathoners run for four h. The problem is they're having to drop their work to keep going. Therefore, their performance is dropped. They're going to have to reduce the workload on the lung.

DEMPSEY: That's an interesting speculation. But I think we tend to do that long before we reach respiratory muscle fatigue. We start playing strategy games with muscles. We switch back and forth with recruitment of respiratory muscles long before we reach so-called fatigue. That's my speculation.

RAVEN: The central inhibition for you, then, is a recruitment of other muscles.

DEMPSEY: That's part of it. Also, I think, in some cases, we actually stop increasing flow rate so much. So you see, I'm not a nonbeliever that the chest wall doesn't get itself in trouble. But I think it's smart enough not to go to the point where it depletes its diaphragm glycogen, for example. I think it starts recruiting other muscles and limiting pressure development *before* that happens.

SUTTON: At extreme altitude, there is evidence that people stop working when their perception of both breathing and muscle fatigue is at the limit. But yet, if you were to look at their arterial PCO_2, they are still able to maintain ventilation. And if you look at peripheral muscle metabolites and energy substrates, there is more than adequate energy available to continue to exercise. Fatigue occurs at a point where there is plenty of available energy. That again supports the idea of central inhibition.

DEMPSEY: Perhaps, and in hypoxia plus heavy exercise you not only have increased ventilatory effort but you also have cerebral hypoxia secondary to the arterial hypoxemia and reduced cerebral blood flow.

4

Temperature Regulation and Prolonged Exercise

ETHAN R. NADEL, PH.D.

INTRODUCTION
 I. HEAT TRANSFER IN THE BODY
 II. HEAT TRANSFER FROM THE BODY
 III. PHYSIOLOGICAL CONTROL OF HEAT TRANSFER RATES
 IV. TEMPERATURE REGULATION DURING PROLONGED EXERCISE
 V. BODY WATER SHIFTS DURING EXERCISE
    A. Effects of Body Fluid Loss
    B. Reflexes That Compensate for Body Fluid Losses
 VI. EFFECTS OF IMPROVED FITNESS AND HEAT ACCLIMATION
SUMMARY
BIBLIOGRAPHY
DISCUSSION

INTRODUCTION

The ability to regulate internal body temperature has provided higher organisms with an important independence from their environments. Since the rates of nearly all physical and chemical reactions are related to the temperature at which the reactions occur, the physiological function of any tissue or organ is linked in general to the temperature of that tissue or organ. Thus, the muscular activity of an ectotherm, which cannot regulate its internal body temperature at all well, is principally a function of the environmental temperature, while an endotherm (homeotherm) is capable of maintaining a range of activities in different thermal environments. By providing for a relatively constant internal body temperature, the temperature regulatory system ensures an internal environment in which reaction rates are relatively high and optimal, with respect to each other.

125

A ready supply of chemically-bound energy is necessary to support the contraction and relaxation processes in skeletal muscle. The contraction process requires energy to provide the crossbridge formation between actin and myosin filaments, and the relaxation process requires energy for the sarcoplasmic membrane to pump calcium ions against their concentration gradient. Since the muscles store the high energy compounds in quantities capable of supporting muscular activity for a few seconds, at best, and the energy equivalents stored in the body can support activity for only a few minutes, the prolongation of exercise for tens of minutes or even hours is made possible only by an integrated organ system response which provides for the resynthesis of the high energy compounds at the same rate as they are used. This integrated response acts to maintain an appropriate rate of fuel and oxygen delivery to the muscles, as well as an appropriate rate of waste removal from the muscles.

In the presence of oxygen, glucose and free fatty acids are degraded to generate chemically bound energy and waste-products. Because of the inefficiency of the energy transfers within the metabolic pathways, heat is generated as one of the waste products. The rate of heat production is a function of the rate of fuel catabolism, with minor differences in the heat production per unit of oxygen uptake due to differences in the mixture of fuels being oxidized. When oxidizing fat exclusively, the heat production is 19.6 kilojoules per liter of oxygen, and when oxidizing glucose exclusively, the heat production is 21.1 kilojoules per liter. Ultimately, according to thermodynamic principles, all of the energy produced and released must be accounted for as heat or as physical work. In sedentary conditions, the rate of heat production of an average sized adult is on the order of 320 to 400 kilojoules per hour. The rate of heat production during exercise is elevated in proportion to the intensity of exercise and can be 4500 to 5500 kilojoules per hour, or in excess of 1000 watts, for extended periods in fit individuals. A thermal load of this order is sufficient to raise the body core temperature by 1.0° C every five to seven minutes if stored in the body; if this were the case, exercise would be limited to relatively brief periods because of the ill effects of excessive hyperthermia. Such a continuous rise in internal body temperature during exercise does not occur because of the high efficiency of the body's temperature regulatory system.

In the following pages, I will describe the means by which heat is transferred from the site of production, principally the contracting skeletal muscles during exercise, to the skin surface, from where it is dissipated to the environment. I will then describe the physiological mechanisms that modulate the rates of heat transfer and the non-thermal factors that act to potentiate or attenuate the rates of transfer in given conditions. Finally, I will describe the characteristics that allow effective temperature regulation during prolonged exercise.

I. HEAT TRANSFER IN THE BODY

In simplest analysis, the rate of heat flux from any body tissue is a function of the temperature gradient between the tissue and the incoming blood, and the rate of blood flow through the tissue. Tissue temperature is related to the rate of tissue metabolism. Inactive skeletal muscle has a relatively low metabolic rate and, therefore, a low rate of heat production, around 2.5 kilojoules per hour for each kilogram of muscle. Inactive muscle is also relatively underperfused. Because of the constancy of both metabolic rate and blood flow in resting muscle, heat flux is relatively stable as well and muscle temperature is generally 33 to 35° C.

During moderately heavy exercise, the rate of heat production in skeletal muscle can be elevated 100-fold, accounting for a heat production of 5000 kilojoules per hour, if we assume the involvement of 20 kilograms of muscle. Thus, immediately after the onset of exercise the rate of heat production greatly exceeds the rate of heat loss from the muscle, resulting in a rapid rise in muscle temperature. Saltin et al. (30) have shown, from indwelling thermocouple measurements, that the active muscle temperature increases at a rate of around 1.0° C per minute during the initial transient of heavy cycle ergometer exercise. However, this high rate of heat storage in muscle is transient. One reason for this is that muscle vascular resistance decreases markedly after the onset of exercise. Increases up to 30-fold in muscle blood flow account for proportional increases in heat flux from the muscle. The second reason is that the initial storage of heat in muscle causes, as just described, an increase in muscle temperature and produces a gradient for heat transfer from muscle to blood. Heat is transferred down the temperature gradient from the active muscle to the blood as the blood passes through the muscle capillaries. As muscle blood flow increases and the temperature gradient reverses, the rate of rise in muscle temperature decreases until a new balance between heat production and heat transfer occurs and muscle temperature becomes steady at an elevated level. Most of the metabolically-generated heat is transferred to the body core by convection in the venous blood, although some of the heat transfer from the muscle occurs by conduction through the tissues to the overlying skin. Thus, the heat flux from the muscle can be determined from the following equation.

$$HF = m_{bl}c\,(T_m - T_{ar}) + h_c\,(T_m - T_{sk})$$

where: HF = heat flux in kJ per min
m_{bl} = muscle blood flow in mL per min
c = specific heat of blood in kJ per (mL °C)
T_m = muscle temperature in °C
T_{ar} = arterial blood temperature in °C
h_c = conductive heat transfer coefficient in kJ per (min °C)
T_{sk} = skin temperature in °C.

Once the heat produced in the contracting muscles is transported to the body core, it must be transported to the skin surface and then to the environment, or the body core temperature will continue to rise. The heat flux from the core to the skin is determined by similar factors as is the flux from the muscle to the core, i.e., the temperature gradient from core to skin and the overall skin conductance. The overall skin conductance is made up of a fixed conductance, which describes the conductive transfer of heat through the body tissues and across the subcutaneous fat layer to the skin surface, and a variable conductance, which describes the convective transfer of heat in the skin circulation. The latter is under physiological control; the ability to vary skin vascular resistance is the primary determinant of the rate of heat transport from the core to the skin. During heavy exercise, skin blood flow can be elevated 20- to 25-fold above the minimal rate. Thus, the ability to elevate skin blood flow during exercise is an essential part of the heat dissipation reflex and is necessary to avoid progressive hyperthermia. However, it should be clear that the heat flux from the body core to the skin is the product of the skin conductance and the temperature difference between the core and the skin; on hot, humid days, when the skin temperature may be quite high because of an inability to evaporate the sweat, even a maximal skin blood flow might not be adequate to provide sufficient heat transport from the core to the skin, and the body core temperature will continue to rise to levels that limit the continuation of exercise.

The heat flux from the body core to the skin can be determined from the following equation.

$$HF = h_{sk}\,(T_{in} - T_{sk}) + h_c\,(T_{in} - T_{sk})$$

where: h_{sk} = overall skin conductance in kJ per (min °C)

(N.B. overall skin conductance is the product of the skin blood flow and the specific heat of blood.)

T_{in} = body core temperature in °C.

(The other definitions are as above.)

Although most of the heat produced in the body is transported to the skin, a certain portion of the internally produced heat can escape the body directly. One means of heat transport from the body core to the environment is by evaporation from the pulmonary system. Mitchell et al. (16) showed that the respiratory evaporative rate during exercise is primarily a function of the rate of pulmonary ventilation, which itself is related to the exercise intensity (at least, at intensities less than 70% of maximal aerobic power). A second means for heat transport from the body core that bypasses the skin occurs when external work is accomplished. In such a case, the work usually can be accounted for as heat. For example, when pedaling against a fixed resistance on a cycle ergometer, around 20% of the metabolically generated energy can be accounted for as heat produced by the friction of the belt against the flywheel. When running on the level, however, there is no net work done on the environment, and all of the metabolically generated energy must be lost from the skin surface or from the pulmonary system.

II. HEAT TRANSFER FROM THE BODY

Figure 4-1 illustrates the avenues of heat transfer from the body core to the skin and from the skin to the environment. Heat ex-

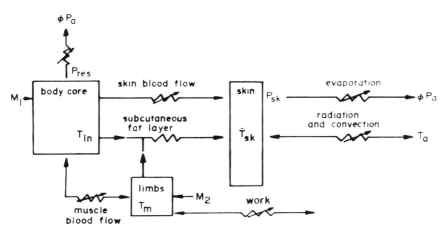

FIGURE 4-1. *A schematic representation of the pathways for heat flow from the body core to the skin to the environment. M_1 and M_2 represent basal and exercise heat production rates, respectively.*

changes from the body by radiation and convection are governed by the respective heat transfer coefficients and the skin to environment temperature gradient. Whereas the transfer coefficient for radiation is constant, the convective heat transfer coefficient increases with increasing air velocity (23), and thus the capacity for heat exchange by convection increases accordingly. It should be clear that on a hot day, when the skin to environment temperature gradient is small (or even in the direction of the skin), the capacity for heat exchange by radiation and convection is likewise small and of minimal value in dissipating the thermal load accompanying exercise.

The body's primary means for dissipating the heat produced during exercise is by the evaporation of sweat. The evaporative rate is a function of the water vapor pressure gradient between the skin and the environment, and independent of the temperature gradient. It is also a function of an evaporative heat transfer coefficient, which, like the convective coefficient, is variable with air movement. The evaporation of 1 gram of water from the skin surface removes around 2.5 kilojoules from the body and, since the sweat glands can deliver up to 30 grams per minute, nearly all of the heat produced during heavy exercise could be dissipated by evaporation in ideal conditions. As with internal heat transport, the ability to modulate the transport of heat from the body to the environment is under physiological control; in this case, the rate of heat transfer depends upon the neuroeffector drive to the sweat glands and the responsiveness of the sweat glands to this drive. However, the effectiveness of transfer is dependent not only on the sweat gland function but also on the characteristics of the environment. If the ambient humidity is high, the water vapor pressure gradient between skin and air will be lower at a given sweating rate, and the evaporative rate will also be lower. In a condition of constant demand, the body wil require an elevated sweating rate to increase the water vapor pressure of the skin to restore the necessary gradient to maintain thermal balance. If the ambient humidity and the ambient temperature are both high, the heat flux capacity from the body is low, and the tendency to store a portion of the heat produced during exercise is great. In such a condition, heavy exercise cannot be prolonged for extended periods.

The heat flux from the body to the environment can be determined from the following equation:

$$HF = (h_{r+c} (T_{sk} - T_a) + h_e (P_{sk} - P_a)A_W/A_D + h_E (P_{res} - P_a) + W$$

where: h_{r+c} = combined radiative and convective heat transfer coefficient in kJ per (min °C)

T_a = ambient temperature in °C

h_e = evaporative heat transfer coefficient in kJ per (min Torr)

P_{sk} = water vapor pressure of skin in Torr

P_a = water vapor pressure of the air in Torr

A_W/A_D = the fraction of body surface area available for heat transfer (ND)

h_E = evaporative heat transfer coefficient in kJ per (min Torr)

P_{res} = water vapor pressure of expired air in Torr

W = rate of external work in kJ per min

(The other definitions are as above.)

With a knowledge of the transfer coefficients and with an ability to measure the relevant environmental and physiological variables, it is possible to make predictions about the thermal balance of an individual in any combination of exercise and environmental conditions. If the body's rate of heat production during exercise exceeds the HF capacity of any of the three equations described above, then the body will store heat, and exercise will not be prolonged. From a physiologist's view, the capacities of the skin circulation and of the sweating mechanism are of primary interest. From the view of a bioengineer, characterization of the heat transfer coefficients and of the environment's capacity for transfer are of primary interest. From the practitioner's point of view, it is important to understand the interactions between the body and the environment to predict the capacity for prolonged exercise and avoid the risk of heat-related illness.

III. PHYSIOLOGICAL CONTROL OF HEAT TRANSFER RATES

As described above, the rate of heat production greatly exceeds the rate of heat dissipation during the first few minutes of exercise, and, consequently, the body core temperature rises. The body has in different loci specialized temperature sensors that direct, in some fashion, the organ system responses that modulate the rates of heat transfer from the body core to the skin and from the skin to the environment. The sensors are free nerve endings that are in particularly high density in the preoptic anterior hypothalamus (11) and over the skin surface (12). The skin temperature sensors provide the thermoregulatory center, also thought to reside within the hypothalamus, with information about the environmental temperature and therefore act as an early warning system in changing conditions. The hypothalamic thermosensors are especially important during exercise, which is one of the few conditions in which the body core temperature increases rapidly.

Thus, the temperature regulatory mechanism evaluates the body's thermal load body by sensing temperature and/or temperature change and directs efferent responses that act to increase the rate of skin blood flow and the rate of sweat secretion and thereby attempt to restore the initial thermal conditions. This model is similar to other negative feedback models that are commonly used to describe physiological systems.

Using this negative feedback model, it is relatively easy to describe the thermal events that occur during exercise. At the onset of exercise, the elevated heat production accompanying muscular contractions causes muscle temperature to rise. The blood perfusing the muscle equilibrates in temperature with the muscle, and the warmed blood returns to the body core, distributing the excess heat throughout the body. The thermal sensors in the hypothalamus respond to the increased temperature, and the regulatory center directs efferent neural traffic to the heat dissipation organs. As internal temperature rises, the threshold temperatures for cutaneous vasodilation and the onset of sweating are surpassed, and the skin blood flow and sweating rate increase in proportion to the increase in body core temperature. Activation of the heat dissipation responses progressively attenuates the rate of rise of internal temperature. At some point, the rate of heat flux from the body core to the environment equals the elevated rate of heat production, and the body core temperature stabilizes at a new level, until some additional perturbation occurs. These events are depicted in Figure 4-2.

The elevated steady state temperature during exercise is the consequence of the temporary inbalance between heat production and dissipation and the rapidity with which the heat dissipation response is activated. An increase in the sensitivity of the sweating response per unit increase of body core temperature would result in a lower steady state body core temperature during a given intensity of exercise, because the absolute heat storage would be less. Likewise, a reduction in the internal temperature threshold for sweating would result in a lower body core temperature during exercise. Physical training and heat acclimatization both induce a "quicker" heat dissipation response to body heating (20), thereby providing a greater margin of safety between operating and limiting temperatures during exercise. Further, in a trained person, the relatively lower body core temperature during exercise calls for a relatively lower skin blood flow, thereby providing a better ability to perfuse contracting muscle (25).

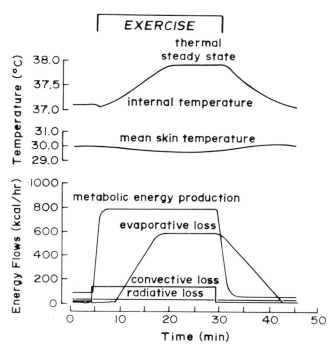

FIGURE 4-2. *Changes in the heat flow rates and the body temperatures during exercise. The thermal steady state is achieved when the rate of heat dissipation balances the rate of heat production. The steady state internal temperature is determined by the "quickness" of the heat dissipation response.*

IV. TEMPERATURE REGULATION DURING PROLONGED EXERCISE

To prolong exercise for tens of minutes or even hours, the heart must simultaneously supply an adequate blood flow to the contracting muscles, to ensure sufficient delivery of oxygen and fuel to meet the energy demand, and an adequate blood flow to the skin, to ensure sufficient delivery of heat to the site of its dissipation to meet the body's thermoregulatory demand. During exercise in cool conditions, the increment in cardiac output above that during rest is proportional to the increment in the muscle metabolic rate. In such conditions, the demand for blood flow to the skin is relatively low and easily met. However, in a warm environment, the drive for an elevated skin blood flow is increased relative to that in a cooler environment, primarily due to the higher skin temperature (26). Thus, in the heat, the combined circulatory demand from muscle and skin is greater at a given intensity of exercise than in a cooler condition. The heart must either deliver adequate blood flow to both muscle and skin or, if the combined demand for flow exceeds the heart's capacity to deliver, one or both of these organs becomes increasingly compromised; accordingly, exercise will be limited to a shorter period and/or performance will be reduced. For example, selective partitioning of the cardiac output to the muscles during heavy exercise in the heat would provide for the maintenance of oxygen delivery but would limit the rate of heat transfer from the body core to the skin, causing the sequestration of heat in the core; ultimately, the effects of hyperthermia would limit exercise. Alternatively, directing an adequate flow to the skin in these same conditions would provide for the maintenance of an adequate rate of heat transfer to resist hyperthermia but would limit oxygen delivery to the muscles; ultimately, the reduced ability to resynthesize the high energy compounds at the required rate would result in an early onset of fatigue and the cessation of exercise. In reality, both skin and muscle blood flows are compromised to some extent during prolonged, heavy exercise in a warm environment (17,19,28).

When environmental temperature exceeds 36° C, all of the metabolic heat of exercise must be dissipated from the body by the evaporation of sweat, because radiative and convective losses cannot occur when environmental temperature is close to or above mean skin temperature. If the evaporative rate is insufficient, body core temperature will rise continuously, and the duration of exercise will be limited. In such conditions, as noted above, the rate of evaporative water loss can exceed 30 grams per minute and therefore approach 2 liters per hour. Since the ill effects of body dehydration begin to occur when body water loss exceeds 3% of body weight (i.e., at around one hour in a 70 kg person), exercise in the heat will be compromised unless the body water content can be restored at a rate that approximates its rate of loss. During exercise in the heat, then, there are really two problems. The body must maintain a sufficiently high sweating rate to provide enough water on the skin surface to evaporate the metabolic load. At the same time, the body cannot allow its water content to fall to too great an extent. Should this occur, a critical depletion in blood volume will lead to a fall in cardiac filling pressure, which requires either compensatory reflex responses that act to maintain the cardiac output and arterial blood pressure or a redistribution in blood flow that leads to compromises in either oxygen delivery to muscle or in heat delivery to skin, or in both. Of major interest to physiologists is which of the regulatory systems predominates in conditions of mutually-exclusive demands and why. Of major interest to athletes is how to avoid the ill effects of a falling blood volume and preserve an optimal performance during exercise in the heat.

V. BODY WATER SHIFTS DURING EXERCISE

During exercise, marked shifts in body water occur due to i) the change in muscle perfusion pressure, which promotes a transient increase in the filtration of fluid out of the vascular compartment and ii) to the gradual redistribution of body water accompanying the evaporative losses from the respiratory and skin surfaces. A loss of plasma water occurs within the first minutes of exercise and is proportional to the intensity of exercise (4). At 90% of maximal aerobic power, this loss can exceed 15% of the plasma volume or more than 400 mL of plasma water. Hawk (10) recognized at the beginning of this century that hemoconcentration occurred accompanying exercise, and Costill (5) showed from muscle biopsy samples that the water content of active muscle was increased immediately following exercise. This observation supports the notion that there is an increased filtration of fluid from the vascular compartment into active muscle as a result of the increased muscle blood flow. Lundvall (13) attributed most of the plasma water egress to osmosis resulting from an elevated tissue osmolality that occurs at the onset of exercise because of hydrogen ion release accompanying excess lactic acid production and increased potassium ion in the extracellular compartment due to the repeated depolarizations of the muscle cells during activity. However, Sjogaard and Saltin (33) concluded, from estimates of extracellular water space in biopsied human muscle tissue, that the movement of water out of the vascular compartment was primarily the consequence of the shift in the hydrostatic, rather than the osmotic, pressure gradient accompanying the increase in muscle blood flow. Most likely, the increases in plasma hydrostatic pressure and tissue osmotic pressure both contribute to the decrease in plasma volume and increase in the water content of active muscle during exercise.

The water lost from the body by the evaporation of sweat is derived from all the body fluid compartments, including the vascular compartment. Adolph (1) reported years ago that water is not drawn equally from all the body spaces. Rather, plasma water losses are somewhat greater (on a relative basis) than are losses from the rest of the body tissues. The relatively greater plasma water loss may be due to the fact that the major cation lost in sweat, sodium, is from the extracellular space, with water following the outward movement of the cations. Plasma water losses are partly compensated for by shifts in water from the other body fluid compartments, but there must be other compensatory adjustments to prevent a fall in the cardiac filling pressure and an associated fall in the heart's ability to maintain an appropriate output.

A. Effects of Body Fluid Loss

A decrease in the circulating blood volume, whether caused by the increase in filtration of fluid from the vascular space, the progressive dehydration that accompanies evaporative losses, or the increase in the volume of blood contained in dilated cutaneous veins, has profound effects on the heart's ability to deliver adequate blood flow to the organs, which require increased flow during exercise. A reduced circulating blood volume causes a lowering of the cardiac filling pressure and, therefore, a lowering of the cardiac stroke volume. To maintain cardiac output and arterial blood pressure, a number of compensatory reflexes must be activated. Rowell et al. (28) showed that during heavy treadmill exercise in a hot environment, the reflex cardioacceleration was not sufficient to compensate for the fall in cardiac stroke volume, and cardiac output was lower than in a cooler environment. In such a condition, the maximum cardiac output must be reduced, and there should be an associated reduction in maximum aerobic power, as well as in performance or tolerance time. Indirect evidence that supports the latter contention is that the rate of blood lactic acid appearance in arterialized venous blood is faster during heavy exercise in the heat than in a cooler environment and the time to exhaustion is shorter, coinciding with the same maximal blood lactic acid concentration (19).

We have shown that individuals artificially rendered hypovolemic (blood volume reduction by the use of diuretics) also suffered an inability to develop sufficient reflex cardioacceleration to provide for the maintenance of cardiac output during moderate exercise in the heat; this was not a problem in the normovolemic state (7,18). In these studies, the cardiac output was reduced by around 2 liters per min (around 20% of the increase from rest) in the hypovolemic condition. Despite the reduction in cardiac output, the heart provided adequate delivery of blood to maintain oxygen delivery to the contracting muscles. However, the rate of heat delivery to the skin was impaired, as demonstrated by the higher internal body temperature, which resulted in part from a lower skin blood flow (18) and venous capacitance (7) in the hypovolemic condition after 30 minutes of exercise. Internal body temperature averaged around $0.4°$ C higher when the volunteer subjects were hypovolemic. The implications for reduced performance should be apparent. A greater rate of heat storage when hypovolemic would result in a more rapid attainment of the tolerance limit of internal body temperature, or a shorter time to exhaustion.

Not only is heat delivery to the skin impaired in dehydration, but dehydration, and its associated effects on the internal environment, also has an important effect on the sweat gland response to an increased body core temperature as well. Greenleaf and Castle (9) and Nielsen (22) both showed that dehydration is accompanied by a higher than normal elevation in body core temperature during a given intensity of exercise. Both suggested that the increased plasma osmolality associated with the plasma water losses may have been responsible for a reduction in the sweating response during exercise. Fortney et al. (6) showed that isotonic hypovolemia had the effect of reducing the sensitivity of the sweating response per unit of body core temperature increase during exercise. Thus, the progressive increase in body core temperature that accompanies progressive dehydration during prolonged exercise could well be a function, at least in part, of a progressive decrease in the sensitivity of sweat gland function. Figure 4-2a provides an illustration of this concept. During exercise when fully hydrated, the steady state body core temperature would be 38.5° C in this illustration, but when dehydrated by 3% of body weight, the decreased sweating sensitivity would force the steady state body core temperature up to 40.0° C.

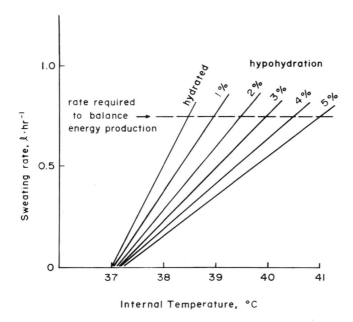

FIGURE 4-2a. *A schematic representation of the effects of progressive dehydration on the sensitivity of the sweating rate response to an increased body core temperature.*

A steadily decreasing sweating sensitivity is a response that acts to conserve body water, but at a constant exercise intensity, which requires a constant rate of heat dissipation, this response results in a steadily increasing body core temperature. The hyperthermia, then, will exacerbate the cardiovascular strain and contribute to a reduced performance or an early termination of exercise.

B. Reflexes That Compensate for Body Fluid Losses

The body has sophisticated reflexes which serve to oppose a fall in arterial blood pressure during heat exposure and exercise. The primary reflexes are those that are triggered by alterations in the activity of intravascular mechanoreceptors located in the cardiopulmonary region and in the carotid and aortic sinuses. The cardiopulmonary (low pressure) reflexes respond to a drop in cardiac filling pressure. These can be thought of as anticipatory in nature, because by ensuring that the filling pressure of the heart is maintained to the greatest extent possible, these reflexes act to prevent (or at least attenuate) a fall in cardiac output, and, hence, arterial blood pressure. These reflexes preserve the ability to maintain exercise performance, albeit at a reduced level. The aortic and carotid (high pressure) reflexes are triggered by a fall in arterial blood pressure and/or pulse pressure. Generally speaking, these are the body's last line of defense against decompensation; by the time these are activated, performance may have already been severely limited.

There are several circulatory responses to exercise that act to maintain an optimal central blood volume but do not necessarily fall into the category of reflexes which are directly responsive to falling blood pressures. These responses are part of the generalized sympathetic nervous system activity accompanying exercise (2), and they participate in the redistribution of cardiac output. For example, the increase in splanchnic vascular resistance has been shown to correspond quite closely to the increase in the relative exercise intensity (27). Splanchnic vasoconstriction can serve to mobilize a large fraction of the 1.5 liters of blood contained in the splanchnic vasculature in extreme conditions (29), making this volume available to the central circulation and thereby helping to maintain the central blood volume.

As described above, when blood volume is artifically contracted by the administration of diuretics, exercise is accompanied by peripheral vasomotor adjustments which tend to stabilize cardiac stroke volume, even if at a lower level than during normovolemic exercise. In our 1980 study (18), these adjustments included an increase in the internal temperature threshold for cutaneous vasodilation, a reduction in the gain of the cutaneous blood flow response per unit of internal temperature increase and a reduction in the maximal attainable skin blood flow. At that time, we thought that these changes were triggered by a reduction in the cardiac filling pressure, but we had no direct evidence for this.

Decreases in cardiac filling pressure are known to cause proportional increases in forearm (skin) vascular resistance (29). An increase in vascular resistance in any vascular bed serves to divert flow away from that organ, opposing the tendency for arterial blood pressure to fall and allowing flow to be maintained in parallel circuits. Further, a reduction in flow to an organ with compliant veins also reduces the venous transmural pressure within that organ and, therefore, the volume of blood held in its veins. Figure 4-3 illustrates the relation between the central venous pressure (CVP) and forearm blood flow in four volunteers exposed to graded lower body negative pressure (LBNP) (34), a maneuver used to simulate the effect of hypergravity and cause the pooling of blood in the lower extremities. During low levels of LBNP (up to −30 Torr), CVP was decreased by more than 6 Torr without any change in the mean arterial or pulse pressures. In response to this decrease in CVP, the forearm

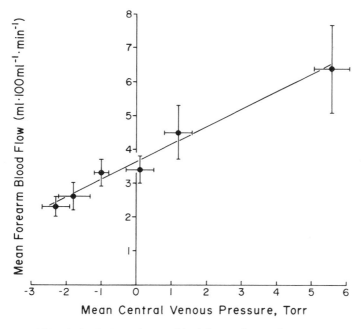

FIGURE 4-3. *The relation between forearm blood flow and central venous pressure during application of lower body negative pressure. Values shown are means and S.E. from four volunteer subjects (21).*

blood flow was lowered from around 6 to around 3 mL per (min 100 mL). We have also shown recently that the forearm arteriomotor elements are responsive to decreases in CVP caused by application of low levels of LBNP during supine exercise (14).

Forearm cutaneous veins in humans have been shown to reflexly constrict during exercise (2). However, it has not been clear whether the forearm veins participate in thermal reflexes or those that are responsive to decreases in the blood pressure (29). We have shown that forearm venous capacitance is relatively lower in the hypovolemic than the normovolemic condition, allowing the conclusion that an increase in the tone of peripheral veins is a response to a lowered central blood volume (7). A decreased cutaneous venous capacitance serves to shift blood centrally at any given venous pressure. It is likely that the forearm venomotor reflex has not been obvious to many, because it does not appear until either a critically low cardiac filling pressure is reached or a fall in arterial blood pressure or pulse pressure occurs. In studies of resting volunteers undergoing periods of LBNP, we found that decreases in forearm venous volume at a given venous pressure during venous occlusion (indicating increases in forearm venomotor tone) were best related to decreases in arterial pulse pressure (34). This relation is shown in Figure 4-4. However, Figure 4-5 shows that we can make a different interpretation for the control mechanism by plotting forearm venous volume against CVP. The latter interpretation is that the veins are relatively unresponsive to changes in CVP above a CVP threshold, but once CVP has fallen below the threshold, the body vigorously defends CVP by a large increase in the gain of the forearm venomotor response per unit fall in CVP. Thus, although it is clear that forearm venomotor tone is among the efferent responses that participate in blood pressure homeostasis, the stimulus for the increase in tone is less well identified. This issue requires further study.

Without regard to the interpretation of the origin of vasomotor and venomotor reflexes during exercise in the heat, it is clear that these reflexes act to prevent a fall in arterial blood pressure in conditions in which central blood volume is reduced (e.g., prolonged exercise in the heat). While acting to shift blood centrally and thereby maintain cardiac filling pressure, these reflexes also act to reduce heat transport to the skin. Thus, we conclude that in conditions of multiple demand, the systems participating in arterial blood pressure regulation predominate over those involved in temperature regulation. Figure 4-6 illustrates these interactions in a multiple loop negative feedback diagram. Since both regulatory systems share a common effector organ (the cutaneous vascular bed), the develop-

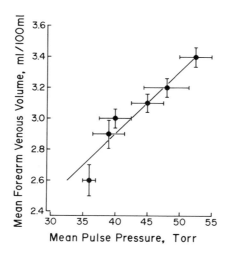

FIGURE 4-4. *The relation between forearm venous volume at a constant venous pressure (during venous occlusion) and arterial pulse pressure during application of lower body negative pressure, as in Figure 4-3 (34).*

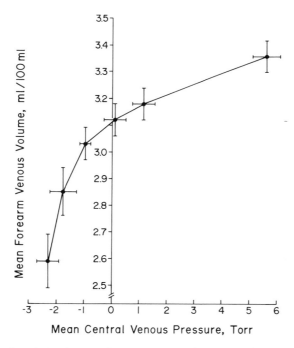

FIGURE 4-5. *The relation between forearm venous volume at a constant venous pressure (during venous occlusion) and central venous pressure during application of lower body negative pressure, as in Figure 4-3 (34).*

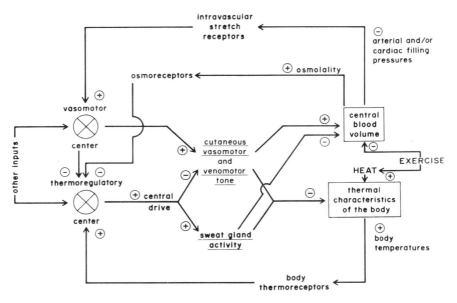

FIGURE 4-6. *A schematic representation of interactions between certain of the systems that participate in the regulation of body temperature and blood pressure, illustrating the shared effector pathway involving cutaneous vasomotor and venomotor tone.*

ment of such a competition must occur when the demand for blood flow from the contracting muscles and the skin exceeds the ability of the heart to deliver. By examining conditions such as this, physiologists are better able to understand the factors leading to the generation of fatigue during prolonged exercise in different environments.

VI. EFFECTS OF IMPROVED FITNESS AND HEAT ACCLIMATION

The benefits of both physical training and heat acclimation on heat tolerance and performance during prolonged exercise have been known for years. In his thorough review, Wyndham (25) provided much evidence that a program of heat acclimation reduces the body heat storage during exercise in the heat. The studies of Piwonka and Robinson (24) and Gisolfi and Robinson (8) demonstrated that trained individuals are better able to dissipate the thermal load of exercise than are their untrained counterparts. More recently, we showed that the sweat glands develop an increased sensitivity during physical training and a lowering of the sweating threshold with heat acclimation (21). Sato and Sato (31) found that sweat glands dissected from physically active people were hypertrophied and had a greater cholinergic sensitivity than those dissected from inactive people. While these adaptations provide for an improved ability to dissipate heat from the skin, the body also must develop means for improved heat transfer from the body core to the skin, in order to be able to resist the ill effects associated with progressive dehydration and the consequent hypovolemia that develops during prolonged exercise, especially exercise in the heat.

Senay et al. (32) showed that heat acclimation stimulated an expansion of the blood volume, primarily by increasing the plasma protein content (which then caused an increase in the plasma water content due to osmotic effects). The precise mechanism for the increased plasma protein content has not been elucidated. A high initial blood volume ensures an adequate filling pressure of the heart, even in the presence of the increased plasma water filtration which accompanies exercise, because of the higher starting volume. Convertino et al. (3) showed that both acclimation and physical training stimulated increases in blood volume, with training resulting in an increase of nearly 500 mL in only eight days. They also found an excellent correlation between total plasma protein content and blood volume and suggested that at least a portion of the new plasma protein was the result of a transient increase in the rate of plasma protein synthesis. This hypothesis has yet to be tested.

The importance of an expanded blood volume was demonstrated recently by Fortney et al. (7). Acute blood volume expansion allowed development of a higher cardiac stroke volume (by 8 mL per beat) and cardiac output (by 1.5 liters per min) during exercise in the heat than in the normovolemic condition. Accompanying the elevated cardiac output was a lower internal body temperature (by 0.25° C) after 30 minutes of exercise. The expanded blood volume permitted a greater heat transfer from the body core to the environment, presumably by allowing a greater distribution of the blood volume to the skin, and thereby contributed to the greater margin of safety from the limiting effects of hyperthermia.

We have also found a striking relation between maximal aerobic power and blood volume (15). The expanded blood volume in fit individuals provides a higher central blood volume during exercise and, by providing for a relatively high cardiac filling pressure, presumably prevents the reduction in heat transfer that occurs when the cardiac filling pressure falls to a critically low level. We need experimental verification of this hypothesis. All the evidence points toward the importance of the initial blood volume as one of the major factors that determine the tolerance of humans to prolonged exercise in the heat. Together with the more responsive sweating mechanism, these adaptations to heat and physical activity provide a greater heat transfer potential and a lower body core temperature during prolonged exercise.

SUMMARY

From the preceding sections one can develop certain principles which apply to the understanding of different tolerances to a combined exercise and environmental thermal load. The total thermal load is related to the exercise intensity (the metabolic energy production), the environmental temperature and the evaporative power of the environment (which is a function of the water vapor pressure of the environment). The ease with which an individual dissipates the total thermal load is a function of the body surface area available for heat exchange, the state of body hydration and the level of physical fitness or heat acclimatization. Because humans operate within a fairly narrow body core temperature range, any factor that alters the rate of heat dissipation from the body during prolonged exercise will have an immediate effect upon both heat storage and the ability to continue. In most cases, humans are concerned with the avoidance of excessive hyperthermia, although hypothermia can become a problem during prolonged exercise in cold or, especially, wet conditions.

The amount of clothing worn during exercise has a great bearing on the ability to dissipate heat. Clothing adds insulation between the skin and the environment and reduces the effective surface area of the skin for heat transfer, thereby reducing the conductance of heat in given conditions. The rate of heat transfer from the skin to the environment depends upon the ambient temperature and humidity and the air velocity. On cool days, most of the heat dissipation from the body will be via convection and radiation. The more one covers the skin, the more one reduces the area for direct heat exchange by these avenues. On cold days it is important to wear layers of clothing to increase the resistance to heat flow from the skin to the environment. It is also best to avoid wetting the clothing, because the evaporation will remove heat from the outer layers and increase the temperature gradient, and, therefore, the heat flow rate, from the skin to the outer layer. Layering can at least provide for dry clothing and reduced heat transfer closest to the skin. On warm days, the major avenue for heat dissipation is the evaporation of sweat. It is important to provide an optimal surface area from which evaporation can occur. Thus, the clothing cover should be minimal.

The progressive loss of body water during prolonged exercise poses a particular problem. As noted above, a redistribution of blood flow away from the skin to ensure an adequate muscle perfusion accompanies progressive dehydration. Further, once the body water loss becomes sufficiently great, the sweating mechanism gradually begins to shut down, and this exacerbates the heat storage problem. To prevent, or at least postpone the events leading to increased heat storage accompanying progressive dehydration, adequate hydration prior to and during prolonged exercise is essential. If hyperthermia and the associated heat-illness symptoms (light-headedness, disorientation, syncope) develop during prolonged exercise, the individual should be removed to a cool environment, and fluid replacement should begin. Humans have a notoriously poor sense of thirst and will not sense the characteristics of developing body fluid depletion; hence, it is essential to anticipate the fluid needs ahead of time to avoid the ill effects associated with dehydration. There is a current need to determine the optimal content of the rehydration fluid. (This topic is discussed elsewhere in this volume.)

Physical training and heat acclimatization not only benefit the individual by endowing a more rapid heat dissipation response to an increasing body core temperature but also endow an expanded blood volume. In given conditions, a volume-expanded individual will have a greater resistance to syncope than an unfit person. Generally speaking, the majority of heat-illness victims are novice runners, the elderly and those with circulatory or respiratory disorders. These are people who have become unfit due to choice or their inability to remain active. People at risk should avoid extremes of activity or heat.

One specific thermoregulatory problem involving exercise that has been observed with increasing frequency is that marathon runners can become markedly hypothermic immediately following the race, even on a mild day. There exists no satisfactory explanation for this phenomenon. Following strenuous running, the heat production declines precipitously at a time when the rate of heat dissipation is still high (due to the evaporation of water remaining on the skin and the high skin blood volume near the skin surface). However, the rate of body core temperature decline is not slowed as it nears the normally-regulated level. It is possible that a certain degree of hypoglycemia, not an uncommon occurrence after a marathon run, interferes with normal body temperature regulation. Problems related to thermoregulatory deficiencies following prolonged, strenuous exercise are not at all well understood and require further study.

BIBLIOGRAPHY

1. Adolph, E.F. Blood changes in dehydration. E.F. Adolph, (ed.) *Physiology of man in the desert*, pp. 10–171, New York: Interscience, 1947.
2. Bevegard, B.S. and J.T. Shepherd. Changes in tone of limb veins during supine exercise. *J Appl Physiol.* 20:1–8, 1965.
3. Convertino, V.A., J.E. Greenleaf and E.M. Bernauer. Role of thermal and exercise factors in the mechanism of hypervolemia. *J Appl Physiol.* 48:657–664, 1980.
4. Convertino, V.A., L.C. Keil, E.M. Bernauer and J.E. Greenleaf. Plasma volume, osmolality, vasopressin and renin activity during graded exercise in man. *J Appl Physiol.* 50:123–128, 1981.
5. Costill, D.L. Sweating: its composition and effects on body fluids. *Ann NY Acad Sci* 301:160–174, 1977.
6. Fortney, S.M., E.R. Nadel, C.B. Wenger and J.R. Bove. Effect of blood volume on sweating rate and body fluids in exercising humans. *J Appl Physiol.* 51:1594–1600, 1981.
7. Fortney, S.M., C.B. Wenger, J.R. Bove and E.R. Nadel. Effect of blood volume on forearm venous and cardiac stroke volume during exercise. *J Appl Physiol.* 55:884–890, 1983.
8. Gisolfi, C., and S. Robinson. Relations between physical training, acclimatization and heat tolerance. *J Appl Physiol.* 26:530–534, 1969.
9. Greenleaf, J.E. and B.L. Castle. Exercise temperature regulation in man during hypohydration and hyperhydration. *J Appl Physiol.* 30:847–853, 1971.
10. Hawk, P.B. On the morphological changes in the blood after muscular exercise. *Am J Physiol.* 10:384–389, 1904.
11. Hellon, R. Hypothalamic neurons responding to changes in hypothalamic and ambient temperatures. J.D. Hardy, A.P. Gagge, and J.A.J. Stolwijk, (eds.): *Physiological and Behavioral Temperature Regulation*. Springfield, IL, Charles C. Thomas, 1970.
12. Hensel, H. Temperature receptors in the skin. J.D. Hardy, A.P. Gagge, and J.A.J. Stolwijk (eds.): *Physiological and Behavioral Temperature Regulation*. Springfield, IL, Charles C. Thomas, 1970.
13. Lundvall, J. Tissue Hyperosmolality as a mediator of vasodilation and transcapillary fluid flux in exercising skeletal muscle. *Acta Physiol Scand.*, suppl. 379:1–142, 1972.
14. Mack, G.W., H. Nose and E.R. Nadel. (In preparation).
15. Mack, G.W., X.R. Shi, H. Nose, A. Tripathi and E.R. Nadel. Diminished baroreflex control of forearm vascular resistance in physically fit humans. *J Appl Physiol.*
16. Mitchell, J.W., E.R. Nadel, and J.A.J. Stolwijk. Respiratory weight losses during exercises. *J Appl Physiol.* 32:474–476, 1972.
17. Nadel, E.R., E. Cafarelli, M.F. Roberts and C.B. Wenger. Circulatory regulation during exercise in different ambient temperatures. *J Appl Physiol.* 46:430–437, 1979.
18. Nadel, E.R., S.M. Fortney and C.B. Wenger. Effect of hydration state on circulatory and thermal regulations. *J Appl Physiol.* 49:715–721, 1980.
19. Nadel, E.R. Effects of temperature on muscle metabolism. *Biochemistry of Exercise*, pp. 134–143. H.G. Knuttgen, J.A. Vogel, J. Poortmans (eds.). Human Kinetics Publications, Champaign, IL, 1983.
20. Nadel, E.R., K.B. Pandolf, M.F. Roberts, et al. Mechanisms of thermal acclimation to exercise and heat. *J Appl Physiol.* 37:515–520, 1974.
21. Nadel, E.R., K.B. Pandolf, M.F. Roberts and J.A.J. Stolwijk. Mechanisms of thermal acclimation to exercise and heat. *J Appl Physiol.* 37:515–520, 1974.
22. Nielsen, C. Effects of changes in plasma volume and osmolality on thermoregulation during exercise. *Acta Physiol Scand.* 90:725–730, 1974.
23. Nishi, Y., and A.P. Gagge. Direct evaluation of convective heat transfer coefficient by napthalene sublimation. *J Appl Physiol.* 29:603–609, 1970.
24. Piwonka, R.W. and S. Robinson. Acclimatization of highly trained men to work in severe heat. *J Appl Physiol.* 22:9–12, 1967.
25. Roberts, M.F., C.B. Wenger, J.A.J. Stolwijk and E.R. Nadel. Blood flow and sweating changes following exercise training and heat acclimation. *J Appl Physiol.* 43:133–137, 1977.
26. Robinson, S. Physiological adjustments to heat. L.H. Newburgh, Ed. *Physiology of heat regulation and the science of clothing*. Philadelphia: Saunders, 193–231, 1949.
27. Rowell, L.B., J.R. Blackmon, R.H. Martin, J.A. Mazzarella and R.A. Bruce. Hepatic clearances of indocyanine green in man under thermal and exercise stress. *J Appl Physiol.* 20:384–394, 1965.
28. Rowell, L.B., H.J. Marx, R.A. Bruce, R.D. Conn and F. Kusumi. Reductions in cardiac output, central blood volume and stroke volume with thermal stress in normal man during exercise. *J Clin Invest.* 45:1801–1816, 1966.
29. Rowell, L.B., J.T. Shepard, F.M. Abboud (eds). Cardiovascular adjustment to thermal stress.

Handbook of Physiology, Section 2, The Cardiovascular System, Vol. III, Peripheral Circulation and Organ Blood Flow, pp. 967–1023. American Physiological Society, Bethesda, 1983.

30. Saltin, B., A.P. Gagge. and J.A.J. Stolwijk. Muscle temperature during submaximal exercise in man. *J Appl Physiol*. 25:679–688, 1968.
31. Sato, K., and F. Sato. Individual variations in structure and function of human eccrine sweat glands. *Am J Physiol*. 245:R203–R208, 1983.
32. Senay, L.C., Jr., D. Mitchell and C.H. Wyndham. Acclimatization in a hot, humid environment: body fluid adjustments. *J Appl Physiol*. 40:786–796, 1976.
33. Sjogaard, G. and B. Saltin. Extra-and intra-cellular water spaces in muscles of man at rest and with dynamic exercise. *Am J Physiol*. 243:R271–R280, 1982.
34. Tripathi, A., G. Lister and E.R. Nadel. Peripheral vascular reflexes elicited during lower body negative pressure. (In Preperation.)
35. Wyndham, C.H. The physiology of exercise under heat stress. *Ann Rev Physiol*. 35:193–220, 1973.

DISCUSSION

BROOKS: How much of the heat generated in your limbs during exercise goes directly to the core? Is it obligatory that it go the core?

NADEL: Most of the heat that is produced during exercise is transferred to the body core by convection in the blood stream.

Some heat is transported by conduction to the skin's surface. It's relatively small. The caveat is that if you're exercising in the water, then, because of the thermal/physical characteristics of water, most of the heat is lost from the skin's surface very rapidly because of the convective heat transfer coefficient of water, which is very high. So, in this case, most of the heat is transported directly from the muscle to the skin to the water environment. Air is a good insulator; water is a good conductor. So that is the caveat. And the rate of heat transfer also depends upon the environmental conditions. For example, people in helium/oxygen environments, people who would work out of diving bells, report different sensations of cold. It's because the thermal conductivity of helium is much greater than nitrogen, and they lose heat much more rapidly. So the thermal neutral point under those conditions is quite different from the environment that we are in now.

BROOKS: For a given metabolic rate in those conditions, would your core temperature be very different?

NADEL: In water it can be. And in extreme environments it can be, yes. Generally speaking, probably not in most types of exercise.

GISOLFI: There was a paper several years ago that looked at the thermal gradient across the femoral artery and femoral vein during exercise. If I'm not mistaken, he didn't see much of a gradient between those two.

NADEL: During the steady state, there's probably not much of a gradient at all. It would probably be only in a transient state where you'd see a regional temperature gradient. Once you've reached the steady state, it should be small. The muscle blood flow is high, and the heat can be transported over a relatively small gradient.

LAMB: Why does the core temperature remain elevated? In many situations, it's obvious that the body would be able to bring it back down to the rest level. Why doesn't it? It is the elevated temperature that's being sensed? Or is it the rate of change in temperature that is being sensed? And you mentioned that there are some sort of receptors. Do you know what they are, where they are?

NADEL: Okay, I'll try to answer these questions in reverse order. The receptors are primarily free nerve endings in the hypothalamus. It's pretty clear that there are thermal receptors distributed in areas other than the hypothalamus. The hypothalamus happens to have an intense concentration of thermal receptors. There are thermal receptors in the spinal cord. There are thermal receptors throughout the body, but the most important receptors, of course, are in the preoptic anterior hypothalamus—the free nerve endings.

LAMB: Is it a rate of change that they're sensing?

NADEL: No. They're sensing absolute temperature. There's been no evidence whatsoever that there are rate sensors within the body core. There are probably rate sensors on the skin surface. It's clear that the dermal sensors respond and act as rate sensors.

TIPTON: Are the spinal thermal receptors regionalized or widely distributed?

NADEL: Know one knows. Let me return to David Lamb's second question is "Why doesn't the temperature come back to the regulated temperature?" During exercise, heat production is high, and the increase in temperature drives the heat loss responses, so that rates of both heat loss and heat production are high. Once heat loss and heat production rates are equal, the temperature is, by definition, steady. If you could increase heat loss to a greater extent, body temperature would come back toward the resting level. As core temperature comes back to the resting level, then heat loss response would fall accordingly. This would result in an unstable condition.

MURRAY: Are the changes in forearm blood flow, so often used to assess the peripheral response to heat exposure, indicative of changes in vascular resistance in other cutaneous beds?

NADEL: Not necessarily, although other vascular beds are used in extreme conditions to maintain arterial blood pressure. I think there are some important pieces of evidence to support that. The older evidence is that splanchnic blood flow is very sensitive to changes in arterial blood pressure. The splanchnic blood flow will decrease at a given exercise intensity if ambient heat is added. Even muscle blood flow can be affected by the total vascular conductance. If you reduce vascular conductance by, for example, using one-legged exercise, this will allow for a greater maximal blood flow. So it turns out that most vascular beds are sensitive to changes in either the filling pressure of the heart or ultimately arterial blood pressure. I like to think of cardiopulmonary receptors as being involved in a type of anticipatory reflex, to help maintain arterial blood flow.

RAVEN: Your studies were done in the supine position. In the upright position, is it possible that the central venous pressure is lower?

NADEL: We can get lower, significantly lower, central venous pressures if we use hypovolemia prior to exercise as a stimulus. We haven't done what I think is probably the key experiment, which is to take the people and exercise them for 2–3 h and try to measure continuously. It's very clear that even if you give people water to drink ad lib during a 3–4 h experiment, they won't drink enough water to maintain body weight. Even if you try to force them, they won't drink enough to maintain body weight. So the assumption is that a certain amount of hypovolemia is occurring. Incidentally, all of these phenomena are amplified if you add ambient heat to the equation.

TIPTON: Are the experiments you do using lower body negative pressure affecting arterial baroreceptors and central sympathetic drive?

NADEL: Yes, if we use high enough negative pressure. I'm certain that low levels of <BNP selectively unload the cardiopulmonary bar-oreceptors and do not effect the arterial baroreceptors.

SUTTON: Always the concern in thermoregulation is just when and why does the system break down. Can you take us that extra step?

NADEL: In a cool environment, the rate of water loss from the body is relatively low. A fit person will start out with much higher blood volume. The point here is that we find a very good relation-ship between maximum aerobic power and blood volume. I don't think it's a benign relationship for many reasons. One of the rea-sons is that it allows for the maintenance of a high central blood volume in conditions in which blood volume is being threatened. So, when someone starts to exercise, there's an effective blood loss because of pooling of blood in dependent veins. Now that may or may not be significant. There's certainly a volume loss because of the filtration of plasma water into the muscle, and that is significant. There is additional volume loss because of the progressive dehy-dration accompanying exercise. In a cool environment, this third phenomenon occurs much more slowly, so thermoregulation may not be threatened in a cool environment before other systems fail. For example, blood glucose or muscle glycogen may run out before the thermoregulatory system is threatened. In a warm environment, the thermoregulatory system might well become the limiting factor because of the loss of body water and the subsequent reflexes which act to maintain arterial blood pressure and allow body temperature to keep climbing. I think that's the key issue here.

SUTTON: Is there any relationship between baroreceptor responsiveness and blood volume?

NADEL: Yes. Just to summarize our work, we think that there's a decreased sensitivity of the cardiopulmonary receptors with increased physical fitness. It may well be, and this is purely hypothetical, that decreased sensitivity of the cardiopulmonary receptors provides a signal for the expansion of blood volume. But I can't tell you whether that's a cause and effect relationship.

MICHELI: We've seen runners cross the finish line at the Boston Marathon between 3 and 4 1/2 h who are surely hyperthermic. They feel warm, and they're sweating, and so forth. But suddenly, about 300 of them, over a period of about a half hour, become hypothermic. They can't seem to bring up their temperature. If you give them 2–3 L of intravenous dextrose and volume, they become thermoregulatory again. What's going on?

NADEL: The later part of the chapter referred to that phenomenon. I think what happens is this: When they finish the marathon, their metabolisms have been high for the prior 3–4 h, and they're losing heat. Their bodies are wet; they're sweating. At the end of the marathon, their metabolic rate suddenly goes down, but they're still losing heat at a very high rate. Probably a lot of these people—this is just guesswork—have a certain amount of hypoglycemia at the end of the marathon, and hypoglycemia may inactivate the temperature regulatory mechanism. Their body temperature will fall, and since there's no protection against that fall, it will keep falling below the normal body temperature. At this point, if you give them dextrose, you're giving them some sugar. I'm not certain whether it's the volume or the sugar that's causing the return to normal thermoregulatory status.

BURKE: There's very little written on the mechanisms of heat loss or heat gain in swimming or cycling or any other prolonged activities. I think too many physiologists think that running is the only prolonged exercise. I think we have a golden opportunity to reach the coach and the practitioner in some other sports that are very concerned with temperature, such as swimming and cycling.

NADEL: I think that's a good suggestion. There's no question that the challenges offered by the environment in swimming are very different from those in the air. The primary protection one has against becoming hypothermic is having a layer of fat underneath the skin. Heat transfer in water moving at 1 1/2 meters per second, is three times higher than in still water. I don't think those differences are trivial.

WEIKER: Clinically, we're seeing a large number of small children being pushed into continuous activity. I've been raised with the idea that children do not dissipate heat as well as adults. I don't know how accurate that is, and I haven't seen it in print.

SHEPHARD: I think Oded Bar-Or promulgated this idea.

BROOKS: Children have very high aerobic capacities per unit of body mass, simply because the body mass is so low. They also have a high surface area to body mass ratio. So, in the heat, they can gain heat more readily. But in daily physical education activities, they seem to dissipate heat pretty well.

CANTWELL: This year is the first time in the Peachtree Road Race that young children won't be allowed to race. They have a separate, shorter chidren's race.

RAVEN: Why did you decide to do that?

CANTWELL: The organizational people were afraid that the kids would get pushed around.

GISOLFI: There is no clear evidence on heat dissipation in children. With regard to older individuals, it's very difficult to show that the impairment in their ability to perfuse the skin or to sweat is not just related to a detraining effect as it would be with a younger individual who's inactive. So I don't think we can conclude that, just because one ages, his thermoregulatory response is inevitably impaired.

NADEL: Sounds as though there's plenty of work to keep us all busy for a while.

5

Endocrine Responses to Prolonged Exercise

John R. Sutton, M.D.

Peter A. Farrell, Ph.D.

INTRODUCTION
  I. ENDOCRINE RESPONSES DURING PROLONGED EXERCISE
  II. ENDOCRINE RESPONSES ASSOCIATED WITH THE PROVISION OF
     FUELS FOR PROLONGED EXERCISE
  III. GLUCOSE TRANSPORT INTO MUSCLE: INSULIN RECEPTORS
  IV. PLASMA GLUCOSE AND PROLONGED EXERCISE
  V. HORMONAL CHANGES RELEVANT TO GLUCOSE HOMEOSTASIS
     A.   Insulin
     B.   Glucagon
     C.   Catecholamines and the Sympathetic Nervous System
     D.   Glucoregulation and the Prevention of Hypoglycemia During Exercise
     E.   Catecholamines and Their Circulatory Effects
  VI. CORTISOL
     A.   The Cortisol Responses to Exercise
     B.   Cortisol Turnover During Exercise
  VII. GROWTH HORMONE
  VIII. REPRODUCTIVE HORMONES
     A.   Gonadotrophins
     B.   Female Gonadal Hormonal Responses to Exercise—Estradiol and
        Progesterone
     C.   Males
  IX. ENDORPHINS AND ENKEPHALINS
     A.   The Effect of Exercise on Endorphins and Enkephalins
     B.   The Role of Endogenous Opiates in the Pituitary Hormonal Responses
        to Exercise
     C.   The Effects of Training (Male vs Female Responses) on Endorphins
  X. FLUID AND ELECTROLYTE BALANCE
     A.   Fluid and Electrolyte Imbalance During Exercise and the Response of
        Renin-Angiotensin-Aldosterone, Vasopressin and Atrial Natriuretic
        Factor
     B.   Hormonal Regulation of Fluids and Electrolytes

XI. WHAT ARE THE IMPLICATIONS OF THE HORMONAL RESPONSES TO
PROLONGED EXERCISE FOR THE PHYSICIAN, THE COACH, AND THE
ATHLETE?
A. Fuel Homeostasis and the Provision of Energy for Exercise
B. The Reproductive Hormones
SUMMARY
BIBLIOGRAPHY
DISCUSSION

INTRODUCTION

The study of endocrine function during exercise is of relatively recent origin and one of the newer fields in the study of exercise. Its evolution depended on the development of sensitive assays capable of measuring the minute quantities of hormones circulating in the blood. In contrast to the measurement of energy substrates which are present in milligram quantities, many hormones circulate in nanogram and picogram quantities and only the development of the radioimmunoassay by Yalow and Berson in 1960 (269) led the way for hormonal quantification in plasma. Studies examining the endocrine responses to exercise have mushroomed. In addition, a dramatically increased number of hormones have been identified, although the importance of many of these during exercise remains to be determined.

In this chapter, we will consider: (1) the endocrine responses during prolonged exercise, (2) the endocrine adaptations to aerobic exercise training, (3) the influence of age and sex on the hormonal responses to exercise, (4) endocrine function as a possible limiting factor to performance of prolonged exercise and (5) the implications for the physician, coach and athlete.

An increase in the plasma concentration of a hormone during exercise usually has been interpreted as an increased hormonal secretion stimulated by exercise. However, this is not necessarily the case. A change in plasma concentration must be interpreted in light of the total physiological exercise response. First, with exercise, there is usually a significant shift of fluid from the circulating compartment and thus, a reduction in plasma volume. This fundamental physiological effect, which begins with the onset of exercise, will result in a significant increase in plasma concentration of all substrates and hormones without any addition of the hormone to the blood compartment or any change in the rate of hormone exiting from this space. Nevertheless, this, a basic physiological phenomenon, is often ignored. The magnitude of the change is often 10% and may be increased further with dehydration. There is a considerable increase in blood volume in athletes compared with non-athletes and thus for a given hormonal concentration, an athlete will have a greater quantity of circulating hormone. If a greater change in hormonal concentration occurs than can be accounted for by the reduction in plasma volume, additional factors need to be considered. An increase in the hormonal production rate is usually responsible for major changes, as occurs with growth hormone. By contrast, a decrease in hormonal metabolism, as seen with many of the steroid hormones such as testosterone, may also be responsible for the increased plasma concentration. In many instances, both of the dynamic changes occur simultaneously and are coupled with the changing plasma volume.

Another important consideration in the biological effectiveness of a hormone concentration is the rate of delivery of that hormone to its target tissue (191). Exercise dramatically increases total blood flow in the body; however, blood flow through specific endocrine glands and tissues is not completely established. Clearly, this is a critical gap in the exercise/endocrine literature.

Many pituitary hormones are secreted in a pulsatile manner. Such rapid and dynamic changes occur following hypothalamic pulsatile secretion. When the effect of an additional stress such as exercise is superimposed, it compounds the interpretation even more. Thus, the timing of exercise experiments must consider if the hormone being investigated is at a peak or nadir in its pulsatile release. There have been a number of recent reviews of hormonal responses to exercise and the reader is referred to the works of Bunt (30), Fotherby and Pal (74), Galbo (82), Harber and Sutton (106), Richter and Galbo (181), Sutton (221), Sutton and Heyes (224), Terjung (241) and Viru (247,248).

The following hormone systems will be covered in this paper:

1. Endocrine responses associated with provision of fuel for exercise:
   -Insulin
   -Glucagon
   -Catecholamines and the sympathetic nervous system
2. Cortisol
3. Growth Hormone
4. Reproductive hormones in females and males:
   -Gonadotrophins-LH and FSH
   -Estradiol
   -Progesterone
   -Testosterone
   -Dihydrotestosterone
5. Endorphins and enkephalins

6. Fluid and electrolyte balance:
   -Renin
   -Angiotensin
   -Vasopressin
   -Atrial Natriuretic Hormone

I. ENDOCRINE RESPONSES DURING PROLONGED EXERCISE

Sources of information about the effects of prolonged exercise on the endocrine system come both from laboratory studies and from studies conducted in the field during competitions. Usually laboratory studies allow a more detailed analysis of the endocrine responses as indwelling intravenous or arterial catheters are used and frequent blood samples may be taken. Thus, the evolution of the hormonal response may be measured together with other related metabolic changes. By contrast, most field studies usually permit taking only a few samples and sampling may be limited to before and after exercise only. Obviously, this limits one's ability to interpret the interrelated changes, as they may be causally related. Any studies designed to determine the mechanism of endocrine changes with exercise and which may require pharmacological intervention such as the use of receptor-blocking/stimulating agents usually need to be performed in a laboratory setting. Such studies must also be interpreted with caution for drug interventions frequently have several effects in addition to the one under study.

II. ENDOCRINE RESPONSES ASSOCIATED WITH THE PROVISION OF FUELS FOR PROLONGED EXERCISE

The continuous production of adenosine triphosphate (ATP) is essential for prolonged exercise and high energy phosphates stored in muscle in the form of ATP or creatine phosphate (CP) will allow muscle contraction to continue only for a matter of seconds. For exercise lasting longer than this, a continuous production of ATP is essential and is derived from the metabolism of fat or carbohydrate and, to a smaller extent, protein. Dr. Gollnick reviews the specific regulation of muscle metabolism (91); our focus in this section is on hormonal changes as they relate to energy supply.

Figure 5-1 shows intracellular and extracellular energy sources. Fat and carbohydrate are present in muscle, and glucose is transported from the liver following glycogenolysis which is under hor-

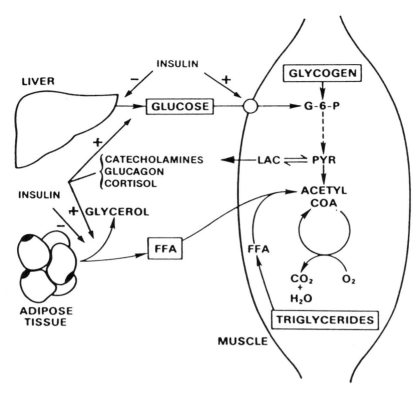

FIGURE 5-1. *Intracellular and extracellular fuel sources during exercise. Fat and carbo-hydrate are present in muscle; glucose is transported from the liver following glycogenolysis. Lipolysis in adipose tissue will release free fatty acids, which are transported in combination with albumin to muscle. Also illustrated in this diagram are the effects of hormones such as catecholamines, glucagon and cortisol (which enhance hepatic glycogenolysis and adipose tis-sue lipolysis) and insulin (which enhances muscle glucose uptake but inhibits hepatic gly-cogenolysis and lipolysis in adipose tissue). (Modified from Richter, E.A. et al, Am J Med. 70:202, 1981.)*

monal regulation (183). Lipolysis in adipose tissue releases free fatty acids (FFA) which are transported in combination with albumin to muscle. Also illustrated in this diagram are the major hormonal ef-fectors of these metabolic changes. In the fasting state, FFA provide the major fuel for muscle (1). This continues with exercise, although the contribution of carbohydrate as an energy source increases with increasing exercise intensity (254,255). With prolonged exercise, the contribution of intramuscular energy sources decreases with in-creasing dependence on blood-borne sources, glucose and FFA (10).

III. GLUCOSE TRANSPORT INTO MUSCLE: INSULIN RECEPTORS

It is apparent that the human organism possesses redundant systems which regulate glucose during exercise. However, the precise basis for the stimulation of glucose transport into muscle during exercise is unknown. In resting muscle, glucose transport occurs by facilitated diffusion and is modulated by insulin. It is also important to note that there is a large species difference in the hormonal control of glucose during prolonged exercise. In dogs, there seems to be a need for at least some circulating insulin during exercise (260). For instance, transport is severely impaired in diabetic animals and is restored to normal by the administration of small quantities of insulin (252). It is possible that insulin in some way maintains the muscle cell membrane so that it can increase glucose transport in response to contractions. Exercise may also enhance the insulin binding to receptor sites on the muscle cell since, in most studies of exercise, insulin concentration itself is either unchanged or diminished (82,134,165). This hypothesis is supported by the observation that in persons with euglycemic hyperinsulinism produced by an insulin-glucose clamp, exercise results in an increase in glucose uptake at the same insulin concentration (207).

The necessity of insulin for glucose transport during exercise in the rat is not so compelling. Plough and colleagues (168) and Wallberg-Henriksson and Holloszy (256) have demonstrated that contracting muscle is capable of significant glucose uptake in the absence of insulin. It is probable that contractions and insulin work synergistically during exercise to increase glucose uptake in man (49,50). Insulin binding to monocytes in response to acute exercise has been reported to both increase (130) and decrease (154). While monocytes are easily accessible, their use in insulin binding studies can be misleading (16,240). In the only human study to our knowledge which measured insulin binding to human muscle during exercise, Bonen et al (16) demonstrated that insulin binding remains unchanged during mild exercise and decreases at dynamic exercise intensities requiring greater than 69% $\dot{V}O_2$ max. This is an intriguing observation since it suggests that insulin binding decreases simultaneously with decreases in circulating insulin. Thus, a more complex regulatory process is emerging and has been well expressed by Roth and Grunfeld (187):

We are accustomed to the notion that hormone concentrations fluctuate widely in response to changes within the organism. With the advent of methods to measure directly the binding of hormone to its receptors, it has become evident that the concentration and affinity of receptors also change rapidly in response to signals from inside and outside the cell. Given that the receptors are at the crossroads between the interior and exterior of the cell, retrospectively it is not surprising that they are so responsive to the environment (187).

IV. PLASMA GLUCOSE AND PROLONGED EXERCISE

Blood glucose regulation during exercise is a balance between peripheral uptake into muscle and output from the liver. These are normally well matched so that plasma glucose remains relatively constant (35), acting as a "fast forward" system with hepatic glucose output responding to need (123). When exercise of moderate intensity (30–60% VO_2 max) continues for an hour, plasma glucose remains within a very narrow range (35). However, if the exercise intensity is lower and the exercise continues longer, plasma glucose will tend to decrease and, in some instances, frank hypoglycemia will develop (70). With more prolonged exercise of even lower intensity for 24 h, serum glucose decreased gradually for the first 10–12 h and thereafter remained constant (270).

In spite of this apparently well-regulated control system to prevent wide swings in plasma glucose, problems do occur. While transient hyperglycemia in normal exercising subjects is of no clinical consequence, hypoglycemia can be important. The first reported incidence of hypoglycemia during prolonged competitive exercise was that of Levine and coworkers who observed a number of such occurrences in well-conditioned athletes during the Boston Marathon (142). In contrast to this was the report of Sutton and coworkers, showing normal and elevated plasma glucose concentrations following the marathon (236). More recently, hypoglycemia has been described in joggers entering fun runs and as these fun runs and marathons are now occurring on an unprecedented scale, it can be seen that hypoglycemia could well be a major medical hazard in such races (Fig. 5-2, 5-3) (221).

In a comprehensive study during prolonged laboratory exercise, Felig and colleagues (70) have demonstrated that hypoglycemia (plasma glucose less than 45 mg·dl^{-1}) occurs in a significant number of subjects. It is interesting to note in their work that on repeated occasions when plasma glucose was maintained at euglycemic levels by the administration of oral glucose, the time to exhaustion and the perceived exhaustion were unaltered. These observations are in apparent conflict with the early work of Christensen and Hansen, who were able to increase performance in exhausted subjects by giving oral glucose (38).

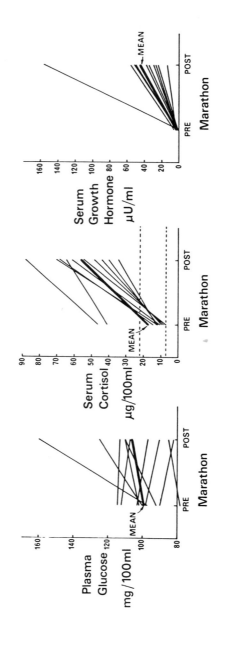

GLUCOSE, CORTISOL AND GROWTH HORMONE – PRE AND POST MARATHON

FIGURE 5-2. *Blood glucose, plasma cortisol and serum growth hormone before and after the marathon in trained athletes. (Reprinted from Sutton, J.R. Sports Medicine, R.H. Strauss (ed.). Philadelphia: W.B. Saunders, 1984, p. 191 with the permission of the editor and publisher.)*

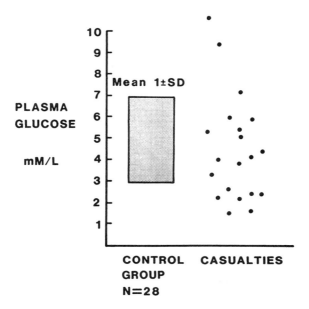

FIGURE 5-3. *Blood glucose following a fun run in patients who "collapsed," compared with 28 control subjects. (Reprinted, credit as in Fig. 5-2.)*

Plasma glucose concentration during exercise depends on a balance between peripheral glucose uptake and hepatic glucose output. Peripheral glucose uptake or glucose disposal will be determined by:

a. Insulin concentration and muscle contractions.
b. Counterregulatory hormone concentrations: catecholamines, cortisol and growth hormone.
c. Changes at the insulin receptor site, in both receptor number and insulin binding affinity to the receptor.
d. Post-receptor changes in muscle: cyclic adenosine monophosphate (cAMP) and rate-limiting enzymes in the glycolytic pathway such as hexokinase, glycogen phosphorylase, phosphofructokinase and pyruvate dehydrogenase may be altered (257).

The regulatory factors for hepatic glucose output are unknown but may be neuronal. Under steady-state conditions of moderate intensity exercise, hepatic glucose output is perfectly matched to peripheral glucose uptake. This is independent of insulin and the counterregulatory hormones, at least in short-term exercise (35,253). However, under most physiological situations of high intensity, short bursts of exercise result in hyperglycemia in which hepatic glucose output exceeds glucose disposal rate. The traditional concept that hepatic glucose output increases in response to increased glucose utilization has recently been challenged. Several reports using both rat (120,210) and human models (127) suggest that glucoregulation may follow a "feed forward" rather than a "feed back" mechanism with increases in glucose production preceding exercise-induced increases in glucose utilization. The hormonal and neural regulators of this proposed mechanism are not yet confirmed, but probably involve central nervous system effects and muscle effects.

V. HORMONAL CHANGES RELEVANT TO GLUCOSE HOMEOSTASIS

Those hormones of paramount importance to glucose homeostasis in short-term exercise are insulin, glucagon, the catecholamines and sympathetic nervous activity. As the duration of exercise becomes more prolonged, cortisol and growth hormone become of greater importance in the metabolic homeostasis of exercise.

A. Insulin

From the isolation of pancreatic insulin in 1922 by Banting and Best (5), forty-one years were to elapse before measurements were made of insulin during exercise. These initial bioassay studies of "insulin-like activity" by Devlin in 1963 demonstrated decreased insulin activity during exercise (53). Recent studies have confirmed this finding, although some have shown no change in insulin concentration. Comprehensive studies of plasma insulin concentration during prolonged work were performed by Pruett (173,174) who has also reviewed the topic of insulin and exercise in diabetic and non-diabetic humans (175,261), as have Vranic and Berger (250).

The metabolic response of insulin to exercise was first studied in 1967 by Schalch (198), using an insulin radioimmunoassay. He reported no change in serum insulin levels during exercise. Several other investigators (118,162,180) made similar observations the following year. Studies by Sutton and colleagues (236) and Sutton (219) revealed different insulin responses between fit and unfit subjects during exercise. The fit subjects tended to have a lower fasting level of insulin and when exercised at the same absolute workload, there was little change in insulin. By contrast, for the same absolute workload, there was a greater depression in plasma insulin in the unfit subjects who were working at a higher intensity of exercise (percentage of $\dot{V}O_2$ max). The intensity of exercise has also been shown to influence insulin metabolism (12). Early studies by Pruett examined the effect of prolonged exercise on serum insulin concentrations (173,174). Her results showed a decrease in serum insulin concentration with prolonged exercise. A number of techniques have been used to investigate the mechanism of the insulin response to exercise. Wright and Malaisse (268) injected rats with guinea pig anti-insulin serum and showed a decrease in the insulin secretion rate following prolonged swimming. Other studies using radio-labelled insulin have failed to show a change in insulin secretion with exercise (162) or showed a decrease (79). Due to the greatly reduced rate of degradation of connecting peptide (C-peptide, which is co-secreted with insulin), it probably serves (with the recognition of specific limitations, (Polonsky and Rubenstein, 169) as a better marker of beta cell secretion than does a change in circulating insulin concentration (59). Several reports demonstrate reductions in C-peptide during prolonged exercise (133).

As with any specific hormonal response to exercise, there are also a number of important interactions with other hormones. In particular, the plasma catecholamines increase with exercise and will concomitantly inhibit insulin secretion. Brisson and coworkers (26), using an alpha-adrenergic blocking drug during exercise, suggested that the decreased insulin secretion during exercise was in fact catecholamine- (alpha-adrenergic receptor-) mediated. Since peripheral norepinephrine concentrations are only a crude estimate of sympathetic nervous system activity, it may be that direct neural input to the pancreas has a greater inhibitory influence on insulin secretion during exercise than does circulating norepinephrine (37). Neuropeptides are also important to beta cell function (2) and these peptides are just beginning to receive attention in terms of exercise-induced alterations in pancreatic function (68).

Although insulin secretion appears to decrease during exercise, some competitors in fun runs or marathons ingest glucose orally prior to exercise to augment insulin secretion when exercise begins. Glucose uptake by muscle will be facilitated and hypoglycemia may occur (43). In addition, when males and females exercise at the same percentage of $\dot{V}O_2$ max, it has been demonstrated that males have a greater decrease in serum insulin concentrations when exercise is continued for 90 min (239).

B. Glucagon

Secreted by the alpha cells of the pancreas, glucagon is important in initiating hepatic glycogenolysis. The first studies to examine the influence of exercise on glucagon secretion suggested that there was a tendency for glucagon to rise with maximum exercise and that unfit subjects may have had a slightly elevated resting glucagon concentration; however, the differences were not statistically significant (236). Subsequent work by Bloom and colleagues (12) confirmed this trend and found a significant difference between trained and untrained subjects, with the untrained having the higher serum glucagon concentration. Nevertheless, the increases with exercise only occurred toward the end of the exercise bouts at the highest exercise intensities. Galbo and coworkers (84) also found that glucagon tended not to rise until the exercise was more prolonged. In contrast to insulin secretion, glucagon does not appear to be mediated by the autonomic nervous system as neither alpha nor beta blockade influenced glucagon secretion during prolonged exercise (84). Tarnopolsky and coworkers (239) showed no difference between female and male responses to exercise when working at the same percentage of $\dot{V}O_2$ max.

Glucagon stimulates hepatic glucose output and this may be important during exercise, particularly in dogs (251,260) and also in rats (182). However, the increase in glucagon concentration during exercise is considerably delayed following the onset of exercise in humans; hence, Bjorkman and coworkers have suggested that glucagon may not be important in hepatic glycogenolysis (9).

C. Catecholamines and the Sympathetic Nervous System

The activity of the sympathetic nervous system and catecholamines was first investigated by measuring urinary excretion of epinephrine and norepinephrine (249). As measurements in plasma became possible in the 1960s, Vendsalu reported increases in plasma catecholamines with exercise (243). Epinephrine is secreted from the adrenal medulla and plays a significant metabolic role, whereas norepinephrine in blood represents an overflow from sympathetic nervous system activity.

Many studies have followed which indicate that epinephrine and norepinephrine secretion are stimulated with exercise, and the greater the intensity of exercise, the greater will be the magnitude of the change (12,81,84). The duration of exercise is also important in determining the magnitude of the catecholamine responses; under field conditions, there is an inverse relationship between plasma epinephrine and norepinephrine and the mileage run (258). A number of other factors also determine the catecholamine responses to exercise. Fleg and coworkers (73) demonstrated that for any relative intensity of work, plasma catecholamines were greater in older rather than younger subjects. Tarnopolsky and colleagues (239) have demonstrated that there was a tendency for a greater epinephrine response in males compared with females performing the same relative intensity of work, but the norepinephrine responses were identical. Furthermore, in females, there is a greater catecholamine response to exercise in the luteal rather than the follicular phase of the menstrual cycle (234), an observation confirmed by Lavoie and colleagues in 1987 (139).

It has been suggested that the mechanisms of the increased plasma catecholamine concentration during exercise and the magnitude of the change with acute high-intensity exercise may be a result of increased catecholamine secretion. Kjaer (126), using tritium-labelled epinephrine in athletes and non-athletes, indicated that the increased epinephrine was due to an increased secretion and that at exhaustion, epinephrine concentration was greater in the trained rather than the untrained subjects despite identical concentrations of glucose and the same heart rate. The norepinephrine response tends to parallel the increase in heart rate rather closely, as documented by Christensen and Brandsborg in 1973 (36). Christensen and Galbo (37) later showed an inverse relationship between plasma norepinephrine and mixed venous oxygen saturation, which was shown by Sutton and coworkers (235) in "Operation Everest II" to be dependent on workload. Although catecholamines have a number of major metabolic effects including the stimulation of lipolysis and hepatic glycogenolysis, an elaborate series of experiments by Gollnick and colleagues (92) demonstrated that adrenomedullectomized rats with ganglion blockade failed to inhibit glycogen depletion in muscle or liver by exercise. However, this approach resulted in an inhibition of adipose tissue lipolysis. Another important metabolic effect of increasing catecholamine secretion during exercise is the inhibition of beta cell insulin secretion from the pancreas. This effect, however, may be mediated by direct neural input to the pancreas (37,122).

Since the degree of sympathetic neural activation varies in different tissues (28,57) future studies on the role of this system during exercise may need to measure activity at or going to specific tissues. The necessity of this approach was recently demonstrated by Victor et al (244) who showed that muscle sympathetic nervous activity in the peroneal nerve of the leg did not change during arm exercise. Thus, dynamic exercise does not elicit a whole-body sympathetic response. Selective neural activation to various tissues may be critical to our understanding of cardiovascular and metabolic responses to prolonged exercise (85).

D. Glucoregulation and the Prevention of Hypoglycemia During Exercise

Taken individually, most of the hormonal changes with exercise are not essential to prevent hypoglycemia. Neither prevention of insulin decrease by insulin infusion (35) nor the glucagon increase by somatostatin infusion (9) will result in hypoglycemia. The beta-adrenergic responses may be somewhat more important as infusion of propranolol, not phentolamine, results in a lower plasma glucose, but not to hypoglycemic concentrations (83,104). Furthermore, hypoglycemia did not develop in exercising patients who had undergone bilateral adrenalectomy and therefore, had lost most of the epinephrine-secreting cells (112).

However, if all the above systems were defective, glucose homeostasis might be in jeopardy. Such a concept was elegantly addressed by Hoelzer and coworkers in 1986 (111). They systematically examined the effects of alpha and beta adrenergic blockade, islet cell clamping (infusion of somatostatin to inhibit insulin and glucagon secretion, with subsequent replacement of insulin and glucagon) and the combination of both these interventions during exercise. They demonstrated that adrenergic blockade, together with islet clamping were required before glucose production was impaired and hypoglycemia resulted (as low as 34 mg·dl^{-1}). They concluded that normally there is sufficient redundancy within the glucoregulatory system to enable glucose production to be matched to glucose utilization, thus preventing hypoglycemia (Fig. 5-4 a-c).

While the intent of this chapter is to describe endocrine changes during prolonged exercise, we would like to briefly review the consequences of chronic exercise on insulin sensitivity. A vast literature exists concerning the effects of acute and chronic exercise on insulin sensitivity. The reader is referred to several reviews which include this topic (83,181,248).

Although much has been learned about exercise training and glucose control using transient glucose challenges (140,210), steady-

HEART RATE (beats/min)

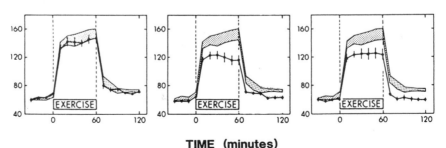

TIME (minutes)

FIGURE 5-4a. *Heart rate response to 60 min exercise at 55–60% $\dot{V}O_2$ max in three different situations, with the control study in the shaded areas. Left panel: Islet clamp study; Middle panel: Adrenergic blockade study; Right panel: Adrenergic blockade + islet clamp study (111).*

GLUCOSE KINETICS:CONCENTRATION

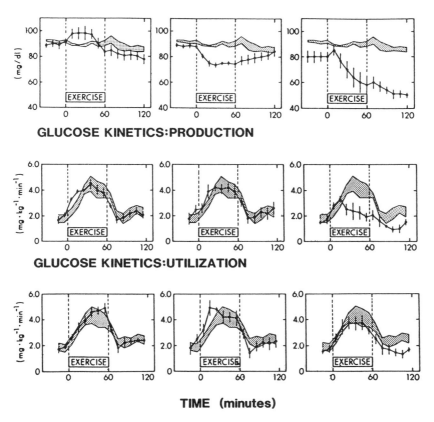

GLUCOSE KINETICS:PRODUCTION

GLUCOSE KINETICS:UTILIZATION

TIME (minutes)

FIGURE 5-4b. *Plasma glucose, glucose production and glucose utilization during 60 min. exercise. Legend as in 5-4a.*

state conditions (glucose clamp techniques) are probably more revealing in terms of identifying insulin/glucose relationships (7). Burstein et al (31) found that metabolic glucose clearance rate was higher at comparable concentrations of hyperinsulinemia in trained subjects 12 h after prolonged exercise than in sedentary controls. This difference was reduced after 60 h of inactivity in trained subjects and no differences between groups were found after 7 days of inactivity. Similar increases in insulin sensitivity using a glucose clamp procedure have been reported in athletes by Sato et al (196); however, the time after the last bout of exercise was not reported. In a rat model, James et al (119) have demonstrated that exercise training results in an increased insulin sensitivity which lasts at least 48 h

INSULIN (μU/ml)

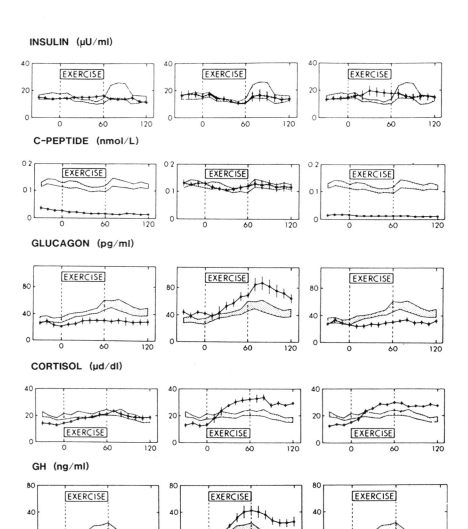

C-PEPTIDE (nmol/L)

GLUCAGON (pg/ml)

CORTISOL (μd/dl)

GH (ng/ml)

TIME (minutes)

FIGURE 5-4c. *Insulin, c-peptide, glucagon, growth hormone, cortisol, epinephrine and nor-epinephrine in 60 min exercise. Legend as in 5-4a. (Figures 5-4a, b and c reproduced from Hoelzer et al, J Clin Invest. 77:212–221, 1986, with permission of author and editor.)*

post-exercise and several reports (119,158) show that muscle glucose uptake accounts for most of this adaptation.

An important question which has been addressed recently (155,156) is whether a single bout of prolonged exercise affects in-

EPINEPHRINE

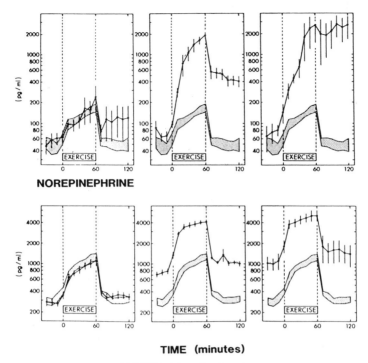

NOREPINEPHRINE

TIME (minutes)

FIGURE 5-4c. *Continued.*

sulin secretion (pancreatic adaptation) and insulin sensitivity (muscle adaptation). These studies (currently reported in abstract form) show that a single bout of prolonged exercise (60 min, 62% $\dot{V}O_2$ max on a cycle ergometer) results in increased insulin sensitivity and responsiveness (glucose disposal at maximally effective steady-state hyperinsulinemia) and this effect lasts at least 2 days, but not 5 days, post-exercise. This group also showed that insulin c-peptide and pro-insulin secretion during sustained hyperglycemia is not altered immediately or 48 h after prolonged exercise. Thus, a single bout of exercise has profound effects on insulin sensitivity, but repeated bouts of exercise (training) may be required to alter pancreatic sensitivity to hyperglycemia.

E. Catecholamines and their Circulatory Effects

Although the catecholamines have significant metabolic effects during exercise apart from the effect on lipolysis, it is their influence on the circulation which dominates. This point was highlighted in a recent study by Rowell and colleagues (190) who exercised subjects at four intensities under two thermal conditions. The increase of epinephrine (E) and norepinephrine (NE) with exercise was related to the intensity of exercise. The increased heat load resulted in little difference in epinephrine secretion. On the other hand, the hotter temperatures markedly increased norepinephrine secretion which paralleled the heart rate response (Fig. 5-5), not linearly, but as the rise in norepinephrine is exponential, so the log norepinephrine concentration is linearly related to heart rate. Thus, the increases in circulating norepinephrine, which depend on the intensity and duration of exercise, also depend on environmental conditions. This increase in norepinephrine plays an important role in blood flow distribution which controls not only oxygen and substrate delivery, but also enhances heat dissipation during prolonged exercise.

The effects of training on the catecholamine response to exercise indicate that at the same absolute exercise intensity, there is a reduction in norepinephrine and epinephrine following a training program. By contrast, as expected, when working at the same relative intensity of exercise post-training, the responses of catecholamines, epinephrine and norepinephrine were not significantly different (108,109,166,267).

An augmented epinephrine response to prolonged exercise has been reported when the endogenous opioid peptide (EOP) system is antagonized (66,99). A similar inhibitory action of EOP has been found during insulin-induced hypoglycemia (20), isometric exercise (137) and during a cold-pressor test (19). Thus, it seems that EOP may modulate the catecholamine response (both E and NE) during times of stress, with the end result being a response which is appropriate to the imposed stress. It should be noted that two reports contradict the above studies; they suggest no involvement of EOP in the endocrine response to exercise. Staessen et al (213) and Brammert and Hokfelt (23) found very little change in the catecholamine response to exercise when naloxone was infused at high or low concentrations. Clearly, more work is required to determine the extent to which EOP modulates specific hormones during and after the stress of exercise.

VI. CORTISOL

A. The Cortisol Responses to Exercise

Although cortisol is also one of the counter-glucoregulatory hormones, we shall include it as a separate section and detail the hypothalamic-pituitary-adrenal regulation of cortisol, as an intact hy-

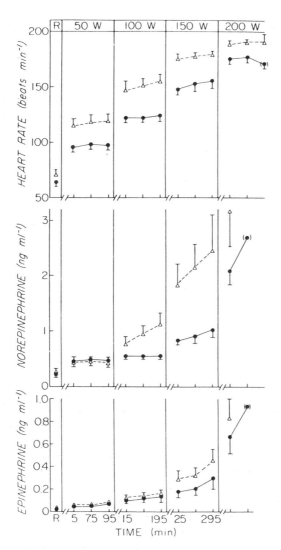

FIGURE 5-5. *Heart rate, norepinephrine and epinephrine responses to different intensities of exercise with body skin temperature held at 30° C (solid dots and lines, ±SE) and at 38° C (open triangles, dashed lines, ±SE). (Reproduced from Rowell et al, J Appl Physiol. 62:647, 1987, with the permission of the authors and editor.)*

pothalamus-pituitary-adrenal axis is essential in this integrated response to exercise. The early studies investigating the effects of exercise on adrenocortical secretion evaluated indirect criteria such as adrenal ascorbic acid cortical depletion, depression of plasma eosinophil count and the measurements of 17 ketosteroids in the urine, to evaluate the response. With the availability of protein binding and radioimmunoassays, an understanding of the plasma cortisol responses began to emerge. It was soon observed that there is considerable variability in the cortisol responses to exercise, depending on the nature of the study performed. Under most circumstances, the changes in plasma cortisol concentration are dependent on the intensity of exercise. Earlier studies by Cornil and colleagues (42) found a decrease in cortisol during short-term moderate exercise, as did Raymond and coworkers (179). It was Davies and Few in 1973 (47) who clearly demonstrated that exercise intensity was important in determining the cortisol response, an observation confirmed by Viru in 1972 (246) and Bloom and coworkers in 1976 (12). Nevertheless, there were some conflicting reports such as those of Kuoppasalmi and coworkers (135) who failed to show any significant increase in cortisol after short-term near-maximal work, as did Wade and Claybaugh (253). The importance of duration of exercise cannot be overlooked. Also, some of the discrepancy in the literature can probably be accounted for by failure to control for the circadian rhythm of cortisol as well as the timing of the experiment after a meal. Brandenberger et al (25) have convincingly demonstrated that if exercise is initiated either after a meal or during an episodic secretory peak, no greater elevation of this steroid will occur.

Sutton and coworkers (236) found extremely high cortisol levels (mean 92 ug $\cdot$ 100 ml^{-1}, with a range of 74–127 µg $\cdot$ 100 ml^{-1}) in 11 subjects following a marathon (Fig. 5-2). Such findings in marathon runners have been supported by the work of Dessypris and coworkers (52) and Newmark and colleagues (160). Many other observations of cortisol responses to field conditions of fun runs and endurance runs usually have shown major increases in plasma cortisol levels. In a fun run during which a number of subjects collapsed, plasma cortisol was elevated in five of six subjects (231). The authors considered the one subject in whom plasma cortisol was in the normal range so unusual that a formal assessment of the hypothalamic-pituitary-adrenal axis was undertaken with insulin hypoglycemia and ACTH stimulation to determine whether the athlete had an impaired adrenal reserve. Current practice would suggest that ACTH and cortisol response to corticotrophin-releasing hormone also be studied. Although measurements of plasma concentrations do give an indication of the magnitude of the change in cortisol, the total integrated response is best obtained by measuring secretion rates or urinary free cortisol, as was performed by Bonen (14). These results demonstrated that the magnitude of the increase in urinary free cortisol with exercise was closely related to the relative intensity of exercise. Brandenberger and Follenius (24) also showed the importance of the duration of exercise in determining the cortisol response and found that even at low work levels, plasma cortisol will rise, provided the exercise period is of sufficient duration.

The importance of the subjects' cardiorespiratory fitness was examined by Sutton and colleagues in 1969 (236); provided that exercise intensity was of the same relative magnitude, i.e. the same percent $\dot{V}O_2$ max, cortisol responses were similar in fit and unfit subjects. By contrast, at the same absolute level of work, fit subjects had no increase in cortisol concentration with submaximal exercise while unfit subjects had any significant increase (219). Hartley and coworkers also failed to show any significant effect of a training program on the plasma cortisol responses to exercise (108,109).

B. Cortisol Turnover During Exercise

The mechanism of the changes in plasma cortisol during exercise are best understood by turnover rate studies in which 3_H-cortisol was administered. At low intensities of exercise, the removal of cortisol from plasma compartment was increased while secretion rate tended to be lower; thus, plasma cortisol concentration fell. By contrast during heavy exercise, in spite of an increased removal rate, secretion increased further; the result was that plasma cortisol concentration was elevated (34,71).

Cortisol secretion is under hypothalamic-pituitary control. The assessment of ACTH during exercise also has indicated a significant increase (32,63,75,86). In what was perhaps the most comprehensive examination of the hypothalamic-pituitary-adrenal axis in runners and non-runners, Luger and colleagues (144) demonstrated the importance of relative intensity of exercise in the determination of cortisol and ACTH responses. They also showed that both ACTH and cortisol tended to be higher during the resting state in highly trained individuals, supporting the findings of Villanueva and coworkers who showed an increase in plasma concentration and cortisol production rate in female runners (245). By contrast, suppression of ACTH with an injection of beta-methasone prior to exercise abolished the cortisol increase with exercise (220) (Fig. 5-6). Thus, it would seem that highly trained runners appear to have a chronic state of hypercortisolism which is particularly heightened before a race, as demonstrated by Sutton and Casey (223) and Luger and coworkers (144) (Fig. 5-7a). These latter scientists went further in evaluating hypothalamic-pituitary-adrenal integrity with an injection of ovine corticotrophin-releasing hormone (CRH). Compared with sedentary and moderately trained individuals, highly trained

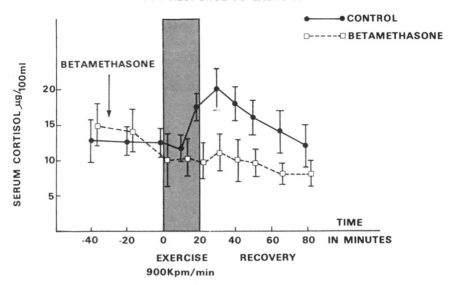

FIGURE 5-6. *Serum cortisol with exercise and the suppression of the increase during exercise by a prior injection of betamethasone to inhibit ACTH, indicating that the increased serum cortisol is due to an increased cortisol secretion (220).*

athletes had a reduced integrated response of ACTH and cortisol response to the same dose of CRH (Fig. 5-7b). Although the authors were unable to determine the mechanism whereby the increased secretion of ACTH with hypercortisolism occurred in the highly trained athletes, they speculated that there might be an increased CRH secretion, as has also been postulated in patients experiencing anorexia nervosa and depression (88,89). Although it has not been studied in great detail, the central role of CRH as it affects the many aspects of pituitary secretion and target organ functions is beginning to be investigated.

VII. GROWTH HORMONE

Growth hormone, as its name implies, is important in human growth but also has a number of other metabolic actions. It consists of 191 amino acids, containing two disulphide bridges. The molecular structure was formally identified by Niall in 1971 (161). The somatotrophe cells occupy approximately 40% of the human pituitary gland and contain about 5–10 mg of growth hormone. Thus,

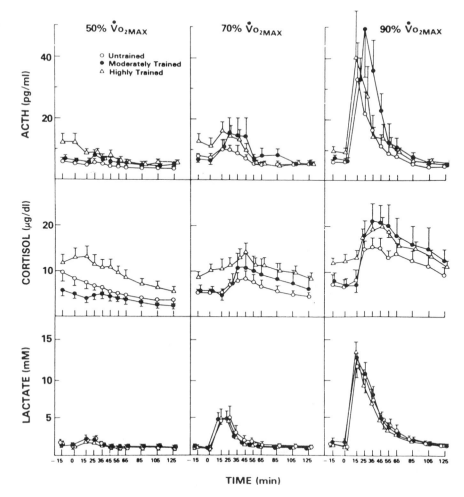

FIGURE 5-7a. *Concentrations of ACTH, cortisol and lactate (mean ±SE) in three groups of subjects (untrained, moderately trained and highly trained) during treadmill exercise at 50%, 70% and 90% VO₂ max. (Reprinted from Luger, A. et al, N Engl J Med. 316:1311, 1987 with the permission of the authors and editors.)*

quantitatively, it is the most abundant of all the pituitary hormones. Growth hormone is released in a pulsatile manner, as are many of the other pituitary hormones. Growth hormone secretion is regulated by growth hormone releasing hormone (GHRH), synthesized in the median arcuate nucleus of the hypothalamus. When stimulated, GHRH causes a release of growth hormone. On the other hand, somatostatin, in the paraventricular nucleus, causes inhibi-

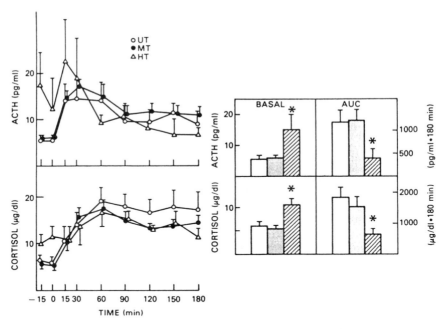

FIGURE 5-7b. *Plasma ACTH and cortisol following administration of ovine corticotrophin-releasing hormone (CRH) (1 ug/kg). Right panel shows basal + ovine CRH-stimulated (time integrated stimulation above base line). Credit as for 5-7a.*
Untrained: (UT) open bars; left
Moderately trained: (MT) stippled bars; middle
Highly trained: (HT) hatched bars; right.

tion of growth hormone secretion when stimulated. Modulation of these two primary regulators of growth hormone secretion can occur via many of the neurotransmitters including the catecholamines, dopamine, serotonin, endorphins and the cholinergic neurones. Resting levels of growth hormone are frequently low, but it is now recognized that growth hormone secretion is pulsatile in nature. The two relatively reproducible physiological stimuli of growth hormone secretion are exercise and sleep. The first studies of growth hormone responses to exercise were conducted by Roth and colleagues in 1963 (188) and Hunter and Greenwood in 1965 (117), whereas the sleep-associated increase in growth hormone is associated predominantly with the first bout of slow-wave sleep, as Takahashi and colleagues reported in 1968 (237). Exercise is as great a stimulus to growth hormone secretion as is sleep; being physiological, it may well be a more appropriate investigation to use for growth hormone deficiency than many of the pharmacological agents (226). The importance of growth hormone pulsatility and the use of 24-h secretion studies for the assessment of growth hormone adequacy have been advocated, although, clearly this involves greater effort and inconvenience for clinicians and investigators (110). Borer and colleagues (17) demonstrated the greatest growth in hamsters with the greatest growth hormone pulse frequency and amplitude.

Factors affecting growth hormone secretion during exercise are the intensity of the exercise and its duration. Sutton and coworkers (236) showed that when taken to exhaustion, both fit and unfit subjects had similar increases in growth hormone concentration but unfit subjects continued to have a prolonged increase in growth hormone secretion for several hours following exercise. When submaximal exercise was performed, the growth hormone response was greater in the unfit subjects at the same absolute work level. This was explored in more detail in studies by Bloom and coworkers (12) who also showed similar responses in growth hormone in fit and unfit subjects when exercising at the same relative intensity. By contrast, when the exercise was of the same absolute magnitude and therefore relatively harder for the unfit subjects, a growth hormone response was seen only in the unfit group (219). Shephard and Sidney (203) indicated the importance of duration and intensity of exercise on the growth hormone response. Following a training program, these workers were also able to demonstrate a greater response in growth hormone in older men (204). The response in females was similar to that in males (230), but the importance of the phase of the menstrual cycle was identified in females with the greater rise occurring in the luteal phase compared with the follicular phase (170). Although the actual stimulation remains unknown, it was postulated by Sutton and colleagues that lactate or the acid-base alteration during exercise might be responsible (236). Data from several sources support this hypothesis, particularly the finding of an augmented growth hormone response when exercise is performed under conditions of acute hypoxia (218). However, this hypothesis was finally put to rest by a number of important observations.

(1) Patients with McArdle's syndrome, in whom no lactic acid is formed during exercise, have an elevation of growth hormone during exercise (Sutton, Toews & Jones, unpublished observations).

(2) In a detailed study in which acid-base balance was manipulated by the administration of ammonium chloride or sodium bicarbonate, subjects were found to have a very different pH during exercise as well as a markedly different serum lactate; the subjects who were the most acidemic had the lowest lactates during exercise while those most alka-

lemic had the highest lactates. However, in spite of marked differences in acid-base balance and lactate concentration, there was an identical growth hormone response to exercise under all conditions (233).

(3) An infusion of L-lactate in resting subjects, reproducing serum concentrations found during moderate-to-heavy exercise, failed to elicit any change in serum growth hormone concentration (233).

The importance to growth hormone secretion of energy substrates on circulating levels of glucose and free fatty acids has been examined by Hansen and colleagues who showed that intravenous glucose suppressed growth hormone rise (102) but Intralipid had no effect (103). The suppressive effects of glucose infusion on the growth hormone response to exercise was shown to be greater in unfit compared with fit subjects (Sutton, 1969, unpublished observations).

The role of various neurotransmitters in influencing growth hormone secretion during exercise has also been examined. Adrenergic receptor blockade was used by Hansen (104) and Sutton and Lazarus (225). Both groups of workers agreed that beta blockade enhanced growth hormone secretion with exercise but while Sutton and Lazarus (225) were unable to demonstrate any significant effect of alpha blockade, Hansen's work (104) showed an inhibition of growth hormone release by exercise during alpha blockade. The importance of serotinergic neurotransmission to growth hormone secretion during exercise was examined by Smythe and Lazarus (206). They were able to demonstrate that cyproheptadine, a serotonin antagonist, minimized growth hormone secretion during exercise.

The role of opioid peptides has been examined recently by several workers; using varying doses of opiate receptor-blocking drugs administered in different ways not surprisingly yielded conflicting results. Naloxone used in low dose had little effect on any hormonal changes (212,227). By contrast, with the exception of one study, high-dose naloxone or naltrexone was shown to augment growth hormone responses to exercise (66,100,149) whereas Moretti and colleagues (159) found the responses abolished completely! There were minor differences in experimental design of these latter studies, so the cause of this apparent discrepancy is unclear. It is uncertain how the individual neurotransmitter works in the regulation of growth hormone secretion, i.e., by affecting somatostatin or GHRH, although a recent study by Borer and coworkers (17) using naloxone and anti-somatostatin anti-serum in hamsters led the authors to conclude that the effects of endogenous opiates are mediated by opposing somatostatin action.

Casanueva and colleagues (33) have suggested that cholinergic neurotransmission may be the final common pathway for many of the stimuli involved in growth hormone secretion. These workers showed complete abolition of the growth hormone response to exercise by prior injections of atropine. They also indicated that many of the drugs such as cyproheptadine and diphenhydramine, which are used to examine serotinergic and histaminergic pathways for growth hormone release, also possess anti-cholinergic properties. Furthermore, reduction of growth hormone secretion in animals treated with reserpine to deplete the aminergic pathways may also not be specific. In addition to depleting brain amines, reserpine also reduces acetylcholine storage.

Growth hormone has many actions including direct effects on adipose tissue, where it increases lipolysis. Growth hormone decreases glucose uptake in the liver, where it will stimulate RNA synthesis, protein synthesis, gluconeogenesis and the production of somatomedin, and in muscle, where increases in amino acid uptake and protein synthesis occur and glucose uptake decreases. The major growth-promoting actions of growth hormone appear to be mediated by somatomedin. There is a delay of several hours between the administration of growth hormone and an observed increase in somatomedin. Although few studies have been done during exercise, Stuart and colleagues (216) (Fig. 5-8) examined subjects for the plasma somatomedin concentration 5–6 hours after a normal stimulus to growth hormone secretion such as exercise, arginine, sleep or insulin hypoglycemia. Although there was a measurable increase in radioimmunoassayable growth hormone, there was very little change in the biologically active somatomedin in response to this single stimulus (215).

VIII. REPRODUCTIVE HORMONES

Two pituitary gonadotrophic hormones, luteinizing hormone (LH) and follicle-stimulating hormone (FSH), regulate gonadal function. Both LH and FSH are controlled in turn by the hypothalamic secretion of gonadotrophin-releasing hormone (GnRH), a decapeptide whose amino acid sequence is identical in all mammals. It is now appreciated that GnRH is secreted in pulses, the frequency and magnitude of which are essential for normal pituitary gonadotrophin secretion, which is also pulsatile.

A. Gonadotrophins

The first studies to examine gonadotrophins during exercise were performed before the pulsatile nature of luteinizing hormone and

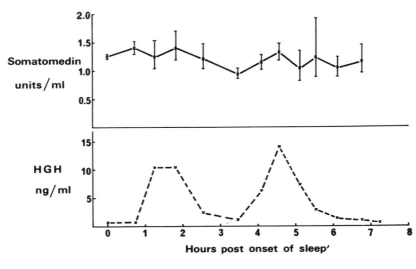

SLEEP STUDY
Normal ♀

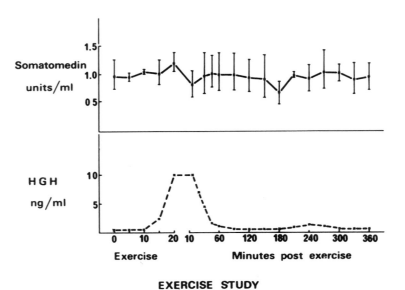

EXERCISE STUDY
Normal ♂

FIGURE 5-8. *Somatomedins with exercise and sleep (216).*

follicle-stimulating hormone secretion was appreciated (148,193,194). Nevertheless, no significant changes were noted during exercise nor were differences between fit and unfit subjects detected (236). These observations were extended to females in 1973 (230) and again, no significant changes were seen, findings which have been confirmed in both men and women on many occasions since. Following a marathon run, Dessypris and colleagues found no significant change in LH (52), nor was there any effect of varying exercise intensity on LH secretion when studied by Kuoppasalmi (135). Similar findings have been noted for FSH responses to exercise. In females, there has been a slight, but biologically minor, increase in FSH levels during exercise in the follicular rather than the luteal phase (124).

The importance of body weight and fat for normal reproductive function is well known, especially in young ballet dancers, who are extremely active (80). Thus, prolonged and intense exercise in females causes a depression rather than a stimulation of reproductive function, as was first reported by Erydeli in 1962 (58). Since that time, many reports of delayed menarche and secondary amenorrhea (46,69,259), shortened or inadequate luteal phases (15,201) and oligomenorehea (142,145) have appeared.

In a detailed cross-sectional study of teenage swimmers, Bonen and coworkers (15) demonstrated a shortened luteal phase, 4.5 ± 0.6 days, as compared with 13.4 ± 1.7 days in a control group of teenagers. During the follicular phase, serum LH concentration was elevated but FSH was depressed. In the luteal phase, estradiol and progesterone were also lower in the swimmers (15) (Fig. 5-9). In an important prospective study of subjects training for the marathon, Prior (171) demonstrated an increased frequency of cycles which were anovulatory or had an inadequate luteal phase. Prior and colleagues (172) also reported the reversibility of infertility and luteal phase insufficiency in a runner who conceived six weeks after ceasing to run. Boyden and colleagues (21,22) also performed a longitudinal training study in 19 healthy and regularly menstruating women who volunteered to participate in an endurance running program designed to enable them to complete a marathon. The subjects trained for more than a year, increasing their mileage from 15.1 ± 4.9 miles·week^{-1} to 63.4 ± 6.9 miles·week^{-1}. Menstrual change was common; 18 of the 19 subjects had oligomenorrhea, but none had amenorrhea. Estradiol decreased and there was a slight but insignificant reduction in LH. However, the most impressive finding was the impairment in LH, and to a lesser extent FSH, responsiveness to injections of GnRH (22). In a more moderate eight-week training program, Bullen and coworkers (29) showed mild ovarian impairment in four of seven subjects, evidenced by a decreased urinary

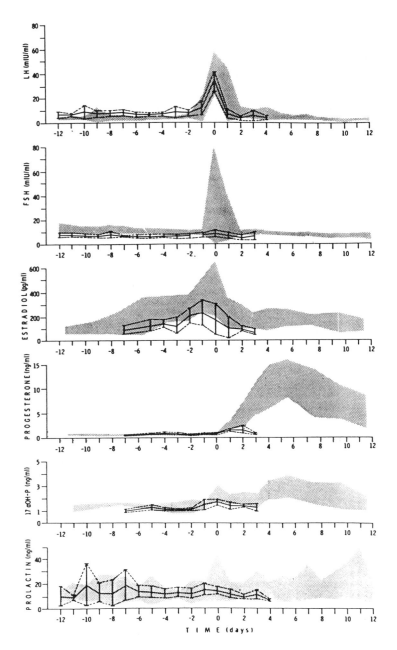

FIGURE 5-9. *Gonadotrophins, prolactin, estradiol, progesterone and 17 alpha-OH progesterone in swimmers with a short or inadequate luteal phase compared with normal control groups (shaded area). (Reprinted from Bonen et al,* J Appl Physiol. *50:545–551, 1981, with permission of the authors and editors.)*

excretion of estradiol and/or progesterone (29). These workers showed no effect of the training program on the reproductive hormonal changes (FSH, LH and estradiol) with exercise.

Initiation of normal menses depends on a pulsatile release of GnRH (195); in 1985, Cumming and colleagues (45) showed almost complete abolition of GnRH, determined by LH pulsatility in six eumenorrheic runners (Fig. 5-10). These workers also reported that other parameters of LH secretion such as pulse frequency, pulse amplitude and area under the LH curve (studied in the early follicular phase) were diminished in the runners, although estradiol was

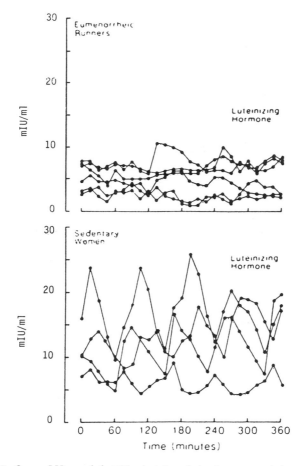

FIGURE 5-10. *Serum LH sampled at 15 min intervals in six eumenorrheic runners showing lack of pulsatility compared with four sedentary controls. (Reproduced from Cumming, D.C. et al, J Clin Endocrinol Metab. 60:810, 1985, with the permission of the author and editor.)*

not significantly different (29.9 ± 5.5 pg·ml^{-1} in runners vs 38.5 ± 2.9 pg·ml^{-1} in controls). The authors concluded that their observations of a hypothalamic defect in athletes who were still menstruating was possibly also the mechanism involved in the more florid primary and secondary amenorrhea in the more susceptible athletes. Thus, "runner's amenorrhea" appears to fit into that class of defect known as "hypothalamic amenorrhea" with abnormalities of GnRH pulsatility (192). Although not all patients with hypothalamic amenorrhea are the same, recent evidence has implicated endogenous opioid inhibition of GnRH pulsatile secretion (199). Infusion of naloxone will increase LH pulse frequency in patients with hypothalamic amenorrhea (178). Long-term use of naloxone, which must be administered intravenously, is impractical, but studies with the oral opiate receptor antagonist naltrexone are presently underway (150). About 65% of athletes who train with long mileage and/or are underweight will recommence menses within one year if they gain weight and reduce their mileage (150).

The search for the male counterpart of exercise-induced hypothalamic amenorrhea has also yielded results. In male athletes undergoing very intense physical training, the very obvious cessation of menses cannot occur, but recently, a suppression of spermatogenesis and testosterone has been documented (4,263). In the most comprehensive study to date, MacConnie and coworkers (145) have demonstrated a subtle hypothalamic-pituitary defect in endurance-trained athletes who were not hypogonadal insofar as they had normal testosterone levels. In this study, the endurance runners had a decreased LH responsiveness to incremental injections of gonadotrophin-releasing hormone when compared with their matched control non-runners (Fig. 5-11). These workers postulated that the difference between their observations and those of Ayers (4) and Wheeler (263) might be that in the latter two studies, severity of exercise training was considerably greater and that their observations (145) represented an intermediate stage in the process of hypothalamic-pituitary-testicular dysfunction. One presumes that the normal physiological pulsatile secretion of LH will also be impaired in such runners.

B. Female Gonadal Hormonal Responses to Exercise—Estradiol and Progesterone

Acute exercise has been found to elevate estradiol and progesterone (124). In this study, for the first time, the importance of the phase of the menstrual cycle was examined and ovulation was confirmed by at least a tenfold increase in plasma progesterone concentration. These observations have been confirmed since by others

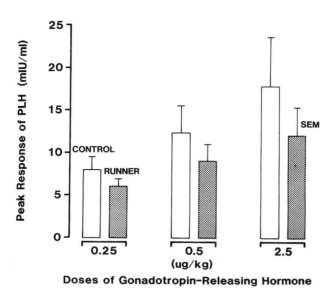

FIGURE 5-11. *Decreased plasma LH response to GnRH in male runners compared with normal controls. Reproduced from MacConnie et al, N Engl J Med. 315:411–417, 1986, with permission of author and editor.)*

(15). Obviously, if there is hypothalamic amenorrhea during endurance exercise, in time, many of the athletes will also become hypoestrogenic with normal levels of prolactin (202). The increase in steroid hormone concentration during exercise was examined by Keizer and coworkers (125) using tritium labelled estradiol; their results showed that a decrease in the metabolic clearance of estradiol occurred during exercise, probably as a result of decreased hepatic blood flow. Plasma testosterone concentration in females, while about one-tenth that of males, nevertheless increases with exercise (230).

C. Males

Androgens, primarily testosterone and dihydrotestosterone, are secreted largely by the testes and to a lesser extent by the adrenal cortex. In a study of the influence of exercise on young athletes, Sutton and coworkers (230) demonstrated a major increase in testosterone. These changes were independent of any changes in LH. These observations have been supported by the more recent findings of Dessypris (52) and Kuoppasalmi (135,136). The contribution of the adrenal cortex to these changes was assessed with a prior injection of beta-methasone to suppress ACTH secretion and while cortisol was inhibited, the androgen responses were unchanged (228).

Catecholamines stimulate the synthesis and secretion of testosterone by the testes and their possible role in other factors causing increases in serum androgens during exercise were examined by the use of alpha and beta blockade, with the result that the plasma androgen concentration remained unchanged (Sutton and Coleman, 1972, unpublished observations).

The increase in serum androgen concentration during exercise independent of LH suggested that this might be related to changes in the metabolism of the hormone and using tritiated testosterone infusion, Sutton and colleagues (229) demonstrated that indeed, this was the case (Fig. 5-12). Not all studies have found increases in testosterone or androgens during exercise. A notable study by Fahey and colleagues (61) examined young subjects, graded them pubertally and looked at the influence of progressive exercise to exhaustion on serum testosterone changes. While there was an increase in testosterone with each pubertal stage, there was only a small, insignificant increase in testosterone with exercise. As mentioned above, during very severe and strenuous exercise, a state of hypothalamic hypogonadism with decreased resting testosterone may occur (263). Endogenous opiates probably have little influence on testosterone increases with exercise; recently, Grossman and colleagues (99) showed no modification of the exercise response using high-dose naloxone in normal subjects.

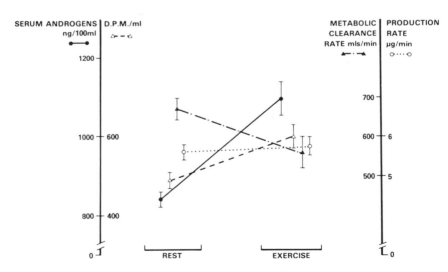

FIGURE 5-12. *Serum androgens, metabolic clearance and production rate of testosterone at rest and during exercise. (Reproduced from Sutton, J.R. et al, 3rd International Symposium on Biochemistry of Exercise, F. Landry and W.A.R. Orban (eds.), Miami, FL: Symposia Specialists Inc., 1978, p. 233, with permission of the editors and publisher.)*

IX. ENDORPHINS AND ENKEPHALINS

The role of endorphins in many physiological responses has been increasingly recognized and the responses to exercise have been discussed in recent reviews (106,222). Although opiates have been used in medicine for several millennia, it was not until the 1970s that technology was sufficiently advanced to examine whether the specific effects of opiates were mediated via opiate-specific receptors. In 1975, Hughes and colleagues (116), using classical pharmacological bioassays, isolated two pentapeptides with opiate-like activity in the pig brain. These were named methionine and leucine enkephalin. (Enkephalin is a Greek word meaning "in the brain.") It was soon recognized that a 91-residue peptide, isolated by Li from the anterior pituitary gland and termed "beta-lipotrophin," contained the methionine enkephalin sequence within its structure. Furthermore, a 31-residue sequence with met-enkephalin at its N-terminal end was also found to have potent opiate activity, more so than in the enkephalins; this was named "beta-endorphin" (endorphin: endogenous morphine). There is a close interrelationship between the enkephalins, endorphins and beta-lipotrophin. Beta-lipotrophin originates from a larger precursor—pro-opiomelanocortin—from which ACTH is also derived. A third class of endogenous opioid peptides—the dynorphins—has now been described. These are extended forms of leucine enkephalin and are among the most potent of the opioid peptides.

Details of the complex bioassays and radioimmunoassays are detailed in the paper by Grossman and Sutton (98). A recent review of endogenous opioid peptides and hypothalamic-pituitary function by Howlett and Rees (114) is seen in the *Annual Review of Physiology*, 1986.

A. The Effect of Exercise on Endorphins and Enkephalins

This has been reviewed in depth recently by Harber and Sutton (106). Most of the studies report that serum concentrations of endogenous opioids, in particular beta-lipotrophin and/or beta-endorphin (B-EP), increase in response to exercise (8,18,32,39,64,75,86, 115,227). Elevations in serum concentrations range from slight to 5-fold above recorded basal concentrations. Few have observed the possibility that the opioids' responses may be intensity-dependent.

Colt and colleagues (39) tested trained long-distance runners and found that in 45% of the subjects, beta-endorphin and beta-lipotrophin plasma concentrations increased during an "easy" run of self-selected pace, whereas 80% of the subjects had elevated beta-endorphin and beta-lipotrophin plasma concentrations after a "strenuous" run of the same distance. In contradiction to this, Farrell and coworkers (64) studied experienced distance runners and found that post-run beta-endorphin and beta-lipotrophin serum concentrations after three different running intensities manipulated on a treadmill did not vary. Recent reports using exercise of varying intensity do not help clarify the question of whether circulating beta-endorphin responds in an intensity-dependent manner. Goldfarb et al (90) found no relationship between percent $\dot{V}O_2$ max and increases in circulating B-EP, while Donevan and Andres (54) found increases in B-EP at workloads above 75% $\dot{V}O_2$ max, but not below that intensity of exercise. During 1 h of exercise at a workload which did not lead to significant peripheral lactate accumulation, DeMeirleir et al (51) found no change in plasma B-EP; however, this same study reports that during exercise to exhaustion (graded increases over a short time interval) significant B-EP accumulates in the blood during exercise and five minutes into recovery. In a recent study by Elias and coworkers (56), an increase was demonstrated in beta-lipotrophin but not in beta-endorphin following acute exercise. The subjects exercised for 20 min at 80% of their predicted maximum heart rates, which would probably be about 70% of their $\dot{V}O_2$ max. Few studies have examined the enkephalin response, but Farrell and coworkers (65,66), and Grossman et al (99) showed no change in trained subjects.

B. The Role of Endogenous Opiates in the Pituitary Hormonal Responses to Exercise

High concentrations of both opioids and their receptors are seen in the median eminence of the hypothalamus and it is not surprising therefore that opiates have been implicated in the regulation or secretion of many pituitary hormones (189). Their influence during exercise, however, is confounded by inappropriate methodology. It is most likely that the changes in hypothalamic concentration of the opiates is most relevant, yet these measurements are impossible to make and it is by implication, using the endorphin antagonist, naloxone, that the role of endorphins on the pituitary hormonal responses to exercise has been obtained. Interpretation is confounded by the exercise protocol, the type and fitness of the individuals studied and the dose of naloxone used. A number of comprehensive studies have analyzed many of the pituitary hormonal responses to exercise, using different doses of naloxone, but have produced variable results. Sutton and coworkers (227), using low-dose naloxone as a single bolus injection, have shown virtually no effect of naloxone on growth hormone, prolactin, TSH, ACTH, beta-lipotrophin or many of the target organ hormones. By contrast, Grossman and colleagues (99), using an 8 mg naloxone bolus followed by an infusion of 5.6 mg·h^{-1}, demonstrated major changes in all the pituitary hormones with an augmentation of prolactin, growth hormone, LH, FSH and ACTH. The one exception to this stimulating effect of naloxone was the observation of a small but statistically significant inhibition of TSH secretion (Table 5-1). More recently, Farrell and coworkers (66), using 50 mg of naltrexone, a long-lasting opioid antagonist administered orally, showed augmentation of the growth hormone, cortisol, glucose and catecholamine responses to exercise.

TABLE 5-1. *Change in circulating hormone with exercise with and without naloxone infusion.*

	SALINE	NALOXONE
Prolactin	123%	198%
G H	263%	802%
L H	57%	104%
F S H	29%	45%
T S H	−30%	−48%
Testosterone	29%	33%
Cortisol	49%	119%
Renin	726%	800%
Aldosterone	216%	298%
Adrenaline	875%	1775%
Noradrenaline	1273%	1372%
MET-enkephalin	32%	2%

From: Grossman, A. et al., (1984)

C. The Effects of Training (Male vs Female Responses) on Endorphins

An augmented effect of 8 weeks training on the endorphin response to exercise was demonstrated by Carr and colleagues (32) in seven females. Studies which have investigated men and women together (87) describe results which show men to have a greater beta-endorphin and beta-lipotrophin response to exercise than women; however, some studies show similar responses in males and females (39,64). There is now general agreement that the endogenous opioid peptides are critically involved in hypothalamic mechanisms governing the release of several pituitary hormones (151). Opioid substances inhibit LH release in adult males (217) and females via the hypothalamic-pituitary axis (194); thus, they may participate in the regulation of gonadotrophin secretion during the menstrual cycle (11,177). Evidence from these reports and others proposes that opioid control throughout the menstrual cycle may vary at different phases of the cycle (62,100,185,262,264).

The effect of training on the endorphin response to subsequent exercise is controversial. A first report by Carr et al (32) suggested that eight weeks of endurance training augments the elevation in circulating beta-endorphin/beta-lipotropin in response to prolonged exercise. Recent data by Howlett et al (115) conflict with this finding since they found no significant change in the B-EP response to prolonged exercise when post-eight week endurance training responses were compared to pre-training responses. The later study agrees with a previous report by Metzger and Stein (153) using treadmill running in rats. It is evident that a fruitful area of research will be the effects of exercise training on the endorphin system. As indicated in previous sections, the adaptation of this peptide system to training may influence endocrine and sympathetic nervous system responses to prolonged exercise.

Some authors have speculated on the role of endorphins in mood alterations consequent to exercise. Studies which have measured mood alterations with exercise and circulating B-EP or enkephalins have failed to show correlational relationships (64,65,67,99,227). Studies which have antagonized EOP during exercise find mood alterations similar to those in control experiments (66,147). One study stands in contrast to this predominant finding. Janal and colleagues (121) found that naloxone (0.8 mg i.v. given twice at 20 min intervals post-exercise) attenuated the elevation in joy and euphoria ratings post-exercise. Plasma beta-endorphin immunoreactivity increased postexercise; however, these increases were not related to mood changes. In summary, most reports fail to support an important role for EOP in mood alterations consequent to exercise. We do not interpret the available data as conclusive in this regard and suggest that better indicators of central nervous system endorphin responses to exercise are required prior to a definitive statement.

Related to this is the question, "do endorphin concentrations measured in the periphery reflect central endorphin activity?". An early indication that there may not be a strong relationship is found in the work of Rossier et al (186) who showed that foot shock in rats causes increases in circulating B-EP with no change in central levels. Metzger and Stein (153) also found elevated circulating B-EP in response to exercise, but no change in the concentration of this peptide in many areas of the brain. More directly related to prolonged exercise is a recent report by Sforzo et al (200) which showed that during two-hour swimming in rats, diprenorphine binding in several brain areas was increased. This group interpreted increased binding as an indication that less endogenous opioid peptides were competing for opioid receptor sites. These central changes occurred simultaneously with marked increases in circulating B-EP. Interestingly, the same trend in binding occurred with one-hour swimming, but the differences were not significantly different from control rats (167). If these findings are verified, it could indicate that opioid action in the brain is dependent upon the duration of exercise and that opioids released peripherally do not enter the central nervous system during prolonged exercise.

X. FLUID AND ELECTROLYTE BALANCE

A. Fluid and Electrolyte Imbalance During Exercise and the Response of Renin-Angiotensin-Aldosterone, Vasopressin and Atrial Natriuretic Factor

The regulation of plasma volume (PV) during a single bout of exercise is complex and depends, among other factors, on exercise intensity and duration. Most commonly, there is a significant reduction in PV with concomitant increases in electrolyte and protein concentrations (40,44,96,242,265), unless the single bout of exercise is prolonged for 8–10 hours (176).

By contrast, most authors have demonstrated that training results in an increase in PV (93,113,128,164). However, a prolonged training period does not appear to be necessary to produce the increase in PV, as Convertino and coworkers (40) have shown that even after three days, a significant elevation in PV occurred. These workers suggested that the training-induced "hypervolemia" was more dependent on the duration of each exercise bout than the total training program. A further subtlety was added by Green and coworkers (93–95) who, using short bursts of supramaximal exercise (120% $\dot{V}O_2$ max), concluded that exercise intensity was an even more important determinant of the hypervolemia than either the length of an individual session or the total duration of the training program.

Thus, it is not surprising that many workers have shown that athletes in a constant state of training have a greater PV than do non-athletes (27,128,205). Such athletes also usually have an increase in red cell mass, but often the increase in PV is proportionally greater resulting in Hb and Hct values which are low or low-normal.

Although the mechanism of hypervolemia is not well understood, it has been observed that total plasma protein increased with training, while plasma protein concentration remained normal (40,129,184). This led Convertino and coworkers (40) to suggest that perhaps an increase in plasma protein, notably albumin, may be the initial factor which gives rise to increased PV, as each gram of protein will, itself, bind 14–15 ml of water (197). For a more detailed review of the various interrelationships of fluid and electrolyte balance in exercise, the reader is referred to the excellent review of Harrison (107).

Any consideration of fluid regulation in exercise requires an appreciation of the Starling force elegantly and precisely documented in 1896 (214). These are expressed mathematically as:

$$F = k \ (P_c - P_i) - (p - i)$$

where F = fluid flow rate

    k = microvascular filtration coefficient, which is equal to the product of the microvascular permeability and microvascular surface area

    P_c = microvascular hydrostatic pressure

    p = plasma colloid osmotic pressure

    i = interstitial fluid colloid osmotic pressure.

In addition to these primary forces in the microvascular bed, there are several intermediate and remote factors which have a bearing on the microvascular fluid flow. Nevertheless, they operate by altering the primary Starling (214) forces and include the following:

-intermediate factors: aortic blood pressure, arterial resistance, venous resistance and right atrial pressure;
-remote factors: norepinephine, which alters arterial resistance and decreases capillary hydrostatic pressure and bradykinin and histamine, which alter the membrane permeability to protein.

B. Hormonal Regulation of Fluids and Electrolytes

Aldosterone is the principal mineralocorticoid involved in sodium regulation. Its secretion is closely linked with that of renin and angiotensin. Exercise at sea level results in a potent increase in renin and aldosterone secretion in both males and females (33,132) and is well demonstrated with prolonged hill walking (157). In females, the phase of the menstrual cycle determines the magnitude of the responses whereby renin, angiotensin and aldosterone all increase to a greater extent in the luteal phase than in the follicular phase (124). The mechanism of secretion of renin is thought to be via beta-adrenergic stimulation. Kotchen and coworkers (132) showed an excellent correlation between catecholamine and renin concentrations. Furthermore, beta receptor blockade greatly diminishes the renin increases (13,105,143). As might be expected, the renin increase will be greater in circumstances of sodium restriction (60,141) and conversely, renin is reduced in response to exercise following a high sodium intake (3). Under most circumstances, the increased renin concentration results in increases in angiotensin (94) and the orderly sequence of events results in an increased secretion of aldosterone (131,146).

A controlled trial with a fixed diet and 6–8 h of hill walking on successive days resulted in marked sodium retention, modest water retention and expansion of the extracellular space (including plasma volume) at the expense of the intracellular space (266). Other studies have shown that these changes were associated with activation of the renin-aldosterone system (157). Although renin is the major stimulus to aldosterone secretion during exercise, under certain circumstances, increases in serum potassium were also implicated (40). Exercise is also a major stimulus to vasopressin (antidiuretic hormone (ADH)) secretion (40,41,97,152,232,253). Although atrial natriuretic factor (ANF) has not been studied in great detail during exercise, preliminary experiments suggest that exercise will also stimulate ANF (163,238). In spite of the fact that the main stimulus to ANF secretion is a distention of the right atrium, no significant increases in right atrial pressure have been reported during exercise (101).

The hormonal responses to heat stress and states of relative dehydration are of particular interest. Under these circumstances, changes which might be expected to mediate internal homeostasis may be put under additional stress. Greenleaf and colleagues (97) found an augmented renin response when exercise was conducted in a hot environment. Studies by Francesconi and coworkers (76,77) showed moderate increases in renin, cortisol, aldosterone and growth hormone during exercise in the heat. Heat acclimatization resulted in expansion of the plasma volume and reduction of the physiological stress of exercise in the heat. Acclimatization also minimized the hormonal response to exercise in the heat (72,76,77) (Fig.5-13). Nevertheless, these are in contrast to the observations of Davies and coworkers (48) who reported that heat acclimatization did not modify the renin and aldosterone responses to exercise in the heat.

The importance of the state of hydration on the hormonal responses to exercise was studied in considerable detail by Francesconi and colleagues (78). The authors examined volunteers under four conditions of hydration: euhydration, 3%, 5% and 7% dehydration. Exercise was prolonged in the heat and in general, there was an increase in plasma renin and aldosterone with exercise and the resting levels of renin-aldosterone, as well as cortisol levels, were higher with more severe degrees of dehydration. Surprisingly, the authors found no difference in responses between 5% and 7% dehydration.

Although we do not have a clear answer in the responses of

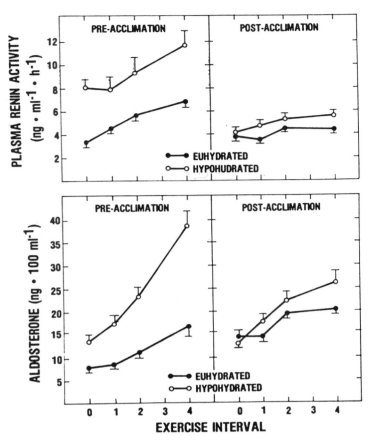

FIGURE 5-13. *The effect of heat acclimatization on the plasma renin and aldosterone responses to exercise in normally hydrated and hypohydrated subjects. (Reprinted from Francesconi et al, J Appl Physiol. 55:1790, 1983, with the permission of the authors and editors.)*

ANF to exercise under thermal and hydration conditions, a clearer picture is emerging of the interrelationship between circulating volume, osmolality, state of hydration and thermal stress, with the hormonal responses attempting to maintain internal homeostasis.

XI. WHAT ARE THE IMPLICATIONS OF THE HORMONAL RESPONSES TO PROLONGED EXERCISE—FOR THE PHYSICIAN, THE COACH, AND THE ATHLETE?

In the past, the major emphasis on hormonal implications for the athlete was the abuse of such hormones as anabolic steroids.

More recently, concerns have been raised regarding the use of growth hormone and in the future, possibly erythropoietin to "blood dope." However, our orientation is the application of physiological and pathophysiological implications from the preceding discussion.

A. Fuel Homeostasis and the Provision of Energy for Exercise

The work of Costill and Miller (43) has shown that when normal healthy athletes take significant carbohydrate immediately prior to exercise, they will have an enhanced insulin response and hypoglycemia may result early in the course of exercise (Fig. 5-14). This has obvious implications for the physician, coach and athlete. Clearly, hypoglycemia can be avoided if a complex carbohydrate such as starch is taken 2–4 h prior to exercise or during exercise itself.

Other considerations for fuel homeostasis concern the many athletes who are diabetics. This topic has been reviewed in considerable detail and practical advice has been given (181,221,250,271).

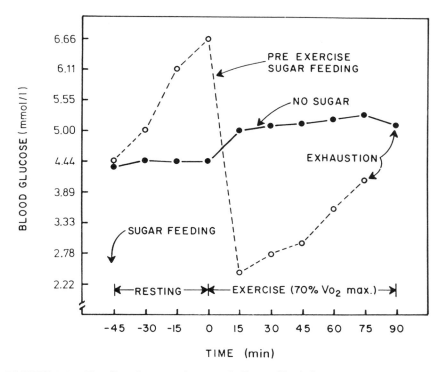

FIGURE 5-14. *The effect of pre-exercise sugar feeding on blood glucose responses to exercise. (Reproduced from Costill, D.L. and J.M. Miller,* Int J Sports Med. 1:2–14, 1980.)

These articles detail the important differences between Type I (juvenile) and Type II (mature) onset diabetics. Of greatest concern, of course, is the Type I diabetic who may require large doses of insulin and careful manipulation of both insulin and diet to prevent the catastrophic changes of sudden hypoglycemia so often noticed in young diabetics. Attention to health, cleanliness, diet and injection site are equally important in the prevention of hypoglycemia and maintenance of optimal health of such athletes. Of slower onset but equally severe consequence is the production of diabetic ketoacidosis. Education of the diabetic athlete will minimize the risk of either of these medical emergencies occurring.

Very few of the other hormonal changes relevant to carbohydrate metabolism have important clinical relevance for the physician, coach or athlete. Excess or diminished cortisol secretion, producing on the one hand Cushing's syndrome and on the other hand Addison's disease, are well known in clinical medicine but have little if any relevance for the athlete. Either condition may be associated with decreased performance and very rarely, hypoadrenal states have been found in athletes. The occasional athlete may be on a short course of high-dose steroids for severe exacerbation of asthma, but it would be unusual for this to result in adrenal suppression or an addisonian-like state. However, short courses of corticosteroids in young active people have resulted in aseptic necrosis of the femoral head and pathological fractures.

There are clinical situations in which there is excessive catecholamine secretion—a pheochromocytoma, often producing abnormalities in carbohydrate metabolism and severe and intermittent hypertension. Such conditions usually result from tumors of the adrenal medulla but also may be associated with tumors anywhere along the sympathetic nerve chain. An excess in growth hormone, if the onset is prior to puberty and the fusion of the epiphyses, will result in gigantism but after puberty, will result in acromegaly. This is usually the result of a tumor of the pituitary gland: chromophobe adenoma. Such tumors are usually slow-growing and the features of acromegaly usually evolve over many years. In the course of the illness, such people may initially have increased strength and do well in competition. However, this is usually short-lived and later a specific skeletal myopathy as well as a cardiomyopathy may develop, rendering the patient weak and prone to develop arrhythmias and cardiac failure. If a person is growth hormone-deficient prior to puberty, he/she will be a dwarf and fall below the third percentile on the growth charts. Such people are not usually athletic.

B. The Reproductive Hormones

This is an interesting and expanding field. Hypothalamic, hypogonadotrophic hypogonadism in athletes is only now being recognized and may be particularly significant in the female for two reasons. If the athlete is hypoestrogenic, there is concern that she also may be infertile and it is not proven whether this infertility is universally reversible. If a state of hypoestrogenism continues for any time, it will predispose the athlete to osteoporosis (55) and some years later, she may have an increased risk of developing fractures, particularly of the hip, spine and distal radius. These conditions in the female are very relevant to the physician, coach and athlete. Although normal menses may resume within one year of ceasing exercise and gaining weight, there may be upwards of 25% of athletes in whom the abnormality remains, with the possibility that they may continue to be infertile.

As our understanding of the mechanisms whereby exercise may induce such changes increases, the importance of good nutrition with adequate calcium in the diet, of maintaining body weight and a normal menstrual cycle is beginning to be appreciated.

While the mechanistic changes affecting the hypothalamus, pituitary and testes may also occur in males and the outcome may also influence fertility, the consequences in terms of the skeleton are less well understood and are not as potentially disastrous as they are in the female who begins adulthood with about 30% less skeletal mass.

SUMMARY

The hormonal changes with severe acute exercise are dramatic but with the exception of the catecholamines, the effects in isolation may be of limited importance. The major role of the norepinephrine response seems to be to maintain circulation. The glucoregulatory hormones serve to prevent hypoglycemia during exercise. There is sufficient redundancy in the system so that unless impairment of more than one of these hormonal regulators occurs, the chance of hypoglycemia is small. Apart from the chance of hypoglycemia, it is the long-term effects of prolonged and intensive exercise which are most dramatic. Evidence is emerging of a significant hypothalamic effect, possibly mediated by endogenous opiates, in which there are subtle changes in hypothalamic pulsatile secretion. The most sensitive hypothalamic hormones appear to be GnRH, CRH and possibly somatostatin. However, it is likely that we will see multiple abnormalities in hypothalamic secretion and the secondary changes of pituitary and endorgans, notably the gonads, during chronic training. This could result in infertility. Although one assumes that all is reversible on cessation or reduction of exercise duration and intensity, that assumption is far from certain. For the female athlete who develops hypothalamic amenorrhea, there may be additional problems if she also becomes hypoestrogenic for a prolonged time. This may lead to eventual osteoporosis and perhaps in later life, fractures of trabecular bone in the lumbar spine and hip, accompanied by considerable pain and disability.

BIBLIOGRAPHY

1. Ahlborg, G., P. Felig, L. Hagenfeldt, R. Hendler and J. Wahren. Substrate turnover during prolonged exercise. *J Clin Invest.* 53:1080–1090, 1974.
2. Ahren, B., G.J. Taborsky and D. Porte, Jr. Neuropeptidergic versus cholinergic and adrenergic regulation of islet hormone secretion. *Diabetologia* 29:827–836, 1986.
3. Aurell, M. and P. Vikgren. Plasma renin activity in supine muscular exercise. *J Appl Physiol.* 31:839–841, 1971.
4. Ayers, J.W., Y. Komesu, T. Romani and R. Ansbacher. Anthropomorphic, hormonal and psychological correlates of semen quality in endurance-trained athletes. *Fertil Steril.* 43:917–921, 1985.
5. Banting, F.G. and C.H. Best. The internal secretion of the pancreas. *J Lab Clin Med.* 7:251–266, 1922.
6. Bealer, S.L., F.J. Haddy, J.N. Diana, G.J. Grega, R.D. Manning, Jr., J.C. Rose and D.S. Gann. Neuroendocrine mechanisms of plasma volume regulation. *Fed Proc.* 45:2455–2463, 1986.
7. Bergman, R.N., D.T. Finegood and M. Ader. Assessment of insulin sensitivity in vivo. *Endocrine Reviews* 6:45–86, 1985.
8. Berk, L.S., S.A. Tan, C.L. Anderson and G. Reiss. Beta-EP response to exercise in athletes and non-athletes. *Med Sci Sports Exerc.* 13:134, 1981.
9. Bjorkman, O., P. Felig, L. Hagenfeldt and J. Wahren. Influence of hypoglucagonemia on splanchnic glucose output during leg exercise in man. *Clin Physiol.* 1:43–57, 1981.
10. Bjornthorp, P., M. Fahlen, G. Grimby, A. Gustafson, J. Holm, P. Renstrom and T. Schersten. Carbohydrate and lipid metabolism in middle-aged physically well-trained men. *Metabolism* 21:1037–1044, 1972.
11. Blankstein, J., F.I. Reyes, J.S.D. Winter and C. Faiman. Endorphins and the regulation of the human menstrual cycle. *Clin Endocrinol.* (Oxford) 14:287–294, 1981.
12. Bloom, S.R., R.H. Johnson, D.M. Park, M.J. Rennie and W.R. Sulaiman. Differences in the metabolic and hormonal response to exercise between racing cyclists and untrained individuals. *J Physiol.* (Lond) 258:1–18, 1976.
13. Bonelli, J., W. Waldhausl, D. Magometschnigg, J. Schwarzmeier, A. Korn and G. Hitzenberger. Effect of exercise and of prolonged oral administration of propranolol on haemodynamic variables, plasma renin concentration, plasma aldosterone and c-AMP. *Eur J Clin Invest.* 7:337–343, 1977.
14. Bonen, A. Effects of exercise on excretion rates of urinary free cortisol. *J Appl Physiol.* 40:155–158, 1976.
15. Bonen, A., A.N. Belcastro, W.Y. Ling and A.A. Simpson. Profiles of selected hormones during menstrual cycles of teenage athletes. *J Appl Physiol.* 50:545–551, 1981.
16. Bonen, A., M.H. Tan, P. Clune and R.L. Kirby. Effects of exercise on insulin binding to human muscle. *Am J Physiol.* 248:E408, 1985.
17. Borer, K.T., D.R. Nicoski and V. Owens. Alteration of pulsatile growth hormone secretion by growth-inducing exercise: Involvement of endogenous opiates and somatostatin. *Endocrinology* 118:844–850, 1986.
18. Bortz, W.M., II, P. Angevin, I.N. Mefford, M.B. Boarder, N. Noyce and J.D. Barchas. Catecholamines, dopamine and endorphin levels during extreme exercise. *N Engl J Med.* 305:466–467, 1981.
19. Bouloux, P.M.G., A. Grossman, S. Al-Damluji, T. Dailey and G.M. Besser. Enhancement

of the sympathoadrenal responses to the cold-pressor test by naloxone in man. *Clin Sci.* 69:365–368, 1985.

20. Bouloux, P.M.G., A. Grossman, N. Lytras and G.M. Besser. Evidence for the participation of endogenous opioids in the sympathoadrenal response to hypoglycaemia in man. *Clin Endocrinol.* 22:49–56, 1985.

21. Boyden, T.W., R.W. Pamenter, P. Stanforth, T. Rotkis and J.H. Wilmore. Sex steroids and endurance running in women. *Fertil Steril.* 39:629–632, 1983.

22. Boyden, T.W., R.W. Pamenter, P. Stanforth, T. Rotkis and J.H. Wilmore. Impaired gonadotrophin releasing hormone stimulation in endurance trained women. *Fertil Steril.* 41:359–363, 1984.

23. Bramnert, M. and B. Hokfelt. Effect of exercise on sympathetic activity and plasma pituitary hormones in naloxone-treated healthy subjects. In: *Central and Peripheral Endorphins: Basic and Clinical Aspects,* E.E. Miller and A.R. Genazzoni, (eds.). New York: Raven Press, 1984, pp 191–194.

24. Brandenberger, G. and M. Follenius. Influence of timing and intensity of muscular exercise on temporal patterns of plasma cortisol levels. *J Clin Endocrinol Metab.* 40:845–849, 1975.

25. Brandenberger, G., M. Follenius and B. Hietter. Feedback from meal-related peaks determines diurnal changes in cortisol response to exercise. *J Clin Endocrinol Metab.* 54:592–596, 1982.

26. Brisson, G.R., F. Malaisse-Lagae and W.J. Malaisse. Effect of phentolamine upon insulin secretion during exercise. *Diabetologia* 7:223–226, 1971.

27. Brotherhood, J., B. Brozovic and L.G.C.E. Pugh. Haemotological status of middle- and long-distance runners. *Clin Sci Mol Med.* 48:139–145, 1975.

28. Brown, M.J., D.A. Jenner, D.J. Allison and C.T. Dollery. Variations in individual organ release of noradrenaline measured by an improved radioenzymatic technique: Limitations of peripheral venous measurements in the assessment of sympathetic nervous activity. *Clin Sci.* 61:585–590, 1981.

29. Bullen, B.A., G.S. Skrinar, I.Z. Beitins, D.B. Carr, S.M. Reppert, C.O. Dotson, M. de M. Fencl, E.V. Gervino and J.W. McArthur. Endurance training effects on plasma hormonal responsiveness and sex hormone excretion. *J Appl Physiol.* 56:1453–1463, 1984.

30. Bunt, J.C. Hormonal alterations due to exercise. *Sports Med.* 3:331–345, 1986.

31. Burstein, R., C. Polychronakos, C.J. Toews, J.D. MacDougall, H.J. Guyda and B.I. Posner. Acute reversal of the enhanced insulin action in trained athletes. Association with insulin receptor changes. *Diabetes* 34:756–760, 1985.

32. Carr, D.B., B.A. Bullen, G.S. Skrinar, M.A. Arnold, M. Rosenblatt, I.Z. Beitins, J.B. Martin and J.W. McArthur. Physical conditioning facilitates the exercise-induced secretion of beta-endorphin and beta-lipotropin in women. *N Engl J Med.* 305:560–563, 1981.

33. Casanueva, F.F., L. Villanueva, J.A. Cabranes, J. Cabezas-Cerrato and A. Fernandez-Cruz. Cholinergic mediation of growth hormone secretion elicited by arginine, clonidine, and physical exercise in man. *J Endocrinol Metab.* 59:526–530, 1984.

34. Cashmore, G.C., C.T.M. Davies and J.D. Few. Relationship between increases in plasma cortisol concentration and rate of cortisol secretion during exercise in man. *J Endocrinol.* 72:109–110, 1977.

35. Chisholm, D.J., A.B. Jenkins, D.E. James and E.W. Kraegen. The effect of hyperinsulinemia on glucose homeostasis during moderate exercise in man. *Diabetes* 31:603–608, 1982.

36. Christensen, N.J. and O. Brandsborg. The relationship between plasma catecholamine concentration and pulse rate during exercise and standing. *Eur J Clin Invest.* 3:299–306, 1973.

37. Christensen, N.J. and H. Galbo. Sympathetic nervous activity during exercise. *Ann Rev Physiol.* 45:139–153, 1983.

38. Christensen, E.H. and O. Hansen. Arbeitsfahigkeit und ernahrung. *Skand Arch Physiol.* 81:160–171, 1939.

39. Colt, E.W.D., S.L. Wardlaw and A.G. Frantz. The effect of running on plasma beta-endorphin. *Life Sciences* 28:1637–1640, 1981.

40. Convertino, V.A., P.J. Brock, L.C. Keil, E.M. Bernauer and J.E. Greenleaf. Exercise training-induced hypervolemia: Role of plasma albumin, renin and vasopressin. *J Appl Physiol.* 48:665–669, 1980.

41. Convertino, V.A., L.C. Keil, E.M. Bernauer and J.E. Greenleaf. Plasma volume, osmolality, vasopressin and renin activity during graded exercise in man. *J Appl Physiol.* 50:123–128, 1981.

42. Cornil, A., A. DeCoster, G. Copinschi and J.R.M. Franckson. The effect of muscular exercise on the plasma cortisol level in man. *Acta Endocrinol.* 48:163–168, 1965.

43. Costill D.L. and J.M. Miller. Nutrition for endurance sports: Carbohydrate and fluid balance. *Int J Sports Med.* 1:2–14, 1980.

44. Costill, D.L., G. Branam, W. Fink and R. Nelson. Exercise induced sodium conservation. *Med Sci Sports* 8:209–213, 1976.
45. Cumming, D.C., M.M. Vickovic, S.R. Wall and M.R. Fluker. Defects in pulsatile LH release in normally menstruating runners. *J Clin Endocrinol Metab.* 60:810–812, 1985.
46. Dale, E., D.H. Gerlach and A.L. Wilhite. Menstrual dysfunction in distance runners. *Obstet Gynecol.* 54:47–53, 1979.
47. Davies, C.T.M. and J.D. Few. Effects of exercise on adrenocortical function. *J Appl Physiol.* 35:887–891, 1973.
48. Davies, J.A., M.H. Harrison, L.A. Cochrane, R.J. Edwards and T.M. Gibson. Effect of saline loading during heat acclimation on adrenocortical hormone levels. *J Appl Physiol.* 50:605–612, 1981.
49. DeFronzo, R.A., E. Ferrannini, Y. Sato, P. Felig and J. Wahren. Synergistic interaction between exercise and insulin on peripheral glucose uptake. *J Clin Invest.* 68:1468–1474, 1981.
50. DeFronzo, R.A., J.D. Tobin and A. Reubin. Glucose clamp technique: A method for quantifying insulin secretion and resistance. *Am J Physiol.* 237:E214–E223, 1979.
51. DeMeirleir, K., N. Naaktgeboren, A. Van Steirteghem, F. Gorus, J. Olbrecht and P. Block. Beta endorphin and ACTH levels in peripheral blood during and after aerobic and anaerobic exercise. *Eur J Appl Physiol.* 55:5–8, 1986.
52. Dessypris, A., K. Kuoppasalmi and H. Adlercreutz. Plasma cortisol, testosterone, androstenedione and luteinizing hormone (LH) in a non-competitive marathon run. *J Steroid Biochem.* 7:33–37, 1976.
53. Devlin, J.G. The effect of training and acute physical exercise on plasma insulin-like activity. *Irish J Med Sci.* 6:423–425, 1963.
54. Donevan, R.H. and G.M. Andres. Plasma B-endorphin immunoreactivity during graded cycle ergometry. *Med Sci Sports Exerc.* 19:229–230, 1987.
55. Drinkwater, B.L., K. Nilson, C.H. Chestnut, III, W. Bremmer, S. Shainholtz and M. Southworth. Bone mineral content of amenorrheic and eumenorrheic athletes. *N Engl J Med.* 311:277–281, 1984.
56. Elias, A.N., K. Iyer, M.R. Pandian, P. Weathersbee, S. Stone and J. Tobis. Beta-endorphin/beta-lipotropin release and gonadotropin secretion after acute exercise in normal males. *J Appl Physiol.* 61:2045–2049, 1986.
57. Esler, M., G. Jennings, P. Korner, P. Blombery, N. Sacharias and P. Leonard. Measurement of total and organ-specific norepinephrine kinetics in humans. *Am J Physiol.* 247:E21–E28, 1984.
58. Erydelyi, G. Gynecologic survey of female athletes. *J Sports Med Phys Fitness* 2:174–179, 1962.
59. Faber, O.K., C. Hagen, C. Binder, J. MarKussen, V.K. Naithani, P.M. Blix, H. Kuzuya, D. Horwitz and A.H. Rubenstein. Kinetics of human connecting peptide in normal and diabetic subjects. *J Clin Invest.* 62:197–203, 1978.
60. Fagard, R., A. Amery, T. Reybrouck, P. Lijnen, E. Moerman, M. Bogaert and A. De Schaepdryver. Effects of angiotensin antagonism on hemodynamics, renin, and catecholamines during exercise. *J Appl Physiol.* 43:440–444, 1977.
61. Fahey, T.D., A. Del Valle-Zuris, G. Oehlsen, M. Trieb and J. Seymour. Pubertal stage differences in hormonal and hematological responses to maximal exercise in males. *J Appl Physiol.* 46:823–827, 1979.
62. Faiman, C., J. Blankstein, F.I. Reyes and J.S.D. Winter. Endorphins and the regulation of the human menstrual cycle. *Fertil Steril.* 36:267–268, 1981.
63. Farrell, P.A., T.L. Garthwaite and A.B. Gustafson. Plasma adrenocorticotropin and cortisol responses to submaximal and exhaustive exercise. *J Appl Physiol.* 55:1441–1444, 1983.
64. Farrell, P.A., W.K. Gates, W.P. Morgan and M.G. Maksud. Increases in plasma beta-EP and beta-LPH immunoreactivity after treadmill running in humans. *J Appl Physiol.* 52:1245–1249, 1982.
65. Farrell, P.A., W.K. Gates, W.P. Morgan and C.B. Pert. Plasma leucine enkephalin-like radioreceptor activity and tension-anxiety before and after competitive running. In: *Biochemistry of Exercise*, H.G. Knuttgen, J.A. Vogel and J. Poortmans (eds.). Champaign, IL: Human Kinetics, 1983, pp 637–644.
66. Farrell, P.A., A.B. Gustafson, T.L. Garthwaite, R.K. Kalkhoff, A.W. Cowley, Jr. and W.P. Morgan. Influence of endogenous opioids on the response of selected hormones to exercise in humans. *J Appl Physiol.* 61:1051–1057, 1986.
67. Farrell, P.A., A.B. Gustafson, W.P. Morgan and C.B. Pert. Enkephalins, catecholamines and psychological mood alterations: Effects of prolonged exercise. *Med Sci Sports Exerc.* 1988. (In press).
68. Farrell, P.A., K.J. Mikines, B. Sonne and H. Galbo. Studies on the influence of endogenous opiates on insulin secretion in rats following exercise using the hyperglycemic clamp technique. *Clin Physiol.* 5:(Suppl 4) Abs. No. 63, 1985.

69. Feicht, C.B., T.S. Johnson, B.J. Martin, K.E. Sparkes and W.W. Wagner. Secondary amenorrhea in athletes. *Lancet* ii:1145–1156, 1978.
70. Felig, P., A. Cherif, A. Minagawa and J. Wahren. Hypoglycemia during prolonged exercise in normal men. *N Engl J Med.* 306:895–900, 1982.
71. Few, J.D. Effect of exercise on the secretion and metabolism of cortisol in man. *J Endocrinol.* 62:341–353, 1974.
72. Finberg, J.P.M. and G.M. Berlyne. Modification of renin and aldosterone: Response to heat by acclimation in man. *J Appl Physiol.* 42:554–558, 1977.
73. Fleg, J.L., S.P. Tzankoff and E.G. Lakatta. Age-related augmentation of plasma catecholamines during dynamic exercise in healthy males. *J Appl Physiol.* 59:1033–1039, 1985.
74. Fotherby, K. and S.B. Pal. Exercise Endocrinology. Berlin: de Gruyter, 1985.
75. Fraioli, F., C. Moretti, D. Paolucci, E. Alicicco, G. Crescenzi and G. Fortunio. Physical exercise stimulates marked concomitant release of beta-endorphin and ACTH in peripheral blood in man. *Experientia* 36:987–989, 1980.
76. Francesconi, R.P., M.N. Sawka and K.B. Pandolf. Hypohydration and heat acclimation: Plasma renin and aldosterone during exercise. *J Appl Physiol.* 55:1790–1794, 1983.
77. Francesconi, R.P., M.N. Sawka and K.B. Pandolf. Hypohydration and acclimation: Effects on hormone responses to exercise/heat stress. *Aviat Space Environ Med.* 55:365–369, 1984.
78. Francesconi, R.P., M.N. Sawka, B. Pandolf, R.W. Hubbard, A.J. Young and S. Muza. Plasma hormone responses at graded hypohydration levels during exercise in heat stress. *J Appl Physiol.* 59:1855–1860, 1985.
79. Franckson, J.R.M., R. Vanroux, R. Leclercq, H. Brunengraber and H.A. Ooms. Labeled insulin catabolism and pancreatic responsiveness during long-term exercise in man. *Horm Metab Res.* 3:366–373, 1971.
80. Frisch, R.E., G. Wyshak and L. Vincent. Delayed menarche and amenorrhea in ballet dancers. *N Engl J Med.* 303:17–19, 1980.
81. Galbo, H. Catecholamines and muscular exercise: Assessment of sympathoadrenal activity. In: *Biochemistry of Exercise IVB,* J.R. Poortmans and G.Niset (eds.). Baltimore: University Park Press, 1981, pp 5-19.
82. Galbo, H. *Hormonal and Metabolic Adaptations to Exercise,* Stuttgart: Thieme Verlag, 1983.
83. Galbo, H., N.J. Christensen and J.J. Holst. Catecholamines and pancreatic hormones during autonomic blockade in exercising man. *Acta Physiol Scand.* 101:428–437, 1977.
84. Galbo, H., J.J. Holst and N.J. Christensen. Glucagon and plasma catecholamine responses to graded and prolonged exercise in man. *J Appl Physiol.* 38:70–76, 1975.
85. Galbo, H., M. Kjaer and N.H. Secher. Cardiovascular, ventilatory and catecholamine responses to maximal dynamic exercise in partially curarized man. *J Physiol.* (Lond), 1987 (In press).
86. Gambert, S.R., T.L. Garthwaite, C.H. Pontzer, E.E. Cook, F.E. Tristani, E.H. Duthie, D.R. Martinson, T.C. Hagen and D.J. McCarty. Running elevates plasma beta-endorphin immunoreactivity and ACTH in untrained human subjects. *Proc Soc Exp Biol Med.* 168:1–4, 1981.
87. Gambert, S.R., T.C. Hagen, T.L. Garthwaite, E.H. Duthie, Jr. and D.J. McCarty. Exercise and the endogenous opioids. *N Engl J Med.* 305:1590–1592, 1981.
88. Gold, P.W., H. Gwirtsman, P.C. Avgerinos, L.K. Nieman, W.T. Gallucci, W. Kaye, D. Jimerson, M. Ebert, R. Rittmaster, D.L. Loriaux and G.P. Chrousos. Abnormal hypothalamic-pituitary-adrenal function in anorexia nervosa: Pathophysiologic mechanisms in underweight and weight-corrected patients. *N Engl J Med.* 314:1335–1342, 1986.
89. Gold, P.W., D.L. Loriaux, A. Roy, M.A. Kling, J.R. Calabrese, C.H. Kellner, L.K. Nieman, R.M. Post, D. Pickar, W. Gallucci, P. Avgerinos, S. Paul, E.H. Oldfield, G.B. Cutler and G.P. Chrousos. Responses to corticotropin-releasing hormone on the hypercortisolism of depression and Cushing's disease: Pathophysiologic and diagnostic implications. *N. Engl J Med.* 314:1329–1335, 1986.
90. Goldfarb, A.H., B.D. Hatfield, G.A. Sforzo and M.G. Flynn. Serum B-endorphin levels during a graded exercise test to exhaustion. *Med Sci Sports Exerc.* 19:78–82, 1987.
91. Gollnick, P.D. Energy metabolism and skeletal muscle function during prolonged exercise. In: *Perspectives in Exercise Science and Sports Medicine,* D.R. Lamb and R. Murray (eds.). Indianapolis: Benchmark Press, 1988.
92. Gollnick, P.D., R.G. Soule, A.W. Taylor, C. Williams and C.D. Ianuzzo. Exercise-induced glycogenolysis and lipolysis in the rat: Hormonal influence. *Am J Physiol.* 219:729–733, 1970.
93. Green, H.J., A. Thomson, M.E. Ball, R.L. Hughson, M.E. Houston and M.T. Sharratt. Alterations in blood volume following short-term supramaximal exercise. *J Appl Physiol.* 56:145–149, 1984.
94. Green, H.J., R.L. Hughson, J.A. Thomson and M.T. Sharratt. Supramaximal exercise after training-induced hypervolemia. I. Gas exchange and acid-base balance. *J Appl Physiol.* 62:1944–1953, 1987.

ENDOCRINE FUNCTION AND PROLONGED EXERCISE **201**

95. Green, H.J., J.A. Thomson and M.E. Houston. Supramaximal exercise after training-induced hypervolemia. II. Blood/muscle substrates and metabolites. *J Appl Physiol.* 62:1954–1961, 1987.
96. Greenleaf, J.E., E.M. Bernauer, H.L. Young, J.T. Morse, R.W. Staley, L.T. Juhos and W. Van Beaumont. Fluid and electrolyte shifts during bed rest with isometric and isotonic exercise. *J Appl Physiol.* 42:59–66, 1977.
97. Greenleaf, J.E., D. Sciaraffa, E. Shvartz, L.C. Keil and P.J. Brock. Exercise training hypotension: Implications for plasma volume, renin, and vasopressin. *J Appl Physiol.* 51:298–305, 1981.
98. Grossman, A. and J.R. Sutton. Endorphins: What are they? How are they measured? What is their role in exercise? *Med Sci Sports Exerc.* 17:74–81, 1985.
99. Grossman, A., P. Bouloux, P. Price, P.L. Drury, K.S.L. Lam, T. Turner, J. Thomas, G.M. Besser and J. Sutton. The role of opioid peptides in the hormonal responses to acute exercise in man. *Clin Sci.* 67:483–491, 1984.
100. Grossman, A., P.J.A. Moult, H. McIntyre, J. Evans, T. Silverstone, L.H. Rees and G.M. Besser. Opiate mediation of amenorrhea in hyperprolactinaemia and in weight-loss related amenorrhea. *Clin Endocrinol.* (Oxford) 17:379–388, 1982.
101. Groves, B.M., J.T. Reeves, J.R. Sutton, P.D. Wagner, A. Cymerman, M.K. Malconian, P.B. Rock, P.M. Young and C.S. Houston. Operation Everest II: Elevated high altitude pulmonary resistance unresponsive to oxygen. *J Appl Physiol.* 63:521–530, 1987.
102. Hansen, A.P. The effect of intravenous glucose infusion on the exercise- induced serum growth hormone rise in normals and juvenile diabetics. *Scand J Clin Lab Invest.* 28:195–205, 1971.
103. Hansen, A.P. The effect of intravenous infusion of lipids on the exercise-induced serum growth hormone rise in normals and juvenile diabetics. *Scand J Clin Lab Invest.* 28:207–212, 1971.
104. Hansen, A.P. The effect of adrenergic receptor blockade on the exercise- induced serum growth hormone rise in normals and juvenile diabetics. *J Clin Endocrinol.* 33:807–812, 1971.
105. Hansson, B.-G. and B. Hokfelt. Long-term treatment of moderate hypertension with penbutolol (Hoe 893d). I. Effects on blood pressure, pulse rate, catecholamines in blood and urine, plasma renin activity and urinary aldosterone under basal conditions and following exercise. *Eur J Clin Pharmacol.* 9:9–19, 1975.
106. Harber, V.J. and J.R. Sutton. Endorphins and exercise. *Sports Med.* 1:154–171, 1984.
107. Harrison, M.H. Effects of thermal stress and exercise on blood volume in humans. *Physiol Rev.* 65:149–199, 1985.
108. Hartley, L.H., J.W. Mason, R.P. Hogan, L.G. Jones, T.A. Kotchen, E.H. Mougey, F.E. Wherry, L.L. Pennington and P.T. Ricketts. Multiple hormonal responses to graded exercise in relation to physical training. *J Appl Physiol.* 33:602–606, 1972.
109. Hartley, L.H., J.W. Mason, R.P. Hogan, L.G. Jones, T.A. Kotchen, E.H. Mougey, F.E. Wherry, L.L. Pennington and P.T. Ricketts. Multiple hormonal responses to prolonged exercise in relation to physical training. *J Appl Physiol.* 33:607–610, 1972.
110. Ho, K.Y., W.S. Evans, R.M. Blizzard, J.D. Veldhuis, G.R. Merriam, E. Samojlik, R. Furlanetto, A.D. Rogol, D.L. Kaiser and M.O. Thorner. Effects of sex and age on the 24-hour profile of growth hormone secretion in man: Importance of endogenous estradiol concentrations. *J Clin Endocrinol Metab.* 64:51–57, 1987.
111. Hoelzer, D.R., G.P. Dalsky, W.E. Clutter, S.D. Shah, J.O. Holloszy and P.E. Cryer. Glucoregulation during exercise: Hypoglycemia is prevented by redundant glucoregulatory systems, sympathochromaffin activation, and changes in islet hormone secretion. *J Clin Invest.* 77:212–221, 1986.
112. Hoelzer, D.R., G.P. Dalsky, N.S. Schwartz, W.E. Clutter, S.D. Shah, J.O. Holloszy and P.E. Cryer. Epinephrine is not critical to prevention of hypoglycemia during exercise in humans. *Am J Physiol.* 251:E104–E110, 1986.
113. Holmgren, A., F. Mossfeldt, T. Sjostrand and G. Strom. Effect of training on work capacity, total hemoglobin, blood volume, heart volume and pulse rate in recumbant and upright position. *Acta Physiol Scand.* 50:72–83, 1960.
114. Howlett, T.A. and L.H. Rees. Endogenous opioid peptides and hypothalamo-pituitary function. In: *Annual Review of Physiology* 48, R.M. Berne (ed.). Palo Alto: Annual Reviews Inc., 1986, pp 613–623.
115. Howlett, T.A., S. Tomlin, L. Ngahfoong, L.H. Rees, B.A. Bullen, G.S. Skrinar and J.W. McArthur. Release of beta-endorphin and met-enkephalin during exercise in normal women: Response to training. *Br Med J.* 288:1950–1952, 1984.
116. Hughes, J., T.W. Smith, H.W. Kosterlitz, L.A. Fothergill, B.A. Morgan and H.R. Morris. Identification of two related pentapeptides from the brain with potent opiate agonist activity. *Nature* 258:577–579, 1975.
117. Hunter, W.M. and F.C. Greenwood. Studies on the secretion of human pituitary growth hormone. *Br Med J.* 1:804–806, 1965.

202 *PERSPECTIVES IN EXERCISE*

118. Hunter, W.M. and M.Y. Sakkar. Changes in plasma insulin levels during muscular exercise. *Proc Physiol Soc.* 110P–112P, Feb., 1968.
119. James, D.E., E.W. Kraegen and D.J. Chisholm. Effects of exercise training on in vivo insulin action in individual tissues of the rat. *J Clin Invest.* 76:657–666, 1985.
120. James, D.E., K.M. Burleigh, E.W. Kraegen and D.J. Chisholm. Effects of acute exercise and prolonged training on insulin response to intravenous glucose in vivo in rats. *J Appl Physiol.* 55:1660–1664, 1983.
121. Janal, M.N., E.W.D. Colt, W.C. Clark and M. Glusman. Pain sensitivity, mood and plasma endocrine levels in man following long-distance running: Effects of naloxone. *Pain* 19:13–25, 1984.
122. Jarhult, J. and J. Holst. The role of the adrenergic innervation to the pancreatic islets in the control of insulin release during exercise in man. *Pflueger's Arch.* 383:41–45, 1979.
123. Jenkins, A.B., D.J. Chisholm, D.E. James, K.Y. Ho and E.W. Kraegen. Exercise-induced hepatic glucose output is precisely sensitive to the rate of systemic glucose supply. *Metabolism* 34:431–436, 1985.
124. Jurkowski, J., E. Younglai, C. Walker, N.L. Jones and J.R. Sutton. Ovarian hormone response to exercise. *J Appl Physiol.* 44:109–114, 1978.
125. Keizer, H.A., J. Poortmans and J. Bunniks. Influence of physical exercise on sex hormone metabolism. *J Appl Physiol.* 50:545–551, 1981.
126. Kjaer, M., N.J. Christensen, B. Sonne, E.A. Richter and H. Galbo. Effect of exercise on epinephrine turnover in trained and untrained male subjects. *J Appl Physiol.* 59:1061–1067, 1985.
127. Kjaer, M., P.A. Farrell, N.J. Christensen and H. Galbo. Increased epinephrine response and inaccurate glucoregulation in exercising athletes. *J Appl Physiol.* 61:1693–1700, 1986.
128. Kjellberg, S.R., U. Rudhe and T. Sjostrand. Increase of the amount of hemoglobin and blood volume in connection with physical training. *Acta Physiol Scand.* 19:146–151, 1949.
129. Koch, G. and L. Rocker. Plasma volume and intravascular protein masses in trained boys and fit young men. *J Appl Physiol.* 43:1085–1088, 1977.
130. Koivisto, V.A., V.R. Soman and P. Felig. Effects of acute exercise on insulin binding to monocytes in obesity. *Metabolism* 29:168–172, 1980.
131. Kosunen, K., A. Pakarinen, K. Kuoppasalmi, H. Naveri, S. Rehunen, C.G. Standerskjold-Nordenstam, M. Harkonen and H. Adlercreutz. Cardiovascular function and the renin-angiotensin-aldosterone system in long-distance runners during various training periods. *Scand J Clin Lab Invest.* 40:429–435, 1980.
132. Kotchen, T.A., L.H. Hartley, T.W. Rice, E.H. Mougey, L.G. Jones and J.W. Mason. Renin, norepinephrine, and epinephrine responses to graded exercise. *J Appl Physiol.* 31:178–184, 1971.
133. Krotkiewski, M., P. Bjorntorp, G. Holm, V. Marks, L. Morgan, V. Smith and G.E. Glurle. Effects of physical training on insulin, connecting peptide (C-peptide), gastric inhibitory polypeptide (GIP) and pancreatic polypeptide (PP) levels in obese subjects. *Int J Obesity* 8:193–199, 1984.
134. Krotkiewski, M. and J. Gorski. Effect of muscular exercise on plasma C-peptide and insulin in obese non-diabetics and diabetics, Type II. *Clin Physiol.* 6:499–506, 1986.
135. Kuoppasalmi, K., H. Naveri, M. Harkonen and H. Adlercreutz. Plasma cortisol, androstenedione, testosterone and luteinizing hormone in running exercise of different intensities. *Scand J Clin Lab Invest.* 40:403–409, 1980.
136. Kuoppasalmi, K., H. Naveri, S. Rehunen, M. Harkonen and H. Adlercreutz. Effect of strenuous anaerobic running exercise on plasma growth hormone, cortisol, luteinizing hormone, testosterone, androstenedione, estrone and estradiol. *J Steroid Biochem.* 7:823–829, 1976.
137. Lam, K.S.L., A. Grossman, P. Bouloux, P.L. Drury and G.M. Besser. Effect of an opiate antagonist on the responses of circulating catecholamines and the renin-aldosterone system to acute sympathetic stimulation by hand-grip in man. *Acta Endocrinol.* 111:152–157, 1986.
138. Lamberts, S.W.J., E.N.W. Janssens, E.G. Bons, P. Uitterlinden, J.M. Zuiderwijk and E. Del Pozo. The met-enkephalin analog FK 33-284 directly inhibits ACTH release by the rat pituitary gland in vitro. *Life Sci.* 32:1167–1173, 1983.
139. Lavoie, J.-M., N. Dionne, R. Helie and G.R. Brisson. Menstrual cycle phase dissociation of blood glucose homeostasis during exercise. *J Appl Physiol.* 1084–1089, 1987.
140. LeBlanc, J., A. Nadeau, M. Boulay and S. Rousseau-Migneron. Effects of physical training and adiposity on glucose metabolism and 125I-insulin binding. *J Appl Physiol.* 46:235–239, 1979.
141. Leenen, F.H.H., P. Boer and G.G. Geyskes. Sodium intake and the effects of isoproterenol and exercise on plasma renin in man. *J Appl Physiol.* 45:870–874, 1978.
142. Levine, S.A., B. Gordon and C.L. Derick. Some changes in the chemical constituents of the blood following a marathon race. *JAMA.* 82:1778–1779, 1924.

143. Lijnen, P.J., A.K. Amery, R.H. Fagard, T.M. Reybrouck, E.J. Moerman and A.F. De Schaepdryver. The effects of beta-adrenoceptor blockade on renin, angiotensin, aldosterone and catecholamines at rest and during exercise. Br J Clin Pharm. 7:175–181, 1979.

144. Luger, A., P.A. Deuster, S.B. Kyle, W.T. Gallucci, L.C. Montgomery, P.W. Gold, D.L. Loriaux and G.P. Chrousos. Acute hypothalamic-pituitary-adrenal responses to the stress of treadmill exercise: Physiologic adaptations to physical training. N Engl J Med. 316:1309–1315, 1987.

145. MacConnie, S.E., A. Barkan, R.M. Lampman, M.A. Schork and I.Z. Beitins. Decreased hypothalamic gonadotropin-releasing hormone secretion in male marathon runners. N Engl J Med. 315:411–417, 1986.

146. Maher, J.T., L.G. Jones, L.H. Hartley, G.H. Williams and L.I. Rose. Aldosterone dynamics during graded exercise at sea level and high altitude. J Appl Physiol. 39:18–22, 1975.

147. Markoff, R.A., P. Ryan and T. Young. Endorphins and mood changes in long distance running. Med Sci Sports Exerc. 14:11–15, 1982.

148. Marshall, J.C. and R.P. Kelch. Gonadotrophin-releasing hormone: Role of pulsatile secretion in the regulation of reproduction. N Engl J Med. 315:1459–1468, 1986.

149. Mayer, G., J. Wessel and J. Kobberling. Failure of naloxone to alter exercise-induced growth hormone and prolactin release in normal men. Clin Endocrinol. (Oxford) 13:413–416, 1980.

150. McArthur, J.W., B.A. Bullen, I.Z. Beitens, M. Pagano, T.M. Badger and A. Klibanski. Hypothalamic amenorrhea in runners of normal body composition. Endocrine Res Comm. 7:13–25, 1980.

151. Meites, J. Relation of endogenous opioid peptides to secretion of hormones. Fed Proc. 39:2531–2532, 1980.

152. Melin, B., J.P. Eclache, G. Geelen, G. Annat, A.M. Allevard, E. Jarsaillon, A. Zebidi, J.J. Legros and C. Gharib. Plasma AVP, neurophysin, renin activity and aldosterone during submaximal exercise performed until exhaustion in trained and untrained men. Eur J Appl Physiol. 44:141–151, 1980.

153. Metzger, J.M. and E.A. Stein. Beta-endorphin and sprint training. Life Sci. 34:1541–1547, 1984.

154. Michel, G., T. Vocke, W. Fish, H. Weicker, W. Schwarz and W.P. Bieger. Bidirectional alteration in insulin receptor affinity by different forms of physical exercise. Am J Physiol. 246:E153–E159, 1984.

155. Mikines, K.J., B. Sonne, P.A. Farrell and H. Galbo. Insulin sensitivity and responsiveness after acute exercise. Med Sci Sports Exerc. 17:242, 1985.

156. Mikines, K.J., P.A. Farrell, B. Sonne and H. Galbo. Glucose dose response curve for plasma insulin after exercise in man. Clin Physiol. (Suppl 4):1985.

157. Milledge, J.S., E.I. Bryson, D.M. Catley, R. Hesp, N. Luff, B.D. Minty, M.W.J. Older, N.N. Payne, M.P. Ward and W.R. Withey. Sodium balance, fluid homeostasis and the renin-aldosterone system during the prolonged exercise of hill walking. Clin Sci. 62:595–604, 1982.

158. Mondon, C.E., C.B. Dolkas and G.M. Reaven. Site of enhanced insulin sensitivity in exercise-trained rats at rest. Am J Physiol. 239:E169–E177, 1980.

159. Moretti, C., A. Fabbri, L. Gnessi, M. Cappa, A. Calzolari, F. Fraioli, A. Grossman and G.M. Besser. Naloxone inhibits exercise-induced release of PRL and GH in athletes. Clin Endocrinol. (Oxford) 18:135–138, 1983.

160. Newmark, S.R., T. Himathongkam, R.P. Martin, K.H. Cooper and L.I. Rose. Adrenocortical response to marathon running. J Clin Endocrinol Metab. 42:393–394, 1976.

161. Niall, H.D. Revised primary structure for human growth hormone. Nat N Biol. (Lond) 230:90, 1971.

162. Nikkila, E.A., M.-R. Taskinen, T.A. Meittinen, R. Pelkonen and H. Poppius. Effect of muscular exercise on insulin secretion. Diabetes 17:209–218, 1968.

163. Nishikimi, T., M. Kohno, T. Matsuura, K. Akioka, M. Teragaki, M. Yasuda, H. Oku, K. Takeuchi and T. Takeda. Effect of exercise on circulating atrial natriuretic polypeptide in valvular heart disease. Am J Cardiol. 58:1119–1120, 1986.

164. Oscai, L.B., B.T. Williams and B.A. Hertig. Effect of exercise on blood volume. J Appl Physiol. 24:622–624, 1968.

165. Pederson, O., H. Beck-Nielsen and L. Heding. Increased insulin receptors after exercise in patients with insulin-dependent diabetes mellitus. N Engl J Med. 302:886–892, 1980.

166. Peronnet, F., J. Cleroux, H. Perrault, D. Cousineau, J. de Champlain and R. Nadeau. Plasma norepinephrine response to exercise before and after training in humans. J Appl Physiol. 51:812–815, 1981.

167. Pert, C.B. and D.L. Bowie. Behavioural manipulation of rats causes alterations in opiate receptor occupancy. In: Endorphins and Mental Health Research, New York: Oxford University Press, 1979, pp 93–104.

168. Plough, T., H. Galbo and E.A. Richter. Increased muscle glucose uptake during contractions: No need for insulin. Am J Physiol. 247:E726–E731, 1984.

169. Polonsky, K.S. and A.H. Rubenstein. C-peptide as a measure of the secretion and hepatic extraction of insulin: Pitfalls and limitations. *Diabetes* 33:486–494, 1984.

170. Prange Hansen, A.A. and J. Weeke. Fasting serum growth hormone levels and growth hormone responses to exercise during normal menstrual cycles and cycles of oral contraceptives. *Scand J Clin Lab Invest.* 34:199–205, 1974.

171. Prior, J.C., K. Cameron, B. Ho Yuen and J. Thomas. Menstrual cycle changes with marathon training: Anovulation and the short luteal phase. *Can J Appl Sports Sci.* 7:173–177, 1982.

172. Prior, J.C., B. Ho Yuen, D. Clement, L. Bowie and J. Thomas. Reversible luteal phase changes and infertility associated with marathon running. *Lancet* ii:269–270, 1982.

173. Pruett, E.D.R. Glucose and insulin during prolonged work stress in men living on different diets. *J Appl Physiol.* 28:199–208, 1970.

174. Pruett, E.D.R. Plasma insulin concentrations during prolonged work at near maximal oxygen uptake. *J Appl Physiol.* 29:155–158. 1970.

175. Pruett, E.D.R. Insulin and exercise in non-diabetic and diabetic man. In: *Exercise Endocrinology,* K. Fotherby and S.B. Pal (eds). Berlin: Walter de Gryter & Co., 1985, pp 1–23.

176. Pugh, L.G.C.E. Blood volume changes in outdoor exercise of 8–10 hour duration. *J Physiol.* (Lond) 200:345–351, 1969.

177. Quigley, M.E. and S.S.C. Yen. The role of endogenous opiates on LH secretion during the menstrual cycle. *J Clin Endocrinol Metab.* 51:179–181, 1980.

178. Quigley, M.E., K.L. Sheehan, R.F. Casper and S.S.C. Yen. Evidence for increased dopaminergic and opiate activity in patients with hypothalamic hypogonadotrophic amenorrhea. *J Clin Endocrinol Metab.* 50:949–954, 1980.

179. Raymond, L., J. Sode and J. Tucci. Adrenocortical responses to exercise. *Clin Res.* 17:523–528, 1969.

180. Reinheimer, W., P.C. Davidson and M.J. Albrink. Effect of moderate exercise on plasma glucose, insulin and free fatty acids during oral glucose tolerance test. *J Lab Clin Med.* 71:429-437, 1968.

181. Richter, E.A. and H. Galbo. Diabetes, insulin and exercise. *Sports Med.* 3:275-288, 1986.

182. Richter, E.A., H. Galbo, J.J. Holst and B. Sonne. Significance of glucagon for insulin secretion and hepatic glycogenolysis during exercise in rats. *Horm Metab Res.* 13:323–326, 1981.

183. Richter, E.A., N.B. Ruderman and S.H. Schneider. Diabetes and exercise. *Am J Med.* 70:201–209, 1981.

184. Rocker, L., K.A. Kirsch, U. Mund and H. Stoboy. The role of plasma proteins in the control of plasma volume during exercise and dehydration in long distance runners and cyclists. In: *Metabolic Adaptation to Prolonged Physical Exercise,* H. Howard and J.R. Poortmans, (eds). Basel: Birkhauser, 1975, pp 238–244.

185. Ropert, J.F., M.E. Quigley and S.S.C. Yen. Endogenous opiates modulate pulsatile LH release in humans. *J Clin Endocrinol Metab.* 52:583–585, 1981.

186. Rossier, J., E.D. French, C. Rivier, N. Ling, R. Guillemin and F.E. Bloom. Foot shock induced stress increases B-endorphin levels in blood but not the brain. *Nature* 270:618–620, 1977.

187. Roth, J. and C. Grunfeld. Endocrine systems: Mechanisms of disease, target cells and receptors. In: *Textbook of Endocrinology,* R.H. Williams (ed). Philadelphia: W.B. Saunders Co., 1981, pp. 34–35.

188. Roth, J., S.M. Glick, R.S. Yalow and S.A. Berson. Secretion of human growth hormone: Physiological and experimental modification. *Metabolism* 12:557–559, 1963.

189. Roth, K.A., E. Weber, J.D. Barchas, D. Chang and J.-K. Chang. Immunoreactive dynorphin-(1-8) and corticotropin-releasing factor in subpopulation of hypothalamic neurons. *Science* 219:189–191, 1983.

190. Rowell, L.B., G.L. Brengelmann and P.R. Freund. Unaltered norepinephrine-heart rate relationship in exercise with exogenous heat. *J Appl Physiol.* 62:646–650, 1987.

191. Roy, M.W., K.C. Lee, M.S. Jones and R.E. Miller. Neural control of pancreatic insulin and somatostatin secretion. *Endocrinology* 115:770–775, 1984.

192. Russell, J.B., D. Mitchell, P.I. Musey and D.C. Collins. The relationship of exercise to anovulatory cycles in female athletes: Hormonal and physical characteristics. *Obstet Gynecol.* 63:452–456, 1984.

193. Santen, B.J. and C.W. Bardin. Episodic luteinizing hormone secretion in man: Pulse analysis, clinical interpretation, physiological mechanisms. *J Clin Invest.* 52:2617–2628, 1973.

194. Santen, R.J., J. Sofsky, N. Bilic and R. Lippert. Mechanism of action of narcotics in the production of menstrual dysfunction in women. *Fertil Steril.* 26:538–548, 1975.

195. Santoro, N., M. Filicori and W.F. Crowley. Hypogonadotropin disorders in men and women: Diagnosis and therapy with pulsatile gonadotropin-releasing hormone. *Endocrine Rev.* 7:11–22, 1986.

196. Sato, Y., Iguchi, A. and Sakamoto, N. Biochemical determination of training effects using

insulin clamp technique. *Horm Metab Res.* 16:483–486, 1984.
197. Scatchard, G., A. Batchelder and A. Brown. Chemical, clinical, and immunological studies on the products of human plasma fractionation. VI. The osmotic pressure of plasma and of serum albumin. *J Clin Invest.* 23:458–464, 1944.
198. Schalch, D.S. The influence of physical stress and exercise on growth hormone and insulin secretion in man. *J Lab Clin Med.* 69:256–269, 1967.
199. Schwartz, B., D.C. Cumming, E. Riordan, M. Selye, S.C. Yen and R.W. Rebar. Exercise associated amenorrhea: A distinct entity? *Am J Obstet Gynecol.* 141:662–670, 1981.
200. Sforzo, G.A., T.F. Seeger, C.B. Pert, A. Pert and C.O. Dotson. In vivo opioid receptor occupation in the rat brain following exercise. *Med Sci Sports Exerc.* 18:380–384, 1986.
201. Shangold, M., R. Freeman, B. Thysen and M. Gatz. The relationship between long-distance running, plasma progesterone and luteal phase length. *Fertil Steril.* 31:130– 133, 1979.
202. Shangold, M.M., M.L. Gatz and B. Thysen. Acute effects of exercise on plasma concentrations of prolactin and testosterone in recreational women runners. *Fertil Steril.* 35:699–702, 1981.
203. Shephard, R.J. and K.H. Sidney. Effects of physical exercise on plasma growth hormone and cortisol levels in human subjects. *Exercise Sport Sci Rev.* 3:1–30, 1975.
204. Sidney, K.H. and R.J. Shephard. Growth hormone and cortisol age differences, effects of exercise and training. *Can J Appl Sports Sci.* 2:189–193, 1977.
205. Sjostrand, T. The total quantity of hemoglobin in man and its relation to age, sex, body weight, and height. *Acta Physiol Scand.* 18:324–336, 1949.
206. Smythe, G.A. and L. Lazarus. Suppression of human growth hormone secretion by melatonin and cyproheptadine. *J Clin Invest.* 54:116–121, 1974.
207. Soman, V.R., V.A. Koivisto, P. Grantham and P. Felig. Increased insulin binding to monocytes after acute exercise in normal man. *J Clin Endocrinol Metab.* 47:216–219, 1978.
210. Sonne, B. and H. Galbo. Carbohydrate metabolism during and after exercise in rats: Studies with radioglucose. *J Appl Physiol.* 59:1627–1639, 1985.
211. Speroff, L. and D.B. Redwine. Exercise and menstrual function. *Phys Sportsmed.* 8:42–50, 1980.
212. Spiler, I.J. and M.E. Molitch. Lack of modulation of pituitary hormone stress response by neural pathways involving opiate receptors. *J Clin Endocrinol Metab.* 50:516–520, 1980.
213. Staessen, J., R. Fiocchi, R. Bouillon, R. Fagard, P. Lijnen, E. Moermon, A. De-Schaepdryver and A. Armery. The nature of opioid involvement in the hemodynamic respiratory and humoral responses to exercise. *Circulation* 72:982–990, 1985.
214. Starling, E. On the absorption of fluids from the connective tissue spaces. *J Physiol.* 19:312–328, 1986.
215. Stuart, M.C. and L. Lazarus. Somatomedins. *Med J Aust.* 1:816–820, 1975.
216. Stuart, M., L. Lazarus and J. Sutton. Somatomedin: Changes following physiological and pharmacological stimuli to growth hormone secretion. *Proc Endocrin Soc Aust.* 15:21, 1972.
217. Stubbs, W.A., A. Jones, C.R.W. Edwards, G. Delitala, W.J. Jeffcoate, S.J. Ratter, G.M. Besser, S.R. Bloom and K.G.M.M. Alberti. Hormonal and metabolic responses to an enkephalin analogue in normal man. *Lancet* ii:1225–1227, 1978.
218. Sutton, J.R. The effect of acute hypoxia on the hormonal response to exercise. *J Appl Physiol.* 42:587–592, 1977.
219. Sutton, J.R. Hormonal and metabolic responses to exercise in subjects of high and low work capacities. *Med Sci Sports* 10:1–6, 1978.
220. Sutton, J.R. Drugs used in metabolic disorders. *Med. Sci. Sports Exerc.* 13:266–271, 1981.
221. Sutton, J.R. Metabolic responses to exercise in normal and diabetic individuals. In: *Sports Medicine,* R.H. Strauss (ed.). Philadelphia: W.B. Saunders, 1984, pp 190–204.
222. Sutton, J.R. Endorphins and the hypothalamic-pituitary-adrenal axis during exercise. In: *Heat Stress,* J.R.S. Hales and D. Richards (eds.). Amsterdam: Elsevier, 1988 (in press).
223. Sutton, J.R. and J.H. Casey. The adrenocortical response to competitive athletics in veteran athletes. *J Clin Endocrinol Metab.* 40:135–138, 1975.
224. Sutton, J.R. and M.P. Heyes. Endocrine responses to exercise at altitude. In: *Exercise Endocrinology,* K. Fotherby and S.B. Pal (eds.). Berlin: de Gruyter, 1984, pp. 239–262.
225. Sutton, J. and L. Lazarus. Effect of adrenergic blocking agents on growth hormone responses to physical exercise. *Horm Metab Res.* 6:428–429, 1974.
226. Sutton, J. and L. Lazarus. Growth hormone in exercise: A comparison of physiological and pharmacological stimuli. *J Appl Physiol.* 41:523–527, 1976.
227. Sutton, J.R., G.M. Brown, P. Keane, W.H.C. Walker, N.L. Jones, D. Rosenbloom and G.M. Besser. The role of endorphins in the hormonal and psychological responses to exercise. *Int. J. Sports Med.* 3(2):xix, 1982.
228. Sutton, J.R., M.J. Coleman and J.H. Casey. Adrenocortical contribution to serum androgens during physical exercise. *Med Sci Sports* 6:72, 1974.

229. Sutton, J.R., M.J. Coleman and J.H. Casey. Testosterone production rate during exercise. In: *3rd International Symposium on Biochemistry of Exercise*, F. Landry and W.A.R. Orban (eds). Miami, Fl.: Symposia Specialists Inc., 1978, pp 227–234.
230. Sutton, J.R., M.J. Coleman, J. Casey and L. Lazarus. Androgen responses during physical exercise. *Br Med J.* 1:520–522, 1973.
231. Sutton, J.R., M.J. Coleman, A.P. Millar, L. Lazarus and P. Russo. The medical problems of mass participation in athletic competition. The "City-to-Surf" race. *Med J Aust.* 2:127–133, 1972.
232. Sutton, J.R., H.J. Green, P. Young, P. Rock, A. Cymerman and C.S. Houston. Plasma vasopressin, catecholamines and lactate during exhaustive exercise at extreme simulated altitude: "Operation Everest II". *Can J Appl Sports Sci.* 11:43P, 1986.
233. Sutton, J.R., N.L. Jones and C.J. Toews. Growth hormone secretion in acid-base alterations at rest and during exercise. *Clin Sci Mol Med.* 50:241–247, 1976.
234. Sutton, J.R., J.E. Jurkowski, P. Keane, W.H.C. Walker, N.L. Jones and C.J. Toews. Plasma catecholamine, insulin, glucose and lactate responses to exercise in relation to the menstrual cycle. *Med Sci Sports* 12:83–84, 1980.
235. Sutton, J.R., J.T. Reeves, P.D. Wagner, B.M. Groves, A. Cymerman, M.K. Malconian, P.B. Rock, P.M. Young, S.D. Walter and C.S. Houston. "Operation Everest II": Oxygen transport during exercise at extreme simulated altitude. *J Appl Physiol.* 1988. (In press).
236. Sutton, J.R., J.D. Young, L. Lazarus, J.B. Hickie and J. Maksvytis. The hormonal response to physical exercise. *Aust Ann Med.* 18:84–90, 1969.
237. Takahashi, Y., D.M. Kipnis and W.H. Daughaday. Growth hormone secretion during sleep. *J Clin Invest.* 23:2079–2090, 1968.
238. Tanaka, H., M. Shindo, J. Gutkowska, A. Kinoshita, H. Urata, M. Ikeda and K. Arakawa. Effect of acute exercise on plasma immunoreactive-atrial natriuretic factor. *Life Sci.* 39:1685–1693, 1986.
239. Tarnopolsky, L., M. Tarnopolsky, J.D. MacDougall, S. Atkinson and J.R. Sutton. Differences in the hormonal and metabolic responses to prolonged exercise in males and females. *J Appl Physiol.* 1988. (In press).
240. Taylor, R., S.J. Proctor, O. James, F. Clark and K.G.M.M. Alberti. The relationship between human adipocyte and monocyte insulin binding. *Clin Sci.* 67:139–142, 1984.
241. Terjung, R. Endocrine responses to exercise. In: *Exercise and Sports Sciences Reviews*, vol. 7, R. Hutton and D. Miller (eds). Philadelphia: Franklin Institute Press, 1979, pp 153–180.
242. Van Beaumont, W., J.E. Greenleaf and L. Juhos. Disproportional changes in hematocrit, plasma volume and proteins during exercise and bed rest. *J Appl Physiol.* 33:55–61, 1972.
243. Vendsalu, A. Studies on adrenaline and noradrenaline in human plasma. *Acta Physiol Scand.* 49 (Suppl 173):1–123, 1960.
244. Victor, R.G., D.R. Seals and A.L. Mark. Differential control of heart rate and sympathetic nerve activity during dynamic exercise. *J Clin Invest.* 79:508–516, 1987.
245. Villanueva, A.L., C. Schlosser, B. Hopper, J.H. Liu, D.I. Hoffman and R.W. Rebar. Increased cortisol production in women runners. *J Clin Endocrinol Metab.* 63:133–136, 1986.
246. Viru, A. Dynamics of blood corticoid content during and after short term exercise. *Endocrinology* 59:61–68, 1972.
247. Viru, A. *Hormones in Muscular Activity.* vol. 1. Hormonal Ensemble in Exercise. Boca Raton, FL: CRC Press, 1985.
248. Viru, A. *Hormones in Muscular Activity.* vol. 2. Adaptive Effect of Hormones in Exercise. Boca Raton, FL: CRC Press, 1985.
249. Von Euler, U.S. and S. Heller. Noradrenaline excretion in muscular work. *Acta Physiol Scand.* 26:183–191, 1952.
250. Vranic, M. and M. Berger. Exercise and diabetes mellitus. *Diabetes* 28:147–163, 1979.
251. Vranic, M. and R. Kawamori. Essential roles of insulin and glucagon in regulating glucose fluxes during exercise in dogs. *Diabetes* 28 (Suppl 1):45–52, 1979.
252. Vranic, M. and G.A. Wrenshall. Exercise, insulin and glucose turnover in dogs. *Endocrinology* 85:165–171, 1969.
253. Wade, C.E. and J.R. Claybaugh. Plasma renin activity, vasopressin concentration, and urinary excretory responses to exercise in men. *J Appl Physiol.* 49:930–936, 1980.
254. Wahren, J. Glucose turnover during exercise in healthy man and in patients with diabetes mellitus. *Diabetes* 28 (Suppl 1):82–88, 1979.
255. Wahren, J., P. Felig, G. Ahlborg and L. Torfeldt. Glucose metabolism during leg exercise in man. *J Clin Invest.* 50:2715–2725, 1971.
256. Wallberg-Henriksson, H. and J.O. Holloszy. Contractile activity increases glucose uptake. *J Appl Physiol.* 57:1045–1049, 1984.
257. Ward, G.R., J.R. Sutton, N.L. Jones and C.J. Toews. Activation by exercise of human skeletal muscle pyruvate dehydrogenase in vivo. *Clin Sci.* 63:87–92, 1982.
258. Ward, M.M., I.N. Mefford, G.W. Black and W.M. Bortz. Exercise and plasma catechol-

amine release. In: *Exercise Endocrinology*, K. Fotherby and S.B. Pal (eds.). Berlin: Walter de Gruyter & Co., 1985, pp 263–294.

259. Warren, M.P. The effects of exercise on pubertal progression and reproductive function in girls. *J Clin Endocrinol Metab.* 51:1150–1157, 1980.

260. Wasserman, D.H., H.L. Lickley and M. Vranic. Interactions between glucagon and other counterregulatory hormones during normoglycemic and hypoglycemic exercise in dogs. *J Clin Invest.* 74:1404–1413, 1984.

261. Webster, B.A., S.R. Vigna and T. Paquette. Acute exercise, epinephrine, and diabetes enhance insulin binding to skeletal muscle. *Am J Physiol.* 250:E186–E197, 1986.

262. Wehrenberg, W.B., S.L. Wardlaw, A.G. Frantz and M. Ferin. Beta-endorphin in hyophyseal portal blood: Variations throughout the menstrual cycle. *Endocrinology* 111:879–881, 1982.

263. Wheeler, G.D., S.R. Wall, A.N. Belcastro and D.C. Cumming. Reduced serum testosterone and prolactin levels in male distance runners. *JAMA.* 252:514–516, 1984.

264. Wildt, L., S. Niesert, G. Wesner and G. Layendecker. Effects of naloxone on LH, FSH and prolactin secretion in hypothalamic amenorrhea. *Acta Endocrinol.* 97 (Suppl 243):52, 1981.

265. Wilkerson, J.E., B. Gutin and S.M. Horvath. Exercise-induced changes in blood, red cell and plasma volumes in man. *Med Sci Sports* 9:155–158, 1977.

266. Williams, E.S., M.P. Ward, J.S. Milledge, W.R. Withey, M.W. Older and M.L. Forsling. Effect of the exercise of seven consecutive days hill-walking on fluid homeostasis. *Clin Sci.* 56:305–316, 1979.

267. Winder, W.W., R.C. Hickson, J.M. Hagberg, A.A. Ehsani and J.A. McLane. Training-induced changes in hormonal and metabolic responses to submaximal exercise. *J Appl Physiol.* 46:766–771, 1979.

268. Wright, P.H. and W.J. Malaisse. Effect of epinephrine, stress and exercise on insulin secretion in the rat. *Am J Physiol.* 214:1031–1034, 1968.

269. Yalow, R.S. and S.A. Berson, Immunoassay of endogenous plasma insulin in man. *J Clin Invest.* 39:1157–1175, 1960.

270. Young, D.R., R. Pelligra and R.R. Adachi. Serum glucose and free fatty acids in man during prolonged exercise. *J Appl Physiol.* 21:1047–1052, 1966.

271. Zinman, B., M. Vranic, A.M. Albisser, B.S. Leibel and E.B. Marliss. The role of insulin in the metabolic response to exercise in diabetic man. *Diabetes* 28 (Suppl 1):76–81, 1979.

DISCUSSION

LAMB: Many athletes believe that consumption of amino acids can stimulate growth hormone release to a much greater extent than exercise alone. Do you believe that this can occur?

SUTTON: We've studied eight subjects with arginine infusion, and, in our experience, the magnitude of the HGH response to arginine is not as great as the exercise response. Amino acids such as tryptophan consumed over long periods may interfere with neurotransmission and actually reduce HGH release. However, I don't actually know what the HGH response would be to prolonged oral doses of amino acids.

TIPTON: What are the nonendocrine stimuli to HGH release? What exercise related factors might play a role in this response? For example, can pain increase HGH levels? How about dietary carbohydrate?

SUTTON: Pain, presumably operating through the hypothalamus, has been known to increase HGH for some years. Hypoglycemia enhances HGH release, and hyperglycemia can suppress it. Oddly, the pituitary contains tremendous amounts of HGH, but we know very little about what causes its release and what its functions are during exercise.

TERJUNG: It seems to me that an important consideration with respect to the possibility of acromegaly development in athletes who use HGH is that long distance runners and cyclists, who presumably experience almost daily surges in HGH during exercise, are not walking around with big jaws and overgrown hands.

SUTTON: But we have to keep in mind that exogenous HGH may cause dramatically greater levels of circulating hormone than any natural stimuli. Most of us suspect that large doses of HGH over a period of months or years may, in fact, result in acromegaly. The irony of acromegaly is that these people, who may be initially very strong, develop a skeletal muscle myopathy with severe weakness and a cardiomyopathy with arrhythmias.

SHERMAN: Do you have any information on whether or not marathoners who become hypoglycemic are those who consume carbohydrates during those races? Have any studies been done on these individuals after these events that would subsequently mark them as having insulin sensitivity problems? Is there any clue why these people respond to exercise with hypoglycemia?

SUTTON: I don't think anyone knows the answer to that.

COYLE: Do you think that many of those who are severely hypoglycemic are just running out of liver glycogen rather than responding to some complex hormonal control of glycogenolysis?

SUTTON: That is the conclusion that we came to, that they have no glycogen storage in the liver.

COYLE: Well, you certainly can't regulate what you don't have.

DAVIS: Weight lifters or power lifters who are using HGH say that they use it in six week cycles, twice a year. Is that enough to elicit acromegaly?

SUTTON: I don't really know, but it seems unlikely to me. Acromegaly, like hypothyroidism, takes a long time to evolve. One of my friends who is an endocrinologist had a wife who was acromegalic, and, quite clearly, she evolved this over a period of about 10 years. One day an old friend who was visiting him asked who was treating his wife's acromegaly? He said, "What do you mean?" When he then went back and looked at the photographs of his wife over the previous 10 years, it was a clear picture. But because the acromegalic change was so subtle, he lived with that person for 10 years and really couldn't notice. The answer to your question is no. Maybe Dick Strauss has some good information on this.

STRAUSS: Well, up until this point, growth hormone has been given for maybe three weeks at a time and then stopped. But with the recombinant growth hormone becoming available, you can pretty well bet that there are at least a few people out there who will take it continuously over several years. So, probably we will see some acromegaly. An even more serious potential problem is the use of growth hormone in children. Pediatricians whom I know are being asked by parents to give growth hormone to their kids during the growth phase in the hope that it will add a couple of inches to the height of a potential basketball player to maybe help get a scholarship for him.

BROOKS: Well, what about the potential use of growth hormone to treat obesity? Isn't that likely to be even a larger problem in the general population?

SUTTON: I'm sure this is so.

STRAUSS: How real is that lipolytic effect of HGH in adults? What you were describing were studies of children who were HGH deficient. Would the same effect occur in adults?

BROOKS: There are people in the San Francisco area who use HGH for control of obesity, but I don't know of any body composition data to verify a positive effect of HGH on lipolysis.

FARRELL: When considering glucose control, one must be very specific about which species one is talking about. If you look at relative importance of the hormones that control glucose in humans versus the rat versus the dog, they're different. John just gave the results from human experiments, but I think there's a lot to be learned from the animal literature. For example, we really need studies on the effects of training on endorphins.

Carr showed that as women became more trained, they exhibited higher beta endorphin responses at the same relative workload. More recently, Howlett and others have shown that if you train women just for seven weeks, the beta endorphin response to the same relative work is somewhat diminished. They also measured methionine enkephalin, and the enkephalin response to the same relative workload in the trained state was completely abolished. They went from a fivefold or eightfold increase in the untrained state to absolutely no increase. This suggests to me that the enkephalin system is probably more trainable than the beta endorphin system. So, if the enkephalin system is very trainable, but the endorphin system isn't, it doesn't really fit with John's work, in which he found a training related change in hypothalamic function with naloxone. This sounds like a beta endorphin effect, so that's confusing. I don't know what's going on but perhaps an animal model could help resolve central opioid adaptations to exercise training.

CANTWELL: John, any comments on the exercising noninsulin-dependent and insulin-dependent diabetic?

SUTTON: The clinical scenario is that for a Type II diabetic, exercise is usually beneficial to glucose regulation and control. The insulin-dependent diabetic, the Type I, can be in real strife, particularly if he is "brittle," because during exercise he must be careful with insulin timing, insulin dosage, and food intake, so he doesn't become frankly hypoglycemic. And if there is any tendency to ketosis, glucose control is often made worse by exercise. It has been suggested that insulin dependent diabetics are not helped significantly with glucose regulation by exercise programs.. While exercise has been advocated as being beneficial, there is little evidence that it helps their glucose control.

FARRELL: The effect of training on glucose control, I think, is also at a crossroads,, because most studies show no change with training in hemoglobin A1C, a good marker of glycemic control over a long period of time. So I think you're very correct in that the exercise story for diabetics really isn't that clear.

SHERMAN: Even though exercise in insulin dependent diabetics doesn't necessarily induce the same changes in insulin sensitivity that it does in normals or noninsulin dependent diabetics, one of the studies shows a reduced requirement for insulin injections to control glucose during the day. Over the long run, since insulin is a very potent atherogenic agent, regular exercise may help reduce the incidence of heart disease in diabetics.

RAVEN: Enkephalins are starting to look like they have major control in the cardiovascular system, perhaps via the sympathetic ganglia. So the enkephalinergic and adrenergic systems are linking up here. I wonder if we've got enough data to address this issue.

FARRELL: If you look at the effects of using the common blockers, naloxone and naltrexone, during exercise, you don't find any effect on heart rate or blood pressure. I think that if you would use blockers that are more delta receptor specific for the enkephalins, then you probably would find changes.

RAVEN: You might not alter heart rate with naloxone, but there is some evidence of changes in contractility.

DAVIS: I think the enkephalin response, if you're talking about blood-borne opiates, is where the research needs to go. There is likely enough enkephalin relation to the adrenal medulla to perhaps react with some of the opiate receptors to cause the physiologic effects. The problem with beta endorphins is that the levels are so low, much lower than any ED 50 response on any of the opiate receptors, that if you are measuring 20 picograms per mL of blood, it's unlikely that there will be any physiological response to that level. So either you need to get to the brain of animals with some kind of specific beta endorphin antagonist and try to look for effects at the hypothalamic level and maybe work up to the human data, or go with the blood enkephalin and see what's happening in the blood that might explain some of these findings.

FARRELL: John, could you comment on what you think is the major reason for insulin being lower during exercise? Is it circulating norepinephrine, or is it direct sympathetic activation of the pancreas?

SUTTON: According to the studies of Galbo, it may well be the latter, I suspect.

6

Nutrition and Prolonged Exercise

W. Mike Sherman, Ph.D.

David R. Lamb, Ph.D.

INTRODUCTION
  I. ENERGY EXPENDITURE OF EXERCISE
    A. Energy Expenditure During Training
    B. Factors Affecting Energy Expenditure
  II. DIETARY PRACTICES OF ATHLETES IN TRAINING
    A. Competitive Athletes
    B. Elite Athletes
    C. Comment on the Dietary Practices of Athletes
  III. FUEL RESERVES OF THE BODY
    A. Protein
      1. Is Protein a Fuel for Prolonged Exercise?
      2. What is the Minimum Recommended Dietary Protein Intake?
    B. Triglycerides
      1. Factors Affecting the Use of Fat as a Fuel During Exercise
      2. Does the Availability of Fat Limit Performance?
    C. Carbohydrates
      1. Muscle Glycogen
        a. Factors Affecting the Utilization of Glycogen During Exercise
        b. Muscle Glycogen as a Limiting Factor During Exercise
      2. Liver Glycogen and Blood Glucose
        a. Maintenance of the Blood Glucose Concentration During Exercise
        b. Incidence of Hypoglycemia During Exercise
    D. Integration of the Use of Fuels During Exercise
  IV. NUTRITION DURING TRAINING
    A. Liver Glycogen Stores
      1. Dietary Carbohydrates and the Replenishment of Liver Glycogen Stores
      2. Carbohydrate Source and Liver Glycogen Synthesis
      3. Competition between Liver and Muscle for Glycogen Synthesis After Exercise

B. Muscle Glycogen Stores
   1. Dietary Carbohydrate Intake and Muscle Glycogen Synthesis
   2. What Is the Optimal Timing of Dietary Carbohydrate Consumption After Exercise?
   3. Exercise Mode and Postexercise Glycogen Resynthesis
   4. Dietary Carbohydrate Source and Muscle Glycogen Synthesis
   5. Does Exercise-Induced Muscle Damage Adversely Affect Muscle Glycogen Resynthesis?
   6. Does Exercise During Recovery from Prior Exercise Adversely Affect Glycogen Resynthesis?
   7. Effects of Different Diets on Training and on Recovery from Training
C. Maintenance of the Carbohydrate Stores During Intense Daily Training

V. NUTRITION DURING THE WEEK BEFORE AN IMPORTANT PERFORMANCE
   A. The Classical Glycogen Supercompensation Regimen
   B. The Modified Regimen for Glycogen Supercompensation
   C. Effect of Glycogen Supercompensation on Performance
   D. Factors Related to Supercompensation
   E. Practical Use of Muscle Glycogen Supercompensation

VI. THE PREEXERCISE MEAL
   A. Glucose Availability During Exercise
   B. The Preexercise Meal and Metabolism During Exercise
   C. Comparison of Fasting and Preexercise Feedings on Metabolism during Exercise
   D. Carbohydrate Source in a Preexercise Meal: Effects on Metabolic Response and Exercise Performance
   E. Effects of Preexercise Glycerol Feedings on Metabolism During Exercise
   F. Effects of Fatty Acids in a Preexercise Meal on Metabolism During Exercise
   G. Effects of Caffeine in a Preexercise Meal on Metabolism During Exercise
   H. Effects of Fasting on Metabolism and Performance
   I. Consumption of the Preexercise Meal

VII. WATER AS A PRIMARY NUTRIENT FOR PROLONGED EXERCISE
   A. Effects of Withholding Water Before or During Prolonged Exercise
      1. Early Experiments
      2. Reduced Plasma Volume and Increased Body Fluid Osmolality
      3. Increased Circulatory Strain
      4. Decreased Sweating Response
      5. Altered Electrolyte Distributions
      6. Altered Hormonal Response to Exercise
      7. Similarity in Gender Responses to Exercise in a Dehydrated State
   B. Effects of Water and Saline Feedings Before and During Prolonged Exercise
      1. Water and Saline Ingestion Before Prolonged Exercise
      2. Water and Saline Feedings Both Before and During Prolonged Exercise
      3. Water and Saline Feedings During prolonged Exercise
      4. Efficacy of Electrolyte Replacement During Prolonged Exercise
   C. Summary of the Effects of Water and Saline Replacement on Homeostasis During Prolonged Exercise

VIII. GASTRIC EMPTYING OF SOLUTIONS CONSUMED BEFORE AND
     DURING PROLONGED EXERCISE
     A. Gastric Emptying Rate During Prolonged Exercise
     B. Gastric Emptying Rate of Carbohydrate-Containing Beverages
  IX. CARBOHYDRATE FEEDINGS DURING PROLONGED EXERCISE
     A. Availability of Glucose Ingested During Exercise
     B. Carbohydrate Ingestion During Prolonged Exercise: Effects on Fatigue
     C. Efficacy of the Ingestion of Fructose or Glucose on Performance During
        Prolonged Exercise
     D. Consumption of Carbohydrate During Exercise
SUMMARY
BIBLIOGRAPHY
DISCUSSION

INTRODUCTION

Evaluation of the diets of athletes has generally demonstrated that when suficient calories are consumed to meet the daily energy expenditure and basal metabolic rate, the diet provides sufficient vitamins and minerals to meet the recommended daily allowance. On the other hand, both elite and nonelite athletes generally consume a diet which is significantly deficient in cabohydrate. It is well documented that the body's carbohydrate stores play an important role in the capacity to perform prolonged intense exercise; when these stores are insufficient, exercise capacity is impaired. Therefore, the major emphasis of this chapter is the maintenance of adequate whole-body carbohydrate stores. Consideration is given to the ingestion of carbohydrates in the daily diet, in the precompetition meal, and immediately before and during competition. In addition, since water is an important constituent of the body for the maintenance of normal function, especially during the stress of exercise, this chapter will consider its role as a nutrient and carbohydrate-delivery agent.

I. ENERGY EXPENDITURE OF EXERCISE

The most basic nutritional concern for athletic performance is the quantity of calories expended in training above that required for normal daily activities and basal metabolic rate. Without the proper balance between energy expenditure and consumption, the athlete's training and competitive capabilities will eventually be hindered by either excessive weight gain or excessive weight loss. Measuring body weight after arising in the morning and voiding is the easiest method the athlete can employ to assess the caloric adequacy of the diet.

A. Energy Expenditure During Training

The normally active but untrained individual will have an energy expnditure of roughly 2,000 to 2,500 kcal·day^{-1} (8.4 to 10.5 MJ·day^{-1}), whereas the athlete undertaking strenuous training for prolonged exercise may have an energy expenditure 1.5 to 3 times higher (22, 79). Unlike their sedentary counterparts whose daily energy expenditure is spread out over the entire day, 30% to 40% of an athlete's daily energy expenditure usually occurs in two to four hours of intense training. The endurance athlete's more concentrated and greater total energy expenditure during the day can impose limitations on the adequacy of the athlete's nutritional intake if normal eating practices are maintained. Assuming an eight hour sleep period, the athlete will have to consume 1.5 to 3 times more calories in 12 to 14 h, compared to the sedentary counterpart, who would have as long as 16 h to compensate for sudden changes in caloric expenditure. The shorter time for ingestion and the higher caloric consumption in athletes who are involved in rigorous training may be partly responsible for the observation of constant "nibbling" patterns of food consumption by such athletes (105).

B. Factors Affecting Energy Expenditure

Total daily energy expenditure in athletes training for prolonged exercise can range from 3,000 to 7,000 kcal·day^{-1} (12.6 to 29.3 MJ·day^{-1}). For activities such as running and walking, the energy expenditure is relatively independent of the velocity of movement, and the total distance or duration of activity can be used to reasonably estimate the caloric cost of the activity. For these activities, estimates of 80 to 110 kcal·mile^{-1} (0.2 to 0.3 MJ·km^{-1}) have been reported (8,113,134). On the other hand, for activities such as cycling, swimming and speed skating, the energy cost for a covered distance is a function of the movement velocity because increased velocity causes increased resistance of air or water, and greater resistance results in a higher caloric expenditure. For example, the energy cost of swimming at 1.5 m·s^{-1} is 2.5-fold greater than swimming at 1.0 m·s^{-1} because of the greater resistance of water at the greater velocity (28). Consequently, the velocity of movement must be taken into account, and it is therefore more difficult to reliably estimate the energy costs of these activities.

During training, caloric expenditure is a function of the amount of oxygen consumed to support the activity. The upper limit of oxygen consumption, the maximal oxygen consumption ($\dot{V}O_2$max), is a function of age, weight, sex, and training state. The $\dot{V}O_2$max for well-trained male athletes is commonly greater than 4.5 L·min^{-1}, with the highest values reported for rowers (6.2 L · min⁻¹) (113,178). Female athletes, because they are smaller, will generally have a $\dot{V}O_2$max which is 20% to 30% lower than that for male athletes (113,178). These values for $\dot{V}O_2$max would provide energy expenditures of between 105 kJ · min⁻¹ (25.1 kcal · min⁻¹) and 73 kJ · min⁻¹ (17.4 kcal · min⁻¹) for males and females, respectively. However, exercise at $\dot{V}O_2$max could last for only a few minutes. Thus, the intensities of exercise used in training or performance of prolonged exercise tasks are below $\dot{V}O_2$max.

In general, there is an inverse relationship between the duration of the activity and the percent of $\dot{V}O_2$max which can be sustained for that activity. This relationship has allowed Brotherhood (22) to develop a table of caloric expenditures for training and performances lasting various durations at different percentages of $\dot{V}O_2$max. This table might serve as a guide for athletes who know their $\dot{V}O_2$max and want to estimate their total caloric expenditure for various training sessions (Table 6-1).

The efficiency of performance will also effect the total caloric expenditure for the activity. Elite athletes commonly have lower oxygen consumption requirements than "good" athletes for completing submaximal exercise tasks at a given pace (134,169). These differences could mean a 15% to 20% difference in caloric expenditure. Therefore, if the athlete can improve movement efficiency during training, both the caloric expenditure during training and the need for dietary calories could be reduced.

TABLE 6-1. *Energy expenditure predictions for competition and training by endurance athletes*

| | Exercise time (hours) | Energy Expenditure | | | | | |
| | | competition | | | training | | |
		%$\dot{V}O_2$max	MJ	(kcal)	%$\dot{V}O_2$max	MJ	(kcal)
Men							
Example:	0.5	89	2.51	(600)	80	2.26	(540)
	1.0	88	4.98	(1190)	77	4.36	(1040)
($\dot{V}O_2$max	2.0	84	9.50	(2270)	73	8.25	(1970)
4.5 L · min⁻¹)	3.0	81	13.75	(3280)	70	11.80	(2840)
Women							
Example:	0.5	86	1.62	(390)	80	1.51	(360)
	1.0	85	3.21	(770)	77	2.90	(693)
($\dot{V}O_2$max							
3.0 L · min₋₁)	2.0	81	6.11	(1460)	73	5.49	(1310)
	3.0	78	8.82	(2110)	70	7.92	(1890)

The data in this table are predicted from the relationship of sustainable relative aerobic power output (% $\dot{V}O_2$max) to exercise time for elite endurance runners (51). They are likely to represent the upper limits of energy expenditure in competition and basic training for most sports activities. Absolute energy expenditure will be determined by individual $\dot{V}O_2$max.

II. DIETARY PRACTICES OF ATHLETES IN TRAINING

Many of the reports on the dietary habits of athletes undergoing heavy training fail to include data on body weight, body composition, intensity, duration, and frequency of training, and estimated daily caloric expenditure. Future reports should certainly include these important variables (56).

The two main factors that dictate caloric consumption during athletic training are the demands of the sport and the size of the individual. On the average, endurance athletes consume 210 $kJ \cdot kg \cdot day^{-1}$ (50.2 $kcal \cdot kg \cdot day^{-1}$) (22), which is probably adequate for most athletes undertaking endurance training. The protein content of endurance athletes' diets averages 15% of the caloric consumption (22). This is the dietary protein content recommended by the American Heart Association (27) and is roughly 1.5 $g \cdot kg^{-1}$ body weight $\cdot day^{-1}$, which is an adequate provision of dietary protein for maintenance of lean tissue (66). The fat content of endurance athletes' diets contains approximately 36% of the caloric consumption. This is slightly higher than the recommended 30% (27), but is less than the 40% fat content of the diet of the general population of the United States (65). The carbohydrate content of the endurance athletes' diet averages 49% of the total caloric consumption; this is 6% lower than recommended by the American Heart Association (27) and between 11% and 21% lower than recommended by sports nutritionists and exercise physiologists (32,166).

A. Competitive Athletes

Burke et al. (24) reported the dietary patterns of elite Australian triathletes undergoing 13, 323, and 75 $km \cdot wk^{-1}$ of swimming, cycling and running, respectively. The athletes weighed 70 kg and had 11% body fat. The subjects consumed an average of 17.14 $MJ \cdot day^{-1}$ (4095 $kcal \cdot day^{-1}$) of which 13%, 27%, and 60% of the calories were derived from protein, fat and carbohydrate, respectively. Analysis of the diets indicated that primarily complex carbohydrates were consumed by the athletes and that nibbling patterns were common. The intake of two minerals (iron, calcium) and five vitamins (Vitamin A, thiamine, riboflavin, niacin, ascorbic acid) by this group exceeded the Australian guidelines for recommended intake. Blood analysis also revealed normal iron status.

Peters et al. (149) surveyed the dietary patterns of 15 male long distance runners competing in a Hawaiian footrace covering 500 km and lasting 20 days. The subjects' average body weight was 70 kg, percent body fat was 9%, and they trained an average of 14 $km \cdot day^{-1}$. During the race the participants consumed an average of 18.45 MJ

(4410 kcal) per day, with protein, fat and carbohydrate providing 10%, 26%, and 49% of the calories, respectively. Interestingly, alcohol consumption during this race also accounted for 15% of the calories consumed. Analysis of the diets for five vitamins (Vitamin A, thiamin, riboflavin, niacin,, ascorbic acid) and four minerals (calcium, magnesium iron, zinc) indicated that the diet provided or exceeded the recommendations for minimal dietary intake (66).

Kirsch et al. (105) examined the feeding patterns of thirteen long-distance runners, eight cyclists and eight sedentary controls who had a daily caloric consumption of 18.88 MJ $\cdot$ day^{-1} (4,400 kcal), 26.28 MJ $\cdot$ day^{-1} (6,500 kcal) and 10.93 MJ $\cdot$ day^{-1} (2,500 kcal), respectively. Their caloric consumptions were 103%, 250%, and 56% greater than estimated basal metabolic rate, respectively. During the four days of study, the subjects remained in energy and water balance. It was observed that the athletes consumed 8 to 10 small meals per day, whereas the sedentary controls consumed three meals per day and one snack. Water consumption occurred in the morning and at noon, but 45% of the fluid intake occurred after 8:00 pm.

Swimming is another sport that requires substantial energy expenditure during training, but which is not often thought of as a prolonged exercise sport. Although many of the events in competition are short, swimmers often undertake arduous twice-daily training. On a light training day, elite swimmers may swim 8,000 to 10,000 m (5 to 6 miles), whereas on a heavy day, 12,000 to 16,000 m (7.5 to 10 miles) is normal. With the energy cost of swimming a given distance being roughly four-times that of running, an elite swimmer must consume a substantial amount of energy during training. For example, a male swimmer might expend 20.8 to 25.0 MJ (5,000 to 6,000 kcal) per day during four h of swimming, whereas a female swimmer might expend 16.7 to 20.8 MJ (4,000 to 5,00 kcal) per day (79). Based on this high caloric consumption, it is expected that swimmers would adopt nibbling eating habits to consume the necessary calories to meet the energy expenditure of daily training. Unfortunately, reliable reports of the eating habits of elite swimmers could not be located in the literature.

B. Elite Athletes

There are a few studies that describe the dietary patterns and contents of "elite" athletes who undergo training for and competition in prolonged exercise. Johnson et al. (101) reported the caloric consumption of six members of the Irish Olympic road cycling squad. The subjects weighed their food for three alternate days during a week and for one weekend day on two separate occasions one year apart. Their average weight and percent body fat, 71 kg and 14%, respectively, were the same for the two measurement periods. Their energy consumption, 16.25 MJ·day^{-1} (3875 kcal·day^{-1}), was also the same for the two measurement periods. The percent of calories derived from protein, fat and carbohydrates averaged 14%, 35%, and 51%, respectively, at both measurement periods. Additionally, their consumption of vitamins and minerals met or exceeded the daily recommended intake. During the year between measurements, the cyclists' training program increased from 480 to 640 km·wk^{-1}.

Recently, Grandjean (Footnote 1) provided information on the dietary patterns of elite males and females training for the 1988 Olympic trials. They trained an estimated 81 to 177 km per week. The males and females weighed an average of 65 kg and 53 kg, respectively, and consumed an average 12.73 MJ (3,042 kcal) per day and 9.81 MJ (2,343 kcal) per day, respectively. The elite males and females consumed the same percentage of calories derived from protein, fat and carbohydrate which were 17%, 33%, and 49%, respectively. This average daily caloric consumption is lower than that recommended for athletes undertaking strenuous daily training, and the percentages of calories derived from carbohydrate, fat, and protein are low, high, and high, respectively.

A nutritional survey of 51 highly trained women runners who qualified for the 1984 Olympic marathon trials and averaged 113 km·wk^{-1} was conducted by Deuster et al. (53). A self-reported three day dietary record (two week days and one weekend day) served as the basis for the diet analysis. This information was provided by the athletes during a period before the trials to exclude the interference of dietary manipulations often practiced by endurance athletes. The mean daily energy consumption was 10.0 MJ (2397 kcal), with 13%, 33%, and 54% of the calories derived from protein, fat, and carbohydrate, respectively. Based on an estimated caloric expenditure of 3.33 MJ (800 kcal) per day for a 6 km training distance and a normal caloric need of 9.2 MJ (2200 kcal) per day for women their age, these athletes were undernourished by roughly 2.5 MJ (603 kcal) per day. This may have contributed to their relatively low 12% body fat. The diet contained adequate contents of calcium, magnesium, iron and copper, but was low in zinc intake. Blood samples indicated marginal iron status. It is likely that if their caloric consumption had been increased, these margnal deficiencies in zinc and iron would have been eliminated.

Grandjean (Footnote 1) recorded the feeding patterns of three elite female cyclists competing in a 12 day cycling stage race (Coors Classic). The total mileage for the stage race was 496 km, with events covering from 0.62 km to 72 km. A nutritionist accompanied the cyclists and weighed all the foods consumed. The women weighed an average of 59 kg and consumed 10.37 MJ·day^{-1} (2,478 kcal·day^{-1}), which is lower than that recommended for women undertaking strenuous training. The average percentages of the calories represented by protein, fat, and carbohydrate were 17%, 33%, and 51%, respectively. Obviously, these women were not self-selecting the recommended content of carbohydrate, fat, and protein during arduous competition.

C.   Comment on the Dietary Practices of Athletes

Based on the recommendations of the American Heart Association (27), the USDA (141), and sports nutrionists and exercise physiologists (32,166), the available scanty evidence indicates that endurance athletes need to increase the amount of carbohydrate and reduce the amount of fat in their diets. Ideally, protein, fat and carbohydrate should contribute 12%, 18% and 70% of the calories consumed (32,166). If caloric consumption meets the caloric expenditure, then available evidence suggests that the minimum recommended daily allowance for minerals and vitamins will be met and exceeded. Thus, vitamin and mineral supplements are probably not necessary for athletes consuming nutritionally adequate diets. Elite athletes in the United States apparently consume diets in which the percentage of calories derived from carbohydrate is grossly inadequate. Further studies are warranted, but they should follow appropriate guidelines to ensure collection of meaningful data (56). Only when the results of such studies become available can improved educational strategies be developed to improve the endurance athletes' diet.

III. FUEL RESERVES OF THE BODY

During prolonged exercise, the fuel depots are mobilized to provide energy for muscular contraction. Of these fuel depots, fat and carbohydrate are the primary substrates used for energy during prolonged exercise. Substantial amounts of protein are utilized for muscular contraction only during prolonged starvation or during prolonged exercise when the carbohydrate reserves are maintained at a low level. Many factors, such as, the duration, intensity, and mode of exercise, influence the relative contributions of these fuels to muscular contraction.

A.   Protein

The major mass of protein in the body is found in muscle tissue. Of the total body weight in a normal man, roughly 20% is protein (14 kg of a 70 kg man). This amount of protein would supply roughly

232 MJ of energy, which, if used as the sole source of energy at an intensity requiring an oxygen uptake of 2.0 L $O_2 \cdot min^{-1}$, would last 93 h (115).

The total body protein content is a function of protein synthesis and degradation. During endurance exercise the rate of protein synthesis declines, but during recovery from such exercise, protein synthesis is increased (17,158). The exact time course and magnitude of these changes and their implications for endurance performance are not known. It is clear that muscle hypertrophy does not occur following endurance training, even though the content of enzyme protein in the muscle increases (92). Although several studies (26,116,117) have demonstrated that the breakdown products of protein increase in the urine, sweat, and serum following a single bout of prolonged strenuous exercise, overall protein synthesis in muscle must slightly exceed degradation during the chronic adaptation to endurance exercise because of the increase in the total muscle protein content. (92).

1. Is Protein a Fuel for Prolonged Exercise? Studies before the early 1970s, using urinary urea excretion as the marker for protein degradation during exercise, generally concluded that protein is not broken down during exercise (see reference 115 for review). These findings led to the interpretation that fat and carbohydrate are the sole contributors to energy production during muscular contraction.

More recent studies using different markers, including radio-labeled tracers of protein metabolism, have suggested that protein may make a small, but important, contribution to the energy expenditure during prolonged exercise. Lemon et al. (117) exercised six subjects for 1 h at 61% at $\dot{V}O_2$max when muscle glycogen was either high or low at the beginning of exercise. They estimated that protein degradation contributed 4.4% of the total energy expenditure when glycogen was high and 10.4% when glycogen stores were low. This equates to an estimated protein degradation rate of 5.8 and 13.7 $g \cdot h^{-1}$ for the high and low glycogen treatments, respectively. These findings suggest that protein degradation might contribute to energy expenditure as the duration of exercise increases and the carbohydrate stores of the body decrease. However, the contribution of protein will not be greater than 15% of the total energy expenditure even under the most severe circumstances (115). Furthermore, no one has suggested any association between the onset of fatigue and the amount of the protein stores or the rate of their breakdown during endurance exercise. Therefore, it is doubtful that protein oxidation is a limiting factor during prolonged exercise.

A more important function of proteins during exercise may be their role in providing amino acid carbon skeletons for the de novo synthesis of glucose in the liver via gluconeogenesis. The most important of these amino acids is alanine. After 40 min of exercise at moderate intensity, the blood alanine concentration is 50% higher than at rest (60). After 4 h at the same intensity, the blood alanine concentration is 3-fold higher than at rest. The extraction of alanine by the liver for gluconeogenesis increases during exercise, whereas the release of alanine by muscle remains relatively constant. Therefore, as the exercise duration at a moderate intensity increases, the arterial alanine concentration decreases. One gram of alanine can provide roughly 0.65 g glucose via gluconeogenesis (155). On this basis, glucose derived from gluconeogenesis from protein precursors might provide 4 g glucose $\cdot h^{-1}$ during moderate exercise. At a light to moderate intensity of exercise, this amount of glucose is significant. However, as the exercise intensity increases, carbohydrate oxidation can increase to a rate greater than 3 g $\cdot min^{-1}$, and de novo glucose production from amino acids plays a very small role in the supply of energy from total body carbohydrate reserves (107).

2. **What Is the Minimum Recommended Dietary Protein Intake?** The minimal protein intake of a sedentary individual should be 0.9 g protein $\cdot kg^{-1}$ body weight $\cdot day^{-1}$ (66). Recent evidence indicates that the average protein intake of endurance trained athletes is 1.0 to 1.5 g protein $\cdot kg^{-1}$ body weight $\cdot day^{-1}$ (22). Because the diets of highly trained athletes might be deficient in certain essential amino acids, Lemon et al. (115) suggested a protein intake of 2.0 g protein $\cdot kg^{-1}$ body weight $\cdot day^{-1}$ by individuals with elevated protein needs. This could be particularly appropriate for endurance athletes because the emphasis on carbohydrates might decrease the athlete's protein intake. It appears, however, that these athletes will be protected from dietary protein deficiency even when there is an increased protein requirement, as long as the caloric intake contains a minimum of 12% to 15% protein.

B. Triglycerides

Fats comprise the largest depot of fuel in the body. In the average 70 kg man with 15% body fat, the 390 MJ (93,179 kcal) of energy in the stored fat would fuel running at 2.0 L $\cdot min^{-1}$ for 157 h (6.5 days) (115,136). The largest deposit of this fat is contained within the adipose tissue; however, muscle also contains its own endogenous triglyceride stores. The triglyceride stores in fast-twitch and slow-twitch skeletal muscle are different. Slow-twitch fibers have a significantly higher triglyceride content (207 mmol $\cdot kg^{-1}$ dry weight) than do fast-twitch fibers (74 mmol $\cdot kg^{-1}$ dry weight) (57). This makes teleological sense, because the slow-twitch fibers are used predominantly during exercise intensities that can be primarily supported by fat metabolism.

   1. Factors Affecting the Use of Fat as a Fuel During Exercise. As the exercise intensity decreases and the duration of the activity increases, the importance of fat as a fuel for muscular contraction increases. After 60 min of exercise at 40% $\dot{V}O_2$max, fat may contribute 40% of the oxidative energy supply, whereas after 4 h of exercise at this intensity, the proportion of the energy supply contributed by fat oxidation has increased to 70% (4). As the exercise intensity increases, however, the contribution of fat oxidation to the energy expenditure decreases. Because diffusion of fatty acids from blood to muscle is slow and rate-limiting for fat oxidation (136) and because the stimulation of endogenous fat utilization by hormones develops slowly (77), fatty acid oxidation in untrained persons not adapted to a high fat diet cannot solely support exercise at intensities greater than 50% $\dot{V}O_2$max (107). Chronic consumption of a high fat diet and endurance training may increase the maximal rate of energy production from fat.

   Fats utilized during prolonged exercise are either blood borne or are in the intramuscular stores. In general, it is believed that fatty acid uptake and oxidation during exercise are proportional to free fatty acid availability (4,82,146). During prolonged exercise, this availability is enhanced by the lowering of blood insulin concentration to relieve an inhibition of lipolysis in adipose tissue by insulin (77). Further lipolysis is stimulated by a gradual rise in the circulating epinephrine concentration (77). The trained individual derives a greater proportion of energy from free fatty acid oxidation, yet after training, the concentration of free fatty acids in the blood during exercise is lower than before training (97,102). Thus, in the presence of a lower lipid mobilization, fat oxidation is enhanced in the trained person. Three factors may contribute to this phenomenon. First, highly trained endurance athletes are known to have a higher proportion of slow-twitch fibers than their untrained counterparts; these slow-twitch fibers have more capillaries (161) to supply fat plus a greater mitochondrial content and oxidative capacity to utilize fat (92). Second, trained individuals have a higher lipoprotein lipase activity in muscle (172). This allows for an increased degradation of plasma triglycerides to free fatty acids in muscle capillaries; these fatty acids can then be used for oxidation by muscle or for the restoration of intramuscular triglyceride stores after exercise (107). A third explanation for increased fat utilization in the trained state with an apparent decrease in fatty acid availability is that training increases the utilization of intramuscular triglycerides. This was recently confirmed by Hurley et al. (97). Although they did not elucidate the mechanism of this adaptation, it is possible that training increases the activity of the type L-hormone-sensitive lipase in humans as has been demonstrated in rats (144).

2. **Does the Availability of Fat limit Performance?** Because body fat reserves are large and because most individuals consume calories during the longest of athletic competitions, the depletion of muscular fat depots has not been identified as a contributor to fatigue. Naturally, during higher intensity exercise, the proportion of fuel oxidation which cannot be supported by protein and fat is made up by the oxidation of carbohydrate, either in the form of muscle glycogen or blood-borne glucose.

C. Carbohydrates

The stores of carbohydrate in the body are not as plentiful as those of fats or proteins. The average man has roughly 8.5 MJ (201 kcal) of energy potentially available from carbohydrate, but since 50% or less is usually used for prolonged exercise, only 5.1 MJ (1218 kcal) are likely to be available from carbohydrates (136). The total body carbohydrate stores available for the generation of energy during exercise are located in the liver or muscle as glycogen, or in the blood as glucose. Because of its large mass, muscle has the most stored glycogen (400 g; 6.7 MJ, 1600 kcal), liver has the next largest amount (70 g; 1.2 MJ, 280 kcal), and a much smaller amount of carbohydrate (2.5 g; 342 kJ, 10 kcal) exists as circulating blood glucose. If carbohydrates were the only source of energy for exercise at 2.0 L $O_2 \cdot min^{-1}$, carbohydrate oxidation would support the energy demands of exercise for roughly two hours. Training for and competition in many athletic events often require efforts longer than three hours. Thus, carbohydrate is not the sole source of energy during prolonged severe exercise. However, unlike fat, carbohydrate metabolism can support high intensity exercise for a substantial period of time; carbohydrate appears to be the preferred fuel for muscle metabolism when the exercise intensity is greater than 65% $\dot{V}O_2$max (162).

1. **Muscle Glycogen.** The muscle glycogen content in untrained sedentary individuals is between 70 and 90 millimoles per kilogram of wet muscle weight ($mmol \cdot kg^{-1}$) (11). The endurance-trained athlete who consumes a mixed diet and rests for a day has a muscle glycogen content of roughly 130 $mmol \cdot kg^{-1}$ (31,168). Unlike the results found for the lipid stores, the fast-twitch and slow-twitch fibers have a similar glycogen content, i.e., 355 and 359 $mmol \cdot kg^{-1}$ dry weight for the slow- and fast-twitch fibers, respectively (57).

a. Factors Affecting the Utilization of Glycogen During Exercise

Intensity of Exercise. As the exercise intensity increases linearly, there is an exponential increase in the rate of muscle glycogen utilization (162). At 50%, 75% and 100% $\dot{V}O_2$max, muscle glycogen is used at rates of 0.7, 1.4, and 3.4 $mmol \cdot kg^{-1} \cdot min^{-1}$ (162). At exercise intensities greater than 90% $\dot{V}O_2$max, exercise has to be stopped before the muscle glycogen stores are depleted; thus, exhaustion must be due primarily to other factors at such high intensities. At exercise intensities less than 60% $\dot{V}O_2$max, individuals can exercise for many hours without depleting the muscle glycogen stores (162). Obviously, at these low exercise intensities, the oxidation of fat is the primary source of energy. At such low intensities, boredom, dehydration, hyperthermia and orthopedic discomfort/injuries are commonly the reasons for fatigue. However, as exercise at 65% to 85% $\dot{V}O_2$max progresses, there is a curvilinear decrease in the muscle glycogen concentration with the greatest decrease occurring in the first 15 to 20 min (88,162). At 65 to 85% $\dot{V}O_2$max, exhaustion is accompanied by the simultaneous depletion of the muscle glycogen stores. In addition, there is a strong relationship between the initial preexercise muscle glycogen concentration and the length of time that exercise can be performed at these intensities (5,12,88) (See Figure 6-1).

Mode of Exercise. The rate of muscle glycogen utilization is about twice as great in the lateral quadriceps during cycling as it is in the

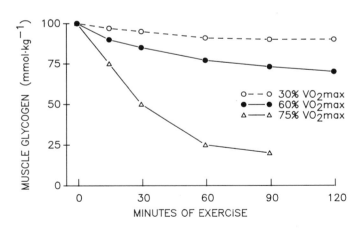

FIGURE 6-1. *Muscle glycogen degradation during exercise at three different intensities. Fatigue coincides with a low muscle glycogen concentration at 75% $\dot{V}O_2$max, whereas other factors contribute to fatigue at 30% and 60% $\dot{V}O_2$max.*

soleus during uphill treadmill running at the same relative intensity (57). During level treadmill running for two hours, the rate of muscle glycogen depletion is greatest in the soleus, intermediate in the gastrocnemius and least in the quadriceps (38). Nevertheless, when running uphill, the absolute rate of glycogen degradation in the quadriceps is increased 3-fold (38). When running on the level for two hours at 70% $\dot{V}O_2$max, glycogen depletion occurs at a faster rate in the slow-twitch fibers than in the fast-twitch fibers (40); this reflects a greater reliance on the slow-twitch fibers during aerobic exercise.

The Environment. A 1.8-fold greater rate of muscle glycogen breakdown occurs during 60 min of cycling at 41° C (15% relative humidity) when compared to the same exercise undertaken in a cold environment (9° C, 55% relative humidity) (63). Thus, the muscle glycogen reserves will be used to a variable amount depending on the environment.

Percent of $\dot{V}O_2$max at Lactate Threshold. Coyle et al.(46) demonstrated that individuals with the same $\dot{V}O_2$max had extremely variable performance times to exhaustion at 89% $\dot{V}O_2$max. The performance time and muscle glycogen utilization were highly correlated ($r = 0.93$, and -0.91, respectively) with the %$\dot{V}O_2$max at lactate threshold. Thus, training to increase the percent of $\dot{V}O_2$max at which the lactate threshold occurs may improve performance during training and competition by decreasing the rate of muscle glycogen breakdown. This will help conserve glycogen so that it will be available during the later stages of exercise.

b. *Muscle Glycogen as a Limiting Factor During Exercise.* Using the information which has been discussed in this chapter, a rough estimation of the time of glycogen depletion for exercise at 70% $\dot{V}O_2$max can be accomplished. During running, one might assume a working muscle mass of 22 kg and a normal muscle glycogen content of 99 mmol $\cdot$ kg^{-1} (136). Therefore, the potentially available muscle glycogen will be 400 g. At 70% $\dot{V}O_2$max, the average rate of muscle glycogen degradation will be 4.5 mmol $\cdot$ kg^{-1} $\cdot$ km^{-1}. Therefore, total depletion of muscle glycogen will theoretically occur at approximately 22 km (13.7 miles) during a marathon. Based on this approximation, it can be seen that it is important to load the muscle glycogen stores maximally before prolonged training and competition.

2. Liver Glycogen and Blood Glucose.

a. *Maintenance of the Blood Glucose Concentration During Exercise.* Liver glycogen is degraded to glucose during exercise, and the glucose is released into the blood to maintain the blood glucose concentration, which is determined by the rate of uptake by glucose-metabolizing tissue and the rate of release of glucose by the liver. As exercise intensity increases to 65% $\dot{V}O_2$max, there is a linear increase in muscle glucose uptake; above 65% $\dot{V}O_2$max, the rate of glucose uptake has presumably plateaued, and further carbohydrate oxidation must be supported by muscle glycogen degradation (152). A recent study (104), however, suggests that the linear relationship between exercise intensity and glucose uptake extends even to maximal intensities. At 50% and 100% $\dot{V}O_2$max the rates of muscle glucose uptake observed were 1.1 and 3.8 mmol·min^{-1}, respectively (104). Nevertheless, at high exercise intensities, muscle glucose uptake and metabolism ordinarily cannot match the necessary energy expenditure, and muscle glycogen is the primary carbohydrate which is metabolized.

During low intensity exercise (30 to 40% $\dot{V}O_2$max), there is a relatively great utilization of fat and low utilization of carbohydrate (47). Thus, the liver glycogen stores will maintain the blood glucose concentration for a long time because the rate of muscle glucose uptake is low. During low intensity exercise, the blood glucose concentration declines slowly and rarely falls below 2.8 mmol·L^{-1} (3,180). Gluconeogenesis accounts for at least half of the liver glucose output during such activity and is an important contributor to the maintenance of the blood glucose concentration (176).

The blood glucose concentration is maintained during the early stages of moderately intensive activity because liver glucose release balances muscle glucose uptake (1). However, as exercise progresses, liver glycogen stores and glucose output decline, while glucose uptake by the muscle remains constant. Accordingly, blood glucose concentration declines because of the imbalance between muscle uptake and liver output (1). During prolonged, moderately intense exercise, gluconeogenesis is accelerated, but this cannot totally compensate for the decline in liver glucose output (1,47). Thus, at 58% $\dot{V}O_2$max, the blood glucose concentration declines to less than 2.5 mmol·L^{-1} after 3.5 h of cycling, whereas it may decline to this level after only 2.5 h of cycling at 74% $\dot{V}O_2$max (1,44,49).

b. Incidence of Hypoglycemia During Exercise. Levine et al.(119) reported blood glucose concentrations less than 2.5 mmol·L^{-1} (i.e., clinical or "frank" hypoglycemia) following a marathon. But not all individuals exhibit hypoglycemia under such conditions. Furthermore, different sensitivities to a lowering of blood glucose exist among individuals (49). Less than 50% of subjects display hypoglycemia when exercised at 60% to 70% $\dot{V}O_2$max for between 2.5 to 3.5 h (1,4,49). Of these, 30% seem to demonstrate fatigue of a central nervous system origin, whereas in the remaining 70% the fatigue can be ascribed to peripheral factors (1,4,49,59).

D. Integration of the Use of Fuels During Exercise

The preceding discussion has indicated that proteins, fats and carbohydrates can serve as fuels during prolonged exercise. The relative contribution of proteins is minimal, and there is no evidence that inadequate protein stores or intake above the recommended daily allowance decreases or increases prolonged performance capacity, respectively. The body stores of fats are plentiful. However, the maximal rate of oxidation of fats cannot totally support exercise at intensities commonly used during training and performance (> 50% $\dot{V}O_2$max). Unfortunately, the muscle, liver, and blood stores of carbohydrate, the primary fuel for training and competition, are limited. An athlete engaging in daily training must be concerned with replenishing the carbohydrate reserves on a daily basis between training sessions. During competition, the athlete must be concerned with optimizing body carbohydrate stores before the race as well as maintaining them during the race.

IV. NUTRITION DURING TRAINING

Because carbohydrate is the major fuel supporting training and competition in prolonged exercise, an athlete must closely monitor the carbohydrate intake in the diet. The carbohydrate and fat contributions to total caloric intake should be increased to 70% and decreased to 15% to 20%, respectively, whereas the protein contribution should remain between 10% and 15%. A high carbohydrate intake will enhance glycogen stores in liver and muscle.

A. Liver Glycogen Stores

1. Dietary Carbohydrate and the Replenishment of Liver Glycogen Stores. In a normal man consuming a mixed diet, the liver glycogen concentration is approximately 270 mmol·kg^{-1} with a range of 87 to 460 mmol·kg^{-1} (94). Since the liver in the average man weighs 1.8 kg, the total glycogen content of liver is roughly 490 mmol (94). The carbohydrate and fat contents of the diet affect liver glycogen, which can be increased to 900 mmol by consumption of a high carbohydrate diet and decreased to 60 mmol after a low carbohydrate diet (94). The average rate of glycogenolysis in the liver is 32 mmol·h^{-1} per entire liver in a rested subject (94). Assuming an average initial liver glycogen content, i.e., 490 mmol, the liver glycogen stores would be empty in 15 h. Thus, an overnight fast will lower the liver glycogen stores and impair performance if exercise greater than two hours is undertaken. Accordingly, to ensure high liver glycogen stores for strenuous prolonged training sessions, as little time as possible should intervene between the final meal and the training session. (See subsequent section on preexercise feedings for limitations). If a workout lasting more than two hours is to be undertaken upon arising, it may be ideal to consume a high carbohydrate diet late in the evening before training.

2. **Carbohydrate Source and Liver Glycogen Synthesis.** Different types of carbohydrates appear to have different effects on liver glycogen synthesis. Nilson and Hultman (139) measured the liver glycogen content of subjects in the postabsorptive state before and after infusion of 5.6 mmol hexose $\cdot$ kg^{-1} body weight $\cdot$ h^{-1} for 4 h. The hexose was either glucose or fructose. The total amount of glucose infused (22.4 g; 90 kcal) was also ingested as a glucose solution to compare the effect of infusion with that of oral ingestion on liver glycogen synthesis. The rate of liver glycogen synthesis was 0.3 mmol glucose units $\cdot$ min^{-1} $\cdot$ kg^{-1} during either the four hour infusion or the oral ingestion of glucose. In contrast, when fructose was infused, the rate of synthesis was increased to 1.1 mmol $\cdot$ min^{-1} $\cdot$ kg^{-1}, 3.7 times the rate of liver glycogen synthesis with glucose. This is similar to the rate of liver glycogen synthesis observed for rat liver in situ (110). This greater rate of liver glycogen synthesis from fructose as compared to glucose is probably related to the significantly greater activity of fructose kinase in the liver when compared to glucose kinase activity (86). Thus, to maximize liver glycogen synthesis, foods should be consumed that have a high fructose content, e.g., fresh fruits.

3. **Competition Between Liver and Muscle for Glycogen Synthesis After Exercise.** Maehlum et al. (123) investigated the effects of cycling exercise to exhaustion at 70% $\dot{V}O_2$max on the postexhaustion disposal of 100 g of ingested glucose. The glucose was consumed during the first 135 min of recovery, and the site of glucose disposal in the exercised group was compared to that of a nonexercised control group. Splanchnic glucose output ranged from 50% to 300% greater during recovery from exercise when compared to control data. Total splanchnic glucose release during recovery was 59 g and 28 g in the exercised and control groups, respectively. Muscle glycogen synthesis occurred at a mean rate of 1.7 mmol $\cdot$ kg^{-1} $\cdot$ h^{-1} in the previously exercised subjects, but the rate of synthesis in control subjects was not reported. The synthesis of muscle glycogen accounted for 55% of the total splanchnic glucose release. Krzentowski et al. (111) suggest that the enhancing effect of prior exercise on splanchnic glucose release is mediated in part by elevated glucagon levels and a reduced insulin release after exercise. Therefore, there is strong evidence that a large proportion of oral glucose ingested after exercise escapes liver retention, allowing muscle gly-

cogen synthesis to occur preferentially over liver glycogen synthesis.

B. Muscle Glycogen Stores

1. Dietary Carbohydrate Intake and Muscle Glycogen Synthesis. Because muscle glycogen stores may limit high intensity exercise, it is important for the athlete to undertake dietary practices that help to ensure normalization of muscle glycogen on a daily basis. Early studies found that at least 48 h were required to restore muscle glycogen after exercise (150,151), but more recent experiments have demonstrated that the muscle glycogen stores can be normalized on a daily basis provided that adequate carbohydrate is consumed in the diet (5,11,31,106).

The studies by Piehl and co-workers (150) in the 1970s were the basis for the early conclusion that at least 48 h were required to restore muscle glycogen to "normal" levels after depletion. Their two hour exercise protocols utilized intermittent work bouts of aerobic exercise and sprints to deplete glycogen in both the slow-twitch and fast-twitch fibers. The muscle glycogen content after the depleting exercise was commonly 23 mmol $\cdot$ kg^{-1} wet weight. The subjects then consumed a 4,000 kcal diet with 60% of the calories derived from carbohydrate (600 g carbohydrate), i.e., 8.6 g carbohydrate $\cdot$ kg^{-1} body weight. The muscle glycogen content at 24 and 34 h after exercise was 76% of the preexercise level (125 mmol $\cdot$ kg^{-1}) and did not return to the preexercise level until 46 h after exercise. Piehl et al. (151) reported similar results in a subsequent study.

The literature is now replete with studies confirming that muscle glycogen can be normalized in 24 h, provided that the diet contains an adequate proportion of carbohydrate. Bergstrom, Hultman & Roch-Norlund (11) had subjects deplete their muscle glycogen stores by cycling to exhaustion. It was found that glycogen was restored to preexercise levels when subjects consumed a diet in which 95% of the calories were derived from carbodydrate (653 g in 2750 kcal). The subjects consumed 9.3 g carbohydrate $\cdot$ kg^{-1} body weight. A similar exercise and dietary regimen (10.6 g carbohydrate $\cdot$ kg^{-1} body weight) was used by Ahlborg et al. (5), who also found that muscle glycogen was restored in 24 h. Subsequently, Kochan et al. (106) confirmed the early repletion of glycogen stores when their subjects consumed 11.3 g carbohydrate $\cdot$ kg^{-1} body weight following cycling exercise.

Muscle glycogen can also be normalized in 24 hours after intermittent exercise. MacDougall et al. (121) had six subjects cycle at 140% $\dot{V}O_2$max for 1 min intervals with 3 min rest periods until work could not be maintained for 30 seconds. The subjects exercised an average of 10.1 min and reduced muscle glycogen to 28% of preexercise levels. Beginning at 2 h after exercise and during the next 24 h, the subjects consumed a diet containing 3020 kcal, 50% of which was carbohydrate (4.8 g carbohydrate $\cdot$ kg^{-1} body weight). Within 24 h, all but one subject had muscle glycogen concentrations equivalent to the preexercise levels. Thus, muscle glycogen can be normalized in 24 h when the mode of glycogen depletion has been either continuous exercise or high intensity intermittent exercise.

Differences in fiber types and their capacities to synthesize glycogen cannot account for the differences in results between the older and more recent studies, because the subjects in most studies had approximately equal distributions of slow-twitch and fast-twitch fibers, and the glycogen synthesis capacity is not different between the fiber types (151). It is possible that the disparities in the time-course of glycogen synthesis can be explained by variable levels of muscle glycogen depletion and variable amounts of carbohydrate consumption on a body weight basis.

The effect of variations in dietary carbohydrate on muscle glycogen synthesis was more closely examined by Costill et al. (31). They required 10 subjects to run 16 km at approximately 80% $\dot{V}O_2$max, after which they ran five 1 min sprints at 130% $\dot{V}O_2$max interrupted by three min rest periods. Muscle glycogen was reduced to 50 mmol $\cdot$ kg^{-1} wet weight immediately after exercise and had changed by -5%, $+51\%$, and $+129\%$ in 24 h when the subjects consumed 2.4, 4.7, and 6.6 g carbohydrate $\cdot$ kg^{-1} body weight, respectively, in two meals during the 24 h period (Fig. 6-2). There was a significant relationship ($r = 0.84$) between the amount of carbohydrate ingested (188 g, 325 g, or 525 g) and the net amount of muscle glycogen synthesized during the 24 h period of study. It should be noted that Costill et al. (31) did not measure the predepletion concentration of muscle glycogen. They suggested that trained athletes have a muscle glycogen concentration which averages 130 mmol $\cdot$ kg^{-1}. Therefore, because the depleting exercise utilized 80 mmol glycogen $\cdot$ kg^{-1} wet weight and because the 70% carbohydrate diet resulted in muscle glycogen synthesis of approximately 80 mmol $\cdot$ kg^{-1} in 24 h, Costill et al. (32) have strongly suggested that the consumption of a 70% carbohydrate diet with 7 g carbohydrate $\cdot$ kg^{-1} body weight will replenish the muscle glycogen stores between daily training sessions.

2. **What is the Optimal Timing of Dietary Carbohydrate Consumption After Exercise?.** The relationship between the amount of carbohydrate ingested and rates of glycogen synthesis and the observation of a hormonal milieu antagonistic to glycogen synthesis (i.e., high glucagon and low insulin) have prompted several inves-

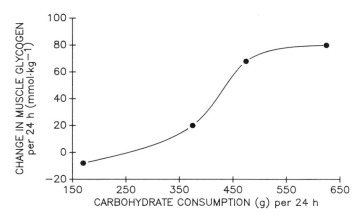

FIGURE 6-2. *The relationship between the amount of carbohydrate consumed in the diet and muscle glycogen synthesis during a 24 h period (31). Muscle glycogen had been reduced to roughly 50 mmol · kg^{-1} before consuming the various diets.*

tigators to examine the optimal timing and amount of glucose ingestion in the hours after exercise to maximize glycogen resynthesis. Maehlum and Hermansen (122) exercised five subjects to exhaustion on a cycle ergometer at 70% $\dot{V}O_2$max. Exercise time was 89 min, and muscle glycogen dropped from 70 to 21 mmol · kg^{-1}. The subjects then fasted for 12 h. During the first 4 h, muscle glycogen increased to 29 mmol · kg^{-1}; however, no further increase in muscle glycogen occurred during the subsequent 8 h of recovery. Because the blood glucose concentration remained constant during recovery, the authors hypothesized that increased gluconeogenesis accounted for the small glycogen synthesis.

Blom et al. (14) investigated the effect of ingesting increasing amounts of carbohydrate during the 8 h immediately following cycling exercise which had reduced muscle glycogen stores to 20 mmol · kg^{-1} wet weight. The subjects consumed 0.7, 1.4, or 2.0 g glucose · kg^{-1} body weight after 0, 2, 4, and 6 h of recovery. This feeding schedule provided between 200 and 600 g carbohydrate (800 to 2400 kcal) during the 8 h period. The rates of muscle glycogen synthesis were 5.3, 4.9, and 5.5 mmol · kg^{-1} · h^{-1}. There was no difference in the rate of muscle glycogen synthesis between these feeding schedules. Another group of subjects performed the same exercise but consumed 0.7 g of either sucrose or fructose per kg body weight after 0, 2, 4, and 6 h of recovery. The rates of glycogen synthesis were 4.74 and 3.24 mmol · kg^{-1} · h^{-1} for the sucrose and fructose feedings, respectively. Thus, the rate of glycogen synthesis when sucrose was consumed was similar to that observed for glucose;

however, the rate with consumption of fructose was only 68% of that observed for glucose or sucrose. Based on these findings, it might be suggested that the maximal rate of glycogen synthesis following exercise is approximately 6 mmol·kg^{-1}·h^{-1} (14).

This estimation by Blom et al. (14) of the maximal rate of postexercise glycogen synthesis is supported by studies of Ivy et al. (Footnote 2), whose subjects cycled at intermittent high and low intensities. In this case, the subjects were fed a glucose solution (2.0 g·kg^{-1} body weight) either 15 min before exercise termination, immediately after, or 2 h after the cessation of exercise. Muscle glycogen was measured at 0, 2, and 4 h after exercise. When glucose was consumed 15 min before or immediately after cessation of exercise, the rate of muscle glycogen synthesis was 7.5 mmol·kg^{-1}·h^{-1}. When glucose was withheld during the initial 2 h following exercise, the rate of muscle glycogen synthesis was three-times lower, i.e., 2.5 mmol·kg^{-1}·h^{-1}. However, when glucose was then provided 2 h after exercise, the rate of muscle glycogen synthesis was increased to 4.1 mmol·kg^{-1}·h^{-1}.

Bonen et al. (16) determined the rate of muscle glycogen synthesis after subjects reduced muscle glycogen to 20% of preexercise levels and then ingested 1.5 g glucose·kg^{-1} body weight 10 min after exercise and again 2 h later. The muscle glycogen concentration was 60% and 70% of the preexercise glycogen concentration by 2 h and 4 h after exercise, respectively. Based on these results and those of Blom et al. (14) and Ivy et al. (Footnote 2), it appears that carbohydrate should be ingested immediately after exercise to optimize muscle glycogen synthesis. The amount consumed should be approximately 0.7 to 2.0 g glucose·kg^{-1} body weight every 2 h. This means that endurance athletes should probably consume high carbohydrate snacks throughout the day between training sessions.

3. **Exercise Mode and Postexercise Glycogen Resynthesis.** The immediate postexercise rate of muscle glycogen synthesis may depend on the mode of exercise used to deplete the muscle glycogen stores. In studies that have used prolonged exercise to deplete muscle glycogen, it is also likely that the liver glycogen stores were depleted. As indicated previously, the rate of muscle glycogen synthesis is very low when carbohydrate is not provided. However, a low rate of glycogen synthesis was not observed during the first 2 h of recovery in subjects that had undertaken high intensity intermittent exercise to deplete muscle glycogen (121). MacDougall et al. (121) found muscle glycogen synthesis rates of 6 mmol·kg^{-1}·h^{-1} in the first 2 h of recovery when their subjects were not fed. Recall that this is approximately the maximal rate of synthesis observed in the prolonged exercise protocols of Ivy et al. (Footnote 2) and Blom

et al. (14). MacDougall et al. (121) theorized that because their exercise task had not depleted the liver glycogen reserves, blood glucose was provided from liver glycogen stores and was used for muscle glycogen synthesis during the 2 h of food deprivation. Further work is required to confirm this hypothesis.

4. Dietary Carbohydrate Source and Muscle Glycogen Synthesis. The type of carbohydrate consumed after glycogen depletion may also slightly affect the rate of muscle glycogen synthesis. Costill et. al. (31) examined the effect of consuming a carbohydrate diet that contained either simple or complex carbohydrates on muscle glycogen synthesis during 48 h after exhaustive running. During the first 24 h, the subjects consumed 9.0 g carbohydrate $\cdot$ kg^{-1} body weight (3700 kcal; 648 g carbohydrate); during the second 24 h, the subjects consumed 5.8 g carbohydrate $\cdot$ kg^{-1} body weight. During the first 24 h, both the simple and complex carbohydrate diets resulted in a total glycogen synthesis of 80 mmol $\cdot$ kg^{-1} wet weight, but during the second 24 h, the complex carbohydrate diet resulted in significantly greater glycogen synthesis (22 versus 8 mmol $\cdot$ kg^{-1}). The authors suggested that this effect of complex carbohydrates was mediated primarily by insulin-induced activation of muscle glucose uptake and glycogen synthesis because complex carbohydrates cause a lower but longer-lasting elevation of blood glucose and insulin than the ingestion of simple carbohydrate (91). Thus, on a daily basis it appears that the consumption of either complex or simple carbohydrates will "normalize" the muscle glycogen reserves between training sessions. However, complex carbohydrates usually provide a better balance of vitamins and minerals than the highly refined simple sugars (6). In fact, the American Diabetes Association recommends that a high percentage of the calories derived from carbohydrate should come from complex carbohydrates (6). Based on the greater synthesis of muscle glycogen while consuming complex carbohydrates during the second 24 h period, complex carbohydrates may be preferred when athletes undertake diet and exercise regimens to supercompensate the muscle glycogen stores.

Because complex carbohydrate foods have a high fiber content, it should be noted that the addition of fiber to the diet lowers postprandial blood glucose concentrations (177). This could adversely affect glycogen resynthesis. Wahren et al. (177) demonstrated that the ingestion of 10 g guar gum (dietary fiber) with 25 g xylose resulted in a significantly lower plasma glucose and insulin response compared to the ingestion of xylose alone. Since these experiments were conducted on sedentary subjects, the exact application to athletics of this effect of fiber on blood glucose during postexercise recovery of muscle glycogen is unclear. However, one might speculate that athletes may benefit from the consumption of low fiber, high carbohydrate diets to maximally resynthesize muscle glycogen.

5. Does Exercise-Induced Muscle Damage Adversely Affect Muscle Glycogen Resynthesis? Sherman et al. (165) observed a slow rate of glycogen synthesis during the week following a marathon when subjects either rested or exercised during that week and consumed a diet containing 12 g carbohydrate per kg body weight during the first 24 h after and 6.8 g carbohydrate per kg body weight during the subsequent days after the marathon. Muscle glycogen was reduced from supercompensated levels (196 mmol $\cdot$ kg^{-1}) to 25 mmol $\cdot$ kg^{-1} by the marathon and had reached a concentration equivalent to that found in rested, trained runners (130 mmol $\cdot$ kg^{-1}) only after five days of recovery from the marathon. Muscle glycogen did not increase substantially during the subsequent four days. This slow rate of synthesis following the marathon may have been related to the muscle damage observed during the days of recovery (89). Kuipers et al. (112) observed a slower rate of muscle glycogen synthesis in muscle that had been damaged by eccentric exercise compared to concentrically exercised muscle. Furthermore, Lash et al. (114) reported a state of insulin resistance 48 h after eccentric running when compared to concentric running.

6. Does Exercise During Recovery from Prior Exercise Adversely Affect Glycogen Resynthesis? Another factor that might potentially impair muscle glycogen synthesis is exercise during the recovery period from prior exercise. Exercise at an intensity requiring carbohydrate combustion is obviously counterproductive to glycogen synthesis. However, it is reasonable to assume that exercise at an intensity which relies primarily on fatty acid oxidation would not affect muscle glycogen synthesis, provided the blood glucose concentration is normal.

Interestingly, this assumption is not supported by the results of Bonen et al. (16). They determined the rate of muscle glycogen synthesis after subjects reduced muscle glycogen to 20% of preexercise levels and then ingested 1.5 g glucose $\cdot$ kg^{-1} body weight 10 min after exercise and again 2 h later. During the total 4 h recovery period the subjects either rested one leg or they exercised one leg to elicit an energy expenditure equivalent to 20% $\dot{V}O_2$max. For both legs, the muscle glycogen concentration had increased to only 26% and 36% of the preexercise concentration at 2 and 4 h after exercise, respectively. Bonen et al. (16) could not explain this very low rate of glycogen synthesis on the basis of their other metabolic measurements and speculated that the maintenance of elevated blood epinephrine after exercise accounted for the impairment of glycogen synthesis.

7. Effects of Different Diets on Training and on Recovery from Training. One study attempted to determine if consumption of a moderate carbohydrate diet affected training capacity on a daily basis (42). Six moderately trained runners undertook three successive days of running 16.1 km at 80% $\dot{V}O_2$max. Muscle biopsies obtained before and after each run were analyzed for glycogen content. During the three days the subjects consumed a self-selected diet reported to contain 40% to 50% of the calories derived from carbohydrate. The average amount of muscle glycogen used for each 16.1 km run on the three days was 30 to 50 mmol·kg^{-1}. The preexercise muscle glycogen concentration for each of the three days was approximately 110, 88, and 66 mmol·kg^{-1} (Fig. 6-3). Although Costill et al. (42) stated that "no consistent pattern was observed with regard to increased levels of fatigue with successive days of exertion," it would be expected that such a pattern might occur because of the relationship between low levels of muscle glycogen and exhaustion found in other studies. Because the content of the diets was not analyzed, it is impossible to determine the amount of carbohydrate consumed per kg body weight for these subjects. Over the three-day period, there was a gradual shift toward increased fat oxidation, as indicated by lower respiratory exchange ratio, lower lactate production, and higher serum free fatty acid concentration. The implications of these results are clear. If adequate carbohydrate is not consumed on a daily basis between training sessions, the preexercise muscle glycogen content will gradually decline; if the task is

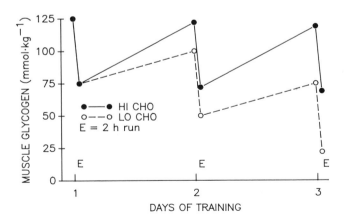

FIGURE 6-3. *Effect of low carbohydrate diet (45% of the calories, open circle) and a high carbohydrate diet (70% of the calories, closed circle) on muscle glycogen during three consecutive days of repeated 2 h running sessions at 70% $\dot{V}O_2$max (32,42).*

one which is limited primarily by the muscle glycogen content, either training or competitive performance will eventually be impaired.

Brooke and Green (20) examined the effect of glucose syrup ingestion on the ability to recover working capacity after previous exhausting exercise. Trained cyclists rode at 70% $\dot{V}O_2$max until a respiratory exchange ratio of 0.73 was reached (work time to this criterion was 155 min). The subjects then rested for 40 min and consumed either a glucose syrup (1490 kJ; 355 kcal), a rice pudding with sucrose added to the same energy value, or a placebo. After the rest, the subjects exercised at 70% $\dot{V}O_2$max until exhausted or until a respiratory exchange ratio of 0.73 was reached. Conservative statistics were used to evaluate the data (replicated Latin Square analysis with Scheffé multiple comparisons). Blood glucose was maintained during exercise for all trials and was significantly elevated during recovery and during exercise for the glucose syrup and pudding/sucrose trials. Significant differences in the mean values for work duration after the 40 min recovery were detected among all treatments. The work times were 1.33 h, 0.97 h, and 0.48 h for the glucose syrup, pudding/sucrose, and placebo trials, respectively. The authors hypothesized that neural factors were involved in the differences between the treatments. However, because muscle glycogen stores were probably significantly reduced by the first exercise task and little synthesis would have occurred during 40 min of recovery, these subjects may have had a high capacity to utilize blood glucose which could have resulted in work enhancement during the glucose syrup and pudding/sucrose trials.

C. Maintenance of the Carbohydrate Stores During Intense Daily Training

It is now clear that the athlete training for and competing in prolonged exercise should consume a diet which contains a high percentage of the calories from carbohydrate. Ideally, 70% of the calories should be provided from carbohydrate, and the caloric consumption should match the daily caloric expenditure. If the diet contains a smaller percentage of calories from carbohydrate during heavy training, there may be a gradual deterioration in training capacity related to a gradual diminution of muscle glycogen. Consumption of high carbohydrate meals should begin as soon as possible after the completion of prolonged exercise, preferably within 30 min, to maximize muscle glycogen synthesis. Exercise during the recovery period should be avoided to maximize muscle glycogen synthesis, however, if exercise is required, extra carbohydrate should be consumed. Furthermore, when exercise has produced muscle soreness and tenderness, there may be an impairment of muscle glycogen synthesis.

V. NUTRITION DURING THE WEEK BEFORE AN IMPORTANT PERFORMANCE

The positive relationship between the preexercise concentration of muscle glycogen and the length of time that intense exercise can be continued has led to experiments designed to determine the optimal methods for maximally increasing muscle glycogen before an important competition. It has been hypothesized that with elevated muscle glycogen, the exercise duration before low muscle glycogen levels cause fatigue can be extended. Muscle that has a maximal concentration of glycogen is often referred to as "glycogen-loaded" or "supercompensated."

A. The Classical Glycogen Supercompensation Regimen

Bergstrom et al. (12) were the first to describe a method to supercompensate the muscle glycogen stores. Six objects consumed a mixed diet (50% of calories derived from carbohydrate) for three days, exercised to exhaustion at 75% $\dot{V}O_2$max, and then consumed a low carbohydrate diet (10% of calories derived from carbohydrate) for three days. Muscle glycogen had decreased from 106 mmol·kg^{-1} to 11 mmol·kg^{-1} after exercise and had increased to only 40 mmol·kg^{-1} three days later. Thereafter, the subjects exercised to exhaustion a second time, consumed a high carbohydrate diet (90% of calories derived from carbohydrate) for three days, and exercised a third time to exhaustion. Muscle glycogen had decreased to 11 mmol·kg^{-1} after the second exercise bout and had increased to 204 mmol·kg^{-1} three days later. The final session of exhaustive exercise reduced muscle glycogen to 24 mmol·kg^{-1}. It is obvious that the low carbohydrate diet (4 g carbohydrate·kg^{-1} body weight) did not stimulate muscle glycogen synthesis, whereas the high carbohydrate diet (36 g carbohydrate·kg^{-1} body weight) markedly increased the muscle glycogen content by 1.9-fold. These different initial muscle glycogen concentrations were highly correlated with the length of time that work could be maintained until exhaustion (r = 0.92), suggesting that elevating the muscle glycogen concentration would enhance this type of performance.

The above results were subsequently confirmed and extended by Ahlborg et al. (5), who used a randomized block design with military cadets as subjects. Group A consumed a mixed diet and then performed exhaustive exercise, after which they consumed a diet containing 95% of the calories from carbohydrate for three days.

Muscle glycogen was 83, 16, and 136 mmol·kg^{-1} before and after exercise and three days later, respectively. Thus, the muscle glycogen content after the high carbohydrate diet was 1.6-fold greater than the preexercise glycogen concentration. Group B consumed a mixed diet, exercised to exhaustion, consumed a low carbohydrate diet for one day (10% of calories from carbohydrate), exercised to exhaustion again, and then consumed a high carbohydrate diet (95% of calories from carbohydrate) for three days. The muscle glycogen content was decreased from 91 to 26 mmol·kg^{-1} by exercise and increased to only 37 mmol·kg^{-1} after three days under the low carbohydrate diet. After the high carbohydrate diet the muscle glycogen content was 165 mmol·kg^{-1} or 1.8-fold higher than the predepletion value. Group C underwent the same treatment as Group B, but consumed the low carbohydrate diet for three days. The muscle glycogen content was decreased from 84 to 20 mmol·kg^{-1} and increased to only 35 mmol·kg^{-1} after the three-day consumption of the low carbohydrate diet. After exercising again to exhaustion and consuming a high carbohydrate diet for three days, the muscle glycogen concentration had increased to 151 mmol·kg^{-1} (1.8-fold higher than the predepletion muscle glycogen concentration).

Based on the observation that exhaustive exercise and maintenance of low glycogen content by a low carbohydrate diet potentiated muscle glycogen synthesis, these authors have advocated the diet and exercise regimen of Group C to supercompensate the muscle glycogen stores. An often overlooked aspect of this particular study is that muscle glycogen was also measured in this group after an additional four days on a high carbohydrate diet. Seven days after the second exercise session, the muscle glycogen content had increased to 205 mmol·kg^{-1} or 2.4-fold higher than the predepletion muscle glycogen concentration.

A report of ineffectiveness of the classical regimen to supercompensate muscle glycogen has been published (174). Trained runners undertook three dietary regimens: 1) six days of a mixed diet (50% of the calories derived from carbohydrate, 6 g·kg^{-1} body weight·day^{-1}) consumed in three daily meals, 2) six days of the same diet consumed in six daily meals, and 3) three days of a low carbohydrate diet (17% of the calories from carbohydrate) followed by three days of a "high" carbohydrate diet (65% of the calories from carbohydrate, 10.5 g·kg^{-1} body weight·day^{-1}). During the first three days the subjects ran for 150 min, 70 min, and 70 min at 70% V̇O$_2$max; they rested for the next three days. Muscle biopsies were obtained after the dietary treatments and were 122, 100, and 122 mmol·kg^{-1}, respectively. The vastus lateralis was biopsied, but this may not be an ideal biopsy site for running exercise (174). This single report of the noneffectiveness of a classical "supercompensation" regimen, however, should not detract from the various other studies which have demonstrated this phenomenon.

B. The Modified Regimen for Glycogen Supercompensation

An apparent problem with exhaustive exercise twice during the week before an important competition for the purpose of reducing muscle glycogen concentration to low levels is that "tapering" for the event may be disrupted. Certainly any time an athlete exercises to exhaustion there is the potential for injury. Additionally, consumption of diets containing less than 10% or greater than 90% of the calories from carbohydrate is not very practical. Most athletes have a difficult time self-selecting diets high in carbohydrate content. Therefore, it was appropriate to determine if a less strenuous exercise and diet regimen would supercompensate muscle glycogen stores. Sherman et al. (168) administered three different dietary treatments to trained runners who followed a standardized tapering exercise regimen. During the six days before a 21 km time trial, the subjects ran at 73% $\dot{V}O_2$max for 90 min, 40 min, 40 min, 20 min, 20 min, and rested, respectively. A muscle biopsy was obtained in the morning on the fourth and seventh days of the experiment and after a time-trial on the seventh day. The three dietary treatments were as follows: 1) control—mixed diet (50% of calories derived from carbohydrate), 2) classical—low carbohydrate diet (25% of calories from carbohydrate) for three days and a 70% carbohydrate diet for three days, 3) modified—the mixed diet for three days and the high carbohydrate diet for three days. During the control trial, muscle glycogen concentrations were 135, 163, and 80 mmol·kg^{-1}, on day 4, day 7 before the time trial, and day 7 after the time trial, respectively. During the classical trial, the corresponding muscle glycogen contents were 80, 210, and 80 mmol·kg^{-1}. During the modified trial, the muscle glycogen contents were 135, 204, and 80 mmol·kg^{-1}. Both the modified and the classical treatments elevated the muscle glycogen content to similarly high supercompensated levels before the time-trial (1.6-fold higher than the muscle glycogen content while consuming the mixed diet) (Fig. 6-4).

Recently Roedde et al. (159) conducted a study to determine if trained athletes had the same capacity for muscle glycogen supercompensation as untrained subjects. Subjects in both groups followed the classical supercompensation regimen, except the high carbohydrate phase contained only 68% of calories from carbohydrate. The trained subjects had higher preexercise glycogen content (115 versus 92 mmol·kg^{-1}), but both groups decreased glycogen to

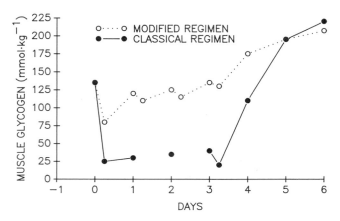

FIGURE 6-4. *Comparison of the "classical" regimen to supercompensate muscle glycogen with the "modified" regimen to supercompensate muscle glycogen during the week before an important competition (168). Note that the "modified" regimen requires "tapering-down" exercise and realistic diets (% of calories from carbohydrate) when compared to the "classical" regimen, which requires exhaustive exercise and extremes of diets.*

a similarly low level (20 mmol·kg^{-1}) after exhausting exercise. By the final day of the high carbohydrate diet, the trained group had a higher glycogen content than the untrained group (174 versus 143 mmol·kg^{-1}), but since this difference is proportional to the difference in glycogen content between the groups before depletion, the authors concluded that the magnitude of the supercompensation effect is the same in trained and untrained subjects (159).

Two apparent problems with this interpretation are that the carbohydrate content of the diet (68%) during the high carbohydrate phase was low compared to other studies and that the supercompensated glycogen concentration was less than that reported in other studies using trained subjects (>190 mmol·kg^{-1}) (159). Because the authors instructed the trained cyclists to taper their exercise to lower levels during the six days preceding the supercompensation week and the muscle glycogen content at the end of that week was merely 115 mmol·kg^{-1}, Roedde et al. (159) suggested that the classical regimen is more effective in supercompensating muscle glycogen than a regimen of tapering. It should be noted, however, that compliance with the tapering schedule was not reported and that during the tapering phase, the subjects were consuming a diet low in carbohydrate (58% of calories). Therefore, the authors' conclusion related to the effectiveness of tapering exercise in muscle glycogen supercompensation is not fully justified.

C. Effect of Glycogen Supercompensation on Performance

Although many studies in the laboratory have confirmed the positive relationship between the preexercise muscle glycogen concentration and endurance performance for cycling and running (5,12,95), the authors are aware of only one study that has evaluated this effect in the field (103). In an experiment employing a repeated measures design and a 30 km time-trial for runners, subjects undertook dietary modification in two trials that resulted in prerace muscle glycogen concentratitons of 94 and 193 mmol·kg^{-1}. All of the subjects finished the race with their best time when they began the race with high concentrations of muscle glycogen. Examination of the split times at 2 km intervals for the two trials revealed that the elevated muscle glycogen concentration did not cause the runners to run faster at the beginning of the race but rather allowed the runners to maintain their optimal pace for a longer period of time. Sherman et al. (168) reported that supercompensation did not improve running performance in a 21 km time-trial, but this is not surprising, because the time-trial was completed in a relatively brief 80 min. It would be of interest to perform additional studies in the field to determine the efficacy of glycogen supercompensation for different activities.

D. Factors Related to Supercompensation

Muscle glycogen supercompensation occurs only in muscles previously "depleted" of their glycogen stores (13). Whether or not complete degradation of glycogen to some low residual quantity is required to maximize this effect is unknown. The maintenance of low muscle glycogen after exercise is facilitated by consumption of a low carbohydrate diet, and this appears to increase the rate of muscle glycogen synthesis. However, the maximal amount of muscle glycogen stored may not be greater than that observed after less stressful regimens of diet and exercise. This suggests that there may be a maximal attainable glycogen concentration, perhaps related to the physical space available in muscle for glycogen storage.

There has been one report of cardiac arrhythmias associated with a "supercompensation" high carbohydrate diet in a middle-aged marathon runner (128). When the marathon runner returned to a normal diet, the arrhythmias ceased. This case report does not prove that consumption of a high carbohydrate will lead to heart problems in athletes. In fact, there is no systematic evidence that glycogen loading regimens are associated with any adverse effects on health.

Muscle glycogen is complexed with water, presumably 3 to 5 g water per gram glycogen (142,143). This association may have implications for energy cost, because body weight may increase by 1 to 4 kg during supercompensation. However, there has been no consistency in the reports of changes in body weight with changes in muscle glycogen concentration (140,141,168). In fact, this relationship between glycogen and water may be highly variable and affected by the rate of synthesis and branching characteristics of the glycogen molecule. The water stored in muscle with glycogen during supercompensation apparently has no detectable beneficial effect on the regulation of body temperature (154). In other words, the extra water released during glycogen breakdown does not noticeably minimize the effects of dehydration during exercise.

It has been suggested that muscle glycogen supercompensation techniques should only be practiced once or twice per competitive season because the high carbohydrate diet loses its efficacy to promote glycogen synthesis (21). However, an order of treatment effect in the studies of muscle glycogen supercompensation has not been reported, and complete depletion of the muscle glycogen stores may not be required to maximally activate glycogen synthesis (108,166,168). Thus, if a high carbohydrate diet is consumed, supercompensation may occur on a daily basis in athletes undertaking severe daily exercise training.

E.   Practical Use of Muscle Glycogen Supercompensation

Although elite athletes who train strenuously and consume high carbohydrate diets may undergo daily muscle glycogen supercompensation, it is still important for both elite and nonelite athletes to undertake a diet/exercise regimen to maximize muscle glycogen stores before an important competition. Such a regimen should include a gradual reduction in the exercise duration and a day of rest during the week before the competition. Additionally, the athlete should ensure that the diet contains at least 70% of the calories from carbohydrate during the three days before the competition. Muscle glycogen supercompensation will not allow an athlete to exercise at a faster rate, but the optimal constant rate will be maintained for a longer period of time because the depletion of muscle glycogen will be delayed.

VI. THE PREEXERCISE MEAL

A prolonged training session or competition after an overnight fast occurs in the presence of significantly depleted liver glycogen stores. If the training or competition relies heavily on blood glucose, performance may thus be hindered after a fast. This has led to experiments on the content of preexercise meals to determine the optimal quantity and timing of such meals to enhance subsequent performance. The optimal type of carbohydrate in the preexercise meal has also been investigated.

A. Glucose Availability During Exercise

Jandrain et al. (100) fed five healthy males 100 g glucose (50% solution, 1.37 $g \cdot kg^{-1}$ body weight) three hours before 4 h of treadmill running at 45% VO_2max. During the 4 h of exercise, 68% of the ingested glucose was oxidized. This shows that glucose consumed 3 h before moderate exercise is available for oxidation by the muscle. These results are similar to those of Ravussin et al. (157), who reported that 41 g of a 100 g glucose load given 1 h before 2 h of cycling at 35% VO_2max were recovered as expired CO_2. They suggested that the ingested glucose represented a readily available energy supply that may have spared muscle glycogen. Furthermore, Ahlborg and Felig (2) found that leg glucose uptake was enhanced during cycling for 4 h at 30% VO_2max when preceded by the ingestion of 200 g glucose (2.7 $g \cdot kg^{-1}$ body weight) 50 min before the start of exercise.

Similar procedures have been used to determine if low muscle glycogen levels at the start of exercise would influence the use of 100 g glucose (1.5 $g \cdot kg^{-1}$ body weight) ingested 1 h before 2 h of cycling at 40% VO_2max (157). After 75 min of exercise, when peak glucose utilization occurred, the subjects with normal glycogen were using principally carbohydrate (65% total energy expenditure), with exogenous glucose representing 24% of the total energy expenditure. On the other hand, the subjects with low glycogen used mainly lipids (70% total energy expenditure), with exogenous glucose representing 20% of the total energy expenditure. Thus, initial muscle glycogen levels did not significantly affect the contribution of exogenous glucose to the total energy metabolism. Although glucose ingested within 1 to 3 h before exercise represents an available energy source during low intensity exercise (<50% VO_2max), it is important to note that after such feedings, blood glucose and insulin concentrations are elevated at the onset of exercise (2,100,157), and, as discussed in the next section, this may be detrimental for exercise at intensities greater than 50% VO_2max.

B. The Preexercise Meal and Metabolism During Exercise

Costill et al. (34) examined the effect of ingestion of 75 g glucose (1.0 $g \cdot kg^{-1}$ body weight) 45 min before exercise at 70% VO_2max on muscle glycogen use and metabolism. Compared to a placebo treatment, there was a 17% greater use of muscle glycogen (34 versus 40 $mmol \cdot kg^{-1} \cdot min^{-1}$) when glucose was consumed. At the start of

exercise preceded by glucose ingestion, the blood glucose and insulin concentrations were 38% and 3.3-fold higher, respectively, than
basal (Fig. 6-5). During exercise, the blood glucose concentration declined from 7 mmol $\cdot$ L^{-1} to 3.5 mmol $\cdot$ L^{-1} in the glucose trial and
increased slightly during the control trial. The amount of total carbohydrate oxidation was 13% greater following the glucose ingestion when compared to the control trial (68 versus 76 g carbohydrate
oxidized per 30 min). Thus, well-trained subjects (VO$_2$max = 59
mL $\cdot$ kg^{-1} $\cdot$ min^{-1}) utilized muscle glycogen and blood glucose at greater
rates when glucose was ingested 45 min before exercise.

Rapid falls in blood glucose concentration have also been reported during exercise at both 75% (109) and 55% VO$_2$max (2) for
30 min and 2 h, respectively, when 75 g glucose (1 g $\cdot$ kg^{-1} body
weight) were consumed 45 min before exercise. In these two studies
(109,2), there was a strong correlation between the preexercise glucose and insulin concentrations and the fall in blood glucose and
insulin during exercise. The rapid fall in blood glucose under these
conditions appears to be primarily mediated by the elevated insulin
concentration (45).

Costill's group (61,83) has published two additional studies in
which the ingestion of glucose (1 g $\cdot$ kg^{-1} body weight) 45 min before
exercise resulted in a rapid decline in the blood glucose concentration. However, there was not an enhanced glycogen breakdown,
nor was there an adverse effect on endurance time to exhaustion

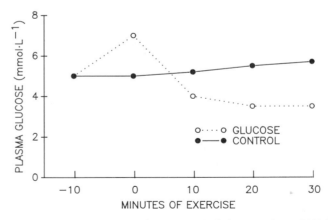

FIGURE 6-5. *Effect of ingesting 75 g glucose 45 min before exercise at 70% VO$_2$max on
the glucose and insulin responses at rest and during exercise (34). When the blood insulin
concentration was elevated at the start of exercise, the blood glucose concentration decreased
significantly and rapidly during subsequent exercise (open circles), whereas, after consuming
a placebo, the blood glucose concentration was maintained during exercise (closed circles).*

(61,83). Levine et al. (118) also reported a normal rate of glycogen breakdown when 30 min of running at 70% $\dot{V}O_2$max was preceded by ingestion of glucose (1 g·kg^{-1} body weight) 45 min before the onset of exercise in fed subjects. Thus, there are no consistently adverse effects of carbohydrate consumption 30–60 min before exercise.

The amount of glucose consumed in a preexercise meal may also affect the subsequent metabolic response during exercise. Devlin et al. (54) fed a low amount of carbohydrate (0.6 g carbohydrate·kg^{-1} body weight) to eight healthy male volunteers 30 min before cycling to exhaustion at 70% $\dot{V}O_2$max. The carbohydrate feeding elevated both the blood glucose and insulin concentrations at the start of exercise when compared to the placebo treatment. Despite these effects on glucose and insulin, performance time to exhaustion (47 versus 53 min), muscle glycogen utilization (50 versus 56 ug·g^{-1}), and total carbohydrate oxidation (118 versus 120 g) were not different between the two treatments. Possible reasons for the discrepancies between the results of Devlin et al. (54) and those of Costill's group (34,61,83) include differences in training states of the subjects differences in insulin sensitivity, quantity of carbohydrate ingested, number of subjects, or statistical analysis. Costill et al. (34) utilized repeated t-tests, which would increase the likelihood of a Type I error, whereas Devlin et al. (54) used more conservative analysis of variance procedures. More recently, several articles have appeared comparing glucose, fructose and placebo as a preexercise supplement with results similar to those of Devlin et al. (54). It should also be pointed out that despite the enhanced glycogen and glucose oxidation during the glucose trial in the initial study by Costill et al. (34), the implications of these metabolic effects for performance capacity cannot be directly ascertained.

Because of the inconsistent effects of glucose feedings 30 to 60 min before exercise, it is impossible to predict whether a particular athlete might experience adverse effects of such a feeding before exercise. However, because there are no reports of significant positive effects of such feedings on performance, it seems reasonable to advise athletes not to consume carbohydrate 30 to 60 min before prolonged exercise.

In contrast to the depressive effects on blood glucose during exercise when carbohydrates are fed 30 to 60 min before competition, preliminary reports indicate that feedings 5 min before exercise can help maintain or elevate blood glucose. Maltodextrin (glucose polymers) feeding (750 mL of a 20% solution) maintained high blood glucose levels relative to a placebo and extended cycling time at 62% $\dot{V}O_2$max by 24% (171). Furthermore, Segal et al. (164) fed 500 mL of an 18% glucose solution immediately before exercise and observed a nonsignificant four min increase in endurance time for intervals of 10 min cycling (74% $\dot{V}O_2$max) interspersed with 20 min rest and repeated to exhaustion. The apparent reason that carbohydrate feedings immediately before exercise do not lower blood glucose during exercise is that increased catecholamine production during the early part of exercise suppresses the release of insulin from the pancreas; thus, less circulating insulin is present to accelerate glucose uptake into tissues.

C. Comparison of Fasting and Preexercise Feedings on Metabolism During Exercise

Dohm et al. (55) and Coyle et al. (45) compared the effects of a high carbohydrate preexercise meal with prolonged fasting on metabolism and performance capacity during exercise. The nine well-trained ($\dot{V}O_2$max $= 61$ ml$\cdot$kg$^{-1}\cdot$min^{-1}) runners used by Dohm et al. (55) either fasted for 24 h or consumed 60 g of carbohydrate (0.9 g$\cdot$kg^{-1} body weight) 2 to 4 h before the start of running at 72% $\dot{V}O_2$max to exhaustion. Exercise capacity appeared to be reduced by the 24 h fast (time to exhaustion 76 versus 82 min), which is in agreement with the reports of Pequignot et al. (147) and Henschel et al. (87). From the start of exercise to roughly half-way through exercise, fasting resulted in a much greater reliance on fat as fuel, as indicated by higher plasma concentrations of free fatty acids, glycerol, and B-hydroxybutyrate, and a lower respiratory exchange ratio. However, at the midpoint of exercise, the differences in the fed treatment and the fasting treatment became less apparent.

Coyle et al. (45) compared the effects of fasting for 16 h with consumption of a high carbohydrate meal (2 g$\cdot$kg^{-1} body weight) in seven well-trained males ($\dot{V}O_2$max $= 65$ ml$\cdot$kg$^{-1}\cdot$min^{-1}) 4 h before the start of 105 min of cycling at 70% $\dot{V}O_2$max. There were no treatment effects on the blood glucose and insulin concentrations at the start of exercise. The authors proposed that the meal was responsible for the differences observed in preexercise muscle glycogen concentrations between the two treatments (163 versus 115 mmol$\cdot$kg^{-1} for the preexercise meal and fasting treatments, respectively); however, glycogen was not determined before the preexercise meal. When the subjects were fed, the first hour of exercise was characterized by an 18% decline in blood glucose, a suppression of the normal increase in blood free fatty acids and glycerol, and a 45% greater rate of carbohydrate oxidation. Thereafter, there were very few differences between the fed and fasted trials, although there was a greater rate of glycogen breakdown during the fed trial (97 mmol·kg^{-1}) as compared to the fasted trial (64 mmol·kg^{-1}). Although the feeding trial resulted in an initially greater reliance on body carbohydrate stores, the effects on performance were not studied.

D. Carbohydrate Source in a Preexercise Meal: Effects on Metabolic Response and Exercise Performance

Another sugar that has been investigated for use in a preexercise meal is fructose. The theoretical rationale for the potential use of fructose is strong. The increases in blood glucose and insulin upon fructose ingestion are only 20% to 30% of those observed after a glucose load (15,50), and plasma glucagon levels remain unchanged after fructose ingestion (15). Because fructose is slowly converted to glucose in the liver (86,127), it might serve as a gluconeogenic precursor and provide a stable supply of fuel for the muscle. Koivisto et al. (109), Levine et al. (118), Fielding et al. (61), and Hargreaves et al. (83) fed fructose (1 g·kg^{-1} body weight) to subjects 30 to 45 min before exercise. With fructose, the blood glucose and insulin concentrations were greater than after ingestion of a placebo but were significantly less than after ingestion of the same amount of glucose. During exercise, the fructose-induced changes in blood concentrations of glucose and insulin closely paralleled those for placebo treatments; however, fructose ingestion resulted in a suppression of free fatty acid release by 40% to 50% (109).

Several experiments have compared the rates of muscle glycogen depletion during exercise preceded by ingestion of a placebo or fructose (1.0 g·kg^{-1} body weight 45 min before exercise). The well-trained subjects of Koivisto et al. (109) cycled for 2 h at 55% $\dot{V}O_2$max, during which time there was no significant difference in muscle glycogen degradation between the two treatments (60% to 65% glycogen decline). Trained runners in the study reported by Fielding et al. (61) ran for 30 min at 70% $\dot{V}O_2$max, during which time there was no difference in the total amount of muscle glycogen breakdown between placebo (26 mmol·kg^{-1}) and fructose ingestion (35 mmol·kg^{-1}). Similar findings were also reported by Hargreaves et al. (83), who studied well-trained cyclists who rode at 75% $\dot{V}O_2$max until exhausted. The amount of muscle glycogen utilized was 93 mmol·kg^{-1} for control and 119 mmol·kg^{-1} for fructose ingestion; time to exhaustion was 93 and 91 min for control and fructose trials, respectively (83).

One study of the effect of fructose ingestion on muscle glycogen breakdown resulted in vastly different results than those reported in the preceding paragraph. Levine et al. (118) had eight well-trained runners consume either a placebo or 75 g fructose ($1 \ g \cdot kg^{-1}$ body weight) 45 min before the start of 30 min of running at 75% $\dot{V}O_2max$. At the start of exercise the blood glucose and insulin concentrations were not different between the two trials. The initial muscle glycogen levels were similar between the treatments ($130 \ mmol \cdot kg^{-1}$), but the amount of muscle glycogen utilized was significantly less for the fructose treatment than for the control treatment (13 versus $28 \ mmol \cdot kg^{-1}$). This represents 54% less muscle glycogen breakdown during the fructose treatment. The fructose treatment apparently provided more energy from blood glucose than did the control trial. The principal difference between the design of the experiment by Levine et al. (118) and the design of other experiments on preexercise fructose feeding is that the subjects of Levine et al. (118) had a high carbohydrate meal 4 h before exercise, whereas subjects in the other studies were fasted. Thus, greater liver glycogen stores may have been advantageous in the study of Levine et al. (118).

Unfortunately, most of the experiments on preexercise fructose ingestion may have employed exercise that was too brief to elucidate an ergogenic effect. It is generally accepted that fructose cannot be directly metabolized by the muscle; its major fate is conversion to glucose and either storage as liver glycogen or release as blood glucose. Because there is a high activity of fructose kinase in the liver and the majority of fructose under normal conditions is converted to liver glycogen (86), it would appear that prolonged exercise that stresses liver glycogen stores and relies heavily on blood glucose is more likely to show a favorable effect of fructose on performance than is exercise of shorter duration.

E. Effects of Preexercise Glycerol Feedings on Metabolism During Exercise

Blood glycerol concentration increases during prolonged exercise, and glycerol is a primary precursor for gluconeogenesis. Because a significant beneficial effect of preexercise glycerol ingestion on exercise performance of rats had been reported (173), Miller et al. (126) studied the effects of preexercise glycerol ingestion on metabolism in men during 150 min of cycling (74% $\dot{V}O_2max$) and on glycogen depletion during 30 min of running (70% $\dot{V}O_2max$). The subjects consumed 1 g glycerol $\cdot kg^{-1}$ body weight or a placebo solution 30 min before an exercise regimen which elevated the blood glycerol concentration at least 10-fold. Although glycerol ingestion delayed the fall in blood glucose during the first 90 min of cycling, the blood glycerol concentration thereafter was not different from the placebo trial. Furthermore, glycerol ingestion did not affect the rate of muscle glycogen degradation. Based on these results, it appears that glycerol cannot undergo gluconeogenesis at a rapid enough rate to serve as a major energy source during strenuous exercise.

F. Effects of Fatty Acids in a Preexercise Meal on Metabolism During Exercise

A significant elevation of blood free fatty acids at the onset of prolonged exercise can reduce carbohydrate oxidation (34). Therefore, Ivy et al. (98) and Decombaz et al. (52) hypothesized that increasing the availability of medium-chain triglycerides at the onset of exercise might spare carbohydrate stores during exercise. Subjects were fed an average of 381 mg medium-chain triglycerides per kg body weight 1 h before exercise at 60% (52) and 70% $\dot{V}O_2$max for 1 h (98). In general, the ingestion of medium-chain triglycerides significantly increased blood ketones, but it did not alter the metabolic response to exercise when compared to a placebo trial (52) or a glucose polymer trial (98). These results suggest that a feeding of medium-chain triglycerides is not a viable method of optimizing energy sources for prolonged exercise.

G. Effects of Caffeine in a Preexercise Meal on Metabolism During Exercise

Caffeine is known to raise the blood free fatty acid concentration, which generally increases energy production from fatty acid degradation (33,34,58). Therefore, it follows that elevation of blood free fatty acids by caffeine ingestion before exercise might spare carbohydrate stores. The effects of ingesting caffeine in amounts equivalent to 6 mg $\cdot$ kg^{-1} body weight (3 cups of coffee) 60 min before exercise have been recently reviewed (156). Many subjects respond with improved endurance, greater work production, and faster race times after drinking caffeinated beverages than after placebo drinks (10,33,58,99). Whether the observed beneficial effect of caffeine on endurance is mediated by sparing muscle glycogen, stimulating the central nervous system, stimulating calcium release from the sarcoplasmic reticulum, or by suppressing intramuscular glycogenolysis is unclear (156). It should be noted that some individuals are hypersensitive to and adversely affected by caffeine; the athletic performance of these persons is likely to suffer under its influence. Therefore, the athlete should initially experiment with the use of caffeine during training sessions well in advance of an important competition. It should be noted that ingestion of large amounts of caffeine could possibly elevate the body caffeine level to those limits of disqualification established by the International Olympic Committee (156).

H. Effects of Fasting on Metabolism and Performance

Another strategy used to spare carbohydrates during exercise is to elevate the blood free fatty acid concentration by prolonged fasting prior to exercise (156). This theory, however, is flawed, because fasting will deplete liver glycogen; if the exercise is to last longer than 90 min, the blood glucose concentration will be lowered and exhaustion may be premature. This theoretical flaw has been recently documented by Loy et al. (120), who exhausted 10 trained cyclists under fed and 24 h fasted conditions. Exhaustion was defined as A) the time when 80% $\dot{V}O_2$max during cycling could not be maintained and B) when subsequently 65% $\dot{V}O_2$max could not be maintained. Despite the 2.2-fold higher blood free fatty acid concentration in the 24-h fasted subjects at the start of exercise, their times to exhaustion were significantly shorter than those for fed subjects. The exercise times to exhaustion at point A) were 90 min and 150 min in the fasted and fed groups, respectively. Total muscle glycogen depletion was the same (70%) for both groups. At exhaustion point B), the blood glucose concentration was lower in the fasted group when compared to the fed group. This observation and the fact that the muscle glycogen concentration in both groups at exhaustion point B) was still 50 to 70 mmol·kg^{-1} supports the interpretation that the individuals in the fasted trial became exhausted because their blood glucose concentration was low. Thus, fasting as a method of elevating the blood free fatty acid concentration is detrimental to training and performance.

I. Consumption of the Preexercise Meal

Although equivocal, the available evidence suggests that the endurance athlete should consume a 70% carbohydrate preexercise meal during the 3 to 6 h period before exercise. Consumption of the preexercise meal during this time will allow the blood insulin concentration to return to normal by the start of exercise and will minimize the deleterious exaggeration of carbohydrate oxidation which might otherwise occur if blood insulin were high at the start of exercise. Because there is a strong positive relationship between training level and the rapidity with which elevated blood glucose concentrations are normalized, the better trained athlete may be able to move the preexercise meal closer to the time of competition and not incur detrimental effects. If fructose is a component of the preexercise meal, it should be a small percentage of the total carbohydrate in the meal, because fructose may cause gastrointestinal distress in some sensitive individuals. Glycerol is not an effective ergogenic aid in a preexercise meal, and caffeine should be used with caution, since the positive effects appear to be individualistic. Prolonged fasting before training or competition should be avoided.

VII. WATER AS A PRIMARY NUTRIENT FOR PROLONGED EXERCISE

Body water is of critical importance to prolonged exercise, especially if the exercise is undertaken in a hot environment. An appropriate volume and distribution of body water is needed during exercise to provide for the optimal dilution of electrolytes, glucose, hormones, proteins, and other dissolved substances in the blood and tissues. Furthermore, water in the blood is required for the delivery of oxygen and nutrients to working muscles and for the transfer of heat from the muscles to the skin to promote heat dissipation by radiation, convection, and evaporation. The evaporation of sweat may be the only route available for heat dissipation in a hot environment, and sweat production may place great demands on body water stores, especially when one considers that sweat rates of 2 $L \cdot h^{-1}$ are possible during prolonged exercise in hot environments. Finally, in the absence of fluid replacement, the loss of water and electrolytes during prolonged exercise can lead to heat exhaustion, heat cramps, and even heat stroke. Thus, water may well be the most important nutrient to be considered for optimizing performance in prolonged exercise.

A. Effects of Withholding Water Before or During Prolonged Exercise

1. Early Experiments. In 1944, Pitts, Johnson, and Consolazio (153) reported data from a series of experiments in which men walked on a treadmill for 1–4 h at 5.6 $km \cdot hr^{-1}$ up a 2.5% grade with or without fluid replenishment (Table 6-2). The environmental temperatures ranged from 32–38° C, the relative humidity was 35–83%, and the subjects were allowed to rest for 10 min each hour. When

TABLE 6-2. *Mean heart rates, rectal temperatures, and sweat rates after 4 h walking at 38° C, 35% R.H. (n = 3-7). (Data extracted from Table 1 in reference (153.)*

Fluid Type	Heart Rate (beats · min⁻¹)	Rectal Temp. (°C)	Sweat Rate (L · h⁻¹)
None	154	38.9	0.76
Water ad lib	143	38.4	0.74
Water each 15 min at SR*	132	38.3	0.80
0.2% NaCl each 15 min at SR*	131	38.3	0.81
3.5% glucose each 15 min at SR*	126	38.1	0.71

*Sweat Rate

the subjects drank nothing during the walks, their rectal temperatures and pulse rates were usually higher and their sweat rates lower than when water, 2% saline, or 3.5% glucose in volumes equivalent to sweat loss were consumed every 15 min or when water was consumed in quantities that just satisfied thirst. These early experiments demonstrated that progressive dehydration during prolonged exercise can adversely affect cardiovascular function, as reflected by elevated heart rates, and temperature regulation, as indicated by high rectal temperatures and reduced sweat rates.

The Pitts, Johnson and Consolazio (153) experiments also suggested that thirst was not an adequate stimulus for the subjects to replace all of the water they lost as sweat. This was confirmed several years later in an experiment reported by Brown (23), in which military recruits attempted to complete a 34 km hike in a desert environment at temperatures ranging from 30–33° C with or without free access to water. Without water, 7 of 13 subjects became exhausted before completing the hike and lost 7.5% of their body weights. When water was provided, only 1 of 9 subjects became prematurely exhausted, but the subjects still lost 4.5% of their body weights during the hike. It is clear that during prolonged manual labor or athletic competition or training one must consume more fluid than that which satisfies thirst if progressive dehydration is to be avoided (93).

2. Reduced Plasma Volume and Increased Body Fluid Osmolality. Even in the absence of significant dehydration during prolonged exercise, some of the plasma volume usually moves out of the capillaries and into the interstitial or intracellular spaces, but progressive dehydration during the exercise increases the overall loss of plasma fluid (36) (Fig. 6-6). For example, Costill et al. (30) measured fluid volume shifts in seven men who cycled for 2 h at 50% $\dot{V}O_2$max in a chamber with a temperature of 38° C and a relative humidity of 46%. After only 10 min of cycling, there was a loss of 4.4% of plasma volume; by the end of 2 h, plasma volume was 9% less than baseline. Another study showed a plasma volume loss of up to 16% in prolonged exercise (37). In competitive athletics, a plasma volume loss of this magnitude means that there is a significant reduction in the volume of circulating blood that is available to meet the increasing demands for blood by muscles for producing force and by skin for dissipating heat.

A loss of plasma volume during exercise is often accompanied by a deterioration in the ability of the exerciser to regulate body temperature. However, it is apparent that there is no clear cause-and-effect association between plasma volume losses and failing temperature regulation; experimentally increasing or reducing plasma

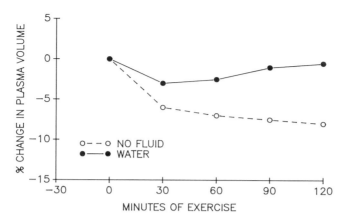

FIGURE 6-6. *Change in plasma volume during 2 h of cycling (50% V̇O₂max) in the heat (38° C, 65% relative humidity) with and without fluid intake during exercise (30).*

volume during exercise does not necessarily result in a systematic improvement or deterioration, respectively, in temperature regulation (70,133). The adverse effects of dehydration on temperature regulation appear to be a complex function of increased body fluid osmolality and decreased plasma volume (70). Thus, even in the absence of a decrease in plasma volume, an increased plasma osmolality caused by dehydration raises the thresholds for initiation of the sweating response and vasodilation in the skin; however a decrease in plasma volume coincident with an increased plasma osmolality additionally causes a reduction in the rate of increase in skin blood flow for a given rise in core temperature and a reduction in the maximal rate of skin blood flow (70,133).

   3.   Increased Circulatory Strain. As plasma volume declines with progressively increasing dehydration and as the cutaneous vascular capacity increases because of greater demands for heat dissipation in prolonged exercise, the circulating blood volume decreases. This leads to a reduction in ventricular filling pressure, a fall in stroke volume, and a compensatory increase in heart rate (25,75,160) (Fig. 6-7) that may be inadequate to prevent a reduction in cardiac output (69,133,160). With increasing dehydration, circulation to the skin decreases to shift a greater percentage of the declining blood volume to the working muscles (69). Unfortunately, this shift of fluids away from the skin reduces the ability of the body to dissipate heat and leads to a progressive increase in heat storage (Fig. 6-8).

   4.   Decreased Sweating Response. Dehydration-induced decrements in plasma volume and increments in body fluid osmolality result in a decreased threshold for sweating onset and a decrease

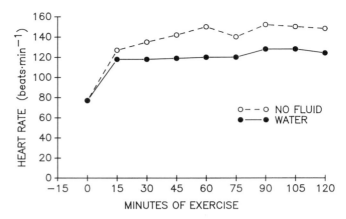

FIGURE 6-7. *Heart rate response to exercise (50% V̇O₂max) in subjects exercising in the heat (32° C, 62% relative humidity) with water or no fluid (75).*

in the rate of sweating for a given increase in core temperature (70,85). This deterioration in sweating leads to a reduced ability to dissipate heat by evaporation and a higher core temperature during prolonged exercise in the dehydrated compared to the hydrated condition (25,43,75,163) (Fig. 6-8).

   5. **Altered Electrolyte Distributions.** Sodium and chloride are the principal electrolytes lost in sweat, but sweat is hypotonic with respect to blood plasma so that sodium, chloride (and potassium) concentrations in plasma are usually elevated by 1% to 4% during

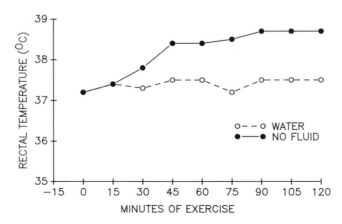

FIGURE 6-8. *Rectal temperature response to exercise (50% V̇O₂max) in subjects exercising in the heat (32° C, 62% relative humidity) with water or no fluid (75).*

prolonged exercise without fluid replenishment (30,35,37,43). Plasma magnesium concentrations either decrease or are unchanged from rest (35). There seem to be no systematic changes with exercise in intracellular concentrations of sodium, chloride, and magnesium in skeletal muscle, perhaps because of variable changes in intracellular water (30,35). When expressed per unit wet muscle weight, potassium concentrations in intracellular water typically decrease by 8% to 10% (30), but all electrolyte changes in muscle during prolonged exercise are very minor when expressed per unit dry weight (35).

6. **Altered Hormonal Response to Exercise.** Relative to a fluid-replenished state, dehydration causes greater elevations in circulating renin activity, aldosterone, cortisol, and vasopressin (18,73,75). The increased renin activity and aldosterone concentrations are associated with decrements in plasma volume, whereas the increased cortisol may be a more generalized response to physiological strain (73). The increased vasopressin is presumably related to increased osmolality of extracellular fluids during prolonged exercise.

7. **Similarity in Gender Responses to Exercise in a Dehydrated State.** The effects of voluntary dehydration (-5% of body weight) 10–15 h in advance of prolonged walking in comfortable, hot/dry, and hot/wet environments are similar for men and women (163). In the hot/wet environment, women had lower sweat rates than men, but dehydration did not significantly reduce sweat rates for either gender in a preacclimation experiment and significantly reduced sweat rate for both genders after a 10-day heat acclimation period (163).

B. Effects of Water and Saline Feedings Before and During Prolonged Exercise

1. **Water and Saline Ingestion Before Prolonged Exercise.** Nielson et al. (138) administered 1 L of water to subjects prior to 1 h of moderately severe exercise and demonstrated that esophageal temperature during exercise was reduced by 0.5° C when compared to a "no fluid" condition. On the other hand, consumption of 1 L of a hypertonic (2%) sodium chloride solution before exercise caused an elevation of core temperature relative to the no fluid condition (138). In another experiment, Nielsen (137) compared the effects on temperature regulation of drinking 1 L of a 2% saline solution or a 2% calcium chloride solution several hours before 1 h of cycling at 40% $\dot{V}O_2$max. They found that the calcium solution caused an earlier onset of sweating, a greater sweat rate, and a lower rise in core temperature, presumably because of the beneficial effects of calcium on hypothalamic function. However, Greenleaf and Brock (80) found that drinking 1 L of a 1.5% solution of calcium gluconate 30–90 min

before 1 h of cycling at 40% to 47% $\dot{V}O_2$max was less effective than either a 0.9% or 1.5% saline solution in maintaining plasma volume during exercise and no better in minimizing increases in core temperature. Thus, there is no reliable evidence that calcium in beverages consumed before exercise is beneficial to temperature regulation or to performance.

2. **Water and Saline Feedings Both Before and During Prolonged Exercise.** Moroff and Bass (130) had subjects drink 2 L of water or abstain from drinking water during 50 min immediately prior to a 90 min treadmill walk in a hot environment. Even though the subjects also consumed 300 mL of water every 20 min during the walk, the prehydrated condition resulted in lower heart rates, increased sweat rates, and lower core temperatures than when no fluids were consumed before exercise. In another experiment, the combination of a 2.7 L water feeding during 60 min of rest before and water consumption sufficient to replace sweat losses every 10 min during 70 min of cycling at 50% $\dot{V}O_2$max resulted in lower rectal temperatures and higher sweat rates than when no fluid was consumed before and isotonic saline was consumed during the exercise (81). Unfortunately, because of the confounding effects of the water versus saline treatments during exercise in this experiment, it is impossible to conclude whether the preexercise water feeding provided any benefit beyond that of the water feeding during exercise.

The investigations cited above studied light to moderate intensities of exercise. In contrast, Gisolfi and Copping (78) tested subjects who ran at 75% $\dot{V}O_2$max for 2 h in the heat. They found no beneficial effect of consumption of 1 L of water 30 min before exercise as long as 200 mL of water was consumed every 20 min during exercise. The fact that most prolonged athletic competition requires exertion at 70% to 80% $\dot{V}O_2$max suggests that the experiment of Gisolfi and Copping (78) more nearly represents what is likely to occur with precompetition hydration than do experiments with light exercise. Accordingly, the premise that preexercise water loading is advantageous to performance is somewhat dubious. On the other hand, there is no reason to suspect that a reasonable regimen of preexercise water consumption will be deleterious to performance. Therefore, we recommend that fluids such as water or moderately concentrated (5–8%) carbohydrate solutions be consumed in volumes of 250–750 mL 5–15 min before undertaking prolonged exercise.

3. **Water and Saline Feedings During Prolonged Exercise.** The early experiments of Pitts, Johnson, and Consolazio (153) on men marching in the desert showed that consumption of water or 0.2% saline or 3.5% glucose to replace sweat loss resulted in lower heart

rates and core temperatures and sometimes greater sweat rates than were noted in a no fluid condition. Francis (75) studied eight men under three different hydration treatments during intermittent exercise consisting of eight 15-min bouts of cycling at 50% $\dot{V}O_2$max interspersed with 5-min recovery intervals. The room air temperature was 32° C, and the relative humidity was 60–65%. During the rest intervals, the subjects either consumed no fluid, water, or an electrolyte solution (20 mM sodium, 10 mM potassium, 1.3% glucose) sufficient to replace sweat losses. In the no fluid condition, plasma volume loss after 2 h was 17.7%; when either fluid replacement beverage was consumed, no significant loss occurred. Similarly, heart rate was 15–20 beats lower, rectal temperature was 1° C lower, and plasma cortisol concentration was significantly reduced when either fluid was consumed during exercise compared to the no fluid condition (See Figures 6-7, 6-8).

In one experiment, four marathon runners ran on a treadmill for 2 h at 70% $\dot{V}O_2$max under each of three conditions: 1) no fluid, 2) 100 mL water every 5 min during the first 100 min, or 3) 100 mL of a glucose-electrolyte beverage (20 mM sodium, 15.3 mM chloride, 2.4 mM potassium, 4.4% glucose) every 5 min for the first 100 min (43). Compared to the no fluid treatment, both fluid replacement regimens significantly lowered rectal temperature and reduced the concentrations of sodium and chloride in plasma.

Candas et al. (25) and Brandenberger et al. (18) compared the effects of five treatments—no fluid, water, a hypotonic beverage (0.4 mM chloride, 0.04% glucose and fructose), an isotonic drink (23.1 mM sodium, 16.7 mM chloride, 3.2 mM potassium, 2.0 mM calcium, 6.8% sucrose), and a hypertonic sugar solution (7.55% glucose, 7.53% fructose) on temperature regulation and cardiovascular function during 4 h of intermittent cycling at a low intensity (mean = 85 W) in a hot environment (34° C, 10° C dew point). Fluid was consumed every 10 min after 70 min of exercise in amounts calculated to replace 80% of sweat losses. Relative to the no fluid condition, all four fluid replenishment regimens decreased rectal temperature, heart rate, plasma protein concentration, plasma osmolality, and losses of plasma volume but did not significantly affect sweat rate or skin temperature (25). Although the hypertonic sugar solution tended to be less effective in minimizing homeostatic disturbances, there were few significant differences attributable to the beverage composition. One exception to this observation was that plasma volume was actually expanded during the isotonic drink treatment, whereas the other beverages only minimized the plasma volume loss found in the no fluid condition. Hormone concentrations in the blood were determined only for the no fluid, water, and isotonic beverage treatments, and both water and the isotonic drink negated the rises in plasma concentrations of cortisol, vasopressin, and renin activity; aldosterone elevations during exercise were significantly blunted only by the isotonic drink (18).

4. Efficacy of Electrolyte Replacement During Prolonged Exercise. Because substantial quantities of sodium and chloride, and to a lesser extent, potassium, are lost in the sweat during prolonged exercise, especially in the heat, many are concerned that this electrolyte loss should be replenished during exercise to maintain the appropriate distribution of electrolytes in the various fluid compartments of the body. However, there is little direct evidence of a beneficial effect of electrolyte replacement for any but a small proportion of endurance athletes. The fact that electrolyte concentrations in plasma usually rise during exercise without fluid replacement (30,35,37,43) indicates that electrolyte supplements are not needed. Furthermore, during repeated exposures to exercise training, the kidneys very effectively conserve sodium and potassium, so that electrolyte balance is usually maintained when an athlete consumes a normal diet, a diet low in potassium (29), or a diet high or low in sodium (7).

However, recent case studies have been reported in which athletes who participated in very prolonged exercise experienced severe hyponatremia, i.e., low plasma sodium concentrations, during exercise (90,140) or up to 7 days after competition (140). These athletes usually consumed large quantities of water or beverages low in electrolytes. Conceivably, ingestion of electrolyte beverages for athletes sensitive to the development of hyponatremia could be effective in obliterating or reducing the severity of hyponatremia. It should also be noted that small amounts of sodium chloride in a beverage enhance palatability. Since palatability determines in large measure how much fluid a person will voluntarily ingest (93), it may well be that electrolytes in sports drinks are important to encourage consumption of as much fluid as possible.

C. Summary of Effects of Water and Saline Replacement on Homeostasis During Prolonged Exercise

Fluid replacement during strenuous prolonged exercise is unquestionably beneficial in minimizing the adverse effects of dehydration on cardiovascular function and temperature regulation. Although not all studies have demonstrated significant improvements in all markers of cardiovascular function and temperature regulation, there is overwhelming cumulative evidence that fluid replacement lowers cardiovascular strain and improves thermoregulation when compared to a condition where fluid is withheld during prolonged exercise. Whether ingestion of fluids before exercise makes a contribution to the maintenance of homeostasis in high intensity, prolonged athletic competition above and beyond that of fluid ingestion only during exercise remains uncertain. The value of electrolytes added to fluids consumed during exercise has yet to be conclusively demonstrated, but individuals susceptible to hyponatremia with water feedings alone may profit from electrolyte supplements. Furthermore, the low concentrations of electrolytes found in athletic beverages (Table 6-3) have not been shown to be harmful and may encourage fluid consumption by enhancing palatability.

VIII. GASTRIC EMPTYING OF SOLUTIONS CONSUMED BEFORE AND DURING PROLONGED EXERCISE

A. Gastric Emptying Rate During Prolonged Exercise

A comprehensive analysis of the literature on gastric emptying and intestinal absorption related to beverages consumed during exercise has been recently published (131), and only highlights of this issue will be addressed in this chapter. The first study of gastric emptying and intestinal absorption of beverages consumed during exercise was that of Fordtran and Saltin (67). They studied the gastric emptying characteristics of water and a glucose-electrolyte solution (13.3% glucose, 0.3% sodium chloride) and the intestinal absorption of six sugar-saline solutions in five subjects at rest and after

TABLE 6-3. *Approximate composition of beverages that may be consumed during prolonged exercise.*

Beverage Type	Sodium (mM)	Potassium (mM)	Sucrose (%)	Glucose (%)	Glucose Polymers (%)	Fructose (%)
Gatorade	20	3.0	4.0	2.0	—	—
Isostar	23	5.0	6.8	0.1	—	0.1
Exceed	10	5.0	—	—	5.0	2.0
Gookinaid ERG	16	10.0	—	5.0	—	—
Body Fuel 450	16	2.0	—	—	4.5	—
Cola Drinks	4	0.1	3.7	6.8*	—	—
Orange Juice	1	52.0	7.0	5.0*	—	—
Apple Juice	2	31.0	2.9	9.0*	—	—
Lemonade	1	5.0	2.6	7.0*	—	—
Tomato Juice	107	62.2	0.8	1.6*	—	—

*A variable mixture of glucose and fructose.

an hour of treadmill running at 70% $\dot{V}O_2$max. They found that gastric emptying rates were slightly reduced during exercise and that exercise effects on water absorption in the intestine were highly variable. Furthermore, gastric emptying rates for the 13.3% glucose solution were substantially slower than those for water.

Subsequently, Costill and Saltin (39) systematically varied the intensity of cycling exercise and the glucose content, temperature, and volume of beverages ingested during cycling. They showed that cycling at intensities up to 60% $\dot{V}O_2$max did not significantly reduce gastric emptying rates; intensities greater than 70% $\dot{V}O_2$max did. Having demonstrated that gastric emptying during moderate intensity exercise was similar to rest, Costill and Saltin (39) tested gastric emptying characteristics of various beverages in resting subjects. One of their findings was that a solution of 2.5% glucose in 34 mM saline had emptied as rapidly after 15 min as the saline alone, whereas 5%, 10% and 15% glucose added to the saline progressively slowed gastric emptying. These findings with measurements of gastric emptying 15–20 min after beverage ingestion were generally confirmed by others (9,19,48,72,96,135).

B. Gastric Emptying Rate of Carbohydrate-Containing Beverages

Gastric emptying of carbohydrate-containing beverages seems to be regulated to provide a fairly constant rate of energy delivery, i.e., 2.0–2.5 kcal · min^{-1}, to the small intestine, regardless of the energy density or osmolality of the ingested beverage (19,96). In other words, after a few minutes of unregulated emptying into the intestine, a solution containing 10% glucose should empty approximately half as quickly as a solution of 5% glucose to deliver energy to the intestine at the same rate. The gastric emptying rate for water is approximately 15 mL · min^{-1} for the first 15 min, that for 5% carbohydrate about 12 mL · min^{-1}, and solutions containing progressively greater amounts of carbohydrate empty progressively more slowly (19). If the maximal rate of energy delivery from the stomach to the intestine is 2.0–2.5 kcal · min^{-1} (120–150 kcal · h^{-1}), approximately 36.0–37.5 g of carbohydrate could be delivered to the intestine per hour. Thus, if a 6% glucose solution were ingested, 600–625 mL would have to be emptied from the stomach each hour to provide maximal rates of energy delivery. At emptying rates of approximately 10 mL · min^{-1} for such a solution, this maximal rate of energy delivery is clearly possible and practical, e.g., with 150–250 mL feedings of a 6% glucose solution every 15–20 min.

Theoretically, the difference between the rates of delivery of water and a 6% glucose solution from the stomach to the intestine would be approximately 275–300 mL $\cdot$ h^{-1}. If water and the glucose solution were absorbed from the intestine at similar rates, it would appear that fluid replenishment would be improved by 275–300 mL/h if one consumed water versus a 6% glucose solution. However, because glucose stimulates water absorption from the intestine (170), this apparent advantage of water over a moderately concentrated glucose solution for fluid replacement may not be real (131).

It should be noted that the previously cited studies of gastric emptying characteristics of ingested beverages did not include measurements during exercise of cardiovascular or thermoregulatory function or performance capacity. Nevertheless, it is widely believed that cardiovascular function, temperature regulation, and exercise performance will be adversely affected during prolonged exercise if ingested beverages contain sugar concentrations greater than 2.5%. This belief is unfounded.

In a study of champion marathoners, Costill et al. (43) found similar and large gastric residues remaining in the stomachs of three of four runners after a 2 h run at 70% $\dot{V}O_2$max, regardless of whether they drank 100 mL water or a glucose-electrolyte beverage (4.4% glucose, 20 mM sodium, 2.4 mM potassium) every 5 min for the first 100 min of the run. More importantly, rectal temperatures, heart rates, ventilation rates, oxygen uptakes, sweat rates, and hemoconcentration values were similar for both drink treatments. Similarly, Owen et al.(145) compared water, a 10% glucose polymer solution, and a 10% glucose solution ingested in volumes of 200 mL every 20 min during treadmill running at 65% $\dot{V}O_2$max for 2 h in a hot environment. They detected no significant beverage effects on gastric emptying, plasma volume changes, rectal or mean skin temperatures or sweat rates. In another comparison of water and beverages containing 5%, 6% or 7.5% carbohydrate, it was found that all carbohydrate beverages improved performance relative to water in a maximal 12-min sprint ride following seven 12-min rides at 70% $\dot{V}O_2$max interspersed with 3-min rest intervals (129). Futhermore, no important beverage-related effects were detected for plasma volume changes, weight loss, oxygen uptake, or gastric emptying. Presumably, the fact that fluid feedings in this experiment were given in relatively small volumes (167 mL) intermittently as opposed to a 400 mL single feeding (39) explained the lack of gastric emptying differences among beverages.

Coupled with numerous other reports (discussed below) that show benefits to prolonged exercise performance when carbohydrate is consumed during exercise, the studies cited in this section show that any differences in gastric emptying that may exist among water and beverages with moderate (5% to 8%) concentrations of carbohydrate are of little importance in determining the efficacy of a beverage for minimizing disturbances in homeostasis and for maximizing performance.

IX. CARBOHYDRATE FEEDINGS DURING PROLONGED EXERCISE

When exercise commences with elevated blood insulin and glucose levels, as might occur if exercise is started within 30–60 min following the ingestion of a glucose meal, there is an exaggerated utilization of glucose that often leads to a rapid lowering of the blood glucose concentration, blunted lipolysis and lipid oxidation, and perhaps an enhanced glycogen breakdown (34). This scenario can be avoided if the carbohydrate solution is ingested immediately before exercise (171) or after exercise has started (99). Exercise stimulates an increase in the blood catecholamine concentration, which suppresses pancreatic insulin release (77,179), thereby minimizing an exaggerated glucose uptake. Thus, if glucose is ingested 5 min before or anytime during vigorous exercise, there will be less of an insulin-induced suppression of lipolysis and fat oxidation, less of an enhancement of glucose uptake and carbohydrate oxidation, and a greater possibility that the carbohydrate feedings might enhance training or competitive performance.

A. Availability of Glucose Ingested During Exercise

Costill et al.(41) reported that a small amount of ^{14}C-glucose appeared in the blood stream within five to seven min after its ingestion during exercise, but the contribution to the total blood glucose pool was very small. As exercise duration and glucose consumption increase, the fraction of blood glucose derived from glucose ingestion increases (41,175). Exogenous glucose concentration in the blood peaks within 30 min after ingestion of a small glucose load during exercise but may take up to 90 min to reach peak concentrations after ingestion of a large glucose meal. Since glucose ingestion is known to suppress glycogenolysis and gluconeogenesis (3), it is conceivable that glucose ingested during exercise might, under the right conditions, replace a large percentage of the endogenous blood glucose as a fuel for exercise. The optimal exercise conditions and feeding schedule, however, have not been elucidated.

B. Carbohydrate Ingestion During Prolonged Exercise: Effects on Fatigue

During training or competition lasting longer than approximately 90 to 150 min, the liver glycogen stores may become depleted, and, as a result, the blood glucose concentration will drop.

Some individuals are especially sensitive to a lowering of blood glucose and exhibit subjective symptoms of central nervous system fatigue that can be prevented by the consumption of glucose during exercise (8). However, these subjects represent only about 25% of a normal subject population (49). On the other hand, there are some subjects who become hypoglycemic but do not exhibit subjective symptoms of central nervous system fatigue during prolonged exercise (1,49,59). Therefore, the contribution of low blood glucose to the mechanism of fatigue is quite variable. However, it is without question that glucose ingestion during exercise can be used to supplement liver glycogen stores during exercise and elevate or maintain the concentration of blood glucose so that training or competitive performance is not compromised by a reduction in blood glucose.

Many of the studies that have examined the effects of glucose feedings during exercise have found a performance-enhancing effect of such treatments. However, the purported mechanisms underlying those effects have differed among studies. Ivy et al. (99) encouraged trained cyclists to maximize work output during 2 h of isokinetic cycling. They were fed 0.21 g glucose $\cdot$ kg^{-1} body weight every 15 min during the first 90 min of exercise. There was no difference in total work output during the 2 h work session, but the subjects receiving glucose were able to exceed their initial work output during the final 30 min of cycling by 11% when compared to the placebo condition. These findings were interpreted to indicate that glucose feedings may be of benefit during prolonged exercise lasting longer than 90 min.

Using these promising findings as the rationale for the positive effect of glucose feedings during exercise, Coyle et al. (49) conducted a study using ten experienced and trained cyclists who were asked to cycle for a minimum of 180 min at 74% $\dot{V}O_2$max. Fatigue was defined as the time at which the work intensity dropped to 10% below 74% $\dot{V}O_2$max. The subjects were fed either a placebo or carbohydrate during exercise. During carbohydrate feedings the subjects were fed a 50% solution containing 1.0 g glucose polymers per kg body weight 20 min after the start of exercise; after 60, 90, and 120 min they were fed a 6% solution containing 0.25 g glucose polymers per kg body weight. In this study, Coyle et al. (49) identified three subjects who did not have a significant reduction in blood glucose during exercise when the placebo was consumed. These three subjects did not derive any benefit from feedings during the glucose polymer trial (time to exhaustion–153 versus 150 min). On the other hand, seven subjects experienced a significant reduction in blood glucose during the placebo trial (4.0 versus 2.9 mmol $\cdot$ L^{-1} at the start of exercise and at fatigue, respectively). During the glucose polymer trial, endurance time was improved by 33 min (126 versus 159 min for placebo and feedings trials, respectively). The authors hypothesized that performance was enhanced in the individuals who were susceptible to a lowering of blood glucose through a mechanism in which the 30% higher blood glucose and 50% higher blood insulin concentrations increased muscle glucose uptake and decreased muscle glycogen utilization, thereby sparing muscle glycogen and improving performance.

More recently, however, Coyle et al. (44) reported that the work-enhancing effect of glucose feedings during exercise for trained cyclists was not accomplished by a sparing of muscle glycogen (Fig. 6-9). Rather, muscle glycogen utilization was the same in both placebo and glucose feedings trials. These results strongly suggest that the glucose feedings resulted in a markedly enhanced glucose uptake that provided sufficient carbohydrate to fuel an additional 1 h of exercise at 70% $\dot{V}O_2$max (180 versus 240 min) in well-trained cyclists. In a similar study, but using trained runners, Fruth and Gisolfi (76) provided 0.31 g glucose $\cdot$ kg^{-1} body weight every 20 min during a run to exhaustion at 70% $\dot{V}O_2$max. All runners completed at least 2 h of exercise, and performance time, though not significantly different, was 16% longer when compared to a placebo trial.

An absence of positive effects of carbohydrate feedings during exercise was reported by Flynn et al. (64). Eight trained cyclists increased muscle glycogen to above normal levels (190 mmol $\cdot$ kg^{-1})

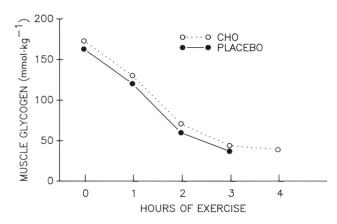

FIGURE 6-9. *Muscle glycogen depletion during cycling at 70% $\dot{V}O_2$max until exhaustion when consuming either a placebo (closed circle) or glucose solution during exercise (open circle) (44). Note that these well-trained cyclists were able to exercise for an additional hour when fed glucose during exercise.*

with a high carbohydrate diet and then cycled for 2 h on an isoki-netic bicycle with the intent to perform as much work as possible during that time. The subjects were fed either a placebo or 0.09 g glucose per kg body weight immediately before exercise and every 20 min thereafter. Although the carbohydrate treatment signifi-cantly elevated blood glucose during exercise when compared to placebo, glycogen depletion was not reduced, and total work was not enhanced by the carbohydrate feedings. The authors suggested that high muscle glycogen concentrations prior to exercise might ne-gate the positive effect of glucose feedings during exercise. How-ever, the subjects in the study of Coyle et al. (44) also began exercise with glycogen concentrations higher than normal. More likely, the lack of a feedings effect in the experiment of Flynn et al. (64) may be associated with the very low amount of carbohydrate consumed by the subjects during the experiment and the relatively short du-ration of exercise (<2 h).

Felig et al. (59) also examined the effect of glucose feedings dur-ing exercise on the development of hypoglycemia and performance time, but their subjects were recreational athletes ($\dot{V}O_2$max = 3.5 L $\cdot$ min^{-1}). Subjects underwent either a placebo trial or glucose trials providing either 0.6 or 1.14 g glucose per kg body weight per h. In the placebo trial, blood glucose fell steadily over time, whereas the glucose trials maintained or elevated blood glucose relative to base-line. Although half of the subjects and two-thirds of the subjects in the low and high carbohydrate feedings trials, respectively, im-proved their mean endurance time by 20 min relative to the placebo treatment, the apparently beneficial effects of carbohydrate feedings were not statistically significant.

The work-enhancing effect of sucrose feedings (chocolate bar) during intermittent exercise was reported in two similar studies by Hargreaves et al. (84) and Fielding et al. (62). In one experiment (84) performance enhancement was associated with glycogen sparing, but not in the other (62). In the experiment of Hargreaves et al. (84), ten trained cyclists exercised for 4 h, during which time they per-formed repeated 20 min bouts of cycling at 50% $\dot{V}O_2$max followed by 10 min of intense intermittent exercise (30 s at 100% $\dot{V}O_2$max followed by 2 min rest). During the last sprint bout, the subjects were timed until exhaustion. The subjects consumed either a pla-cebo or candy bars immediately before and at varying intervals dur-ing exercise (total sucrose = 172 g $\cdot$ 4 h^{-1}). Compared to the placebo trial, blood glucose was maintained at a higher concentration after 2 h of exercise with hourly sucrose feedings, and total glycogen de-pletion was 25% less during the carbohydrate feeding trial (126 ver-sus 101 mmol $\cdot$ kg^{-1}). Sprint performance during the final sprint effort was 45% longer during the carbohydrate treatment (127 s versus 87 s).

In contrast, the subjects of Fielding et al. (62) consumed 86 g sucrose · h^{-1} on either an hourly or half hourly basis. The blood glucose concentration declined during exercise for the placebo and the hourly feeding treatments but was maintained when carbohydrate was consumed every half-hour. In spite of these differences in the blood glucose concentration, the rates of muscle glycogen degradation were the same between trials. Sprint performance was enhanced when carbohydrate was ingested every half-hour.

In summary, many, but not all, published studies show that carbohydrate feedings during prolonged exercise can improve performance. Unfortunately, the mechanism underlying this improvement remains unresolved.

C. Efficacy of the Ingestion of Fructose or Glucose on Performance During Prolonged Exercise

Massicotte et al. (124) examined the oxidation of glucose or fructose during 180 min of cycling at 50% $\dot{V}O_2$max. Trained subjects consumed 0.22 g carbohydrate per kg body weight every 20 min during exercise. The blood glucose concentration (5.2 mmol · L^{-1}) was maintained with glucose or fructose but declined slightly during exercise with the placebo treatment (4.2 mmol · L^{-1}). Fat utilization was highest with the placebo, but significantly greater for fructose than for glucose. Fructose, however, was less available for oxidation during exercise; 56% of the ingested fructose was oxidized compared to 75% of the ingested glucose. The total carbohydrate oxidation was less for glucose (174 g) and fructose (173 g) than for control (193 g). During this experiment, both glucose and fructose maintained the blood glucose concentration, but fructose increased fat oxidation when compared to glucose. The net effect, however, was that endogenous carbohydrate (muscle glycogen) oxidation was the same for the glucose and fructose trials. Performance was not monitored in this experiment.

Recently, Flynn et al. (64) compared the effects of various loads of glucose and fructose on glycogen breakdown and exercise performance during 2 h of isokinetic cycling during which the trained subjects were asked to perform as much work as possible. The absence of beneficial effects for glucose versus placebo were reviewed previously. In one fructose trial, a solution of 5.0% maltodextrins and 5.0% fructose (0.18 g per kg body weight) was provided before exercise and every 20 min during exercise; a second fructose trial of 7.7% maltodextrins and 2.3% fructose was supplied with the same feeding schedule and consumption. The subjects began these trials with elevated muscle glycogen (190 mmol·kg^{-1}). On average, the two fructose solutions elevated blood glucose more during exercise than either glucose or placebo treatments. However, there was no difference in the amount of muscle glycogen utilized for the exercise tasks nor in the total work performed during the 2 h experiment. It is likely that either the carbohydrate consumption was inadequate or the exercise duration was too short in this experiment for the beneficial effects of carbohydrate ingestion during exercise to be exhibited.

Murray et al. (132) studied the effect of ingestion of a 5% glucose polymer solution, 6% glucose·sucrose, 7% glucose·fructose, and a placebo on performance during 1.6 h of intermittent cycling exercise of varying intensity (55% to 100% $\dot{V}O_2$max) using recreational athletes. After 1 h of steady-state exercise at 55% and 65% $\dot{V}O_2$max, there was no difference in the subjects' ability to perform 480 revolutions at 80% $\dot{V}O_2$max between the treatments. After an additional 0.6 h of submaximal exercise, however, the subjects were able to perform the second high intensity work task an average of 42 s faster when consuming the 6% and 7% carbohydrate beverages compared to control. No differences in performance among the carbohydrate beverage treatments were detected.

Some subjects experience gastrointestinal distress when consuming fructose. Every subject in the study by Fruth and Gisolfi (76) complained of and experienced nausea, gas, and diarrhea during exercise while consuming fructose. Fruth and Gisolfi (76) fed five trained runners 0.31 g fructose·kg^{-1} body weight or a placebo every 20 min during running to exhaustion at 70% $\dot{V}O_2$max. All subjects ran longer than 2 h, but running time was 13% less during the fructose trial when compared to the placebo. It should be noted, however, that when small amounts of fructose are combined with glucose or glucose polymers, gastrointestinal problems are observed in only 2% of the subjects (76).

D. Consumption of Carbohydrate During Exercise

Carbohydrate ingestion during exercise at high intensity (65% to 75% $\dot{V}O_2$max) lasting longer than 90 min often enhances performance. A carbohydrate source sufficient to provide 0.5–1.5 g of carbohydrate per kg body weight should be consumed in volumes of 500–1000 mL immediately before or shortly after exercise begins. Thereafter, 150–250 mL carbohydrate beverages should be ingested every 15 to 30 min as a 5% to 8% solution providing at least 0.2 g carbohydrate per kg body weight per h. Feeding schedules such as this can significantly extend the time to exhaustion in well-trained athletes and in lesser trained subjects. The mechanism underlying improved performance appears to be mediated via either a sparing of muscle glycogen or a maintenance of high blood glucose concentrations during prolonged exercise. The literature suggests that sucrose, glucose, and glucose polymers are similarly effective in enhancing performance and that fructose in athletic beverages should be limited to concentrations of approximately 2% to 3% to minimize gastrointestinal disturbances.

SUMMARY

Athletes undertaking prolonged exercise expend significantly more calories than their sedentary counterparts. Although the scanty dietary information on athletes indicates that men meet the increased energy expenditure by increasing caloric consumption, women often appear to eat less than required to maintain body weight. When the caloric consumption meets the daily energy expenditure, the minimum dietary requirements for vitamins and minerals are usually met or exceeded. However, athletes need to increase the carbohydrate content of their diets from an average of 45% to 50% of the calories to at least 60% and preferably 75%. This is especially important for the athlete who undertakes daily strenuous training. It is very apparent that water consumption is vital for the maintenance of prolonged exercise capacity. Furthermore, increasing the muscle glycogen stores by supercompensation regimens, consumption of a high carbohydrate preexercise meal, and consumption of carbohydrate during prolonged exercise have all been shown to enhance endurance performance. Therefore, strategies should be devised to provide adequate water and carbohydrates during training and performance.

BIBLIOGRAPHY

1. Ahlborg, G., and P. Felig. Lactate and glucose exchange across the forearm, legs, and splanchnic bed during and after prolonged leg exercise. *J Clin Invest.* 69:45–54, 1982.
2. Ahlborg, G., and P. Felig. Substrate utilization during prolonged exercise preceded by ingestion of glucose. *Am J Physiol.* 233:E188–E194, 1977.
3. Ahlborg, G., and P. Felig. Influence of glucose ingestion on fuel hormone response during prolonged exercise. *J Appl Physiol.* 41:683–688, 1976.
4. Ahlborg, G., P. Felig, L. Hagenfeldt, R. Hendler, and J. Wahren. Substrate turnover during prolonged exercise in man: splanchnic and leg metabolism of glucose, free fatty acids, and amino acids. *J Clin Invest.* 53:1080-1090, 1974.
5. Ahlborg, B., J. Bergstrom, J. Brohult, L.-G. Ekelund, E. Hultman, and G. Maschio. Human muscle glycogen content and capacity for prolonged exercise after different diets. *Foersvarsmedicin.* 3:85–99, 1967.
6. American Diabetes Association: Principles of nutrition and dietary recommendation for individuals with diabetes mellitus. *Diabetes Care.* 2:520–523, 1979.
7. Armstrong, L.E., D.L. Costill, W.J. Fink, D. Bassett, M. Hargreaves, I. Nishibata, and D.S. King. Effects of dietary sodium on body and muscle potassium content during heat acclimation. *Eur J Appl Physiol.* 54:391–397, 1985.

8. Astrand, P.-O., and K. Rodahl. *Textbook of Work Physiology.* New York: McGraw Hill, 1986.
9. Barnes, G., A. Morton, and A. Wilson. The effect of a new glucose-electrolyte fluid on blood electrolyte levels, gastric emptying and work performance. *Austral J Sci Med Sport.* 16:25–30, 1984.
10. Berglund, B., P. Hemmingsson. Effects of caffeine ingestion on exercise performance at low and high altitudes in cross-country skiers. *Intl J Sports Med.* 3:234–236, 1982.
11. Bergstrom, J., E. Hultman, and A.E. Roch-Norlund. Muscle glycogen synthase in normal subjects: basal values, effect of glycogen depletion by exercise and of a carbohydrate-rich diet following exercise. *Scand J Clin Lab Invest.* 29:231–236, 1972.
12. Bergstrom, J., L. Hermansen, and B. Saltin. Diet, muscle glycogen and physical performance. *Acta Physiol Scand.* 71:140–150, 1967.
13. Bergstrom, J., and E. Hultman. Muscle glycogen synthesis after exercise: An enhancing factor localized to the muscle cells in man. *Nature.* 210:309–310, 1967.
14. Blom, P.C.S., N.K. Vollestad, and L. Hermansen. Diet and recovery processes. In: *Physiological Chemistry of Training and Detraining,* P. Marconnet, J. Poortmans, and L. Hermansen (Eds.). New York: S. Karger, 1982, pp. 148–161.
15. Bohannon, N.V., J.H. Karam, and P.H. Forsham. Endocrine response to sugar ingestion in man. *J Am Diet Assoc.* 76:555–560, 1980.
16. Bonen, A., B.W. Ness, A.N. Belcastro, and R.L. Kirby. Mild exercise impedes glycogen repletion in muscle. 58:1622–1629, 1985.
17. Booth, F.W., W.P. Nicholson, and P.A. Watson. Influence of muscle use on protein synthesis and degradation. In: *Exercise and Sport Science Reviews,* R.L. Terjung (Ed.). Philadelphia: Franklin Institute Press, 1982, vol 10, pp. 27–48.
18. Brandenberger, G., V. Candas, M. Follenius, J.P. Libert, and J.M. Kahn. Vascular fluid shifts and endocrine responses to exercise in the heat: effect of rehydration. *Eur J Appl Phsiol.* 55:123–129, 1985.
19. Brener, W., T.R. Hendrix, and P.R. McHugh. Regulation of the gastric emptying of glucose. *Gastroenterology* 85:76–82, 1983.
20. Brooke, J.D., and L.F. Green. The effect of a high carbohydrate diet on recovery following prolonged work to exhaustion. *Ergonomics.* 17:480–497, 1974.
21. Brooks, G.A., and T.D. Fahey. *Exercise Physiology: Human Bioenergetics and Its Applications.* New York: John Wiley & Sons, 1984.
22. Brotherhood, J.R. Nutrition and sports performance. *Sports Medicine* 1:350–389, 1984.
23. Brown, A.H. Dehydration exhaustion. In: *Physiology of Man in the Desert,* E.F. Adolph and associates. New York: Interscience Publishers, 1947, pp. 208–225.
24. Burke, L.M., and R.S.D. Read. Diet patterns of elite Australian male triathletes. *Physician and Sports Medicine.* 15:140–155, 1987.
25. Candas, V., J.P. Libert, G. Brandenberger, J.C. Sagot, C. Amoros, and J.M. Kahn. Hydration during exercise: effects on thermal and cardiovascular adjustments. *Eur J Appl Physiol.* 55:113–122, 1986.
26. Cerny, F.J. Protein metabolism during two hour ergometer exercise. In: *Metabolic Adaptations to Prolonged Exercise,* H. Howald, and J. Poortmans (Eds.). Birkhauser Verlag: Basel, 1975, pp. 232–237.
27. Committee on Nutrition, American Heart Association. *Circulation.* 58:762A–766A, 1978.
28. Costill, D.L., J. Kovaleski, D. Porter, J. Kirwan, R. Fielding, and D. King. Energy expenditure during front crawl swimming: Predicting success in middle-distance events. *Intl J Sports Med.* 6:266–270, 1985.
29. Costill, D.L., R. Cote, and W. Fink. Dietary potassium and heavy exercise: effects on muscle water and electrolytes. *Am J Clin Nutr.* 36:266–275, 1982.
30. Costill, D.L., R. Cote, W.J. Fink, and P. Van Handel. Muscle water and electrolyte distribution during prolonged exercise. *Int J Sports Med.* 2:130–134, 1981.
31. Costill, D.L., W.M. Sherman, W.J. Fink, C. Maresh, M. Witten, and J.M. Miller. The role of dietary carbohydrates in muscle glycogen resynthesis after strenuous running. *Am J Clin Nutr.* 34:1831–1836, 1981.
32. Costill, D.L., and J.M. Miller. Nutrition for endurance sport: Carbohydrate and fluid balance. *Int J Sports Med.* 1:2–14, 1980.
33. Costill, D.L., G.P. Dalsky, W.J. Fink. Effects of caffeine ingestion on metabolism and exercise performance. *Med Sci Sports Exer.* 10:155–158, 1978.
34. Costill, D.L., E.F. Coyle, G. Dalsky, W. Evans, W. Fink, and D. Hoopes. Effects of elevated plasma FFA and insulin on muscle glycogen usage during exercise. *J Appl Physiol.* 43:695–699, 1977.
35. Costill, D.L., R. Cote, and W.J. Fink. Muscle water and electrolytes following varied levels of dehydration in man. *J Appl Physiol.* 40:6–11, 1976.
36. Costill, D.L., G. Branam, D. Eddy, and W.J. Fink. Alteration in red cell volume following exercise and dehydration. *J Appl Physiol.* 37:912–916, 1974.

37. Costill, D.L., and W.J. Fink. Plasma volume changes following exercise and thermal dehydration. *J Appl Physiol.* 37:521–525, 1974.
38. Costill, D.L., E. Jansson, P.D. Gollnick, and B. Saltin. Glycogen utilization in the leg muscles of men during level and uphill running. *Acta Physiol Scand.* 94:475–481, 1974.
39. Costill, D.L., and B. Saltin. Factors limiting gastric emptying during rest and exercise. *J Appl Physiol.* 37:679–683, 1974.
40. Costill, D.L., P.D. Gollnick, E. Jansson, B. Saltin, and B. Stein. Glycogen depletion in human muscle fibers during distance running. *Acta Physiol Scand.* 89:374–383, 1973.
41. Costill, D.L., A. Bennett, G. Branam, and D.O. Eddy. Glucose ingestion at rest and during prolonged exercise. *J Appl Physiol.* 34:764–769, 1973.
42. Costill, D.L., R. Bowers, G. Branam, and K. Sparks. Muscle glycogen utilization during prolonged exercise on successive days. *J Appl Physiol.* 31:834–838, 1971.
43. Costill, D.L., W.F. Kammer, and A. Fisher. Fluid ingestion during distance running. *Arch Environ Health.* 21:520–525, 1970.
44. Coyle, E.F., A.R. Coggan, M.K. Hemmert, and J.L. Ivy. Muscle glycogen utilization during prolonged strenuous exercise when fed carbohydrate. *J Appl Physiol.* 61:165–172, 1986.
45. Coyle, E.F., A.R. Coggan, M.K. Hemmert, R.C. Lowe, and T.J. Walters. Substrate usage during prolonged exercise following a preexercise meal. *J Appl Physiol.* 59:429–433, 1985.
46. Coyle, E.F., A.R. Coggan, M.K. Hemmert, and T.J. Walters. Glycogen usage and performance relative to lactate threshold. *Med Sci Sports Exer.* 16:20, 1984 (abstract).
47. Coyle, E.F., and A.R. Coggan. Effectiveness of carbohydrate feeding in delaying fatigue during prolonged exercise. *Sports Medicine.* 1:446–458, 1984.
48. Coyle, E.F., D.L. Costill, W.J. Fink, and D.G. Hoopes. Gastric emptying rates of selected athletic drinks. *Res Quart.* 49:119–124, 1978.
49. Coyle, E.F., J.M. Hagberg, B.F. Hurley, W.H. Martin, III, A.A. Ehsani, and J.O. Holloszy. Carbohydrate feeding during prolonged strenuous exercise can delay fatigue. *J Appl Physiol.* 55:230–235, 1983.
50. Crapo, P.A., O.G. Kolterman, and J.M. Olefsky. Effects of oral fructose in normal, diabetic, and impaired glucose tolerance subjects. *Diabetes Care.* 3:575–582, 1980.
51. Davies, C.T.M., and M.W. Thompson. Physiological responses to prolonged exercise in ultramarathon athletes. *J Appl Physiol.* 61:611–617, 1986.
52. Decombaz, J., M.-J. Arnaud, H. Milon, H. Moesch, G. Philippossian, A.-L. Thelin, and H. Howald. Energy metabolism of medium-chained triglycerides versus carbohydrates during exercise. *Eur J Appl Physiol.* 52:9–14, 1983.
53. Deuster, P.A., S.B. Kyle, P.B. Moser, R.A. Vigersky, A. Singh, and E.B. Schoomaker. Nutritional intakes and status of highly trained amenorrheic and eumenorrheic women runners. *Fertility & Sterlility.* 46:636–643, 1986.
54. Devlin, J.T., J. Calles-Escandon, and E.S. Horton. Effects of preexercise snack feeding on endurance cycle exercise. *J Appl Physiol.* 60:980–985, 1986.
55. Dohm, G.L., R.T. Beeker, R.G. Israel, and E.B. Tapscott. Metabolic response to exercise after fasting. *J Appl Physiol.* 61:1363–1368, 1986.
56. Durnin, J.V.G.A., and A. Ferro-Luzzi. Conducting and reporting studies on human energy intake and output: Suggested standards. *Human Nutr & Appl Nutr.* 37A:141–144, 1983.
57. Essen, B. Intramuscular substrate utilization during prolonged exercise. *Ann NY Acad Sci.* 301:30–44, 1977.
58. Essig, D., D.L. Costill, and P.J. Van Handel. Effects of caffeine ingestion on utilization of muscle glycogen and lipids during leg ergometer cycling. *Intl J Sports Med.* 1:86–90, 1980.
59. Felig, P., A. Cherif, A. Minagawa, and J. Wahren. Hypoglycemia during prolonged exercise in normal men. *N Engl J Med.* 306:895–900, 1982.
60. Felig, P. Amino acid metabolism in exercise. *Ann NY Acad Sci.* 301:56–63, 1977.
61. Fielding, R.A., D.L. Costill, W.J. Fink, D.S. King, J.E. Kovaleski, and J.P. Kirwan. Effects of preexercise carbohydrate feedings on muscle glycogen use during exercise in well-trained runners. *Eur J Appl Physiol.* 56:225–229, 1987.
62. Fielding, R.A., D.L. Costill, W.J. Fink, D.S. King, M. Hargreaves, and J. Kovaleski. Effect of carbohydrate feeding frequencies and dosage on muscle glycogen use during exercise. *Med Sci Sports Exer.* 17:472–476, 1985.
63. Fink, W.J., D.L. Costill, and P.J. Van Handel. Leg metabolism during exercise in the heat and cold. *Eur J Appl Physiol.* 34:183–190, 1975.
64. Flynn, M.G., D.L. Costill, J.A. Hawley, W.J. Fink, P.D. Neuffer, R.A. Fielding, and M.D. Sleeper. Influence of selected carbohydrate drinks on cycling performance and glycogen use. *Med Sci Sports Exer.* 19:37–40, 1987.
65. Food and nutrient intakes of individuals in one day in the United States, Spring 1977. Nationwide Food Consumption Survey 1977–78 USDA, Washington, D.C. Preliminary Report No. 2, Sept. 1980.

66. Food and Nutrition Board. *Recommended Dietary Allowances.* 9th ed. Natl. Acad. Sci., Washington, 1980.
67. Fordtran, J.S., and B. Saltin. Gastric emptying and intestinal absorption during prolonged severe exercise. *J Appl Physiol.* 23:331–335, 1967.
68. Fortney, S.M., E.R. Nadel, C.B. Wenger, and J.R. Bove. Effect of blood volume on sweating rate and body fluids in exercising humans. *J Appl Physiol.* 51:1594–1600, 1981.
69. Fortney, S.M., C.B. Wenger, J.R. Bove, and E.R. Nadel. Effect of blood volume on forearm venous flow and cardiac stroke volume during exercise. *J Appl Physiol.* 55:884–890, 1983.
70. Fortney, S.M., C.B. Wenger, J.R. Bove, and E.R. Nadel. Effect of hyperosmolality on control of blood flow and sweating. *J Appl Physiol.* 57:1688–1695, 1984.
71. Foster, C., D.L. Costill, and W.J. Fink. Effects of preexercise feedings on endurance performance. *Med Sci Sports Exer.* 11:1–5, 1979.
72. Foster, C., D.L. Costill, and W.J. Fink. Gastric emptying characteristics of glucose and glucose polymers. *Res Quart Exerc Sport.* 51:299–305, 1980.
73. Francesconi, R.P., M.N. Sawka, and K.B. Pandolf. Hypohydration and heat acclimation: plasma renin and aldosterone during exercise. *J Appl Physiol.* 55:1790–1794, 1983.
74. Francesconi, R.P., M.N. Sawka, K.B. Pandolf, R.W. Hubbard, A.J. Young, and S. Muza. Plasma hormonal responses at graded hypohydration levels during exercise-heat stress. *J Appl Physiol.* 59:1855–1860, 1985.
75. Francis, K.T. Effect of water and electrolyte replacement during exercise in the heat on biochemical indices of stress and performance. *Aviat Space Environ Med.* 50:115–119, 1979.
76. Fruth, J.M., and C.V. Gisolfi. Effects of carbohydrate consumption on endurance performance: fructose versus glucose. In: *Nutrient Utilization during Exercise,* E.L. Fox (Ed.). Columbus, Ohio: Ross Laboratories, 1983, pp. 68–77.
77. Galbo, H., E.A. Richter, J. Hilsted, J.J. Holst, N.J. Christensen, and J. Henriksson. Hormonal regulation during prolonged exercise. *Ann NY Acad Sci.* 72–80, 1977.
78. Gisolfi, C.V., and J.R. Copping. Thermal effects of prolonged treadmill exercise in the heat. *Med Sci Sports Exer.* 6:108–113, 1974.
79. Grandjean, A.C. Nutrition for swimmers. *Clin Sports Med.* 5:65–76, 1986.
80. Greenleaf, J.E., and P.J. Brock. Na+ and Ca2+ ingestion: plasma volume-electrolyte distribution at rest and exercise. *J Appl Physiol.* 48:838–847, 1980.
81. Greenleaf, J.E., and B.L. Castle. Exercise temperature regulation in man during hypohydration and hyperhydration. *J Appl Physiol.* 30:847–853, 1971.
82. Hagenfeldt, L. Turnover of individual free fatty acids in man. *Federation Proc.* 34:2236–2240, 1975.
83. Hargreaves, M., D.L. Costill, W.J. Fink, D.S. King, and R.A. Fielding. Effect of preexercise carbohydrate feedings on endurance cycling performance. *Med Sci Sports Exer.* 19:33–36, 1987.
84. Hargreaves, M., D.L. Costill, A.R. Coggan, W.J. Fink, and I. Nishibata. Effect of carbohydrate feedings on muscle glycogen utilization and exercise performance. *Med Sci Sports Exer.* 16:219–222, 1984.
85. Harrison, M.H., R.J. Edwards, and P.A. Fennessy. Intravascular volume and tonicity as factors in the regulation of body temperature. *J Appl Physiol.* 44:69–75, 1978.
86. Heinz, F. Metabolism of fructose in the liver. *Acta Med Scand* (suppl.) 542:27–33, 1972.
87. Henschel, A., H.L. Taylor, and A. Keys. Performance capacity in acute starvation with hard work. *J Appl Physiol.* 6:624–633, 1954.
88. Hermansen, L., E. Hultman, and B. Saltin. Muscle glycogen during prolonged severe exercise. *Acta Physiol Scand.* 71:129–139, 1967.
89. Hikida, R.S., R.S. Staron, F.C. Hagerman, W.M. Sherman, and D.L. Costill. Muscle fiber necrosis associated with human marathon runners. *J Neurol Sci.* 59:185–203, 1983.
90. Hiller, W.D.B., M.L. O'Toole, F. Massimino, R.E. Miller, and R.H. Laird. Plasma electrolyte and glucose changes during the Hawaiian Ironman Triathlon (abstract). *Med Sci Sports Exer.* 17:219, 1985.
91. Hodges, R.E., and W.A. Krehl. The role of carbohydrates in lipid metabolism. *Amer J Clin Nutr.* 17:334–346, 1965.
92. Holloszy, J.O., and E.F. Coyle. Adaptations of skeletal muscle to endurance exercise and their metabolic consequences. *J Appl Physiol.* 56:831–838, 1984.
93. Hubbard, R.W., B.L. Sandick, W.T. Matthew, R.P. Francesconi, J.B. Sampson, M.J. Durkot, O. Maller, and D.B. Engell. Voluntary dehydration and alliesthesia for water. *J Appl Physiol.* 57:868–875, 1984.
94. Hultman, E. Liver as a glucose supplying source during rest and exercise with special reference to diet. In: *Nutrition, Physical Fitness and Health,* J. Parizkova, and V.A. Rogozkin (Eds.). Baltimore: University Park Press, 1978, pp. 9–30.
95. Hultman, E. Studies on muscle metabolism of glycogen and active phosphate in man with special reference to exercise and diet. *Scand J Clin Lab Invest.* 19 (suppl. 94):1–63, 1967.

96. Hunt, J.N., J.L. Smith, and C.L. Jiang. Effect of meal volume and energy density on the gastric emptying of carbohydrates. *Gastroenterology* 89:1326–1330, 1985.

97. Hurley, B.F., P.M. Nemeth, W.H. Martin, III, J.M. Hagberg, G.P. Dalsky, and J.O. Holloszy. Muscle triglyceride utilization during exercise: effect of training. *J Appl Physiol.* 60:562–567, 1986.

98. Ivy, J.L., D.L. Costill, W.J. Fink, and E. Maglischo. Contribution of medium and long chain triglyceride intake to energy metabolism during prolonged exercise. *Int J Sports Med.* 1:15–20, 1980.

99. Ivy, J.L., D.L. Costill, W.J. Fink, and R.W. Lower. Influence of caffeine and carbohydrate feedings on endurance performance. *Med Sci Sports Exer.* 11:6–11, 1979.

100. Jandrain, B., G. Krzentowski, F. Pirnay, F. Mosora, M. Lacroix, A. Luyckx, and P. Lefebvre. Metabolic availability of glucose ingested 3 h before prolonged exercise in humans. *J Appl Physiol.* 56:1314–1319, 1984.

101. Johnson, A., P. Collins, I. Higgins, D. Harrington, J. Connolly, C. Dolphin, M. McCreery, L. Brady, and M. O'Brien. Psychological, nutritional, and physical status of Olympic road cyclists. *Brit J Sports Med.* 19:11–14, 1985.

102. Karlsson, J., L.-O. Nordesjo, and B. Saltin. Muscle glycogen utilization during exercise after physical training. *Acta Physiol Scand.* 90:210–217, 1974.

103. Karlsson, J., and B. Saltin. Diet, muscle glycogen, and endurance performance. *J Appl Physiol.* 31:203–206, 1971.

104. Katz, A.S. Broberg, K. Sahlin, and J. Wahren. Leg glucose uptake during maximal dynamic exercise in humans. *Am J Physiol.* 251:E65–E70, 1986.

105. Kirsch, K.A., and H. von Amelin. Feeding patterns of endurance athletes. *Eur J Appl Physiol.* 47:197–208, 1981.

106. Kochan, R.G., D.R. Lamb, S.A. Lutz, C.V. Perrill, E.M. Reimann, and K.K. Schlender. Glycogen synthase activation in human skeletal muscle: effects of diet and exercise. *Am J Physiol.* 236:E660–E666, 1979.

107. Koivisto, V.A. The physiology of marathon running. *Sci Prog Oxf.* 70:109–127, 1986.

108. Koivisto, V., M. Harkonen, S.-L. Karonen, P.H. Groop, R. Elovainio, E. Ferrannini, L. Sacca, and R.A. Defronzo. Glycogen depletion during prolonged exercise: influence of glucose, fructose or placebo. *J Appl Physiol.* 58:731–737, 1985.

109. Koivisto, V., S.-L. Karonen, and E.O. Nikkila. Carbohydrate ingestion before exercise: comparison of glucose, fructose, and sweet placebo. *J Appl Physiol.* 51:783–787, 1981.

110. Krebs, H.A., N.W. Cornell, P. Lund, and L.R. Hems. Some aspects of hepatic metabolism. In: Regulation of Hepatic Metabolism, F. Lundquist and N. Tygstrup (Eds.). Copenhagen: Munksgaard, 1974, pp. 549–557.

111. Krzentowski, G., F. Pirnay, A.S. Luyckx, N. Pallikarakis, M. Lacroix, F. Mosora, and P.J. Lefebvre. Metabolic adaptations in post-exercise recovery. *Clin Physiol.* 2:277–288, 1982.

112. Kuipers, H., H.A. Keizer, F.T.J. Verstappen, and D.L. Costill. Influence of prostaglandin-inhibiting drug on muscle soreness after eccentric exercise. *Int J Sports Med.* 6:336–349, 1985.

113. Lamb, D.R. *Physiology of Exercise: Responses & Adaptations.* New York: MacMillan, 1984.

114. Lash, J.M., W.M. Sherman, S. Bloomfield. Muscle soreness: glucose and insulin response. *Med Sci Sports Exer.* 19:S75, 1987 (abstract).

115. Lemon, P.W.R., K.E. Yarasheski, and D.G. Dolony. The importance of protein for athletes. *Sports Med.* 1:474–484, 1984.

116. Lemon, P.W.R., D.G. Dolony, and B.A. Sherman. Effect of intense prolonged running on protein metabolism. In: *Biochemistry of Exercise*, H.G. Knuttgen, J.A. Vogel, and J. Poortmans (Eds.). Champaign, Illinois: Human Kinetics Publishers, 1983, vol. 13, pp. 362–372.

117. Lemon, P.W.R., and J.P. Mullin. Effect of initial muscle glycogen levels on protein catabolism during exercise. *J Appl Physiol.* 48:624–629, 1980.

118. Levine, L., W.J. Evans, B.S. Cadarette, E.C. Fisher, and B.A. Bullen. Fructose and glucose ingestion and muscle glycogen use during submaximal exercise. *J Appl Physiol.* 55:1767–1771, 1983.

119. Levine, S.A., B. Gordon, and C.L. Derick. Some changes in the chemical constituents of the blood following a marathon race: with special reference to the development of hypoglycemia. *J Am Med Assoc.* 82:1778–1779, 1924.

120. Loy, S.F., R.K. Conlee, W.W. Winder, A.G. Nelson, D.A. Arnall, and A.G. Fisher. Effects of 24-hour fast on cycling endurance time at two different intensities. *J Appl Physiol.* 61:654–659, 1986.

121. MacDougall, G.R. Ward, D.G. Sale, and J.R. Sutton. Muscle glycogen repletion after high-intensity intermittent exercise. *J Appl Physiol.* 42:129–132, 1977.

122. Maehlum, S., and L. Hermansen. Muscle glycogen concentration during recovery after prolonged severe exercise in fasting subjects. *Scand J Clin Lab. Invest.* 38:557–560, 1978.

123. Maehlum, S., P. Felig, and J. Wahren. Splanchnic glucose and muscle glycogen metabolism after glucose feeding during postexercise recovery. *Am J Physiol.* 235:E255–E260, 1978.

124. Massicotte, D., F. Peronnet, C. Allah, C. Hillaire-Marcel, M. Ledoux, and G. Brisson. Metabolic response to [13C]glucose and [13C]fructose ingestion during exercise. *J Appl Physiol.* 61:1180–1184, 1986.

125. Maughan, R.J., and C.E. Fenn, M. Gleeson, and J.B. Leiper. Metabolic and circulatory responses to the ingestion of glucose polymer and glucose/electrolyte solutions during exercise in man. *Eur J Appl Physiol.* 56:356–362, 1987.

126. Miller, J.M., E.F. Coyle, W.M. Sherman, J.M. Hagberg, D.L. Costill, W.J. Fink, S.E. Terblanche, and J.O. Holloszy. Effect of glycerol feeding on endurance and metabolism during prolonged exercise in man. *Med Sci Sports Exer.* 15:237–242, 1983.

127. Miller, M., J.N. Craig, W.R. Ducker, and H. Woodward, Jr. The metabolism of fructose in man. *Yale J Biol Med.* 29:335–360, 1956.

128. Mirkin, G. Carbohydrate loading: a dangerous practice. *J Am Med Assoc.* 223:1511–1512, 1973.

129. Mitchell, J.B., D.L. Costill, J.A. Houmand, M.G. Flynn, W.J. Fink, and J.D. Beltz. Effects of carbohydrate ingestion on gastric emptying and exercise performance. *Med Sci Sports Exer.*, 1988 (in press).

130. Moroff, S.V., and D.E. Bass. Effects of overhydration on man's physiological responses to work in the heat. *J Appl Physiol.* 20:267–270, 1965.

131. Murray, R. The efficacy of consuming carbohydrate-electrolyte beverages during and following exercise. *Sports Medicine,* 4:322–351, 1987.

132. Murray, R., D.E. Eddy, T. Wakasugi-Murray, J.G. Seifert, G.L. Paul, and G.A. Halaby. The effect of fluid and carbohydrate feedings during cycling exercise in the heat. *Med Sci Sports Exer.,* 19:597-604, 1987.

133. Nadel, E.R., S.M. Fortney, and C.B. Wenger. Effect of hydration state on circulatory and thermal regulation. *J Appl Physiol.* 49:715–721, 1980.

134. Nagle, F.J., and D.R. Bassett. Metabolic requirements of distance running. In: *Limits of Human Performance,* D.H. Clarke and H.M. Eckert (Eds.). Champaign, Illinois: Human Kinetics Publishers, 1985, pp. 19–30.

135. Neufer, P.D., D.L. Costill, W.J. Fink, J.P. Kirwan, R.A. Fielding, and M.G. Flynn. Effects of exercise and carbohydrate composition on gastric emptying. *Med Sci Sports Exer.* 18:658–662, 1986.

136. Newsholme, E.A. The regulation of intracellular fuel supply during sustained exercise. *Ann NY Acad Sci.* 301:81–91, 1977.

137. Nielsen, B. Effect of changes in plasma Na+ and Ca++ ion concentration on body temperature during exercise. *Acta Physiol Scand.* 91:123–129, 1974.

138. Nielsen, B., G. Hansen, S.O. Jorgensen, and E. Nielsen. Thermoregulation in exercising man during dehydration and hyperhydration with water and saline. *Int J Biometeor.* 15:195–200, 1971.

139. Nilson, L.H.: and E. Hultman. Liver and muscle glycogen in man after glucose and fructose infusion. *Scand J Clin Lab Invest.* 33:5–10, 1974.

140. Noakes, T.D., N. Goodwin, B.L. Rayner, T. Branken, and R.K.N. Taylor. Water intoxication: a possible complication during endurance exercise. *Med Sci Sports Exer.* 17:370–375, 1985.

141. Nutrition and Your Health—Dietary Guidelines for Americans. USDA—DHEW, Washington, D.C. Home and Garden Bulletin, No. 232, 1980.

142. Olsson, K.E., and B. Saltin. Variations in total body water with muscle glycogen changes in man. *Biochem Exerc Med Sports.* 5:159–162, 1969.

143. Olsson, K.E., and B. Saltin. Variations in total body water with muscle glycogen changes in man following exercise. *Acta Physiol Scand.* 80:11–18, 1970.

144. Oscai, L.B. Type L hormone-sensitive lipase hydrolyzes endogenous triacylglycerols in muscle in exercised rats. *Med Sci Sports Exer.* 15:336–339, 1983.

145. Owen, M.D., K.C. Kregel, P.T. Wall, and C.V. Gisolfi. Effects of ingesting carbohydrate beverages during exercise in the heat. *Med Sci Sports Exer.* 18:568–575, 1986.

146. Paul, P. FFA mobilization of normal dogs during steady-state exercise at different workloads. *J Appl Physiol.* 28:127–132, 1970.

147. Pequignot, J.M., L. Peyrin, and G. Peres. Catecholamine-fuel interrelationships during exercise in fasting man. *J Appl Physiol.* 48:109–113, 1980.

148. Pernow, B., and B. Saltin. Availability of substrates and capacity for prolonged heavy exercise in man. *J Appl Physiol.* 31:416–422, 1971.

149. Peters, A.J., R.H. Dressendorfer, J. Rimar, and C.L. Keen. Diets of endurance runners competing in a 20-day road race. *Physician and Sports medicine.* 14:63–70, 1986.

150. Piehl, K. Time course for refilling of glycogen stores in human muscle fibers following

exercise-induced glycogen depletion. *Acta Physiol Scand.* 90:297–302, 1974.

151. Piehl, K., S. Adolfsson, and K. Nazar. Glycogen storage and glycogen synthase activity in trained and untrained muscle of man. *Acta Physiol Scand.* 90:779–788, 1974.

152. Pirnay, F., M. LaCroix, F. Morosa, A. Luyckx, and P. Lefebvre. Glucose oxidation during prolonged exercise evaluated with naturally labeled (13C) glucose. *J Appl Physiol.* 31:416–422, 1977.

153. Pitts, G.C., R.E. Johnson, and F.C. Consolazio. Work in the heat as affected by intake of water, salt and glucose. *Am J Physiol.* 142:253–259, 1944.

154. Plyley, M.J., D.L. Costill, and W.J. Fink. Influence of glycogen "bound" water on temperature regulation during exercise. *Can J Appl Sport Sci.* 5:5, 1980 (abstract).

155. Poortmans, J.R. Protein turnover and amino acid oxidation during and after exercise. *Med Sport Sci.* 17:130–147, 1984.

156. Powers, S.K., and S. Doss. Caffeine and endurance performance. *Sports Medicine.* 2:165–174, 1985.

157. Ravussin, L., P. Pahus, A. Dorner, M.J. Arnaud, and E. Jequier. Substrate utilization during prolonged exercise preceded by ingestion of 13C-glucose in glycogen depleted and control subjects. *Pflugers Arch.* 382:197–202, 1979.

158. Rennie, M.J., R.H.T. Edwards, S. Krywawych, C.T.M. Davies, D. Halliday, and D.J. Millward. Effects of exercise on protein turnover in man. *Clin Sci.* 61:627–639, 1981.

159. Roedde, S., J.D. MacDougall, J.R. Sutton, and H.J. Green. Supercompensation of muscle glycogen in trained and untrained subjects. *Can J Appl Sport Sci.* 11:42–46, 1986.

160. Rowell, L.B., H.J. Marx, R.A. Bruce, R.D. Conn, and F. Kusumi. Reductions in cardiac output, central blood volume and stroke volume with thermal stress in normal man during exercise. *J Clin Invest.* 45:1801–1816, 1966.

161. Saltin, B., J. Henriksson, E. Nygaard, P. Anderson, and E. Jansson. Fiber types and metabolic potentials of skeletal muscle in sedentary man and endurance runners. *Ann NY Acad Sci.* 301:3–29, 1977.

162. Saltin, B., and J. Karlsson. Muscle glycogen utilization during work of different intensities. In: *Muscle Metabolism during Exercise*, B. Pernow, and B. Saltin (Eds.). New York: Plenum Press, 1971, 289–300.

163. Sawka, M.N., M.M. Toner, R.P. Francesconi, and K.B. Pandolf. Hypohydration and exercise: effects of heat acclimation, gender, and environment. *J Appl Physiol.* 55:1147–1153, 1983.

164. Segal, K., A. Nyman, J.G. Kral, P. Bjorntorp, D.P. Kotler, and F.X. Pi-Sunyer. Effects of glucose ingestion on submaximal intermittent exercise. *Med Sci Sports Exer.* 17:205, 1985 (abstract).

165. Sherman, W.M., D.L. Costill, W.J. Fink, F.C. Hagerman, L.E. Armstrong, and T.F. Murray. Effect of a 42.2-km footrace and subsequent rest or exercise on muscle glycogen and enzymes. *J Appl Physiol.* 55:1219–1224, 1983.

166. Sherman, W.M. Carbohydrates, muscle glycogen, and muscle glycogen supercompensation. In: *Ergogenic Aids in Sport*, M.H. Williams (Ed.). Champaign, Illinois: Human Kinetics Publishers, 1983, pp. 3–26.

167. Sherman, W.M., M.J. Plyley, R.L. Sharp, P.J. VanHandel, R.M. McAllister, W.J. Fink, and D.L. Costill. Muscle glycogen storage and its relationship with water. *Intl J Sports Med.* 3:22–24, 1982.

168. Sherman, W.M., D.L. Costill, W.J. Fink, and J.M. Miller. The effect of exercise and diet manipulation on muscle glycogen and its subsequent use during performance. *Int J Sports Med.* 2:114–118, 1981.

169. Sjodin, B., and J. Svedenhag. Applied physiology of marathon running. *Sports Medicine.* 2:83–99, 1985.

170. Sladen, G.E., and A.M. Dawson. Interrelationships between the absorptions of glucose, sodium and water by the normal human jejunum. *J Clin Sci.* 36:119–132, 1969.

171. Snyder, A.C., D.R. Lamb, T.S. Baur, D.F. Connors, and G.R. Brodowicz, Maltodextrin feeding immediately before prolonged cycling at 62% VO$_2$max increases time to exhaustion. *Med Sci Sports Exer.* 15:126, 1983 (abstract).

172. Taskinen, M.-R., E.A. Nikkila, S. Rehunen, and A. Gordin. Effect of acute vigorous exercise on lipoprotein lipase activity of adipose tissue and skeletal muscle in physically active men. *Artery* 6:471–483, 1980.

173. Terblanche, S.E., R.D. Fell, A.C. Juhlin-Dannfelt, B.W. Craig, and J.O. Holloszy. Effects of glycerol feeding before and after exhausting exercise. *J Appl Physiol.* 50:94–101, 1981.

174. Tremblay, A., J. Sevigny, M. Jobin, and C. Allard. Diet and muscle glycogen in vastus lateralis of runners for the marathon. *J Can Dietetic Assoc.* 41:128–135, 1980.

175. Van Handel, P.J., W.J. Fink, G. Branam, and D.L. Costill. Fate of 14C glucose ingested during prolonged exercise. *Intl J Sports Med.* 1:127–131, 1980.

176. Wahren, J. Glucose turnover during exercise in man. *Ann NY Acad Sci.* 301:45–55, 1977.

177. Wahren, J., A. Juhlin-Dannfelt, O. Bjorkman, R. DeFronzo, and P. Felig. Influence of fiber ingestion on carbohydrate utilization and absorption. *Clin Physiol.* 2:315–321, 1982.
178. Wilmore, J.H. The application of science to sport: Physiological profiles of male and female athletes. *Can J Appl Sport Sci.* 4:103–115, 1979.
179. Wright, P.H., and W.J. Malaisse. Effects of epinephrine, stress and exercise upon insulin secretion by the rat. *Am J Physiol.* 214:1031–1034, 1968.
180. Young, D.R., R. Pelligra, J. Shapira, R.R. Adachi, and K. Skretingland. Glucose oxidation and replacement during prolonged exercise in man. *J Appl Physiol.* 23:734–741, 1967.

FOOTNOTES

1. Ann C. Grandjean, Chief Nutrition Consultant, USOC, Swanson Center for Nutrition, 502 S. 44th Street, Room 3007, Omaha, Nebraska 68105.
2. John L. Ivy, Exercise Physiology Laboratory, Bellmont 222, University of Texas, Austin, Texas 78712.

DISCUSSION

COYLE: Maybe this is a good time to address the idea that athletes have diets which are grossly inadequate in carbohydrates. That's a strong statement. You were saying that athletes normally get an average of 50% of calories in carbohydrates, which would amount to, if a person consumed 3,600 calories per day, about 450 grams of carbohydrates per 24 hours. You are recommending that they ingest about 70% of the calories in carbohydrates, which would put them up around 600. I have the feeling also that many athletes I see are suboptimal in carbohydrates; they are dragging and they feel stale, and that may be related to inadequate stores. But, do you really think that you can say with confidence that most athletes are grossly inadequate in dietary carbohydrate?

SHERMAN: I think they're often deficient. They're certainly often suboptimal. Based on the fact that nutritionists and exercise physiologists have been recommending high contents of carbohydrates in diets for a number of years now, the carbohydrate content remains too low. Perhaps stronger language is necessary to try to drive that point home.

Another interesting point is that there is some evidence that suggests that damage to muscle tissue, perhaps invoked by prolonged distance running, especially by eccentric contractions, is another important consideration in the muscle's capacity to resynthesize glycogen. Even when marathon runners consume relatively high amounts of carbohydrates, the rate of muscle glycogen synthesis is relatively slow.

MURRAY: What is the mechanism by which hard training or injury appears to diminish the rate at which glycogen is resynthesized?

SHERMAN: I don't think the mechanism has been elucidated. If you force an individual or an animal to traumatize the muscles, specifically to disrupt the sarcolemma, resynthesis of muscle glycogen is slowed. This may be because resynthesis is linked to hormone receptor binding events; with trauma, the effect of insulin on glucose uptake is impaired, thus resulting in decreased synthesis of muscle glycogen, because the primary fate of glucose after depletion in muscle is glycogen synthesis.

Let's switch over to the topic of pre-exercise meals. There are many studies related to the timing of the preexercise meal. I think one of the studies which is most frequently cited is the study by Costill, in which the subjects consumed 75 gm of glucose 45 minutes before exercise at 70% of $\dot{V}O_2$max, and muscle glycogen and glucose were followed for 30 minutes of exercise. That was compared to a control trial where they consumed a placebo solution. They found with the glucose feeding a dramatic drop in the blood glucose concentration at the start of exercise, and the insulin concentration was about 4-fold higher than basal. In addition, they found roughly a 17% increase in muscle glycogen utilization over placebo. This suggests that the consumption of a high carbohydrate meal 45 minutes before exercise of that intensity may not be good for athletes. It's important to point out, though, that if this type of meal is consumed right before exercise starts or after exercise has commenced, the insulin and glucose response is blunted, i.e., you don't see a drop in blood glucose or increased muscle glycogen utilization during exercise.

COYLE: It's my interpretation that the practical application of these studies has been overstated in the last few years. We had subjects who exercised longer than 30 minutes—we had them going one hour and 45 minutes—and we found that the glucose/insulin alterations were transient phenomena.

GISOLFI: I wonder what would happen if you first did a glucose tolerance test on subjects and then did this type of experiment. Perhaps we would be able to identify individual susceptibilities.

NADEL: It may be true that most people can tolerate the ingestion of carbohydrates 45 minutes or an hour before exercise, but there are going to be people who can't.

COYLE: Perhaps trained subjects are more likely to experience this reaction because their increased insulin sensitivity drives blood glucose down. Also, they are able to activate a larger muscle mass during exercise; it may be as simple as that.

MURRAY: In addition to all of the other qualifications that have been previously mentioned, it is important to keep in mind that most of these preexercise feeding studies fed very large carbohydrate doses of 400 calories or more. Perhaps comparatively smaller pre-exercise doses don't evoke this response. After all, most athletes never consume 100 grams of pure glucose prior to exercise. They either consume a meal of mixed nutrients or a much smaller dose of carbohydrate.

BROOKS: So, Mike, when all is said and done, what is your recommendation for a pre-game meal: a high-carbohydrate meal three to four hours before?

SHERMAN: Yes, that's the recommendation we make.

BROOKS: What form of carbohydrate?

SHERMAN: I think it primarily depends on the athlete. If you have well-trained athletes, I think they're going to handle simple carbohydrates fine. Complex carbohydrates would somewhat reduce the glycemic response, and those might be a little better from that standpoint, but it's going to take longer to digest them, and some athletes might run into problems with gastrointestinal distress.

BROOKS: It used to be, some time ago, that athletes would have things like toast and eggs or potatoes and a small steak. Since their schedules weren't as hectic, those athletes might have been as well prepared as they are today.

SHERMAN: That's a good point. Training schedules certainly are hectic nowadays, and that may well be taking a toll. Ed Coyle has some data showing that the swimmers at the University of Texas are reporting in the morning with very low blood glucose concentrations.

COYLE: Swimmers are chronically starved. By simply having them eat 200 gm of carbohydrate before they go to bed, they come back feeling better with higher blood glucose the next morning.

BURKE: The same problem arises with cyclists. They constantly seem to have food in their stomachs. They are just so fatigued that they have to keep eating a little bit at a time. They just don't have the energy to eat three big meals a day.

GISOLFI: What about the reverse, the concept that we should diet or starve ourselves for 8 to 12 hours before competition?

BROOKS: It's my recollection that, with humans, exercise performance is curtailed under these circumstances.

LAMB: Several studies indicate that drinking either water or maybe a dilute electrolyte solution before going into exercise seems to be useful. But Carl Gisolfi has a study that didn't show any advantages of pre-hydration over simply drinking during the exercise. So the question that I have is, do we really know whether superhydration before exercise in athletic situations helps?

NADEL: If you drink free water, then the body will protect itself against becoming hypotonic, so that water will just be filtered from the kidneys. If you're going to drink before exercise, I would guess you would have to take electrolytes with the water. If you don't do that, the water will just pass through. In studies we've done on rehydration following exercise, subjects rehydrate better—with better plasma volume restoration—if they consume an electrolyte solution, i.e., about half normal saline, following exercise. The question is, does this hold before or during exercise, and I think it does.

GISOLFI: It does. If you ingest a glucose and electrolyte solution, you defend the plasma volume during exercise more than if you would just give water.

TIPTON: Because of the electrolytes?

GISOLFI: Well, it was a glucose-electrolyte solution, so I'm not sure.

SUTTON: A number of people are now reporting hyponatremia following endurance exercise. What should we recommend?

EICHNER: I know a physician who was taking care of a heat stressed runner who was drinking water for two hours until the runner got headaches and was confused. His plasma sodium was 120 mEq/L. He was evidently fine during the race; it was after the race when problems developed. In the medical tent he just drank ice water, and it drove his sodium down.

SHERMAN: It is beginning to be clear that carbohydrate consumption during exercise can, in fact, improve performance. The interpretation of some of the data strongly suggests that the reason subjects are able to exercise longer with carbohydrate feeding is high glucose availability. The glucose ingestion does play a major role as an ergogenic aid during prolonged exercise.

DAVIS: A common belief is that a 2.5% carbohydrate solution, based on the time of gastric emptying, is best. That recommendation is based on the possibility of decreased fluid absorption associated with beverage containing more than 2.5% carbohydrate. I strongly believe solutions higher than 2.5% carbohydrate are okay. They provide carbohydrates that are necessary for performance, and they don't impair fluid replenishment or thermoregulation.

7

Psychological Factors and Prolonged Exercise

ROD K. DISHMAN, PH.D.

FRANK J. LANDY, PH.D.

INTRODUCTION
  I. RESPONSES TO TRAINING IN TOP ATHLETES
     A.   The Challenge
     B.   A Role for Psychology
     C.   Psychological Monitoring of Training for Prolonged Exercise
     D.   Psychological Models of Training Stress
 II. ACUTE AND CHRONIC RESPONSES TO EXERCISE IN NON-ATHLETES
     A.   Mental Stress Tolerance
          1.   Acute Responses Within Individuals
          2.   Group Comparisons on "Fitness"
          3.   Experimental Study
          4.   Endorphin Research in Humans
          5.   Monoamine Research in Humans
          6.   Comparative Studies
     B.   Stress-Behavior Risks Associated with Prolonged Exercise
          1.   Eating Disorders and Prolonged Exercise
          2.   Exercise Abuse
          3.   A Model of Motivation for Exercise Dependence
     C.   Anxiety
          1.   Acute Tension Reduction
          2.   Associated Chronic Changes
          3.   Exercise as Treatment
          4.   The Biology of Anxiety and Exercise
     D.   Depression
          1.   Associated Chronic Changes
          2.   Exercise as Treatment
          3.   The Biology of Depression and Exercise
     E.   Sleep Disorders
          1.   Quasi-Experimental Studies
          2.   Possible Mechanisms

III. CORRELATES OF PERFORMANCE DURING ACUTE EXERCISE
    A.   Personality and Prolonged Exercise Performance
    B.   Perception During Prolonged Exercise Performance
    C.   Cognition During Prolonged Exercise Performance
IV. ADHERENCE TO PROLONGED EXERCISE IN PREVENTIVE MEDICINE
    A.   Prescriptions for Adherence
    B.   Behavioral Problems with Intensity Prescriptions
        1.   Limitations of Training HR
        2.   Problems of Self-Regulation
V. MOTIVATION MODELS FOR THE STUDY OF PROLONGED EXERCISE
    A.   Expectancy Theory
        1.   Exercise Examples: Top Athletes
        2.   Exercise Examples: Outcomes for Non-Athletes
        3.   Exercise Examples: Adherence in Preventive Medicine
    B.   Goal Setting:
        1.   Exercise Examples: Top Athletes
        2.   Exercise Examples: Outcomes for Non-Athletes
        3.   Exercise Examples: Adherence in Preventive Medicine
VI. LIMITATIONS OF RESEARCH DESIGN AND METHODOLOGY
    A.   Sample Size
    B.   Conflicting Results
VII. IMPLICATIONS FOR APPLIED RESEARCH AND PRACTICE
BIBLIOGRAPHY
DISCUSSION

INTRODUCTION

Psychological variables influence, and are influenced by, human performance in measurable and predictable ways (22,23,67,183,186). This chapter examines what is currently known about how such factors apply to the understanding of prolonged exercise. Few studies of prolonged exercise have used psychological methods. Therefore, we will also include studies of less intensity and duration that have clear implications for prolonged exercise. Specific attention is paid to (1) responses to training in top athletes, (2) acute and chronic responses to exercise in non-athletes, (3) correlates of performance during acute exercise, (4) adherence to prolonged exercise in preventive medicine, and (5) motivation models for the study of prolonged exercise. These topics are chosen because they categorize the available research in sport psychology that appears to have direct implications for prolonged exercise. Other areas, such as competition and applied interventions, while important, are not included, because research in these areas using prolonged exercise is not yet sufficient for review (68).

Limitations of research design and methodology and implications for applied research and practice will also be addressed in final sections, so that an understanding of what is known and what needs more study can be clarified. Where possible, recommendations for further research and practical application are offered; this is challenging, however, because research traditions, theories, and methods have not been uniformly applied to psychological questions of practical impact in prolonged exercise. Scientists will be encouraged that the psychology of prolonged exercise remains a fruitful area of study, while athletes and practitioners will likely be perplexed that the quantity and quality of past research yields so few verified principles of application.

I. RESPONSES TO TRAINING IN TOP ATHLETES

A. The Challenge

Mathematical models suggest that world endurance records are far below the limits of human physiology. Analysis of record-setting amateur performances from 1924 through 1972 revealed near linear rates of acceleration, ranging from 5% to 15%, at all distances (241) (Fig. 7-1). Most remarkable, however, was not the collective increase in speed, but the increase across distances of what has been termed *specific endurance* (the ability to sustain work of high power). The 1985 marathon record of Carlos Lopes, to illustrate, was run at 331.7 meters per minute. This is comparable to the 326.3 meter per minute pace of Great Britain's Charles Lawes when he established the mile record in 1864, yet the 26.2 mile marathon distance reveals Lopez to have a specific endurance more than 26.2 times that of Lawes (Fig. 7-2). For trends projected by these data to hold true across the next forty years (e.g., by the year 2025 the 10,000 meters would be run in 24 min, 31 s and the marathon in 1 h, 53 min, 13 s), specific endurance will, in many cases, need to be doubled from the 1972 values. More recent data have yielded a similar picture (Fig. 7-3). A time vs. distance plot of world running records immediately prior to the 1980 Summer Olympic Games in Moscow predicted that for a world class male runner to gain 1% in speed at any distance, he must be able to travel 13% farther at his previous top speed. A 100% increase in specific endurance, by this equation, yields but a 5% increase in speed (228).

Reigel (228) presents a least-squares power function to describe human endurance where time (min) = distance (km) × a (regression derived constant)$^{b(\text{fatigue exponent})}$. The fatigue factor is defined as the rate at which mean velocity decreases with increased distance and time needed to complete a given race. By this calculation men and women have identical fatigue factors for running and swimming, while the speed and specific endurance of women are much less than those of men. World record endurance performances can be

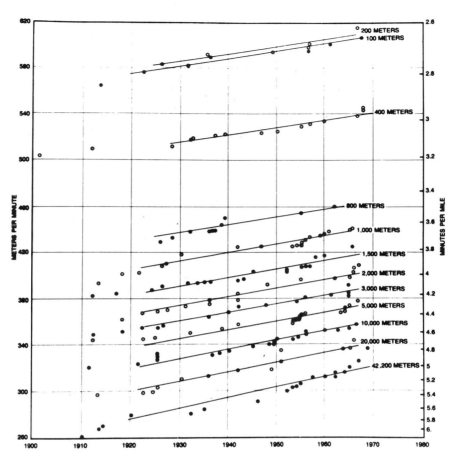

FIGURE 7-1. *Improvement in speed in footracing at metric distances from 1924 to 1972. Each circle represents a new record at each distance. The sloping lines show the increase in speed in meters per min and mins per mile. From Ryder, H.W., H.J. Carr and P. Herget, 1976. Future performance in footracing.* Scientific American, 234 *(6), p. 113. Reprinted with permission.*

compared between men and women in running for distances from 1500 m to the marathon and in swimming for distances of 400, 800, and 1500 m. For swimming times common to both sexes, these range from 4 to 15 min; women attain approximately 94% the speed of men. Across the longer common time span of two h for running, the champion women runners have developed about 90% of the speed of elite men across a distance range of 1.5 to 42.2 kilometers, where men and women share common speeds (a range roughly from 5.4 m·s^{-1} to 6.2 m·s^{-1}), women have shown a specific endurance

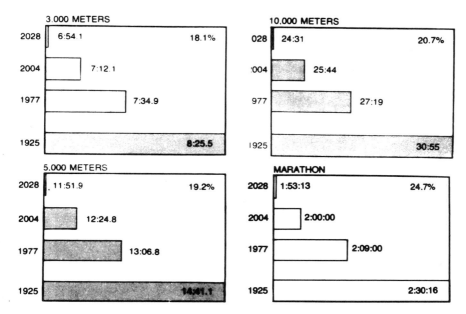

FIGURE 7-2. *Projections of future performance in footracing based on increased mean speed for each event since 1925. The percentage shown with each distance event reflects the improvement in time from a 1925 record to the projected record for 2028. From Ryder, H.W., H.J. Carr and P. Herget, 1976. Future performance in footracing.* Scientific American, *234 (6), pp. 118–119. Reprinted with permission.*

of approximately 20%. This indicates they have done one-fifth the work of men at these speeds.

B. A Role For Psychology

How much of this discrepancy is psychological in origin? Norway's Ingrid Kristiansen, current women's world record holder in the marathon at just over 2 h, 21 min, illustrates the challenge of endurance training (Fig. 7-4). She has bested by over 33% the women's top, marathon time of the mid-1960s, three and one-half h. By the calculations above, Kristiansen first had to be capable of running at the old record-setting pace for more than four times the distance. Surely, female biology has not changed this much in twenty years. Social motivation probably has. Increased participation and training among women may account for much of this increase in marathon speed. During the same period, the marathon mark for males has improved about 3%.

The basis for a time vs. distance curve describing human performance has been recognized and debated for many years in ap-

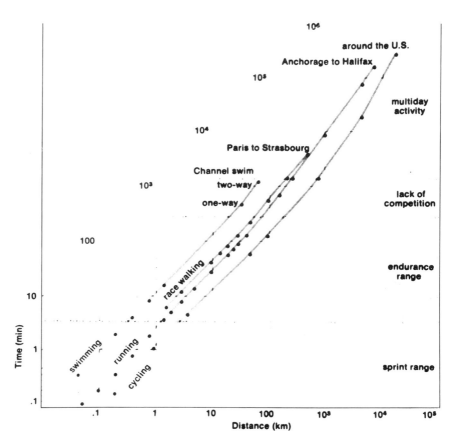

FIGURE 7-3. *World records in 1979 for swimming, race walking, running and cycling. Time is represented as a simple power function of distance. From Riegel, P.S., 1981. Athletic records and human performance.* American Scientist, 69 *(3), p. 286. Reprinted with permission.*

plied physiology and physics (126,164,166,202,237,273,274). Despite ongoing controversy over optimal curve fitting equations, the mathematical models of running performance collectively place physiological adaptability in a role that appears subordinate to behavioral and pathological barriers to endurance training. Ryder et al. (241) noted that the impact of increased specific endurance can be masked by the tradition of running races at a fixed distance against time rather than at a fixed pace for distance. Implicated are the willingness and the ability of athletes to tolerate a training volume sufficiently stressful to produce record potentiating gains in physiology (181). Ryder et al. (241) support this likelihood by noting that two-

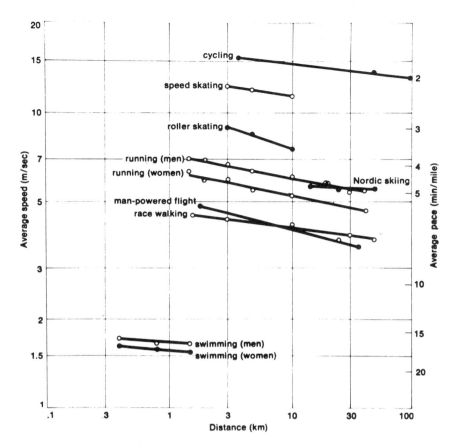

FIGURE 7-4. *Comparisons of speed versus distance plots for 1979 world records for men and women in different events. From Riegel, P.S., 1981. Althletic records and human performance.* American Scientist, 69 (3), p. 287. *Reprinted with permission.*

thirds of the record holders they studied never established another record. Twenty-five percent set a new record at a different distance, but only 20% bested their personal standard at a given distance. Ryder et al. suggested:

> The champions stop not at a given speed but when they set a record. Succeeding champions do the same. They telescope . . . all the achievements of the great runners of the past and then stop with a gold medal. . . . Since it is the medal and not the speed that stops them, the speeds they reach cannot be considered in any way the ultimate physiological limit. (p. 114) . . . "At present the

PSYCHOLOGICAL FACTORS AND PROLONGED EXERCISE **287**

factor limiting record performance may be pathological or psychological, but it is not physiological" (p. 119).

These perspectives raise a number of intriguing questions for sports medicine and exercise science. How, in fact, do psychological or pathological factors interact with physiological adaptations during endurance training? For the most part, however these questions have gone unasked. During the past sixty years, a great deal has been learned about physiological changes induced by acute and chronic exercise within a wide range of environmental parameters and across pathological, normal, and elite populations. Yet, by comparison, virtually nothing has been learned about the role of psychological factors in regulating these changes or pathologic responses to exercise (58,67). Those who do study behavioral barriers to exercise performance adopt an acute rather than a chronic perspective and almost exclusively rely on psychometric methods that rarely include biologic measurements (60).

The aspiring endurance athlete appears confronted with two distinct, though intertwined, problems of adaptation. Biological changes must be evoked to satisfy the increasing metabolic requirements of a necessarily faster pace, but a homeostatic integrity must be maintained that permits these changes to occur. The hypothetical negatively accelerating chronic response of physiological systems to proportionate increases in training strain is clinically well known. As athletes move to their unknown limits, a progressively greater stress gives a progressively smaller yield (Fig. 7-5).

By this function, effective training requires a chronic behavioral response that *positively* accelerates across time. Thus, a zone of limitation seems unavoidably imposed if training motivation cannot cover the area described by the divergence of the biological and behavioral functions described hypothetically in Fig. 7-5. The need for behavioral strain exceeds the incentives and reinforcers available to provide it. There is also reason to believe that, in some instances, motivation to adapt can impose behavioral strain that exceeds the physiological ability to adapt. Yet, the systematic study of training motivation in endurance athletes has been neglected.

C. Psychological Monitoring of Training for Prolonged Exercise

In a series of cross-sectional and prospective studies with endurance athletes (runners, wrestlers, rowers, swimmers), Morgan (189) and colleagues have repeatedly found successful athletes (defined by Olympic and national team selection or consensus elite status) to possess profiles of mood states (POMS) indicative of positive mental health. At the outset of training or the team selection pro-

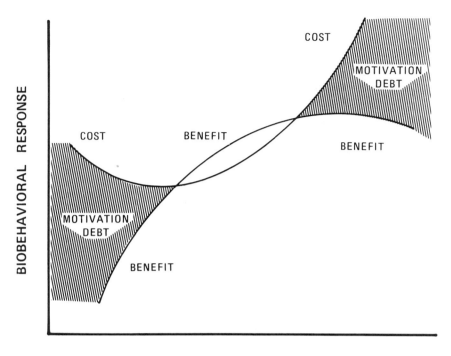

BIOBEHAVIORAL RESPONSE

EXERCISE VOLUME

FIGURE 7-5. *Hypothetical dose response curve for integrated psychological, motivational, and biomedical response to chronic training for prolonged exercise.*

cess, eventually successful athletes show less tension, depression, anger, fatigue, and confusion, and more vigor than their unsuccessful peers or population norms; Morgan has coined this the "iceberg profile." Similarly, athletes on the U.S. Alpine ski team who were dropped from the team were more likely (40%) to be clinically depressed (Zung scale) at the outset of the ski season than were those (15%) not dropped from the team, while initial psychological wellbeing was negatively associated with subsequent health problems (177) (Fig. 7-6).

Morgan et al. (191) have also reported that increased total mood disturbance assessed by the POMS correlates with performance decrements, believed attributable to overtraining, among collegiate swimmers across the season. Conversely, as training volume decreases with tapering, mood disturbance lessens. Cases are common where an initial iceberg profile inverts among swimmers who present themselves to the university health service with symptom complaints. Comparable observations have been reported among U.S. Olympic speed skaters (115) (Fig. 7-7). Skaters were monitored six-months prior to the trials for the 1980 Winter Games, at the end of summer conditioning, and immediately prior to and after the trials. Athletes subsequently selected for the team demonstrated decreasing depression and increasing vigor across the training period, peaking at the trials. By comparison, the athletes not selected showed more labile mood shifts and maintained a reduced vigor from pre-training levels.

Personality may play a role in psychological adaptation to training. Among male and female contenders for the 1984 U.S. Olympic speedskating team, those scoring high on our psychometric test of self-motivation (73) showed less total mood disturbance and missed

The "Iceberg" Profile

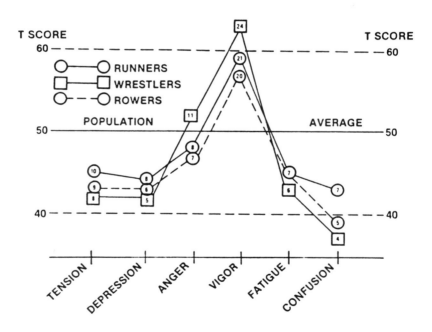

PROFILE OF MOOD STATES (POMS)

FIGURE 7-6. *Psychological characteristics illustrating the "iceberg profile" for elite U.S. runners, wrestlers, and rowers assessed by the Profile of Mood States (POMS). From Morgan, W.P. 1985. Selected psychological factors limiting performance: a mental health model. In D.H. Clarke and H.M. Eckert (eds). Limits of Human Performance (p. 76). Champaign, IL: Human Kinetics Publishers. Reprinted with permission.*

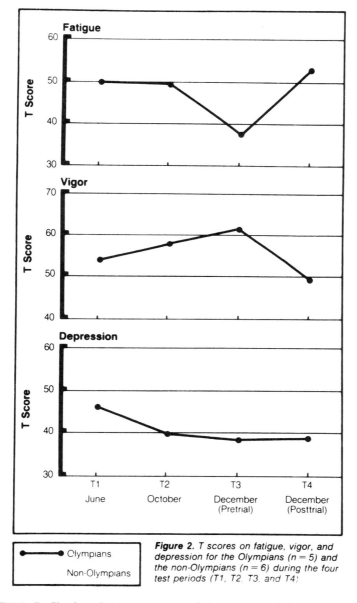

Figure 2. T scores on fatigue, vigor, and depression for the Olympians (n = 5) and the non-Olympians (n = 6) during the four test periods (T1, T2, T3, and T4)

FIGURE 7-7. *Profile of mood states responses on fatigue, vigor, and depression scales among Olympic caliber speedskaters during training for the 1980 winter games. From Gutmann, M.C., M.L. Pollock, C. Foster and D. Schmidt, 1984. Training stress in Olympic speed skaters: a psychological perspective.* The Physician and Sportsmedicine, 12, *(12), p. 51. Reprinted with permission.*

fewer non-injury related training sessions across the training period (151) (Fig. 7-8). These data are consistent with the hypothetical training response described in Fig. 7-5 and suggest that an inappropriate behavioral response to training can be predicted to some degree by an incongruous motivational profile that can be measured at the outset of training. This profile may have potential as a marker for pathological responses during training that are assessable by psychometric means.

Case reports suggest that the overtrained or stale athlete typically presents symptoms nearly identical to those of the clinical patient suffering a reactive depression. When staleness occurs in athletics, it typically is associated with an objective performance decrement, and reduced training or complete rest is required. Thus, prevention is highly desirable. Psychometric approaches to preventing staleness can compare interindividual responses to a known clinical range and intraindividual variability. Transient responses can be contrasted with a typical or baseline response obtained in the absence of training stress. Needed are studies of training for pro-

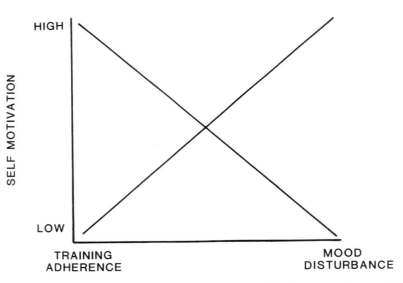

1984 OLYMPIC SPEEDSKATING HOPEFULS

FIGURE 7-8. *Candidates for the 1984 U.S. Olympic speedskating team who were highly self-motivated missed fewer days of training for non-injury reasons and had less total mood disturbance (assessed by the Profile of Mood States) when compared with low self-motivated contenders. Adapted from D. Knapp et al. 1984. Self-motivation among 1984 Olympic Speedskating hopefuls and emotional response and adherence to training. Medicine and Science in Sports and Exercise (abstract) 16(2): p. 114.*

longed exercise that combine assessments of psychometric, neuroendocrine, and immune responses to establish dose-response relationships. These might then permit predictions of risk for overtraining, aid prevention, or enhance recovery.

D. Psychological Models of Training Stress

In addition, studies of exercise overtraining may benefit from attention to prevailing psychological models of occupational stress. Two models seem particularly applicable and are compatible with the biobehavioral model presented in Fig. 7-5. These are the Person-Environment Fit Model of French and the Job Strain Model of Karasek (161). The former is illustrated in Fig. 7-9. In this model, stress is represented in box G, labeled the subjective person-environment fit. Environmental events are not viewed as universal stressors. Rather, their stress impact depends on perceptions or evaluations made by the individual. These evaluations are not only estimates of the demands stemming from the environment but also estimates by the individual of personal ability and motivation to meet those demands. The model suggests two protective mechanisms against stress: social support and ego defense. If these mechanisms do not operate effectively, the model assumes that stresses will produce strains that may include poor performance, psychosomatic disorders, and dissatisfaction. This model provides an interesting perspective on the traditional biobehavioral models of athletic overtraining, in terms of how an athlete's personality may mediate staleness. Particularly of interest in light of Knapp's work with Olympic speedskaters (Fig.

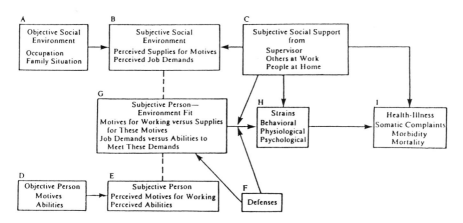

FIGURE 7-9. *The Person-Environment Fit Model of occupational stress. From Cooper, C. and R. Payne 1978.* Stress at work. *New York: John Wiley and Sons (p. 83). Reprinted with permission.*

PSYCHOLOGICAL FACTORS AND PROLONGED EXERCISE **293**

7-8) is the correlation previously observed between self-motivation and ego-strength (73). This suggests self-motivated athletes may have better defense mechanisms against perceived stress, and this view would be conceptually consistent with research on psychological hardiness as a mediator of the stress-illness relationship (153).

A more recent extension of job stress models by Karasek (143) is illustrated in Fig. 7-10. Karasek suggests that equally or more important than perceived environmental stress or job demands is the extent to which the individual perceives control over important decisions about the job and its environment (Fig. 7-10). Figure 7-10 illustrates various combinations of job demands and constraints or latitudes in decision making. High demand-low decision latitude yields highest strain, whereas high demand-high latitude enhances personal adaptability because personal actions can be invoked to reduce strain. This model has particular appeal for elite athletes in training for prolonged exercise, because the concrete biological demands of athletic conditioning may make it difficult for athletes to adjust perceived abilities or motives sufficiently to compensate for task demands. If so, perceived control over training decisions might enhance stress coping. Each model offers numerous testable hypotheses regarding the psychology of training adaptations to prolonged exercise training among top athletes.

II. ACUTE AND CHRONIC RESPONSES TO EXERCISE IN NON-ATHLETES

Studies of acute and chronic psychological responses to prolonged exercise have mostly been conducted with non-athletes, and these studies comprise the bulk of the sport psychology literature relevant for understanding the outcomes of prolonged exercise. Although inferences to top level performers are not possible, the existing literature helps frame questions for future research that can bear on human adaptability to prolonged exercise from a perspective of public health. It is important to quantify the psychological effects of prolonged exertion in the population. Toward this purpose, topical areas that characterize the extent literature are described. These include (1) mental stress tolerance, (2) stress-behavior risks associated with prolonged exercise, (3) anxiety, (4) depression, and (5) sleep disorders.

A. Mental Stress Tolerance

The effective levels of acute exercise intensity, chronic training, or physical fitness to promote a generalized tolerance to mental stress have not yet been quantified, but studies collectively support the

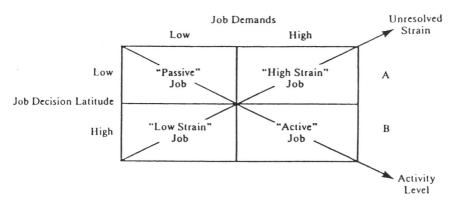

FIGURE 7-10. *Job demand-decision control model of job strain. From R.A. Karasek, Jr.* *1979. Job demands, job decision latitude, and mental strain: Implications for job redesign.* Administrative Science Quarterly, 24: *p. 288. Reprinted with permission.*

contention that physical fitness is associated with relatively low physiological reactivity or quicker recovery from psychosocial stress. Studies on which this conclusion is based are described next.

1. Acute Responses Within Individuals. Neurologic and neuroendocrine responses to cold and sound stressors were reduced after an acute run among experienced runners (55), but EMG, HR, and skin conductance responses to mental arithmetic in the sedentary have not differed when arousal levels were manipulated by smoking, perceptual conflict (a vigilance tack) or bicycle exercise at 60% of maximum heart rate (238). Other reports among conditioned males suggest that visual evoked brain potentials (38) and brainstem auditory evoked responses show reduced latencies following acute runs of 10–18 miles, but no change in EEG visual evoked potentials 1.5 to 8.5 h followed a marathon (106). These studies used a within subject design, so selection bias cannot be determined, and cause cannot be solely attributed to prolonged exercise. Thus, the degree to which acute responses to mental stress, as a function of fitness, depends on training status or physical activity experience requires further study, where these variables are controlled or manipulated.

The method of choice for manipulating exercise and mental stress interactions is not clear, however, because of the known dissociation of cortical, spinal, and muscular indices of neurologic activation from neuroendocrine response under various stress conditions (28,134,263). There are also large individual differences in response to a standard mental stressor. For example, while serum catecholamine and lactate reliably show a dose response to graded exercise that is made relative in intensity according to exercise tolerance (i.e., $\dot{V}O_2max$), different hormones, including cortisol, prolactin, and beta-endorphin, vary widely within and between individuals with repeated exercise testing (47,135). Furthermore, acute studies do not examine the effects that chronic exercise training may have.

2. **Group Comparisons on "Fitness".** Early attempts to estimate training effects have relied on cross-sectional comparisons of groups differing in fitness level. Highly fit, trained individuals have shown an earlier and larger initial climb in plasma catecholamines and prolactin in response to mental stress and a more rapid recovery to baseline than the untrained (258). This could be interpreted as better stress adaptability. Among high fit subjects, heart rate and state anxiety responses can be similar to low fit subjects during mental stress, but more fit subjects have faster heart rate recovery and lower state anxiety after mental stress is removed (258). High self-reported weekly aerobic activity has also been associated with lower heart rate, systolic blood pressure, and myocardial preejection period in response to a shock-avoidance task (165). Studies consistently show quicker cardiovascular and electrodermal recovery from psychological stress among metabolically fit subjects (45,134,145,146,258). Cross-sectional study with intact groups also suggests that aerobic fitness may interact with personality (e.g., Type A Behavior Pattern) to influence physiological response (e.g., blood pressure and heart rate recovery) to behavioral or psychological stress (139,158).

3. **Experimental Study.** Cross-sectional results have not yet been confirmed by experimental designs, however. Differences in psychophysiological responsivity between subjects in existing fitness categories may stem from intrinsic sources other than activity history, and $\dot{V}O_2max$ does not indicate state of training. Training studies with initially unfit individuals have only recently appeared, and they provide mixed findings (101,146,215,234,254,257). Training gains have not, however, been documented by an increase in measured $\dot{V}O_2max$. The few longitudinal studies have relied on heart rate changes to measure fitness, and these confound fitness with dependent measures of psychophysiological reactivity that also are based on heart rate. It is thus necessary in studies of exercise training and mental stress tolerance to induce changes in metabolic tolerance to exercise in an experimental design or to quantify training status (i.e., activity history). This is needed in future studies, so that the roles of training and fitness adaptations to prolonged exercise in mental stress tolerance can be determined.

The social, cognitive, and neurobiological mechanisms for these changes also require elucidation. Prevalent models for understanding these mechanisms have been based on neurobiological approaches and focus on endorphin and monoamine systems in human and comparative studies.

4. Endorphin Research in Humans. Acute endurance exercise does consistently increase plasma levels of beta-endorphin and leu-enkephalin in human beings (118). Although an early study found that naloxone (a drug that blocks endorphins from receptor binding) increased the perception of pain after running (116), a smaller naloxone dose in another study did not block mood elevation from a running session (174). More recently, Farrell et al. (90) administered a blinded dose of naltrexone (50 mg) prior to a 30 min exercise bout at 70% of $\dot{V}O_2$max. Despite endorphin blockade, subjective tension was reduced following the exercise session, thus evidence does not support a correlated change of cognitive and physiological variables to exercise stress.

If endorphins regulate exercise moods, blockade of their chemical action by a competing drug should prevent the mood swing. Controversy over an effective dose for blockade remains. However, other studies that have measured mood and plasma endorphins in experienced runners show that both are elevated after acute exertion, but mood is not predicted by beta-endorphin or leu-enkephalin responses (87,88) (Fig. 7-11). Recent research (90) indicates that while serum catecholamines increase during acute exertion of high intensity (85% $\dot{V}O_2$max), leu-enkephalin remains unchanged; catecholamines and leu-enkephalins are co-secreted in response to various

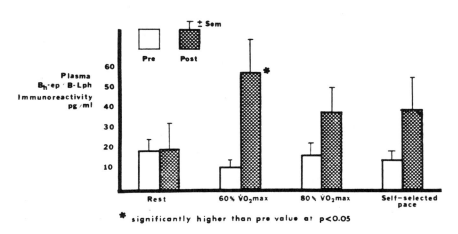

FIGURE 7-11. *Plasma beta-endorphin, beta-lipotrophin immunoreactivity before and after 30 min of treadmill running at 3 intensities. From P. Farrell et al. 1982. Increases in plasma B-endorphin and B-lipotrophin immunoreactivity after treadmill running in humans.* Journal of Applied Physiology: Respiratory, Environmental, and Exercise Physiology, *52(5): p. 1247. Reprinted with permission.*

other stressors. Endorphin levels also vary greatly across individuals at the same relative exercise intensity. Thus, they apparently cannot be predicted by prescribing workout intensity according to a percentage of aerobic fitness ($\dot{V}O_2$max) in the same way as can many other responses to exercise. Moreover, endorphins found in the blood of exercising humans can come from several tissues other than the brain (e.g., the pituitary and adrenal glands), and their importance for brain function and mood is unknown. Plasma levels also do not distinguish between changes in neuronal release, reuptake, or site of action.

   5.   **Monoamine Research in Humans.** Altered levels or dysregulation of the metabolism of monoamines (principally norepinephrine, serotonin, and dopamine) remain prominent models of affective disorders (223). Because of the reliable acute increase in plasma norepinephrine with intense prolonged exercise, speculation has arisen over the role of acute and chronic exercise in the treatment and study of affective disease, principally depression. Most studies in this area have assayed urinary or plasma MHPG (3-methoxy-4-hydroxy phenylglycol), which is a major metabolite of norepinephrine. Although just 20% to 60% of MHPG found in urine is estimated to originate in brain tissues, urinary levels are believed to correspond with brain and spinal fluid changes. Acute exercise studies of depressed patients have shown both increased MHPG (12,80,224) and unchanged MHPG (276,277), with no corresponding change in clinical diagnosis. These studies have used low levels of unquantified exercise. Studies that have quantified acute exercise relative to exercise tolerance have sampled nondepressed subjects and shown increased plasma MHPG, with no change in urinary MHPG (110,132,218,278). It is believed, however, that sulphated MHPG, rather than total MHPG, is reflective of brain function, and one exercise study has shown increased sulphate subfraction of MHPG, even though total MHPG was unaltered (132).

   Chronic studies of prolonged exercise training and MHPG response have not been conducted, but cross-sectional comparison of fitness groups based on $\dot{V}O_2$max differences have shown no MHPG differences (264,265,266); psychological factors were, however, associated with norepinephrine metabolites.

   6.   **Comparative Studies.** Based on available studies and techniques, advances in human exercise neurobiology will probably require the use of newer imaging technologies, such as magnetic resonance and positron emission tomography, to describe the origin, direction, and psychological significance of brain neurotransmitter changes that accompany prolonged exercise. Animal research using rat models of exercise neurobiology represents a promising alter-

native approach in mechanism research, because it permits direct assessment and experimental manipulation of stress and neurobiological response (196). Ethics and technology currently restrict this in human research. Our recent study (70) shows that untrained emotionally labile and emotionally stable rats do not differ in treadmill performance, so the effect of exercise training on their behavioral and neurobiological responses can be compared without selection bias on emotionality.

To determine the mechanisms of generalized stress adaptations from exercise, it is also necessary to distinguish between metabolic, subjective and cortical/spinal arousal responses and their neural and endocrine pathways within the sympathetic nervous system. Because accomplishing this with human beings may exceed current experimental techniques, comparative studies of stress in animals can be informative. To illustrate, corticosterone levels are higher than normal in rats who suffer stress-induced gastric lesions (267), whereas serotonin levels in the midbrain, cortex, and hippocampus are lower compared with non-lesioned controls (125). Both cases seem to reveal biochemical markers of neuroendocrine stress that can be influenced by exertion. Acute swimming (9) and chronic running (30), for example, elevate rat brain serotonin in non-lesioned rats, whereas chronically exercised rats suffer less progressive ulceration than sedentary cohorts following reserpine induced gastric lesions (141). Also, rats that spontaneously ran after exposure to unpredictable, uncontrollable electric shock showed lower plasma corticosterone and cholesterol than their sedentary cohorts (267). Collectively, these findings are indicative of psychoendocrine adaptations to exercise that might be generalized across stress modalities. Future studies might concentrate on how emotional systems in the brain (e.g., limbic structures) are involved with neurologic and neuroendocrine regulation during exercise and other stressors. Again, endorphin and monoamine systems represent attractive targets for study.

Studies indicate that norepinephrine, serotonin, and endorphins can be increased and decreased following acute exercise (9,10,17,111,217,272,289), but a recent report shows paradoxical changes in brain and plasma beta-endorphin following acute exercise in the rat (250). Chronic studies of training responses to prolonged exercise of 30 min to two h, five days per week for eight weeks have shown increased brain norepinephrine (30,31,48).

The meaning for human psychology of exercise-related changes in levels or regional distribution of neurotransmitters in animals remains unclear, however. Moreover, the extant neurophysiological literature using the rat has typically confounded exercise stress with cold in swimming studies and electric shock in running studies. In most cases, exercise stress (e.g., speed or duration) is controlled by the experimenter, yet uncontrollability is a powerful hormonal inducer in the rat. Thus, future studies should quantify or control other stressors during exercise in order to clarify the unique impact of exercise.

B. Stress-Behavior Risks Associated with Prolonged Exercise

Although the psychological risks associated with prolonged exercise have not been experimentally studied nor quantified in epidemiological studies, they appear small in contrast to the benefits that accrue with exercise (65). Nonetheless, it is important to quantify risks, and future studies should build on early questions raised over eating disorders and exercise abuse and the motivational processes that underlie exercise dependence.

1. **Eating Disorders and Prolonged Exercise.** Clinical study (295) has suggested that excessive exercisers, particularly runners, present signs and symptoms analagous to the anorectic. These include a common family history, socioeconomic class and pressures; preoccupation with food and leanness; and personality traits of anger suppression, asceticism, denial of medical risk, introversion, and perfectionism. Although exercise is promoted as a healthy alternative to restrictive dieting among the weight conscious, the concern raised is the possibility that exercise commitment could lead to anorexia for some personalities or could exacerbate an existing eating disorder.

While there are undoubtedly anorectics who are compulsive exercisers, research (18,65) reveals for the vast majority that exercise commitment and anorexia nervosa are separate entities. In fact, there are case reports (154) of effective treatment of anorexia by combining psychotherapy with running. Although anorectics often boost the impact of food restriction by hyperactivity, their fitness ($\dot{V}O_2$max) is very low compared to committed exercisers, while stress hormone profiles differ between the groups. Anorectics often have elevated scores on standard tests of psychopathology, while habitual participants in prolonged exercise usually score in the normal range of the same tests and show mood profiles that indicate positive mental health (18,67). Although we have observed a significant correlation between a psychometric estimate of eating disorder proneness (Eating Disorder Inventory) and low weekly/caloric intake in runners and wrestlers, this was not of clinical significance (61).

Although some studies of small samples of ballerinas, gymnasts, and wrestlers show higher than expected rates of eating problems, how long they persist and whether they represent goal-appropriate behaviors for the sport, rather than medical or psychological pathology, is not established (65). In most cases the eating behaviors of athletes and habitual exercisers do not appear to signal anorexia nervosa or bulimia.

2. **Exercise Abuse.** There are case reports, however, of excessive involvement or dependence with exercise training. Morgan (185) described eight cases of "running addiction," where commitment to running exceeded prior commitments to work, family, social relations, and medical advice. Similar cases have been labeled as positive addiction, runner's gluttony, fitness fanaticism, athlete's neurosis, and obligatory running (65). Little is understood, however, about the origins, diagnostic validity, or the mental health impact of abusive exercise.

However, the inability or unwillingness to interrupt and taper involvement in a prolonged exercise training program or replace a preferred form of exercise with an alternative, when this decision is indicated by medical need or vocational or social responsibilities, may reflect an emotional problem with clinical meaning. The few studies that show psychopathology in habitual runners (242), indicate that exaggerated emphasis on exercise or fitness abilities can manifest a pre-morbid proneness to problems of an imbalanced and insecure self-concept. For most people, however, the benefits of prolonged exercise exceed the risks of abuse.

3. **A Model of Motivation for Exercise Dependence.** Understanding exercise abuse or dependence is important for quantifying and managing risks associated with prolonged exercise training. Exercise dependence has, however, also been proposed as a model for understanding exercise motivation in the population (59,62). Because theoretical models of exercise dependence have not been tested (282), one that is promising will be discussed here. Solomon (261) has presented data supporting an opponent process theory of acquired motivation that has appeal for explaining emotional and motivational responses accompanying prolonged exercise. Fig. 7-12 and 7-13 illustrate fundamental responses predicted by the model.

It is proposed that there is a two-phase process underlying emotional behavior. The primary phase is excitatory and is initiated by presentation of a stimulus. The secondary phase is initially inhibitory in response to the first phase and is called the opponent or slave process. The model suggests there are limits to deviation from emotional or hedonic neutrality that are acceptable to an individual, and when they are exceeded, the inhibitory opponent process is evoked to return excitation to an acceptable level. This is typically an over-compensation, not merely a return to baseline. When external stimulation ends, so, too, does the primary process, shortly

Primary Process

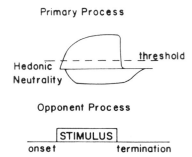

Opponent Process

FIGURE 7-12. *Underlying opponent processes after few presentations. From F.J. Landy 1978. An opponent process theory of job satisfaction.* Journal of Applied Psychology 63: *p. 538. Reprinted with permission.*

followed by a slower decay in the opponent process. These mechanisms purportedly operate identically for positive and aversive stimuli, and while the opponent or slave process is weak and slow during early stimulus presentations, it becomes faster and stronger with repeated experience. Thus, an initially pleasurable or unpleasurable event loses its impact and time course upon repetition, while the opponent process grows in impact and time course.

For example, if the initial reaction to prolonged exercise is negative (it is painful), the opponent process would be positive, i.e., relief upon cessation. The relief would be initially mild, appear slowly and disappear quickly. If exercise persists over many trials, the primary response to the actual exercise should become less aversive and the opponent process response following exercise more positive, i.e., a quicker onset and slower decay. Thus an individual could become dependent on exercise in pursuit of the pleasurable opponent process. Conversely, if the initial exercise experience is positive and the opponent response aversive, an individual will similarly be

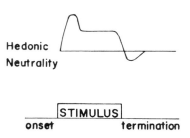

FIGURE 7-13. *Manifest hedonic (emotional) response after few stimulus presentations. From F.J. Landy 1978. An opponent process theory of job satisfaction.* Journal of Applied Psychology 63: *p. 538. Reprinted with permission.*

motivated to increase exposure to a positive primary process that is dampened with experience and to avoid the non-exercising opponent-process state, which is aversive and is strengthened with repetition. In each case, the model has appeal for both cognitive and physiological approaches to the study of antecedants and consequences of prolonged exercise, but it remains untested in the exercise sciences (282).

C. Anxiety

The importance of developing behavioral skills for coping with anxiety is reinforced by estimates that less than one in four of the 13 million sufferers of anxiety will seek professional treatment (252). Periodic exercise provides an effective option for controlling some forms of anxiety in some people. It can be comparable or preferred to other cognitive and somatic alternatives, such as biofeedback, hypnotic suggestions, meditation, progressive relaxation, and distracting rest, and may share anxiety-reducing components found in other therapies and coping behaviors. Prolonged exercise may help manage anxiety by (a) regulating the autonomic nervous system, (b) distracting anxiety ruminations, or by (c) relabeling the cognitive appraisal of arousal symptoms.

1.   Acute Tension Reduction. Rhythmic endurance-type exercise of moderate and vigorous intensities using at least one half of the body's muscle mass is accompanied by reduced tension, when tension is measured neurophysiologically. This effect has been seen for individuals who experience clinically-elevated symptoms, but it also occurs in those who are asymptomatic. Walking, jogging, cycling, and bench stepping for 5 to 30 min at 40% (in young, middle aged and elderly men and women) to 60% (in young adults) of maximum heart rate are associated with acute reductions in skeletal muscle action-potential, when it is measured by resting electromyograms in biceps brachii, Hoffman reflex, and achilles tendon reflex (53,54). These changes can persist up to one h following cessation of the exercise. Twenty min of aerobic exercise at 40% or 75% of $\dot{V}O_2$max has yielded a 13% and 22% reduction, respectively, in Hoffman reflex activity among men aged 20 to 45 years (33). In asymptomatic adults, transient increases in alpha brain wave activity measured by electroencephalograms can also occur after submaximal stationary bicycle rides (86) (see Fig. 7-14).

Local tension reduction with exercise seems to be specific to skeletal muscle, but the effect is not dependent on fusimotor feedback from sensory receptors in muscle (53). For these reasons, reduced muscle tension with exercise seems to reflect a central (corticospinal) relaxation effect, but this hypothesis has not been tested.

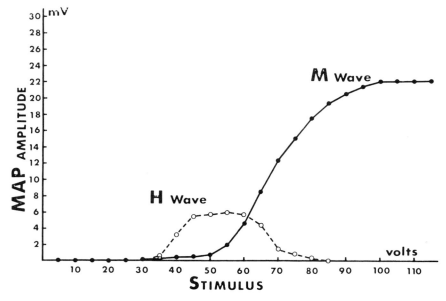

FIGURE 7-14. *Plot of the stimulus-response curves for "M" and "h" waveforms describing a typical H/M ratio of the Hoffman reflex which decreased following acute prolonged exercise of 40% and 80% VO₂max. From H.A. deVries et al. 1981, Tranquilizer effect of exercise.* American Journal of Physical Medicine 60 (2): p. 61. Reprinted with permission.

Generalization to other muscle groups where clinical symptoms of tension occur (e.g., frontalis) is not, however, reliable for either trait anxious or non-anxious individuals. Exercise has been as effective in reducing EMG tension as Meprobamate, a now obsolete sedative (50), and yields effects that are comparable to biofeedback but are no greater than distracting rest (52) or sauna (51).

These studies indicate that a neurological relaxation response can accompany acute aerobic exercise. However, personality and life history influence the neurophysiological patterns people experience during stress. Because of this, exercise responses will also vary (54,55,86,158,256).

2. Associated Chronic Changes. Similar reductions in tension occur following chronic exercise in animals when tension is measured by behavior (279,290) and for human beings when subjective anxiety is assessed. Endurance athletes, such as distance runners, rowers, and wrestlers, report lower state anxiety at rest than do others of the same age (189). Because endurance athletes are not lower than average in trait anxiety (85), this finding may indicate an exercise effect more so than an intrinsic characteristic. Also, endurance athletes typically report increased anxiety when they must interrupt their conditioning program (230,280). These cross-sectional data offer weak inference about causality, but they suggest that the low anxiety characteristic of habitual exercisers is due to activity.

Self-selection may, however, influence the degree to which anxiety reductions will occur with exercise. In one study (247), habitual joggers reported fewer bodily symptoms (e.g., tension) but more cognitive symptoms (e.g., worry) of anxiety than did a group of meditators. Because exercisers and meditators each chose their activity, and a measure of trait anxiety was used, this study supports the view that exercise is a preferred coping behavior for certain types of people. Exercise might also facilitate reduction of somatic symptoms more so than cognitive aspects of anxiety. One cross-sectional study of a large sample (43) found that treadmill endurance during graded exercise testing was inversely related to somatic symptoms in certain patients, while others who were inactive and unfit complained of physical symptoms, but were not subjectively tense. None of these cross-sectional comparisons of static groups determined whether exercise leads to reduced anxiety or if low anxious people choose to be active. Two recent studies, however, have shown that reduced state anxiety following 20 min of bicycle exercise at 65% of $\dot{V}O_2$max (71) or 20 min of treadmill running at 80% of HR max (26) is reliably seen for trained individuals, but not for the untrained. A recent prospective experiment (172) comparing exercise training and cognitive-behavior modification found that both were effective for reducing anxiety, but neither had an advantage for cognitive or somatic symptoms. In an uncontrolled study comparing chronic exercise and meditation, subjective stress was decreased in both conditions, but resting EEG was unchanged (249).

Other prospective studies of group change, nonequivalent control group comparisons, and randomized experiments confirm that exercise can reduce state anxiety. Both acute and chronic exercise of vigorous intensities consistently are associated with a reduction in state anxiety following graded and continuous treadmill exercise and exercise in natural settings (14,184). These effects can last as long as four to six h but are quite variable during this time (196). Changes in trait anxiety following chronic exercise training are much less reliable. An equal number of studies show decreases and no change, while a few show increase (65).

These studies do not, however, account for the mitigating impact of other personality traits and life stressors on exercise effects and do not contrast the pattern of chronic response to exercise against a chronic baseline life stress response. Exercise might not make people better, but it could keep them from getting worse.

3. **Exercise as Treatment.** Exercise effects may not be different from other effective interventions. Experimental study has shown, for example, that both chronic exercise and cognitive anxiety management training (AMT) can reduce state anxiety and systolic blood pressure among self-referred patients with anxiety disorders, but only AMT reduced trait anxiety (167). Exercise can be as effective as group counseling in reducing anxiety, but benefits seen after a few months may not persist (269). Exercise can also be as effective as meditation or distracting rest (6). Thus, it appears that exercise is best viewed as one method for intermittent coping with daily events or thoughts that provide an anxiety response. Exercise is less likely to alter anxiety traits or persistent sources of stress.

Recent data, however, suggest that anxiety reduction following acute exercise is related to activity history (26,71). Also, the effects of exercise on subjective anxiety are not reliable for mild exercise intensities, and it appears that an intensity exceeding 70% of $\dot{V}O_2$max or age-adjusted HRmax for at least 20 min is needed to insure an acute reduction. Reductions in neuromuscular signs of anxiety may, however, occur at an intensity as low as 40% of $\dot{V}O_2$max (33) (Fig. 7-15).

4. **The Biology of Anxiety and Exercise.** A maximal aerobic effort can lead to a temporary increase in state anxiety, but this should not be a clinical concern because trait anxious individuals (184) experience normal anxiety during graded exercise testing. Despite reports that intravenous injections of sodium lactate can induce panic attacks in anxiety neurotics (173), exercise intensities that elevate blood lactate four to five times above resting levels have not led to anxiety attacks or elevated state anxiety in either anxiety prone or normal individuals (71,184). Moreover, case data (78,203,210,211), show that chronic exercise can be an effective adjunct for treating phobias. These disrepancies probably reflect the unique metabolic and acid-base state induced by exercise, compared with buffered lactate injection, and the problems in distinguishing between generalized anxiety disorders, panic disorder, and phobias. Although peripheral biochemical correlates of fitness and exercise responsivity are related to subjective anxiety (216), current evidence does not clarify the biology of anxiety reduction that accompanies prolonged exercise.

D. Depression

The roots of depression are often viewed as a disregulation of either cognitive (11) or neurobiological processes (223). Because 30% of the 10 million Americans who suffer depression will not seek professional treatment (252), the potential usefulness of exercise as

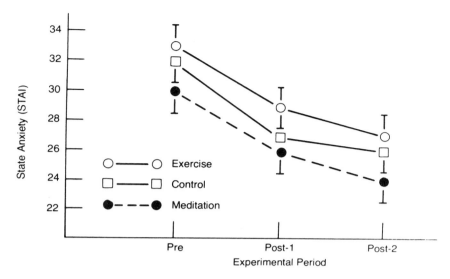

FIGURE 7-15. *State anxiety before and following control conditions, Benson's relaxation response, and 20 mins of walking at 70% of* $\dot{V}O_2$. *From Bahrke, M.S. and W.P. Morgan 1978. Anxiety reduction following exercise and meditation.* Cognitive Therapy and Research 2: p. 326. *Reprinted with permission.*

a self-help behavior is enhanced. The usefulness of exercise is likely, however, to depend on the *cause* of the depression as much as its symptoms. Various hypotheses have been put forth to explain why exercise might have antidepressant properties (113). These include (a) generalizable feelings of achievement, (b) feelings of self-control or competence, (c) symptom relief or distraction, (d) substitution of good habits for bad ones (i.e., those that are self-edifying replace those that are self-destructive), (e) development of patience, and (f) consciousness alterations. These concepts apply mainly to moderate nonpsychotic depression.

An antidepressant effect might also stem from neurobiological changes with exercise. These include regulation of the sympathetic tone of the autonomic nervous system and changes in the release, binding, or uptake of neurotransmitters, such as norepinephrine, dopamine, serotonin, GABA, endorphins and enkephalins. These hormones help regulate mood and nervous system functions (127,223). After exercise, several are elevated in the plasma of human beings and are altered in the brains of rats and mice. Altered cerebral circulation and metabolism have also been implied as a mood elevator (65).

Exercise might also be effective for reducing depression that is superimposed on medical or surgical illness by rehabilitating the physical disorder (e.g., cardiac rehabilitation) and rebuilding physical self-confidence for safe exertion and a return to normal life roles.

1. Associated Chronic Changes. Studies confirm that chronic aerobic exercise can be associated with reductions in clinical and psychometric symptoms of moderate unipolar depression. These can parallel increased fitness ($\dot{V}O_2$max) (77,113,144,179), but they can also occur when fitness changes are not measured or reported (150,193,270). The MMPI depression scale has discriminated between middle aged men who are highly fit and active and those who are unfit and sedentary (168), but cross-sectional contrasts like this cannot determine if low depression precedes, follows, or interacts with exercise training or fitness. Also, fitness has been unrelated to depression (MMPI) and urinary metabolites of catecholamine neurotransmitters during resting conditions and occupational stress (265).

However, a recent controlled experiment from Norway reported by Martinsen (193) has shown a direct, though small, correlation between increased aerobic fitness (Astrand-Ryhming) and symptom abatement for patients suffering major depressive episode (DSM III). This was strongest for males and appeared to reflect real fitness gains more so than changes in the autonomic nervous system. Whether fitness contributed to the antidepressant effect or merely accompanied increases in activity as the depression subsided was not tested (Fig. 7-16).

Although several exercise training studies of healthy adults and college students show significant decreases in psychometric depression (32), this is not a reliable result among individuals that begin exercise within the normal range on standard depression tests. Randomized experimental trials across 20 weeks (198) and two years (271) show no change from initially normal scores. This suggests that when changes are seen for normal subjects in non-randomized studies, they reflect an expectancy effect, a self-esteem bias, or a mood elevation that is not part of clinical depression or cannot be measured by the scales used.

2. Exercise as Treatment. Exercise effects can, however, be comparable to conventional psychotherapy or counseling and meditation-relaxation techniques used for treating moderate psychiatric depression (13,150,193). In one 12-month follow up of randomly assigned psychiatric outpatients, 11 of 12 effectively treated with running therapy were still asymptomatic, while one-half of those who had received traditional psychotherapy had returned for treatment. In a replication study, treatment gains after 12 weeks were comparable between running therapy and meditation training; in each

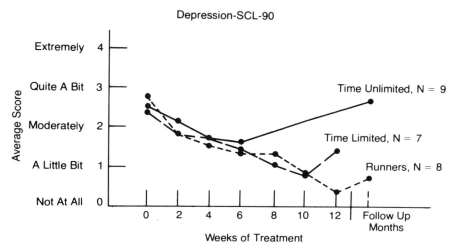

FIGURE 7-16. *Changes in symptoms of depression in psychiatric outpatients accompanying two types of psychotherapy and running therapy. From J. Greist et al. 1978. Running through your mind.* Journal of Psychosomatic Research *22: p. 278. Reprinted with permission.*

case gains were greater than in group psychotherapy and remained so nine months following treatment (150).

Uncontrolled clinical trials have also shown that symptoms of depression are alleviated among cardiac patients following chronic exercise rehabilitation (144,253,270). In a randomized trial, improvements seen after three months were lost by one year (269). Fitness training does, however, contribute to exertional self-confidence among cardiac patients, and this is consistent with symptom reduction in depressive disorders that are secondary to medical/surgical illness. Because these findings occur reliably in group outpatient programs, but not in physician-encouraged home rehabilitation (83,178), social reinforcement within an exercise setting may be equally or more important than exercise training. Studies of cardiac patients scoring within the normal range on psychometric tests of depression at the outset of training show no change following cardiopulmonary exercise programs of three-month (236), six-month (204), and two year durations (271).

3. **The Biology of Depression and Exercise.** None of the biochemical hypotheses previously discussed that implicate monoamines in the mechanism of antidepressant effects of prolonged exercise has been confirmed. There is also presently no evidence that exercise training can be an effective intervention with severe or bipolar depressions, and little is known about the optimal volume or

mode of exercise needed for symptom abatement. Though not well studied, there seem to be, however, no medical complications with exercise for patients using lithium or tricyclic antidepressants (193).

E. Sleep Disorders

Exercise is also believed to have sleep promoting effects. Prolonged exercise may regulate sleep by increasing the need for energy conserving rest or restorative tissue repair due to increasing metabolic demands. It is also believed that exercise can regulate the autonomic nervous system in ways that offset the hyperarousal often characteristic of anxiety and depression.

1. Quasi-experimental Studies. Many studies show that acute exercise may cause increased slow wave sleep (SWS) on the exercise evening (128). When the exercise is of vigorous intensity (e.g., 50% to 70% VO_2max) and continued to exhaustion, the increase in SWS occurs early in the night's sleep and is accompanied by a decrease in rapid eye movement (REM) sleep (34). While these effects can occur for untrained, but moderately active, individuals, the most consistent SWS changes are seen for trained athletes (128). Modifications in SWS are believed to result from the greater energy expenditure in an exercise session by athletes. The few acute studies of ultraendurance runs, however, show mixed results (251,283).

The SWS of trained athletes, under typical conditions, seems consistently to benefit from acute exercise, but is disrupted by abstention from training (5). It is not established, however, that sleep-related effects are due to habitual activity history rather than to intrinsic personality or biological characteristics that might predispose athletes both to chronic exercise and to enhanced SWS after acute exercise. Acute comparisons of fit and unfit subjects show that differences in sleep cycles between the groups are not dependent on daily exercise (214, 284, 285). This implies that sleep is more responsive to chronic changes in energy expenditure than to daily variations. However, SWS is not affected by increased training in the already trained, and convincing prospective training studies of initially low fit individuals have not been conducted.

2. Possible Mechanisms. It has been proposed that SWS is more dependent on metabolic needs, whereas REM sleep is more a function of personality and behavior patterns. If so, longitudinal studies of exercise effects should consider individual differences in addition to fitness status. The question of mechanisms whereby exercise may facilitate sleep remains unresolved, but both energy expenditure and central nervous system characteristics or changes are probably involved. Acute rhythmic exercise, such as running, fits psychophysiologic criteria for a relaxation response, and recent evidence of an endogenous pyrogenic effect during vigorous running (37) is consistent with comparative research showing neuroleptic and serotonergic responses to heating of the hypothalamus. Each change has been implicated in aiding sleep (156). Recent study also suggests that body heating during exercise plays a key role in acute SWS changes among highly fit females who are normal sleepers (129). Findings collectively suggest that the increased body temperature that accompanies running might facilitate sleep through a relaxation response, but this requires experimental study.

III. CORRELATES OF PERFORMANCE DURING ACUTE EXERCISE

A. Personality and Prolonged Exercise Performance

Research on personality as an influence on performance has a long history in sport (85,189), but most studies have lacked theoretical direction, sampled convenient intact groups, and examined sports not involving prolonged exercise. Psychological traits can predict behaviors and psychological states with relatively high accuracy across a narrow range of settings or with less accuracy when a broad spectrum of conditions is considered. Although it is likely that psychological states are most linked with endurance performance, the prediction of the occurrence of these states is of importance to athletes and coaches. This prediction is the goal of personality research.

The usefulness of personality for understanding and predicting human performance has been reported. Kane (142) found male British sprinters and throwers to be more extraverted than distance runners, and introversion among marathon runners has been detected in the United States using various measures among males (109,192). Female marathoners were observed in one report to be more extraverted than their male cohorts (182), and the prevalence of extraversion among elite male distance runners has also been reported (197).

In general, athletes of both sexes are extraverted compared with population norms (85). Because theories of extraversion and supporting human performance research predicts that extraverts tend to be sensation-seeking, stimulus reducing individuals, there is intuitive appeal to a role for extraversion in sport. The mixed evidence regarding the prevalence of extraversion among endurance athletes renders the importance of extraversion for prolonged exercise unclear. One study has reported that extraversion is negatively correlated with perceived exertion during bicycle ergometry of 150–200 w (187). Although perceived exertion during graded submaximal cycling and treadmill running predicts physical working capacity (190,294), the validity of extraversion for predicting prolonged exercise performance has not been reported.

Psychometric correlates of extraversion have also been examined among endurance athletes and as concomitants of prolonged exercise. Cross-sectional studies of static groups have reported that contact power athletes (football players and wrestlers) demonstrate higher pain tolerance for radiant heat than non-contact athletes (tennis players) (240) and that endurance athletes (cross-country runners) tend to psychophysically augment a size stimulus (Petrie method), tolerate less pain (ischemic shin pressure), and perceive the passage of time as more rapid, when compared with contact athletes and non-athletes (239). Later work suggested that perceived exertion during an acute bout of exercise at a standard intensity was related to perceptual styles, such as field dependence-independence and perceptual augmentation-reduction (231,232).

These cross-sectional studies imply that perceptual styles may provide a performance advantage or disadvantage in prolonged exercise, and case anecdotes have recently extended this idea to attentional styles among endurance swimmers (206) and cyclists (138) and to cognitive-attentional strategies among distance runners (197). Yet the limiting role of perception and cognition during prolonged exercise has received little research attention and remains unclear.

B. Perception During Prolonged Exercise Performance

Most studies of psychophysical responses during exercise have employed category ratings of perceived exertion (RPE) (24) during short bouts of graded or submaximal treadmill and bicycle exercise under controlled laboratory conditions. A few field studies of swimming and endurance running have also appeared (35,137). Category ratings of RPE yield a linear or a negatively accelerating function with power output and $\dot{V}O_2$ L·min^{-1}, but when RPE is assessed by classical ratio scaling techniques, it follows a power function comparable to that found for other sensory modalities. Reductions in perceived exertion at a standard power output following exercise training parallel reduced physiological responses, while RPE at comparable pre-to-post training relative exercise intensities remain unchanged. Under various short-term exercise conditions, particularly graded exercise, RPE covaries with heart rate, $\dot{V}O_2$ L·min^{-1} and with other physiological correlates of exertional stress having both established and unestablished sensory analogues. These correlates include ventilatory minute volume, respiration rate, skin and body temperature, muscle and blood lactate, blood pH, respiratory exchange ratio rate pressure product, serum cortisol and urinary and serum catecholamines (212) (Fig. 7-17).

Some controversy has arisen regarding the most predominant sensory inputs to RPE, and support has been advanced for either a central systemic control model, based largely upon cardiorespiratory stress, or a peripheral model, based on localized discomfort. More recent evidence suggests that neither "univariate" model offers an adequate description; this is consistent with the theoretical view that perceived exertion may be a part of both a homeostatic and a "comfort-sensory" system. For example, ratings of perceived exertion are known to vary during prolonged constant work, despite a physiological steady state (188). Moreover, this interpretation is reinforced by a retrospective psychometric study of subjective symptomatology during prolonged bicycle exercise to voluntary exhaustion (mean of

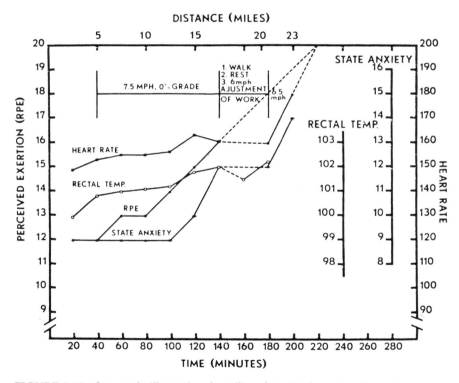

FIGURE 7-17. *Case study illustrating the utility of perceived exertion for predicting prolonged exercise performance during a treadmill simulation of a marathon. From Morgan, W.P. 1981. Psychophysiology of self-awareness during vigorous physical activity.* Research Quarterly for Exercise and Sport, *52: p. 412. Reprinted with permission.*

PSYCHOLOGICAL FACTORS AND PROLONGED EXERCISE **313**

36 min) at 56% of $\dot{V}O_2$max under neutral ambient conditions (148) (Fig. 7-18). Separate clusters of mood related exertional symptoms emerged, including factors related to fatigue, task aversion, and motivation to perform. This study did not, however, demonstrate the degree to which the subjective symptoms limited performance.

In addition, during graded exercise and short bouts of submaximal exercise, normal relationships between RPE and HR can readily be perturbed by various interventions, including beta-blockade, ambient temperature changes, vibrating shock, and hypnotic suggestion. Although neuromuscular sensation appears to dominate RPE at low exercise intensities, and ventilatory measures dominate RPE at high intensities ($>70\%$ $\dot{V}O_2$max), RPE remains proportional to % $\dot{V}O_2$max throughout the exercise intensity spectrum (212). However, during prolonged exercise (20–30 min) at roughly 80% of $\dot{V}O_2$max there is a dissociation of RPE from the serum beta-endorphin response (88), from the leu-enkephalin response (88,89,90), from $\dot{V}O_2$ ($ml \cdot kg^{-1} \cdot min^{-1}$), and the respiratory exchange ratio (130).

It seems clear that any model of RPE that relies predominantly on physiological mediators of the exercise-perception relationship will be inadequate, since system correlates of exercise serve only to identify the type of physical stress imposed. Thus, it should not be surprising to observe that different subjective weightings are assigned to different physiological indices of stress under different exercise demands. In multiple regression models, using physiological variables alone as predictors of RPE, at most, 60% to 70% of the variance in RPE has been explained.

The measurement variability in perceived exertion highlights the fallacy of attempts to quantify a subjective sensation with objective measures alone. That is, a certain amount of interindividual variation in subjective estimates of exercise demands can be dismissed at a physiological level due to differences in fitness or physical tolerance for a standard exercise stimulus, but the objective stress of the activity actually differs in such a case. On the other hand, physiological variation is not as effective in explaining intraindividual variation in effort sense. Although day-to-day fluctuation in exercise tolerance might be explained as physiological or biochemical variation, it is reasonable to suppose that cognitive and affective variables also play a major psychobiological role in such changes (99).

In addition, the previously noted relationships between psychological traits of extraversion and neuroticism and mood states of anxiety and depression are consistent with the view that psychologically-induced stress may confound accurate perception of metabolic stress during exercise. However, the predictive and explanatory potentials of psychobiological paradigms of exercise perception

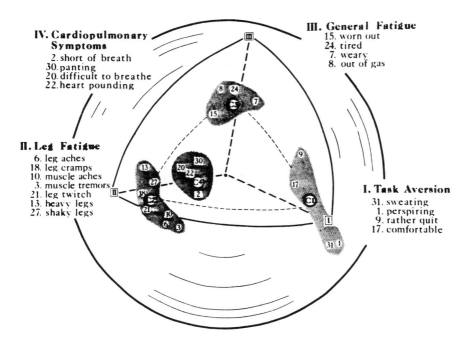

IV. Cardiopulmonary
Symptoms
2. short of breath
30. panting
20. difficult to breathe
22. heart pounding

III. General Fatigue
15. worn out
24. tired
7. weary
8. out of gas

II. Leg Fatigue
6. leg aches
18. leg cramps
10. muscle aches
3. muscle tremors
21. leg twitch
13. heavy legs
27. shaky legs

I. Task Aversion
31. sweating
1. perspiring
9. rather quit
17. comfortable

FIGURE 7-18. *Geometric cluster analysis of subjective adjective response to prolonged bi-cycle exercise at an intensity of 56% of $\dot{V}O_2max$. From P.C. Weiser, R.A. Kinsman and D.A. Stamper 1973. Task-specific symtomatology changes resulting from prolonged sub-maximal bicycle riding.* Medicine and Science in Sports 5(2) p. 83. *Reprinted with per-mission.*

have received limited attention in the study of perceived exertion. Moreover, social psychological study has been essentially nonexis-tant. The predominant physiological model employed in the study of effort sense during the past two decades has yet to add to the understanding of psychological limitations to prolonged exercise.

Recently, we have examined how variables related to perceived discomfort might expand the usefulness of perceived exertion in predicting prolonged exercise performance. Our recent study of pre-ferred exertion (i.e., self-selected power output) during a 20 minute bicycle ride indicated that task aversion, $\dot{V}O_2max$, serum lactate, and state anxiety predicted 78% of the variance in power output. State anxiety, a masculine gender role orientation, Type A behavior, and trait anxiety predicted % $\dot{V}O_2max$ at the end of the ride; these psy-chometric variables accounted for variability in % $\dot{V}O_2max$ that was not explained by serum lactate, activity history (kcal $\cdot$ kg^{-1}-wk^{-1}), and ventilatory threshold (91) (Fig. 7-19 and 7-20).

PREFERRED EXERTION
BICYCLE RIDE (N = 24)

KPM at 20 min

Task Aversion $R^2 = .45$, $p < .005$
$\dot{V}O_2$ max (ml • kg^{-1} • min^{-1}) $R^2 = .57$, $p < .001$
Lactate at 20 min (mmol/l) $R^2 = .68$, $p < .001$
Post-ride State Anxiety $R^2 = .78$, $p < .001$

FIGURE 7-19. *Predictive model of power output during a 20 min stationary bicycle ride at self-selected preferred exertion. The dependent variable is self-selected watts (KPM at constant power) after 20 min of cycling. The predictive model shows significant increases in explained variance with setwise inclusion of the predictor variables.*

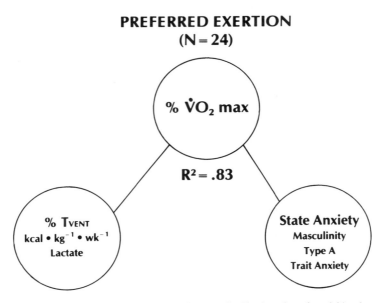

PREFERRED EXERTION
(N = 24)

FIGURE 7-20. *Psychobiologic model of predictors of self-selected preferred bicycle exertion in watts expressed as % $\dot{V}O_2$max. The psychological variables explained variance in % $\dot{V}O_2$max not explained by the physiological variables, and the combined model was most effective; 83% of preferred exertion was explained.*

C. Cognition During Prolonged Exercise Performance

Years ago, it was reported that pre-event anticipatory increases in heart rate accounted for 59% of the total heart-rate adjustment during footracing among young girls (259). In a related laboratory study, hypnotically imagined exercise induced an elevation in heart rate that was 57% of that measured (42 bpm above rest) during an actual 10-minute treadmill bout at 3 mph and 5% grade (15). Morgan (186) has reported in a recent review that hypnotic suggestions of light and heavy work made to resting subjects have increased oxygen consumption by 92 to 409 ml · min^{-1}, ventilatory minute volume by 4.0 to 19.3 L · min^{-1}, heart rate by 10 to 40 bpm, and cardiac output by 4.7 L · min^{-1}. Studies of hypnotically hallucinated exercise during rest have also demonstrated elevations in blood lipids and several of the stress hormones that help regulate metabolic adjustments during exercise (Fig. 7-21).

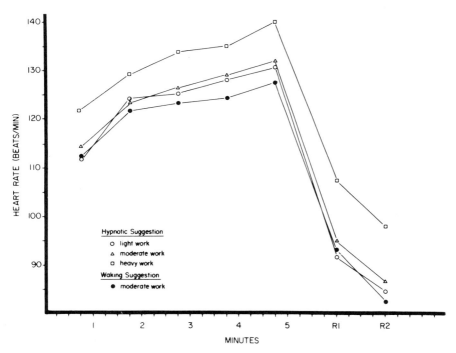

FIGURE 7-21. *Heart rate during and following bicycle ergometer exercise performed at an intensity of 100 watts under waking control (closed circles) and hypnotic suggestions of light (open circles), moderate (triangles), and heavy (squares) exercise. From W.P. Morgan et al. 1973. Perceptual and metabolic responsivity to standard bicycle ergometry following various hypnotic suggestions.* The International Journal of Clinical and Experimental Hypnosis 21(2): p. 95. Reprinted with permission.

Similar results can occur during exercise. Morgan, Raven, Drinkwater and Horvath (199) have shown that during five min of stationary bicycling at a constant power of 100 watts, hypnotic suggestions of heavy exercise can result in increased perceptions of exertion, a 15 beats · min^{-1} increase in heart rate, and a 15 L increase in ventilatory minute volume when contrasted with waking control responses at the same intensity (Fig. 7-22 and 7-23). Similarly, at a constant power of 100 watts, when hypnotic suggestions of five min of "uphill" exercise followed 10 min of suggested "level" exercise, a significant evaluation in perceived exertion occurred. This was accompanied by an increase in minute ventilation of 10 liters above control conditions (914). In the waking state, imagined emotions of anger and fear have augmented the typical increases in heart rate (by 12 to 19 bpm) and systolic blood pressure (by 12 to 13 mmHg) that accompany light bench stepping (40 cm for 1 min) (248). Conversely, studies inducing standardized relaxation procedures during exercise have reported reductions in oxygen consumption of 4% (0.763 to 0.730 L · min^{-1}) (13) and 9% (0.800 to 0.720 L · min^{-1}) (103) during continuous (8- and 10-minute) stationary bicycling (heart rates were constant at 95 and 115 bpm) in nonathletes and 12% (36.7 to 32.1 mL · kg^{-1} · min^{-1}) (296) during continuous (20-minute) treadmill run-

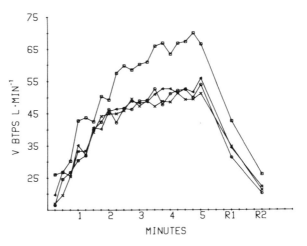

FIGURE 7-22. *Ventilatory min volume during and following bicycle ergometer exercise performed at an intensity of 100 watts under waking control (x) and hypnotic conditions involving suggestions of light (open circles), moderate (triangles), and heavy (squares) work. From W.P. Morgan et al. 1973. Perceptual and metabolic responsivity to standard bicycle ergometry following various hypnotic suggestions.* The International Journal of Clinical and Experimental Hypnosis *21(2): p. 95. Reprinted with permission.*

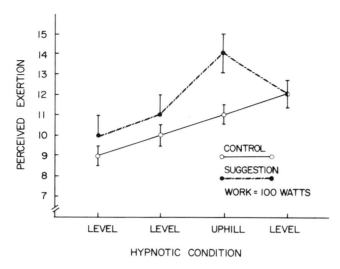

FIGURE 7-23. *Ratings of perceived exertion during bicycle ergometer exercise performed at an intensity of 100 watts under waking control and hypnotic suggestions of level and uphill exercise. Adapted from W.P. Morgan et al. 1976. Hypnotic perturbation of perceived exertion: ventilatory consequences.* The American Journal of Clinical Hypnosis *18(3), p. 188. Reprinted with permission.*

ning (50 percent $\dot{V}O_2$max) in crosscountry athletes. Procedures for gas measurement were not, however, described in the latter study.

The magnitude of these reductions is not, however, consistent with studies employing more prolonged or intense exercise, and it is doubtful that a psychological state can alone increase the acute metabolic efficiency of an experienced runner to an extent that approximates the total variability in efficiency seen among both competitive (12%) and recreational (17%) runners (40). The practical performance or medical significance of these types of metabolic changes would appear to be restricted to ultra-endurance events, hostile environments (e.g., temperature and humidity extremes), and patients with cardiopulmonary or metabolic disorders. In each case, emotional stress could compound, or psychological skills might ease, existing strain to a meaningful extent. The observation that imagined work can produce a physiological arousal similar in form and approaching the magnitude of actual prior exercise of light or moderate intensities is consistent with a potentiating effect for thoughts, emotions, and perceptions on performance.

Among young untrained adults, motivating conditions or contrived performance expectations can typically lead to a 5% to 15% transient increase in muscular force and endurance (67). Although psychological factors are routinely implicated in physiological models of muscular fatigue, studies of the mechanisms by which this association might be explained have not been reported. In a field/laboratory study (220) biofeedback (EMG) assisted increases in resting neuromuscular tension spanning a discrete ordinal range of low (0.5–1.0 μV), moderate (4.5–5.5 μV), and high (9.5–10.5 μV) amplitudes were associated in a negative monotonic fashion with both force and precision of subsequent voluntary muscle contraction, but described a biphasic function (V relationship) with fatigue, in small muscle groups of their wrist flexors. Although CNS influences may play a role in fiber recruitment (firing rate and pattern) and fatigue during prolonged exercise (36,244), to our knowledge this has not been studied in humans by psychological methods (123).

Elite male distance runners have been shown to report less perceived exertion and consume less oxygen at a standard treadmill speed when compared with collegiate runners. They also reported a tendency to dissociate thoughts and feelings of exertion during competition (198). Subsequently, in an experimental design, use of the Bensonian relaxation technique has increased self-limited treadmill endurance by 20% among healthy young males, even in the absence of measurable metabolic or biochemical changes (195). This effect has not, however, been replicated in a field test of prolonged exercise (291). However, in field performance tests and symptom-limited treadmill tests where expired gases are measured, 12% to 18% of aerobic power has been accounted for by psychological traits related to motivation (57,72). Such results argue strongly for a psychology of human performance that might be systematically altered (Fig. 7-24,7-25,7-26).

IV. ADHERENCE TO PROLONGED EXERCISE IN PREVENTIVE MEDICINE

Estimates indicate that only 10% to 20% of the American adult population participate in fitness activities with sufficient intensity and regularity to meet ACSM training guidelines for fitness (29,268). Just 20% to 30% of eligible employees will regularly use worksite fitness facilities, while less than half the users exercise at fitness-inducing levels (96). In supervised exercise programs for preventive medicine, it is typical that one-half of participants drop out, while compliance with an exercise prescription by regular attenders varies from 30% to 80% (208). These statistics suggest that existing fitness standards (3) and prescriptions (2) present excessive behavioral challenges for some segments of the adult population (Fig. 7-27).

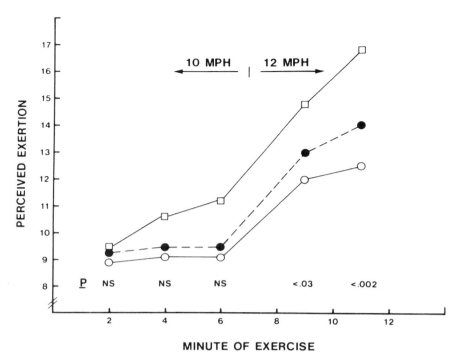

FIGURE 7-24. *Ratings of perceived exertion in elite marathon (open circles) and middle-long distance (closed circles) runners and college middle distance runners (squares). From W.P. Morgan and M.L. Pollock 1977. Psychologic characterization of the elite distance runner. Annals of the New York Academy of Sciences 301: p. 395. Reprinted with permission.*

A. Prescriptions for Adherence

Findings from the Ontario Exercise Heart Collaborative Study (OEHCS) (209) suggest that compliance among post-myocardial infarction patients is no better for low intensity, low frequency exercise (one day · week^{-1} at less than 50% $\dot{V}O_2$max) than for fitness increasing activity (three to five days · week^{-1} at 60% to 80% of $\dot{V}O_2$max). Conversely, several studies with obese adolescents and adults and middle-aged and elderly individuals of normal weight typically indicate higher compliance with lower intensity prescriptions (75). Adults who lack positive attitudes toward controlling their health and do not view exercise as a healthy behavior are likely to select low frequency, low intensity exercise when given the choice, or they tend to drop out of intensive fitness programs (59). The sedentary also tend to view exercise as requiring too much time and effort (75,208), and they report excessive subjective fatigue even when ex-

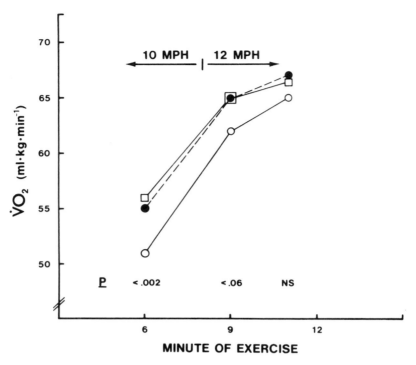

FIGURE 7-25. *Mean oxygen consumption of elite marathon (open circles) and middle-long distance (closed circles) runners and college middle distance runners (squares). From W.P. Morgan 1985. Psychogenic factors and exercise metabolism: a review.* Medicine and Science in Sports and Exercise, *17: p. 315. Reprinted with permission.*

ercise intensity is adjusted for fitness level (133). Even among sedentary who intend to increase their activity, one-half will fail to do so; perceptions of excessive time and exertion demands (107) and lack of confidence about the ability to carry out a fitness program (243) are common barriers that apparently dilute intentions to be active.

These findings imply that the volume of exercise that promotes adherence remains to be identified. A recent study of obese adolescents found that weight loss due to increased routine activity (i.e., movement games and walking) was not only comparable but was maintained longer than the weight loss induced by a traditional fitness regimen (82). Similar findings were obtained in a population-based study in northern California. Among 1,400 adults studied for one year, twice as many added moderate physical activity (walking, climbing, gardening, etc.) to their weekly routines (26% of men and 33% of women) than added vigorous fitness activities (11% of men

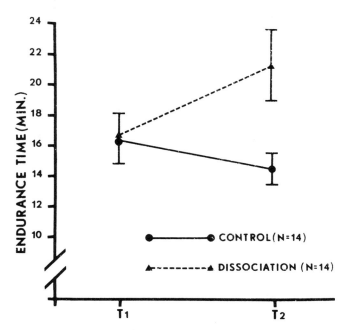

FIGURE 7-26. *Increase in mean endurance time during treadmill walking at 80% of* $\dot{V}O_2$*max under a control condition and a condition of cognitive dissociation based on Benson's meditation strategy. Adapted from W.P. Morgan et al. 1983, Facilitation of physical performance by means of a cognitive strategy.* Cognitive Therapy and Research, *7(3): p. 260. Reprinted with permission.*

and 5% of women). Notably, six times as many women preferred walking over a traditional fitness regimen. While 50% of those adopting a vigorous fitness plan quit, just 25% (women) and 35% (men) discontinued a moderate activity routine (243).

Because epidemiologic studies demonstrating that a health protection effect is associated with prolonged exercise have defined physical activity by job classification or caloric expenditure rather than by fitness, the health significance of fitness thresholds remains unclear. Another study suggests that self-choice of activity can increase adherence to prolonged exercise (281). Thus, an expanded view of what is an appropriate set of activity type, intensities, frequencies, and durations may be justified on behavioral and epidemiologic grounds.

For certain patient groups, a restricted prescription may still be needed to reduce cardiopulmonary or orthopedic risks. However, it has long been recognized by clinical experts that there are many plans that can achieve similar fitness outcomes. Recently Haskell

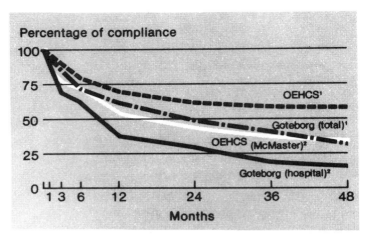

FIGURE 7-27. *Compliance rates in two long-term clinical trials of exercise and rehabilitation following myocardial infarction, Ontario Exercise Heart Collaborative Study (OEHCS) and Goteborg, Sweden. From Oldridge, N.B. 1982. Compliance and exercise in primary and secondary prevention of coronary heart disease: a review.* Preventive Medicine *11: p. 62. Reprinted with permission.*

and colleagues (122) have recommended a minimum expenditure of 4 calories per kilogram of body weight per exercise session for the previously sedentary. Years ago Balke (7), suggested that a total caloric cost per activity session that equalled 10% of daily metabolic expenditure would provide an effective standard within which various specific plans might be prudently implemented. The motivational importance of encouraging variety has long been assumed exercise clinicians (Fig. 7-28).

B. Behavioral Problems with Intensity Prescriptions

The general problem of exercise compliance is addressed in more detail elsewhere (75,175,208). However, participants can adhere to an exercise program (i.e., attend the recommended number of sessions for the specified amount of time) but fail to comply with the prescribed intensity. Also, the intensity prescription might at times be behaviorally inappropriate. Intensity prescriptions have particular significance not only because they influence cardiovascular risks among some patient groups and determine fitness adaptations, but also because they can be aversive and create barriers to motivation. Increases in a person's exertion level seem more resistive to interventions than do increases in frequency or duration. Studies using behavior modification techniques to increase physical activity have focused more on frequency or duration of exercise than intensity or

Summary of variables that may determine the probability of exercise

Determinant	Changes in probability	
	Supervised program	Spontaneous program
Personal characteristics		
Past program participation	+ +	
Past extra-program activity	+	
School athletics, 1 sport	+	0
School athletics, >1 sport		+
Blue-collar occupation	– –	–
Smoking	– –	
Overweight	– –	
High risk for coronary heart disease ..	+ +	
Type A behavior	–	
Health, exercise knowledge	–	0
Attitudes	0	+
Enjoyment of activity	+	
Perceived health	+ +	
Mood disturbance	– –	– –
Education	+	+ +
Age	00	–
Expect personal health benefit	+	
Self-efficacy for exercise		+
Intention to adhere	0	0
Perceived physical competence	00	
Self-motivation	+ +	0
Evaluating costs and benefits	+	
Behavioral skills	+ +	
Environmental characteristics		
Spouse support	+ +	+
Perceived available time	+ +	+
Access to facilities	+ +	0
Disruptions in routine	– –	
Social reinforcement (staff, exercise partner)	+	
Family influences		+ +
Peer influence		+ +
Physical influences		+
Cost		0
Medical screening	–	
Climate	–	
Incentives	+	
Activity characteristics		
Activity intensity	00	–
Perceived discomfort	– –	–

KEY: + + = repeatedly documented *increased* probability; + = weak or mixed documentation of *increased* probability; 00 = repeatedly documented that there is *no change* in probability; 0 = weak or mixed documentation of *no change* in probability; – = weak or mixed documentation of *decreased* probability; – – = repeatedly documented *decreased* probability. Blank spaces indicate no data.

FIGURE 7-28. *Summary of personal, environmental, and physical activity characteristics that have been found to be associated with supervised and free-living exercise programs. From R.K. Dishman, J.F. Sallis, and D.R. Orenstein, 1985. The determinants of physical activity and exercise.* Public Health Reports, *100: p. 161. Reprinted with permission.*

type, and the increases seen in weekly caloric expenditure have typically been less than half that believed necessary to reduce health risk (62).

   1. Limitations of Training HR. Various indicators of exertional strain (e.g., caloric cost, %$\dot{V}O_2$max ventilatory or lactate breakpoints) are used for exercise intensity prescriptions, but heart rate is most practically feasible and widespread. Heart rate prescriptions present some problems, though. Even when variability due to age, training status, and testing mode is accounted for, idiosyncratic differences in measured heart rate maximum (HRmax) remain that are of clinical significance (171). When the more common procedure of age-predicted HR max (220 bpm minus age) is used, even greater errors occur. Heart rate is also altered by emotional states and medications. For these reasons, exclusive reliance on heart rate for testing and prescription can lead to overestimates and underestimates of a presumably optimal metabolic strain for some individuals. Hence, the clinical observation that participants given age predicted heart ranges frequently complain they are too easy or too late is not surprising.

   Several exercise clinicians (35,221) have suggested using ratings of perceived exertion (RPE) as a complement to heart rate prescriptions. Reports show RPE can be a better estimate of $\dot{V}O_2$max than is HR alone (207) and that a prediction model combining HR and RPE is a better measure of voluntary working capacity than either measure alone (190,294). However, studies of how the two might be weighted to optimize a metabolic training prescription are not available.

   Borg (1973) earlier proposed that the model RPE $\times$ 10 = HR could be effective, but several clinicians (35,221) report clinical observations that a correction factor of 20 to 30 bpm must be added (i.e., [RPE $\times$ 10] + 20 to 30 bpm = HR) for RPEs of 11 to 13 and heart rates within typical training ranges of 130 to 160 bpm. Similarly, Burke and Collins (35) and Pollock (221) have observed among experienced adult joggers that RPEs of 11 to 16 correspond to heart rates ranging from 144 to 174 in healthy adults and cardiac patients from about 16 to 60 years of age. Because study has shown that subjects can reproduce a treadmill pace using previous RPEs when HRs were 150 bpm or above and RPEs were 12 or higher (260), perceived exertion holds some practical promise for improving intensity prescriptions among some people (Fig. 7-29).

   This is reinforced by a recent study (79) of 20 untrained college women. On bicycle ergometry, nine subjects exceeded ventilatory threshold at 75% of HR reserve. This proportion increased to 13 to 15 subjects at 80% and 85%, respectively, of HR reserve or, corre-

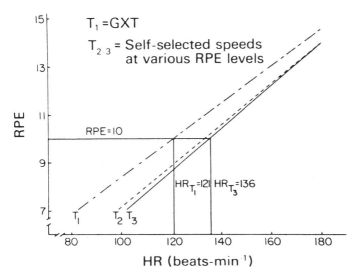

FIGURE 7-29. *Linear regression of heart rate as a function of self-selected treadmill speed (T_1 and T_2) reproduced from perceived exertion of exercise intensity during T_1. From M.A. Smutok. G.S. Skrinar, and K.B. Pandolf 1980. Exercise intensity: subjective regulation by perceived exertion.* Archives of Physical Medicine and Rehabilitation, *61(12): p. 571. Reprinted with permission.*

spondingly 70% and 75% of $\dot{V}O_2$max. Because 75% of HR reserve is a widespread exercise intensity prescription for college women, these findings suggest excessive perceived strain may result when only a heart rate prescription is employed with untrained subjects. This is supported by the observation by Purvis and Cureton (226) that ventilatory threshold is associated with RPEs of 13 to 14. A rating of 13 corresponds with a subjective category of "somewhat hard." It seems unlikely that sedentary individuals will find prolonged exercise reinforcing at intensities well above ventilatory or lactate thresholds.

2. Problems of Self-Regulation. There are also random and motivated errors when a prescribed training heart rate range is self-regulated by the patient. Chow and Wilmore (42) found, during four daily 15 minute sessions of self-paced treadmill jogging, that without feedback, adult males were able to remain in a prescribed training range (60% to 70% $\dot{V}O_2$max) only 25% of the time sampled. Allowing subjects to periodically monitor pulse rate increased accuracy to 55%, while using RPE gave a similarly low accuracy of 48.5%. Average error for the heart rate monitoring group was just 2.6 bpm above the prescribed group mean, and error for RPE was 5 bpm below. However, 60% of control subjects receiving the prescription instructions typical of adult fitness programs exercised at a mean heart rate during each session that was outside their individually prescribed ranges. In our recent study (74), the mean error between prescribed and attained target heart rate on the first day of jogging following a typical prescription (60% HR reserve) based on measured heart rate maximum was +23 bpm. Subjects who had been given RPE instructions during treadmill testing had a mean error of +3 bpm; however, the standard deviation was 19 bpm. This suggests that the prescribed target of 140 bpm could have been behaviorally inappropriate for some subjects. Most subjects who overshot target heart rate were still exercising below 75% of heart rate reserve (Fig. 7-30).

Though little is known about the impact preferred levels of exertion have on prescription compliance, it is unlikely that prescriptions based on HR and RPE will optimize compliance for some individuals. Farrell et al. (87) have observed during continuous treadmill running that trained runners choose exercise at an intensity approximately 75% of $\dot{V}O_2$max, even though their perceived exertion

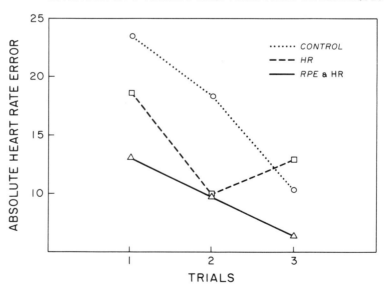

ABSOLUTE HEART RATE ERROR USING THREE FEEDBACK TECHNIQUES

FIGURE 7-30. *Absolute heart rate error during field trials using feedback of heart rate or heart rate combined with ratings of perceived exertion to regulate exercise training heart rate. From R.K. Dishman, et al., 1987. Using perceived exertion to prescribe and monitor exercise training heart rate.* International Journal of Sports Medicine, 8: p. 211. *Reprinted with permission.*

at this level (11.5 on the Borg scale) is significantly greater than that at 60% $\dot{V}O_2$max but not different from 80% $\dot{V}O_2$max. Surprisingly, beta-endorphin/beta-lipotropin immunoreactivity was greatest at the lowest (60% $\dot{V}O_2$max) exercise intensity. This may indicate that the slower, less preferred pace was psychologically more stressful to the experienced runner (Fig. 7-31).

Other study suggests that some types of individuals are motivated to exceed conventional prescriptions. Ewart et al. (84) found that 33% of subjects high in exercise self-efficacy (high confidence in the ability to exercise) tended to overshoot training heart rate prescriptions (70% to 85% HR max), and this is consistent with common clinical observations that some individuals are overmotivated for the exercise prescribed. Those who undershot (25% of the sam-

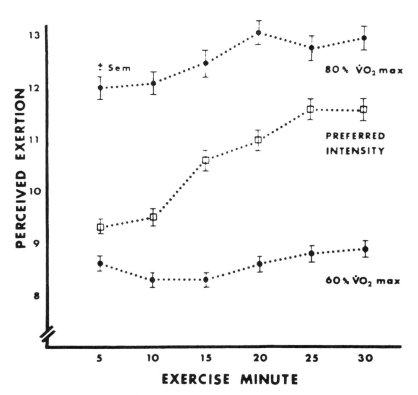

FIGURE 7-31. *Borg category ratings of perceived exertion during 30 min of treadmill running at 3 intensities. From P. Farrell, et al., 1982. Increases in plasma B-endorphin/B-lipotropin immunoreactivity after treadmill running in humans.* Journal of Applied Physiology: Respiratory, Environmental, and Exercise Physiology, 52(5): p. 1247. *Reprinted with permission.*

ple) the training prescription tended to overestimate their self-monitored HR. Similarly, Rejeski, et al. (227) found that cardiac patients scoring high on the Type A job involvement scales of the Jenkins Activity Survey trained in the upper range of their HR prescriptions and had greater than expected increases in maximum exercise level achieved after training, even though they were irregular in attendance at the supervised exercise sessions. This is consistent with a population based study in Belgium (149) showing that Type A males (Jenkins Activity Survey) tend to exercise at higher weekly energy levels during leisure time than do Type B's. Although the construct validity of the Jenkins Activity Survey as a measure of coronary disease risk, has been increasingly questioned, it may have practical use as a motivational measure in exercise studies.

V. MOTIVATION MODELS FOR THE STUDY OF PROLONGED EXERCISE

To this point, and throughout the chapter, variables have been discussed that might facilitate, modify or suppress prolonged exercise. Motivation is a construct that has been traditionally invoked by psychologists to explain individual differences in the initiation, direction, intensity, persistence, and termination of behavior. It is appropriate to consider possible contributions of the construct of motivation to the consideration of prolonged exercise.

Motivational theories can be placed into one of five classes (161). These classes include need theory, behaviorist theory, balance theory, expectancy theory and goal setting theory. Need theory suggests that individuals have physical and psychological needs that, in turn, create drives. These drives (e.g., hunger, competition) are the major mechanisms of motivation. Behaviorist theory (particularly the traditional radical behaviorism of B. F. Skinner), suggests that behavior is initiated, directed and modulated by the extent to which reinforcements have become associated with behavior patterns. In fact, radical behaviorism, though it purports to address the five parameters of motivated behavior described above (i.e., initiation, direction, intensity, etc.) rejects the construct of motivation as unnecessary. Balance theory is a cognitive approach to motivation based on the notion that psychological discrepancies (e.g., between self-image and images held by others) create tension. This tension is uncomfortable and the individual engages in actions to relieve this tension. Thus, the tension is considered to be a major mechanism of motivation. Expectancy theory is based on the premise that individuals have preferences for outcomes of behavior and that they form beliefs about the probability that a given action will lead to a preferred (or non-preferred) outcome. Goal setting theory suggests that individuals are motivated by hard specific goals that they have set or have accepted from others.

A review of the recent motivation literature suggests that need theory, behaviorist theory, and balance theory have failed to generate the empirical support that is required of a viable approach to understanding the construct of motivation (162). In contrast, the general approach and premises of both the expectancy theory and the goal setting theory have been supported by empirical research. To be sure, this research has been conducted predominantly in work settings and educational settings, but the principles and predictions seem to fit the context of prolonged exercise quite well. This is probably because these theories emphasize the understanding of effort expenditure—one of the major dependent and independent variables in the study of prolonged exercise. In this section, these two theories are considered in greater detail. The goal is to add some coherence to the widely scattered empirical literature in the prolonged exercise research domain. Although these models are based on cognitive variables, other more biobehavioral models (e.g., Solomon's opponent process model discussed earlier) may apply as well.

A. Expectancy Theory

The expectancy theory resulted from a combination of the field theoretic approach of Kurt Lewin and the early work on cognitive expectations done by people such as Helen Peak and Julian Rotter. The basic propositions are relatively simple. The theory says that each individual develops affective orientations toward alternative outcomes in their environment. The orientations are called valences and are seen to operate much like the valences in chemical elements. Positively viewed outcomes attract the individual, and negatively viewed outcomes repel. A critical postulate of this proposition is that each individual has unique valences for outcomes. What is positive to one person may be negative to another. The second proposition of the expectancy theory is that each individual holds certain beliefs that a particular action will lead to a particular outcome. For example, if good health is desired as an outcome, one might believe that this outcome is more probable as a result of participation in prolonged exercise. If, on the other hand, one believes that exercise inevitably leads to injury, the outcome of good health is less probable. Even though in both instances good health is positively valent, a difference exists in the belief that exercise will or will not achieve that outcome. As a result, the former case is more likely and the latter case is less likely to engage in prolonged exercise.

There are several important mechanisms to note in the model illustrated in Fig. 7-32. First, expectancy theory attempts to explain the forces that influence the expenditure of energy. In other words, the theory predicts effort rather than performance. To be sure, effort is a critical component of performance, but performance is influenced by additional variables, such as ability. In addition, the model is multiplicative rather than additive. This means that if either the value for valence or the value for expectancy is 0, no effort will be expended. One variable cannot make up for the other if the individual sees no likelihood of an action resulting in a desired outcome. A final important mechanism of the model is the comparison that an individual makes among possible outcomes in terms of preference or valence. The theory is a within-individual theory rather than a between-individuals theory. This means that a comparison of your valence for an outcome, such as public recognition, and my valence for that same outcome is largely irrelevant. What *is* relevant is a comparison of your valence for public recognition vs. your valence for satisfying social relations. It is the latter comparison that is likely to be more informative with respect to whether an athlete goes to the track to practice rather than joining friends who are going to a movie.

By determining the various outcomes that individuals hold with respect to action-outcome probabilities, expectancy theory has been effective in predicting how energy is expended (161,162). Although specific versions of the valence-expectancy model (222,287) have not been applied in the area of exercise and sport psychology, the issue of effort expenditure seems sufficiently similar to other settings in which the valence-expectancy theory has been applied to warrant serious consideration from the sport psychology community. In addition, many of the studies that have been conducted that relate to the motivation for engaging in prolonged exercise would seem to implicitly suggest just such a model. As we noted earlier, the rapid increase in best times for female marathon runners suggests that something other than training methods, equipment or biology is implicated in the improvement. It is likely that both the valences and the expectancies of potential participants have been modified in the past decade. Since male and female recognition and prize money are equal in most world class events now, women are more likely to (accurately) perceive a relationship between effort and outcome than in earlier decades. In addition, as more women begin to compete, performances begin to take on a "standard" appearance rather than an "extraordinary" one. Once again, this would imply a change in expectations that would lead to more participation and higher levels of performance.

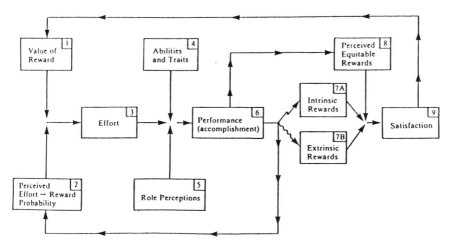

FIGURE 7-32. *A valence-instrumentality-expectancy model of performance motivation. From L.W. Porter and E.E. Lawler, 1968.* Managerial attitudes and performance. *Homewood, IL: Irwin-Dorsey. Reprinted with permission.*

1. Exercise Examples: Top Athletes. It is likely that valences and expectancies also enter into world-record performances as well. Consider the observations of Ryder et al. (241) that champions seem to "stop" after setting a record and are not likely to improve on their own world-record time. Valence-expectancy theory would seem to provide a framework for understanding this phenomenon. In the first place, once an individual holds a record, there would be a reduced valence for holding a "better" record. The amount of recognition will not change. In the professional running circuit, most of the substantial economic rewards come from winning, not from setting records (although many race directors are now adding substantial bonuses for race, national and world records). Similarly, since the amount of effort necessary to improve on the past record is likely to be exponentially related to the actual improvement, the "cost" is substantial compared to the benefit.

Finally, it may very well be that individuals see that it is unlikely that an extraordinary effort will yield a new record, since they are all too well aware of the effort necessary to set the old record. The point that we are making here is that there has been little systematic effort to discover the valences and expectancies of athletes (elite or non-elite) engaged in competitive exercise. We will have more to say about this shortly, when we consider the issue of goal setting.

PSYCHOLOGICAL FACTORS AND PROLONGED EXERCISE **333**

2. Exercise Examples: Outcomes for Non-Athletes. In the area of potential exercise pathology, there is another potential application for the valence-expectancy theory. It is clear that many victims of anorexia nervosa and bulimia are also engaged in prolonged exercise (aerobics, running, swimming, etc.) as an adjunct mechanism for achieving weight loss. It would seem equally clear that these individuals value "thinness" above many other outcomes and have firm beliefs regarding the relationship between exercise and weight loss. It would be useful to examine the valence-expectancy differences between normals and anorectics (matched with respect to exercise volume), in order to illustrate the central role of beliefs and valences in behavior and effort. Similarly, in less pathological populations, it would be illuminating to contrast valences and beliefs with respect to the relative effectiveness of dieting vs. exercise in weight loss. In naive subjects, there is a common misconception that small amounts of exercise yield substantial caloric expenditures. This may account for the high drop-out rate in many voluntary or self-monitored exercise programs geared toward weight loss. When initial efforts yield less than spectacular results, it is likely that expectancies regarding the effect of exercise on weight loss are radically altered (i.e., lowered). These alterations, in turn, are likely to reduce effort expenditure.

Another area of pathology that has been considered (and will be treated more substantially later in the chapter) is anxiety. Most individuals who suffer from anxiety symptoms have a high valence for a symptom-free lifestyle. Seldom do individuals enjoy their symptoms. As a result, it would appear that the variable of interest in such situations would be the belief or expectancy that prolonged exercise would lead to a diminution (albeit a temporary one) of symptoms. The work of individuals such as deVries et al. (53,54) and Farmer, Olewine, and Comer (86) suggests that such an effect is likely in some cases. Once again, there would seem to be value in exploring the expectancies that are held by those suffering from symptoms defining anxiety with regard to the effects of exercise on these symptoms. In a sense, the discussion of the role of beliefs in pathological behavior parallels the work of people like Beck (11), who accept the central role of cognitions in behavior. Nevertheless, the valence-expectancy model is somewhat broader than the framework underlying therapeutic intervention. This is probably the result of having developed the model in non-pathological environments.

It has been reported that endurance athletes become anxious when their conditioning program is interrupted (230,280). This is understandable from a valence-expectancy framework. There is a clear expectancy that interruption will lead to deconditioning and that deconditioning will lead to poor performance. As a result, there is a relatively strong force on the athlete to continue training in spite of injury or illness. When this becomes impossible, the individual exhibits the classic symptoms of blocked goal-attainment (i.e., frustration). From the valence-expectancy framework, it would seem important to identify new actions that would lead to positively valent outcomes. This is the logic underlying alternative training for injured athletes. Runners who experience pain related to weight-bearing or impact-related activities are encouraged to cycle or swim; swimmers with shoulder pain are encouraged to cycle or run, etc. As before, the critical area for research exploration would be the belief system held by the individual athlete regarding the relationship between these alternative activities and valued outcomes.

   3.   Exercise Examples: Adherence in Preventive Medicine. Some literature related to adherence statistics in fitness programs suggests that standards may be set too high and that this is the cause for low adherence and/or high drop-out rates in such programs. This is consistent with recent findings by Sallis et al. (243) that community adults are more likely to adopt and maintain moderate routine physical activity than fitness-inducing regimens. The implications would be that standards should be lowered. The valence-expectancy theory might suggest an alternative explanation. It might be argued that those who drop out or fail to maintain a prescribed schedule of exercise are those who do not believe that they can carry out the activity with sufficient skill to yield the desired results or that activity will lead to the desired outcome. If this is the case, lowering the expected standards is not likely to change behavior because the expectancy remains low. Oldridge et al. (209) found that postmyocardial infarction patients were no more likely to adhere to a low intensity, low frequency exercise program than to a more demanding one. Expectancies might be a central explanatory mechanism in understanding this result. It may be that these patients believe that even modest levels of exercise might do them harm rather than good. If this were the case, the issue would be one of discrepant valences between therapist and patient, rather than discrepant expectancies. The use of variations on the expectancy theory in decision-making interventions to increase exercise adherence is well described elsewhere by Wankel (288).

   Furthermore, the research of Epstein et al. (82) and Thompson and Wankel (281) suggests that an individually-chosen (or preferred) activity might elicit higher compliance rates than an imposed program. This is consistent with the valence-expectancy theory, since a self-selected activity would (by definition) have a higher expectancy value associated with it. This would suggest that an individual should be permitted to nominate one or more preferred activities, and the therapist should then develop a frequency/intensity program for that activity. It is often assumed that one should determine the preferred level of exertion for an individual before developing an exercise program. Instead, to create an exercise program that will encourage adherence it may be that one needs to know more about the preferred activity and the expectancy that this activity will lead to a desired outcome.

Although recent findings suggest that valence-expectancy models such as those described may predict interest in prolonged exercise or adoption of an exercise program but not its maintenance (147), implications of valence-expectancy concepts illustrate the useful role that a theoretical framework might play in trying to understand the barriers to and results of prolonged exercise from a motivational perspective. Further, they highlight the possibility that cognitive variables—and in particular expectancies and valences—play a central role in accounting for variance in effort expenditure and performance that remains unexplained by other physical and physiological variables.

B.   Goal Setting

Recently, goal-setting mechanisms have been suggested as major controlling influences in both effort expenditure and performance levels. This research has been reviewed by Locke et al. (170). The major proposition of the theory is simple and straightforward: specific hard goals will lead to higher performance and greater effort than either no goals or general (e.g., "do your best" goals). There is impressive empirical support for this position in the literature of industrial psychology, particularly with respect to effort expenditure. One version of the goal setting model appears in Fig. 7-33 (161).

As was the case with the valence expectancy model, there are some striking instances in the sport and exercise literature that suggest the suitability of this model for understanding the dynamics of prolonged exercise and performance (161).

   1.   Exercise Examples: Top Athletes. Earlier, we cited the work of Ryder et al. (241) illustrating that individuals seem to be more motivated to win rather than to achieve a particular speed in running. Ryder et al. made this observation to argue that physiological variables most likely do not impose limits on improved performance. It has often been noted that it is more difficult to break a world record without serious competition (i.e., to run against the clock). In fact, this principle is responsible for the presence of "rabbits" in running events whose role it is to increase the early pace

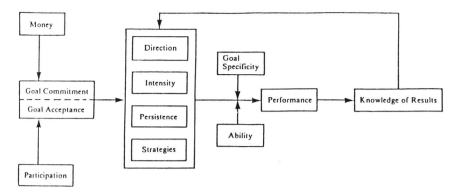

FIGURE 7-33. *A goal setting model of performance motivation. From F.J. Landy, 1985. The Psychology* of Work Behavior *(3rd Ed.). Homewood, IL: Dorsey Press, p. 339. Reprinted with permission.*

of the race. Winning a competitive event is a real and specific hard goal. Further, a person in front of or behind you provides immediate and continuous feedback, allowing you to change strategy, modulate intensities, etc. Similarly, in training, it is virtually universal for coaches to provide specific goals for "hard" workouts. This is most apparent in speed or interval training for runners or swimmers (e.g., a runner might be given a target time of 58 seconds for a series of 400 meter interval sprints).

2. **Exercise Examples: Outcomes for Non-Athletes.** This same goal-setting mechanism might be responsible for the differences noted between the psychological effects of exercise in cardiac patients belonging to either a group outpatient program or a home rehabilitation program. In a study of these two groups (83,178), more reliable and positive effects were found for the group outpatient subjects. It is possible that the group outpatient condition had specific goals and the home rehabilitation program was of the "do your best" variety. It is also probable that feedback was more immediate and informative in the group outpatient program.

3. **Exercise Examples: Adherence in Preventive Medicine.** Bandura and Cervone (8) demonstrated the efficacy of goals and feedback in an exercise setting. Subjects in the study performed a bicycle ergometer task in one of four conditions: goals only: feedback only, goals and feedback, or control. Effortful performance increase was twice as great (60% vs 30%) in sessions following feedback for subjects in goal conditions compared to subjects in no goal conditions (with feedback), feedback only conditions (with no goals), and control conditions. The experimental task lasted only five min

(as did the baseline pre-experimental session). This would not conform to our definition of prolonged exercise in the current volume. Nevertheless, the implications are clear. Similar results might be expected for longer exercise periods. Indeed, Martin et al. (176) have reported that rigid, long-term goals, but flexible daily goals promote exercise adherence. Because, however, goal setting in this study was imbedded in a multiple component cognitive behavior modification intervention, its unique effects cannot be evaluated.

At this time, there is little systematic research or application of the goal-setting theory in sports and exercise. The studies available show mixed results (8,117,291), but they have studied short-term muscular endurance rather than prolonged exercise. Task specificity appears important to consider in future studies, because the exertion demands of prolonged exercise are strikingly different from the industrial-organization tasks studied in the goal-setting literature and because recent goal-setting theory recognizes the task demands in explaining human performance (102). Nevertheless, the observations made above, coupled with the encouraging empirical support for the goal-setting theory in other settings, and the recent study of Bandura and Cervone (8) and Hall et al. (117) suggest a potential role for the goal-setting theory in sports and exercise research when prolonged exertion is of interest.

VI. LIMITATIONS OF RESEARCH DESIGN AND METHODOLOGY

Two analytic issues have some important implications for future research directions and activities in the area of prolonged exercise. These two issues involve the prevalence of small samples in sport and exercise research and the interpretation of conflicting research findings.

A. Sample Size

In the literature reviewed in the current chapter, it is not uncommon to see experimental and control groups in sizes of 10 to 20, or within-subject designs with 15 subjects. This presents a serious problem for many reasons. First, it is likely that we are seeking small to modest effects (compared to training variables or physiological variables) when we examine the psychological influences and outcomes in prolonged exercise studies. As a result, we often need substantial sample sizes (in some common instances greater than 100) to detect such effects. Statistically, the issue is referred to as one of "power." Low power (i.e., diminished possibility of detecting true effects or differences) results in two different kinds of errors. First, one is more likely to (often inappropriately) discard a reasonable hypothesis and, in effect, discredit a theory with low power rather than with high power. As an example, one might contrast exercise therapy with a control condition and conclude that exercise therapy is not efficacious because there was no difference detected between an experimental group (n = 10) and a control group (n = 20). Second, one is more likely to accept (again, inappropriately) the absence of a difference between two groups as evidence in support of a theoretical position. For example, one might be tempted to draw a parallel between a clinical syndrome (e.g. anorexia) and an exercise history (e.g., high frequency activity patterns) because there was no difference in responses to a standard personality profile between the clinical group (n = 10) and the exercise group (n = 20). Once again, the deck is stacked against finding a difference as a result of low power. It might be argued that this is simply the nature of the subject populations in this type of research; it is difficult or impossible to construct large samples. In fact, it is simple enough to determine exactly what sample size is necessary for any level of power desired or effect size anticipated, but power of the statistical test used in a study is seldom reported in sport psychology research. In many instances, the sample sizes would have been achievable. More importantly, the laws of inference being used by researchers are unsympathetic to the practical difficulties of research. Regardless of why the sample size is small, the two types of errors described above are having a major impact on the direction of research and theory in sports and exercise domains.

B.   Conflicting Results

A second analytic issue that affects the extent to which theory and research can advance in the field relates to the common observation that research in the same area using the same variables and theories often yields results in conflict with existing research or findings. It is tempting to see this as the raw material for the research enterprise. From this perspective, we should simply continue to gather data and replicate results until one side "wins". An alternative approach is to test the hypothesis that these conflicting results actually result from some well-known and easily-controlled statistical artifacts. As an example, assume that we have developed a new psychological measure to predict time to exhaustion at an exercise intensity of 80% of VO_2max. In an attempt to demonstrate the efficacy of this new measure, several dozen researchers around the country set out to compare the new test with actual performance during treadmill ergometry. After the studies are completed, we find that the correlations between our psychological test and performance range from $+.82$ to $+.23$ with a mean of $+.50$ and a standard deviation (in this case a standard error) of .16—a substantial range. It is likely the test would be dismissed as imprecise and of little use. An examination of the studies that were conducted might, however, be quite illuminating. We would probably find that the number of subjects used in the studies varied from 15 to 125, that the range of performance within the two tests (the psychological test and the treadmill test) varied by as much as 4:1 between studies, and finally, that the reliability of the measurements varied from study to study as a result of the experimental procedures, experimenters, etc. Each of these three variables (sample size, range restriction, reliability) can be shown to affect the variability of results across studies. In addition, each of these factors can be statistically controlled. As a result, we might actually find that all of the observed variability among studies is the product of these three variables. This would permit us to make a more definitive statement about the relationship between the two variables of interest.

It is our impression that many areas of psychological investigation in the sport and exercise literature can be characterized by this variability of sample size, range and reliability. As a result, we suggest that meta-analytic strategies be applied to several of these areas, in an attempt to resolve disputes and reduce apparent discrepancies. The procedures are relatively simple and are well documented in recent texts by Hedges and Olkin (124) and Glass, McGaw, and Smith (105). These techniques have proven very useful in identifying underlying consistencies in wide ranges of social and behavioral research settings. For example, we noted earlier that there was much inconsistency in results and methods in studies of how exercise or aerobic fitness influence mental stress tolerance. Crews and Landers (46) recently examined these inconsistencies by meta-analysis of 92 effect-size estimates from 34 studies of 1,449 subjects. They conclude that the average effect size was approximately one-half of one standard deviation and that differences across studies on potential moderating factors, including those that described exercise, subjects, research design, or measures of stress did not influence the effect size seen.

Although this analysis helps clarify how characteristics of past research can have an impact the association seen, it is important to note also the major limitation of meta-analysis; its results clarify, but cannot improve upon, past research. As we noted earlier, a randomized experimental study in which a measured increase in $\dot{V}O_2max$ is demonstrated is the required design to test the hypothesis that aerobic fitness influences tolerance for stressors other than exercise. Because such a study has not been reported, the impact of its advance in research design and measurement of effect size in a meta-analysis cannot be evaluated. In addition, if physical activity rather than fitness is to be an independent variable, then physical activity must be quantified. But quantification of physical activity has also not been considered in the mental stress tolerance literature. Thus, meta-analysis cannot address it. Thus, meta-analysis cannot be viewed as a panacea for inadequate research, but as a guide to better research. Even so, we suggest that in some areas of sport psychology, it may be better to delay additional studies that replicate digressive designs or methods and, instead, take a careful and critical look at the results we have in hand right now. Such a strategy would seem often to be a more effective practice of the scientific enterprise.

VII. IMPLICATIONS FOR APPLIED RESEARCH AND PRACTICE

(1) Mathematical models of time and distance relationships among top level athletes suggest that increased performance in prolonged exercise requires a training volume that will place many athletes at risk for pathological adaptations. Although incidence, prevalence, and etiology of overtraining and staleness is not yet known, psychological monitoring of chronic training responses has shown promise for detecting risk. Although training adaptation is likely a complex medical and psychobiological process, psychological models that consider how athletes appraise environmental demands and how they perceive personal ability and personal control over training and competitive decisions may help explain chronic training stress. Based on these theoretical models and sport research, the personality of an athlete may moderate training stress, but social support appears to be equally important. Applied interventions that consider these factors may eventually prove useful for prevention or recovery when athletes are at risk for pathological adaptations to prolonged exercise.

(2) Only 20% of the 29 million American adults who suffer a mental health problem during a six month period will seek professional care. Because anxiety and depression are the most prevalent problems, evidence showing that prolonged exercise is associated with reduced anxiety and depression is timely for public health interventions. Evidence also suggests that aerobic fitness is associated with enhanced sleep and with reduced physiological reactivity to mental stressors. The National Institute of Mental Health consensus panel on exercise has concluded that several psychological benefits are associated with prolonged exercise. The social, cognitive, or neurobiological mechanisms responsible for these associated changes and the predictability of the changes remain unclear, however.

Prolonged exercise consistent with American College of Sports Medicine (ACSM) guidelines for fitness training appears to be appropriate, although the relative importance or necessity of increased fitness or activity level has not been demonstrated, and most studies have not used precise measures of fitness or physical activity in experimental designs. In a few studies, exercise has been as effective as meditation and tranquilizing medication for treating tension and anxiety. Reports of mental health risks associated with high levels of exercise involvement also have not used experimental methods or precise measures of physical activity.

Based on current evidence, mental health risks of exercise for the public appear to be far outweighed by potential health benefits. Future research should study other species and human subjects of both sexes, and various levels of age, fitness, and activity history, using randomized placebo experiments. In addition, explanatory models from social, psychological, cognitive, and neurobiological orientations should be simultaneously contrasted in order to predict and understand the causality of mental health outcomes associated with prolonged exercise in both supervised and free-living settings.

(3) Early research suggested that personality factors related to motivation and perception were associated with prolonged exercise performance, but controversy surrounding the correlational methods used and the weak associations seen render available studies of little practical impact. In a similar way, the many studies showing that perceived exertion is related to power output and physiological responses during prolonged exercise have not shed light on how perceived exertion influences performance. Future studies should examine how perceived discomfort and preferred exertion relate to perceived exertion and performance using predictive and experimental designs.

Experimental manipulations of cognitive variables during exercise of short duration (about one to five min) and low intensity (approximately 100 watts or at a heart rate of 100 beats $\cdot$ min^{-1}) have led to small changes in oxygen consumption, ventilatory minute volume, heart rate, and blood pressure that could have an impact on performance during prolonged exercise. But only a single study has demonstrated that an applied cognitive intervention can enhance performance during prolonged exercise (80% to 90% $\dot{V}O_2$max). This area offers great promise for practical application, but there simply have not been enough studies conducted on prolonged exercise using acceptable research designs to permit conclusions.

(4) When ACSM guidelines for fitness training are used as the standard for participation, drop out rates from supervised programs remain high (about 50%), and the prevalence of prolonged exercise

in the population remains low (about 10%). While the determinants of the adoption and maintenance of activity programs likely come from complex interactions among characteristics of the individual participant, the social environment, and the exercise setting, it may be important also to consider exercise plans or prescriptions that complement existing fitness guidelines to better fit some population segments and types of individuals. This possibility is reinforced by recent population-based research showing that health-related moderate activity, such as walking and vigorous gardening, has higher adoption and maintenance rates than do fitness regimens. The potential health effectiveness of activity alternatives to prolonged exercise bears epidemiologic scrutiny. Personality and self-perception also appear to influence the degree to which individuals effectively regulate exercise intensity prescriptions. Perceived exertion may represent one adjunct to traditional heart rate prescriptions that can have practical impact on improving intensity compliance in supervised settings.

(5) Most psychological research germane to prolonged exercise has lacked a clear theoretical orientation to explain or predict results and guide applied interventions. Valence-expectancy and goal-setting models were discussed in detail to illustrate how cognitive psychology might interpret present findings and form hypotheses for new research. These theoretical approaches also implicate technologies for applied interventions that can be tested for effectiveness in prolonged exercise performance. So, much of the clear potential in this area remains unfulfilled. Future study must, however, compensate for past shortcomings. Experimental designs should have adequate statistical power and should include precise measures of psychology and exercise that stem from theory from the practical performance problems of athletes, and from health concerns in the population.

ACKNOWLEDGMENTS

Thanks go to Daniel M. Landers, Arizona State University for his comments on an earlier draft and Donna Smith, University of Georgia for processing the manuscript under an extreme time press.
Sections of this paper have relied heavily on earlier reviews by the authors (58,60,65,66,67,160,161,162).

BIBLIOGRAPHY

1. Allen, M., J. Thierman, and D. Hamilton. Naloxone eye reverse the miosis in runners— implications for an endogenous opiate test. *Can. J. Appl. Sport Sci.*, 8:98–103, 1983.
2. American College of Sports Medicine. *Guidelines for graded exercise testing and exercise prescription* (3rd ed.). Philadelphia: Lea and Febiger, 1986.
3. American College of Sports Medicine. The recommended quantity and quality of exercise

for developing and maintaining fitness in healthy adults. *Medicine and Science in Sports*, 10:7–10, 1978.

4. Appenzeller, D., J. Standefer, J. Appenzeller et al. Neurology of endurance training: endorphins. *Neurol.*, 30:418–419, 1980.
5. Baekeland, F. Exercise deprivation. *Archives of General Psychiatry*, 22:365–369, 1970.
6. Bahrke, M.S. and W.P. Morgan. Anxiety reduction following exercise and meditation. *Cognitive Therapy and Research*, 2:323–333, 1978.
7. Balke, B. Prescribing physical activity. In: A. Ryan and F. Allman (eds) Sports Medicine. Academic Press, New York, 1974.
8. Bandura, A. and D. Cervone. Self-evaluative and self-efficacy mechanisms governing the motivational effects of goal systems. *Journal of Personality and Social Psychology*, 45:1017–1028, 1983.
9. Barchas, J.O. and D.X. Freedman. Brain amines: Response to physiological stress. *Biochem. Pharmacol.*, 12:1232–1235, 1981.
10. Barta, A., K. Yashpal and J.L. Henry. Regional redistribution of B-endorphin in the rat brain: the effect of stress. Proceedings of the Canadian College of Neuropsychopharmacology, 44:1981.
11. Beck, A.T. *Cognitive therapy and the emotional disorders*. New York: International Universities Press, 1976.
12. Beckman, H., M.H. Ebert, R. Post, and E.K. Goodwin. Effects of moderate exercise on urinary MHPG in depressed patients. *Pharmaopsychiatry*, 12:351–356, 1979.
13. Benson, H., T. Dryer, and C.H. Hartley. Decreased VO_2 consumption during exercise after elicitation of the relaxation response. *J. Human Stress*, 4:38–46, 1978.
14. Berger, B.G. and D.R. Owen. Mood alteration with swimming. *Psychosomatic Medicine*, 45:425–433, 1983.
15. Berman, R., E. Simonson, and W. Heron. Electrocardiographic effects associated with hypnotic suggestion in normal and coronary sclerotic individuals. *J Appl Phys.*, 7:89–96, 1954.
16. Blair, S.N., et al. Changes in coronary heart disease risk factors associated with increased treadmill time in 753 men. *Am. J. Epidemiol.*, 118:352–359, 1983.
17. Bliss, E.L. and J. Ailion. Relationship of stress and activity to brain dopamine and homovanillic acid. *Life Sciences*, 10:1161–1169, 1971.
18. Blumenthal, J.A., S. Rose, and J.L. Chang. Anorexia nervosa and exercise: Implications from recent findings. *Sports Medicine*, 2:237–247, 1985.
19. Blumenthal, J.A., R.S. Williams, and T.L. Needels. Psychological changes accompany aerobic exercise in healthy middle-aged adults. *Psychosomatic Medicine*, 44:529–536, 1982.
20. Blumenthal, J.A., R.S. Williams, and R.B. Williams et al. Effects of exercise on the Type A (coronary prone) behavior pattern. *Psychosomatic Medicine*, 42:289–296, 1980.
21. Blumenthal, J.A., D.D. Schocken, T.L. Needels et al. Psychological and physiological effects of physical conditioning on the elderly. *Journal of Psychosomatic Research*, 26:505–510, 1982.
22. Boff, K.R., L. Kaufman and J.P. Thomas. *Handbook of perception and human performance: Vol. 2, Cognitive processes and perception.* New York: Wiley-Interscience, (eds.) (1986).
23. Boff, K.R., L. Kaufman and J.P. Thomas. *Handbook of perception and human performance: Vol. 1, Sensory processes and perception.* New York: Wiley-Interscience, (eds.), 1986.
24. Borg, G.A.V. Perceived exertion: a note on history and methods. *Medicine and Science in Sports*, 5:90–93, 1973.
25. Bortz, W.M., P. Angwin, I.N. Mefford et al. Catecholamines, dopamine, and endorphin levels during extreme exercise. *New England Journal of Medicine*, 305:466–467, 1981.
26. Boutcher, S.H. and D.M. Landers. Mood states of nonrunners and runners after vigourous exercise, (In Press).
27. Brisson, G.R., P. Diamond, D. de Carufel et al. Influence of trait anxiety upon blood LH and testosterone levels under resting and working conditions in young adult males. *Med. Sci. Sport Exer.*, (abstract), 13:74, 1981.
28. Brooke, S.T. and B.L. Long. Efficiency of coping with a real-life stressor: a multimodal comparison of aerobic fitness. *Psychophysiology*, 24:173–180, 1987.
29. Brooks, C.M. Adult participation in physical activities requiring moderate to high levels of energy expenditure. *The Physician and Sportsmedicine*, 15(4):119–132, 1987.
30. Brown, B.S., T. Payne, C. Kim, G. Moore, P. Krebs, and W. Martin. Chronic response of rat brain norepinephrine and serotonin levels to endurance training. *Journal of Applied Physiology*, 46:19–23, 1979.
31. Brown, B.S. and W. Van Huss. Exercise and rat brain catecholamines. Journal of applied Physiology, 34:664–669, 1973.
32. Brown, R.A., D.E. Ramirez, and J.M. Taub. The prescription of exercise for depression. *The Physician and Sportsmedicine*, 6:34–45, 1978.
33. Bulbulian, R. and B.L. Darabos. Motor neuron excitability: the Hoffman reflex following

exercise at high and low intensity. *Medicine and Science in Sports and Exercise*, 18:697–702, 1986.

34. Bunnell, D.E., W. Bevier and S.M. Horvath. Effects of exhaustive exercise on the sleep of men and women. *Psychophysiology*, 20:50–58, 1983.

35. Burke, E.J. and M.L. Collins. Using perceived exertion for the prescription of exercise in healthy adults. In R.C. Cantu (ed.) *Clinical Sports Medicine*. Lexington, MA, pp. 93–105, 1984.

36. Burke, R.E. Motor units: Anatomy, physiology, and functional organization. In *Handbook of Physiology. The Nervous System*. Motor Control. Bethesda, MD: Am. Physiol. Soc., Vol. II:345–422, 1981.

37. Cannon, J.G. and M.J. Kluger. Endogenous pyrogen activity in human plasma after exercise. *Science*, 220:617–619, 1983.

38. Carlow, T.J., O. Appenzeller and M. Rodriguez. Neurology of endurance training: visual evoked potentials before and after a run. *Neurology*, 28:390, 1978.

39. Carr, D.B. B.A. Bullen, G.S. Skrinar et al. Physical conditioning facilitates the exercise induced secretion of betaendorphin and beta-lipotropin in women. *New England Journal of Medicine*, 305:560–563, 1981.

40. Cavanagh, P. and R. Kram. The efficiency of human movement—a statement of the problem. *Medicine and Science in Sports and Exercise*, 17:304–307, 1985.

41. Chodzko-Zajko, W.J. and A.H. Ismail. MMPI interscale relationships in middle aged male subjects before and after an eight month fitness program. *Journal of Clinical Psychology*, 40:163–169, 1984.

42. Chow, R.J. and J.H. Wilmore. The regulation of exercise intensity by ratings of perceived exertion. *J Cardiac Rehab.*, 4:382–387, 1984.

43. Collingwood, T.R., I.H. Bernstein and D. Hubbard. Canonical correlation analysis of clinical and psychological data in 4,351 men and women. *Journal of Cardiac Rehabilitation*, 3:706–711, 1983.

44. Colt, E.W. S.L. Wardlaw, and A.G. Frantz. The effect of running on plasma beta-endorphin. *Life Sci.*, 28:1637–1640.

45. Cox, J.P. J.F. Evans and J. L. Jamieson. Aerobic power and tonic heart rate response to psychosocial stressors. *Personality and Social Psychology Bulletin*, 5:160–163, 1979.

46. Crews, D.J. and D.M. Landers. A meta-analytic review of aerobic fitness and reactivity to psychosocial stressors. Medicine and Science in Sports and Exercise, 19(suppl.):S114–S120, 1987.

47. Davis, H.A., G.C. and J.R. Bassett. Serum cortisol response to incremental work in experienced and naive subjects. *Psychosom. Med.*, 43:127–132, 1981.

48. de Castro, J.M. and G. Duncan. Operantly conditioned running: Effects on brain catecholamine concentrations and receptor densities in the rat. *Pharmacology, Biochemistry and Behavior*, 23:495–500, 1985.

49. deVries, H.A. Immediate and long-term effects of exercise upon resting muscle action potential. *Sports Med. and Phys. Fit.* 8:1–11, 1968.

50. deVries, H.A. and G.M. Adams. Electromyographic comparison of single doses of exercise and meprobromate as to effects on muscular relaxation. *American Journal of Physical Medicine*, 51:130–141, 1972.

51. deVries, H.A. P. Beckman, H. Huber and L. Dieckmeir. Electromyographic evaluation of the effects of sauna on the neuromuscular system. *Journal of Sports Medicine and Physical Fitness*, 8:1–11, 1968.

52. deVries, H.A. R. Burke and R.T. Hooper. Efficacy of EMG biofeedback in relaxation training. *American Journal of Physical Medicine*, 56:75–81, 1977.

53. deVries. H.A., C.P. Simard, and R. A. Wiswell et al. Tranquilizer effect of exercise. *American Journal of Physical Medicine*, 60:57–66, 1981.

54. deVries, H.A. R.A. Wiswell, and R. Bulbulian et al. Tranquilizer effect of exercise. *American Journal of Physical Medicine*, 60:57–66, 1981.

55. Dienstbier, R.A., J. Crabbe, and G.U. Johnson et al. Exercise and stress tolerance. In M.H. Sacks and M.L. Sachs (eds) *Psychology of Running*. Champaign, Il: Human Kinetics Publishers, pp. 192–210, 1981.

56. Dimsdale, J.E. and J. Moss. Plasma catecholamines in stress and exercise, *JAMA*, 243–340–342, 1980.

57. Dishman, R.K. Aerobic power, estimation of physical ability, and attraction to physical activity. *Research Quarterly for Exercise and Sport*, 49:285–295, 1978.

58. Dishman, R.K. Behavioral barriers to health-related physical fitness (pp. 48–83). In L. K. Hall and C. Meyer (ed.) *Epidemiology, behavior-change and rehabilitation in chronic disease*. Champaign, Il: Human Kinetics Publishers, 1988.

59. Dishman, R.K. Compliance/adherence in health-related exercise. *Health Psychology*, 1:237–267, 1982.

60. Dishman, R.K. Contemporary sport psychology. In R. Terjung (ed.) *Ex. and Sport. Sci.*

Rev., Philadelphia, Franklin Institute Press, 1982.

61. Dishman, R.K. Eating disorders and exercise commitment among athletes and habitual runners. Paper presented at the American Psychological Association Meeting, Washington, D.C., August 25, 1986.

62. Dishman, R.K. Exercise adherence and habitual physical activity. In W.P. Morgan and S.N. Goldston (Ed.). *Exercise and Mental Health*. Washington, D.C., Hemisphere Publishing Corp., 1987.

63. Dishman, R.K. *Exercise Adherence: Its Impact on Public Health*. Champaign, IL: Human Kinetics Publishers, 1988.

64. Dishman, R.K. Identity crises in North American sport psychology: academics in professional issues. *Journal of Sports Psychology*, 5:123–134, 1983.

65. Dishman, R.K. Medical psychology in exercise and sport. *Med Clin N Am.*, 69:123–143, 1985.

66. Dishman, R.K. Mental health. In V. Seefeldt (Ed.). *Physical activity and well-being* (pp. 304–341). Reston, VA: American Alliance for Health, Physical Education, Recreation, and Dance, 1986.

67. Dishman, R.K. Psychological aids to performance. In R.H. Strauss (Ed.) *Drugs and Performance in Sports* (pp. 121–146), Philadelphia, W.B. Saunders Co., 1987.

68. Dishman, R.K. Psychology of sports competition. In A.J. Ryan and F.L. Allman (Eds.) *Sports Medicine* (2nd Ed.) New York: Academic Press, (In Press).

69. Dishman, R.K. Stress management procedures. In M. Williams (Ed.) *Ergogenic Aids in Sport.* Human Kinetics: Champaign, IL, 275–320, 1983.

70. Dishman, R.K., R. Armstrong, M. Delp, R. Graham and A. Dunn. Open field behavior is not related to treadmill performance in exercising rats. Manuscript submitted to *Phys and Behavior*.

71. Dishman, R.K., R. Farquhar, K. Cureton, and M. Collins. Anxiety responses to preferred levels of prolonged exercise in trained and untrained men. Manuscript submitted for publication, The University of Georgia, Athens, 1988.

72. Dishman, R.K., R.G. Holly and E.S. Schelegle. Psychometric, perceptual, and metabolic predictors of self-limited submaximal and maximal treadmill performance (abstract). *Medicine and Science in Sports and Exercise*, 17(2):198–199, 1985.

73. Dishman, R.K. and W. Ickes. Self-motivation and adherence to therapeutic exercise. *J Behav Med.*, 4:421–438, 1981.

74. Dishman, R.K. R. Patton, J. Smith R. Weinberg and A.W. Jackson. Using perceived exertion to prescribe and monitor exercise training heart rate. *International Journal of Sports Medicine*, 8:208–213, 1987.

75. Dishman, R.K., J. Sallis and D. Orenstein. The determinants of physical activity and exercise. *Public Health Reports*, 100:158–171, 1985.

76. Doctor, R. and B.J. Sharkey. Note on some psychological and subjective reactions to exercise and training. *Percept. and Mot. Skills*, 32:233–237, 1971.

77. Doyne, E.S. D.L. Chambless and L.E. Beutler. Aerobic exercise as a treatment for depression in women. *Behavior Therapy*, 14:434–440, 1983.

78. Driscoll, R. Anxiety reduction using physical exertion and positive images. *Psychological Record*, 26:87–94, 1976.

79. Dwyer, J. and R. Bybee. Heart rate indices of the anaerobic threshold. *Medicine and Science in Sports and Exercise*, 15:72–76, 1983.

80. Ebert, M.H., R. M. Post, and F.K. Goodwin. Effect of physical activity on urinary M.H.P.G. excretion in depressed patients. *Lancet*, 2:766, 1972.

81. Ekblom, B., and A.N. Goldbarg. The influence of training and other factors on the subjective rating of perceived exertion. *Acta Physiol Scand.*, 83:399–415, 1971.

82. Epstein, L.H. R.R. Wing, R. Koeske et al. A comparison of lifestyle change and programmed exercise on weight and fitness changes in obese children. *Beh. Therapy*, 1982.

83. Erdmanm R.A. and H.J. Duivenvoorden. Psychologic evaluation of a cardiac rehabilitation program: A randomized clinical trial in patients with myocardial infarction. *Journal of Cardiac Rehabilitation*, 3:696–704, 1983.

84. Ewart, C.K., K.J. Stewart and R.E. Gillilan et al. Usefulness of self-efficacy in predicting overexertion during programmed exercise in coronary artery disease. *Am. J. Cardio.*, 57:557–561, 1986.

85. Eysenck, H.J., D.K.B. Nias and D.N. Cox. Sport and personality. *Advances in Behavioral Research and Therapy*, 4:1–55, 1982.

86. Farmer, P.K. D.A. Olewine, D.W. Comer et al. Frontalis muscle tension and occipital alpha production in young males with coronary prone (Type A) and coronary resistent (Type B) behavior patterns. *Medicine and Science in Sports and Exercise* (abstract), 10:51, 1978.

87. Farrell, P.A., W.K. Gates, M.G. Maksud and W.P. Morgan. Increases in plasma B-endorphin/B-lipotropin immunoreactivity after treadmill running in humans. *Journal of Ap-

plied *Physiology:* Respiratory, Environmental, and Exercise Physiology, 52:1245–1249, 1982.

88. Farrell, P.A. W.K. Gates, W.P. Morgan and C.B. Pert. Plasma leucine enkephalin-like radioreceptor activity and tension-anxiety before and after competitive running. In H.G. Knuttgen, J.A. Vogel, and J. Poortmans (Eds). *Biochemistry of Exercise.* Champaign, IL: Human Kinetics Publishers, pp. 637–644, 1983.

89. Farrell, P.A. A.B. Gustafson, T.L. Garthwaite, R.K. Kalkhoff, A. W. Cowley and W.P. Morgan. Influence of endogenous opioids on the response of selected hormones to exercise in man. *Journal of Applied Physiology,* 61:1051–1057, 1987.

90. Farrell, P.A. A.B., Gustafson, W.P. Morgan and C.B. Pert. Enkephalins, catecholamines, and psychological mood alterations: effects of prolonged exercise. *Medicine and Science in Sports and Exercise,* 19:347–353, 1987.

91. Farquhar, R. R.K. Dishman, K. Cureton and M. Collins. Physiological and perceptual correlates of preferred exertion. Unpublished data, The University of Georgia, 1987.

92. Feltz, D.K. and R.R. Albrecht. Psychological implications of competitive running. In M.R. Weiss and D. Gould (ed.) *Sport for Children and Youth:* 1984 Olympic Scientific Congress Proceedings. Champaign, IL: Human Kinetics Publishers, 1985.

93. Feltz, D.L. and M.E. Ewing. Psychological characteristics of elite young athletes. *Medicine and Science in Sports and Exercise,* 1987.

94. Feltz, D.L. and R.R. Albrecht. Psychological implications of competitive running. In *Sport for Children and Youths,* The 1984 Olympic Scientific Congress Proceedings, Vol. 10: M. Weiss and D. Gould (Eds)., Champaign, IL: Human Kinetics, 225–230, 1986.

95. Feltz, D.L. et al. The effect of prolonged exercise on circulating enkephalins, catecholamines and psychological mood alterations. *Medicine and Science in Sports and Exercise,* 1987.

96. Fielding, J.E. Effectiveness of employee health improvement programs. *JOM,* 24:907–916, 1982.

97. Folkins, C.H. and W.F. Sime. Physical Fitness training and mental health. *American Psychologist,* 35:373–389, 1981.

98. Fraioli, F., C. Moretti, D. Paolucci et al. Physical exercise stimulates marked concomitant increase of beta-endorphin and adrenocorticotropic hormone (ACTH) in peripheral blood in man. *Experientia,* 36:987–989, 1980.

99. Frankenhauser, M. Behavior and circulating catecholamines. *Brain Res.,* 31:241–262, 1971.

100. Gambert, S.R., T.L. Garthwaite, C.H. Pontzen et al. Running elevates plasma beta-endorphin immunoreactivity and ACTH in untrained human subjects. *Proc. Soc. Exp. Biol. Med.,* 168:1–4, 1981.

101. Garber, C.E., S.F. Siconolfi, P. Beaudin and R.A. Carleton. The effects of regular exercise on circulatory reactivity to mental stress. *Medicine and Science in Sports and Exercise* (abstract), 16:139, 1984.

102. Garland, H. A cognitive mediation theory of task goals and human performance. *Motivation and Emotion,* 9:232–260, 1985.

103. Gervino, E.V. and A. E., Veazey. The physiologic effects of Benson's Relaxation Response during submaximal aerobic exercise. *J. Cardiac Rehabilitation,* 4:254–261, 1984.

104. Gibbons, L.W. S.N. Blair, K.H. Cooper and M. Smith. Association between coronary heart disease risk factors and physical fitness in healthy adult women. *Circulation,* 67:977–983, 1983.

105. Glass, G.V., B. McGaw and M.L. Smith. *Meta-Analysis in Social Research.* Beverly Hills, CA: Sage Publications, 1981.

106. Gliner, J.A., J.A. Matsen-Twisdale, S.M. Horvath and M.B. Maron. Visual evoked potentials and signal detection following a marathon race. *Medicine and Science in Sports,* 11:155–159, 1979.

107. Godin, G., R.J. Shepard, and A. Colantonio. The cognitive profile of those who intend to exercise but do not. *Public Health Reports,* 101:521–526, 1986.

108. Goldfarb, A.H., B.D. Hatfield, G.A. Sforzo, and M.G. Flynn. Serum B-endorphin levels during a graded exercise test to exhaustion. *Medicine and Science in Sports and Exercise,* 19(2):78–82, 1987.

109. Gotang, A., T. Clitsome, and T. Kostrubala. A psychological study of 50 sub-3-hour marathoners. *Annals of the New York Academy of Sciences,* 301:1020–1028, 1977.

110. Goode, D.J., H. Dekirmenjian, H.T. Meltzer and J.W. Maas. Relation of exercise to MHPG excretion in normal subjects. *Arch Gen Psychiatry,* 29:391–396, 1973.

111. Gordon, R., S. Spector, A. Sjordsma and S. Udenfriend. Increased synthesis of norepinephrine in the intact rat during exercise and exposure to cold. *Journal of Pharmacology and Experimental Therapy,* 153:440–447, 1966.

112. Gould, D., T. Horn and J. Spreemann. Sources of stress in junior elite wrestlers. *J of Sport Psy.,* 5:159–171, 1983.

113. Griest, J.H., M.H. Klein, R.R. Eischens, M. Faris, A. Gurman and W.P. Morgan. Running as a treatment for depression. *Comprehensive Psychiatry,* 20:41–54, 1979.

114. Gruber, J. Physical activity and self-esteem development in children: A meta-analysis. In G.A. Stull and H.M. Eckhardt (Eds.), *Effects of Physical Activity on Children:* Papers of the American Academy of Physical Education, 19:30–48. Champaign, IL: Human Kinetics Publishers, 1986.
115. Gutmaan, M.L., M.L. Pollock, C. Foster and D. Schmidt. Training stress in Olympic speedskaters: a psychological perspective. *The Physician and Sportsmedicine*, 12(12):45–57, 1984.
116. Haier, R.J., B.A. Quaid and J.S. Mills. Naloxone alters pain perceptions after jogging. *Psychiatry Research*, 5:231–232, 1981.
117. Hall, H.K., R.S. Weinberg and A. Jackson. Effects of goal specificity, goal difficulty, and information feedback on endurance performance. *Journal of Sport Psychology*, 9:43–54, 1987.
118. Harber, V.J. and J.R. Sutton. Endorphins and exercise. *Sports Medicine*, 1:154–171, 1984.
119. Harris, D.V. The psychology of the female runner. In B.L. Drinkwater (Ed.) *Female Endurance Athletes*, 59–74, 1986.
120. Hartley, A.A. and J.T. Hartley. In response to Stones and Kozma: Absolute and relative declines with age in champion swimming performances. *Experimental Aging Research*, 10:151–153, 1984.
121. Hartley, A.A. and J.T. Hartley. Performance changes in champion swimmers aged 30 to 84 years. *Experimental Aging Research*, 10:141–147, 1984.
122. Haskell, W.L., H.J. Montoye and D. Orenstein. Physical activity and exercise to achieve health-related physical fitness. *Public Health Reports*, 100:202–212, 1985.
123. Hatfield, B. and D. Landers. Psychophysiology of sport. *Exercise and Sport Sciences Reviews*, 15:200–245, 1987.
124. Hedges, L.V. and I. Olkin. *Statistical Methods for Meta-Analysis*. Orlando, FL: Academic Press, 1985.
125. Hellhammer, D.H., J.N. Hingtgen and S.A. Wade. Serotonergic changes in specific areas of rat brain associated with activity-stress lesions. *Psychosomatic Medicine*, 45:115–122, 1983.
126. Hill, A.V. The physiological basis of athletic records. *Lancet*, 21:409–428, 1925.
127. Hippius, H. and G. Winokur. (Eds.) *Psychopharmacology* 1: *Clinical psychopharmacology*. Amsterdam: Excerpta Medica, 1983.
128. Horne, J.A. The effects of exercise upon sleep: A critical review. *Biological Psychology*, 12:241–290, 1981.
129. Horne, J.A. and V.J. Moore. Sleep EEG effects of exercise with and without additional body cooling. *Electroencephalography and Clinical Neurophysiology*, 60:33–38, 1985.
130. Horstman, D.H., W.P. Morgan, A. Cymerman and J. Stokes. Perception of effort during constant work to self-imposed exhaustion. *Perceptual and Motor Skills*, 48:1111–1126, 1979.
131. Howard, J.H., D.A. Cunningham and P.A. Rechnitzer. Physical activity as a moderator of life events and somatic complaints: A longitude study. *Canadian Journal of Applied Sport Sciences*, 9:194–200, 1984.
132. Howlett, D.R. and F.A. Jenner. Studies relating to the clinical significance of urinary 3-methoxy-4-hydroxyphenylethylene glycol. *British Journal of Psychiatry*, 132:49–54, 1978.
133. Hughes, J.R., R.S. Crow, D.R. Jacobs, M.B. Mittlemark and A.S. Leon. Physical activity, smoking, and exercise-induced fatigue. *Journal of Behavioral Medicine*, 7:217–230, 1985.
134. Hull, E.M., S.H. Young, and M.G. Ziegler. Aerobic fitness affects cardiovascular and catecholamine responses to stressors. *Psychophysiology*, 21:353–360, 1984.
135. Hyyppa, M.T., S. Aunola and V. Kuusela. Psychoendocrine responses to bicycle exercise in healthy men in good physical condition. *International Journal of Sports Medicine*, 7:89–93, 1986.
136. Ismail, A.H. and A.M. El-Naggar. Effect of exercise on cognitive processing in adult male. *J Hum Ergol.*, 10:83–91, 1981.
137. Jackson, A.W., R.K. Dishman, S. LaCroix, R. Patton and R. Weinberg. The heart rate, perceived exertion, and pace of the 1.5 mile run. *Medicine and Science in Sports and Exercise*, 13:224–228, 1918.
138. Jacobs, A. Sport psychology, In E.R. Burke (Ed.) *The Science of Cycling*. Champaign, IL: Human Kinetics Publishers, Inc., 1986.
139. Jamieson, J.L. and N.F. Lavoie. Type A behavior, aerobic power, and cardiovascular recovery from a psychosocial stressor. *Health Psychology*, 6:361–371, 1987.
140. Jasnoski, M.L., D.S. Holmes, S. Solomon, and C. Aguiar. Exercise, changes in aerobic capacity, and changes in self-perceptions: An experimental investigation. *Journal of Research in Personality*, 15:460–466, 1981.
141. Johnson, T.H., D.G. Tharp. The effect of chronic exercise on reserpine-induced gastric ulceration in rats. *Medicine and Science in Sports*, 6:188–190, 1974.
142. Kane, J.E. Psychological correlates of physique and physical abilities. In E. Jokl and E. Simon (Eds.). *International Research in Sport and Physical Education*, 85–94. Springfield, IL: Charles C. Thomas Publishers, 1964.

143. Karasek, R.A., Jr. Job demands, job decision latitude, and mental strain: implications of job redesign. *Administrative Science Quarterly*, 24:285–308, 1979.
144. Kavanagh, T., R.J. Shephard, J.A. Tuck, and S. Quershi. Depression following myocardial infarction: The effects of distance running. *Annals of the New Nork Academy of Sciences*, 301:1029–1038, 1977.
145. Keller, S. Physical fitness hastens recovery from emotional stress. *Medicine and Science in Sports and Exercise*, 12:118, 1980.
146. Keller, S. and P. Seraganian. Physical fitness level and autonomic reactivity to psychosocial stress. *Journal of Psychosomatic Research*, 28:279–287, 1984.
147. Kendzierski, D. and V.D. LaMastro. Reconsidering the role of attitudes in exercise behavior: a decision theoretic approach. *Journal of Applied Social Psychology*, (In Press).
148. Kinsman, R.A., P.L. Weiser and D.A. Stamper. Multidimensional analysis of subjective symptomatology during prolonged strenuous exercise. *Ergonomics*, 16:211–226, 1973.
149. Kittel, F., M. Kornitzer, G. Debacker et al. Type A in relation to job stress, social and bioclinical variables: The Belgian physical fitness study. *Journal of Human Stress*, December, 37–45, 1983.
150. Klein, M.H., J. H. Greist, A.S.Gurman, R.A. Neimeyer, D.P. Lesser, N.J. Bushnell and R.E. Smith. A comparative outcome study of group psychotherapy vs. exercise treatments for depression. *International Journal of Mental Health*, 13(3–4), 148–177, 1985.
151. Knapp, D., M. Gutmann, C. Foster et al. Self-motivation among 1984 Olympic speed-skating hopefuls and emotional response and adherence to training. *Medicine and Science in Sports and Exercise* (abstract), 16:114, 1984.
152. Kobasa, S.C., S. Maddi, and M.C. Puccetti. Personality and exercise as buffers in the stress-illness relationship. *Journal of Behavioral Medicine*, 5:391–404, 1982.
153. Kobasa, S.C., S.R. Maddi, M.C. Puccetti and M.A. Zola. Effectiveness of hardiness, exercise, and social support as resources against illness. *Journal of Psychomatic Research*, 29:525–533, 1985.
154. Kostrubala, T. *The Joy of Running*. New York: J.B. Lippincott, 1976.
155. Kowal, D.M., J.F. Patton, and J.A. Vogel. Psychological states and aerobic fitness of male and female recruits before and after basic training. *Aviation, Space, and Environmental Medicine*, 49:603–606, 1978.
156. Krueger, J.M., J. Walter, C.A. Ginarello, S.M. Wolff and L. Chedid. Sleep promoting effects of endogenous pyrogens (interleukin 1). *American Journal of Physiology*, 246:R994–R999, 1984.
157. Kupfer, D.J., D.E. Sewitch, L.H. Epstein, C. Bulik, C.R. McGowen and R. Robertson. Exercise and subsequent sleep in male runners: failure to support the slow wave sleep-mood-exercise hypothesis. *Neuropsychobiology*, 14:5–12, 1985.
158. Lake, B.W., E.C. Suarez, N. Schneiderman and N. Tocci. The type A behavior pattern physical fitness, and psychophysiological reactivity. *Health Psychology*, 4:169–187, 1985.
159. Lamb, D.R. *Physiology of Exercise* (2nd Ed). New York, Macmillan Publishing Company, 1984.
160. Landy, F.J. An opponent process theory of job satisfaction. *Journal of Applied Psychology*, 63:533–547, 1978.
161. Landy, F.J. *The psychology of work behavior* (3rd ed.). Homewood, IL: Dorsey Press, 1985.
162. Landy, F.J. and W.S. Becker. Motivation theory reconsidered. *Research in Organizational Behavior*, 9:1–38, 1987.
163. Lichtman, S. and E.G. Poser. The effects of exercise on mood and cognitive functioning. *Journal of Psychosomatic Research*, 27:43–52, 1983.
164. Lietzke, M.H. An analytical study of world and Olympic racing records. *Science*, 120, 333–339, 1954.
165. Light, K.C., P.A. Obrist, and S.A. James. Self-reported exercise levels and cardiovascular responses during rest and stress. *SPR Abstracts, Psychophysiology*, 21:586, 1984.
166. Lloyd, B.B. World running records as maximal performances. *Circulation Research*, Supplement 1, 20–21:218–226, 1967.
167. Lobitz, W.C., H.L. Brammel and S. Stoll. Physical exercise and anxiety management training for cardiac stress management in a non-patient population. *Journal of Cardiac Rehabilitation*, 3: 683–688, 1983.
168. Lobstein, D.D., B.J. Mosbacher and A.H. Ismail. Depression as a powerful discriminator between physically active and sedentary middle-aged men. *Journal of Psychosomatic Research*, 27:69–76, 1983.
169. Locke, E.A. and G.P. Latham. The application of goal setting to sports. *Journal of Sport Psychology*, 7: 205–222, 1985.
170. Locke, E.A., K.N. Shaw, L.M. Saari and G.P. Latham. Goal setting and task performance: 1969–1980. *Psychological Bulletin*, 90:125–152, 1981.
171. Londeree, B. and M.L. Moeschberger. Effect of age and other factors on maximal heart

rate. *Research Quarterly for Exercise and Sport*, 53:297–304, 1982.

172. Long, B.L. Aerobic conditioning and stress inoculation: A comparison of stress-management interventions. *Cognitive Therapy and Research*, 8:517–522, 1984.

173. Margraf, J., A. Ehlers and W.T. Roth. Sodium lactate influsions and panic attacks: A review and critique. *Psychosomatic Medicine*, 48:23–51, 1986.

174. Markoff, R.A., P. Ryan and T. Young. Endorphins and mood changes in long-distance running. *Medicine and Science in Sports and Exercise*, 14:11–15, 1982.

175. Martin, J.E. and P. Dubbert. Exercise applications and promotion in behavioral medicine: Current status and future directions. *Journal of Consulting and Clinical Psychology*, 50:1004–1017, 1982.

176. Martin, J.E., P.M. Dubbert, A.D. Kattell, J.K. Thompson, J.R. Raczynski, M. Lake, P.O. Smith, J.S. Webster, T. Sikova, and R.E. Cohen. The behavioral control of exercise in sedentary adults: Studies 1 through 6. *Journal of Consulting and Clinical Psychology*, 52:795–811, 1984.

177. May, J.R. and T. Veach. A psychological study of health, injury, and performance in athletes on the U.S. Alpine Ski Team. *The Physician and Sportsmedicine*, 13(10):111–116, 1985.

178. Mayou, A. A controlled trial of early rehabilitation after myocardial infarction. *Journal of Cardiac Rehabilitation*, 6:387–402, 1983.

179. McCann, I.L. and D.S. Holmes. Influence of aerobic exercise on depression. *Journal of Personality and Social Psychology*, 46:1142–1147, 1984.

180. McGowen, C.R., R.J. Robertson and L.H. Epstein. The effect of bicycle ergometer exercise at varying intensities on the heart rate, EMG, and mood state responses to a mental arithmetic stressor. *Research Quarterly for Exercise and Sport*, 56:131–137, 1985.

181. Michael, E. and S. Horvath. Psychological limits in athletic training. In F. Antonelli (Ed.). *Proceedings of the International Society of Sport Psychology World Congress in Sport Psychology*, Rome, Italy, 1965.

182. Mikal, K.V. Extraversion in adult runners. *Perceptual and Motor Skills*, 57:143–146, 1983.

183. Morgan, W.P. Affective beneficence of vigorous physical activity. *Medicine and Science in Sports and Exercise*, 17:94–100, 1985.

184. Morgan, W.P. Anxiety reduction following acute physical activity. *Psychiatric Annals*, 9:141–147, 1979.

185. Morgan, W.P. Negative addiction in runners. *The Physician and Sportsmedicine*, 7:57–70, 1979.

186. Morgan, W.P. Psychogenic factors and exercise metabolism: a review. *Medicine and Science in Sports and Exercise*, 17:309–317, 1985.

187. Morgan, W.P. Psychological factors influencing perceived exertion. *Medicine and Science in Sports*, 5:97–103, 1973.

188. Morgan, W.P. Psychophysiology of self-awareness during vigorous physical activity. *Research Quarterly for Exercise and Sport*, 52:385–427, 1981.

189. Morgan, W.P. The trait psychology controversy. *Research Quarterly for Exercise and Sport*, 50, 50–76, 1980.

190. Morgan, W.P. and G. Borg. Perception of effort in the prescription of physical activity. In T. Craig (Ed.) *The Humanistic and Mental Health Aspects of Sports, Exercise and Recreation.* American Medical Association, Chicago, p.126–129, 1976.

191. Morgan, W.P., D.R. Brown, J.S. Raglin, P.J. O'Connor and K.A. Ellickson. *Psychological monitoring of overtraining and staleness.* British Journal of Sports Medicine, (In Press).

192. Morgan, W.P. and D. Costill. Psychological characteristics of the marathon runner. *Journal of Sports Medicine and Physical Fitness*, 12:42–46, 1972.

193. Morgan, W.P. and S.N. Goldston. *Exercise and Mental Health.* Washington, D.C.: Hemisphere Publishing, (Eds.) 1987.

194. Morgan, W.P., K. Hirota, G.A. Weitz et al. Hypnotic perturbation of perceived exertion: Ventilatory consequences. *Am J Clin Hypn.*, 18:182–190, 1976.

195. Morgan, W.P., D.H. Horstman, A. Cymerman and J. Stokes. Facilitation of physical performance by means of a cognitive strategy. *Cog There Res.*, 7:251–264, 1983.

196. Morgan, W.P., Olson, E.B. and N.P. Pedersen. A rat model of psychopathology for use in exercise science. *Medicine and Science in Sports and Exercise*, 14:91–100, 1982.

197. Morgan, W.P. and M.L. Pollock. Psychologic characterization of the elite distance runner, *Ann NY Acad Sci*, 301:382–402, 1977.

198. Morgan, W.P. and M.L. Pollock. Physical activity and cardiovascular health: Psychological aspects. In F. Landry and W.A.R. Orban (Eds.), *Physical activity and human well-being.* Miami, FL: Symposia Specialists, Inc., 1978.

199. Morgan, W.P., P. Raven, B. Drinkwater and S.M. Horvath. Perceptual and metabolic responsivity to standard bicycle ergometry following various hypnotic suggestions. *International Journal of Clinical and Experimental Hypnosis*, 21:86–93, 1973.

350 *PERSPECTIVES IN EXERCISE*

200. Morgan, W.P., J.A. Roberts and A.D. Feinerman. Psychological effect of chronic physical activity. *Medicine and Science in Sports*, 2:213–217, 1970.
201. Morgan, W.P., J.A. Roberts and A.D. Feinerman. Psychological effect of acute physical activity. *Arch. Phys. Med. and Rehab.*, 52:422–425, 1971.
202. Morton, R.H. Comment on "An analysis of world records in three types of locomotion." *European Journal of Applied Physiology*, 53:324–327, 1984.
203. Muller, B. and H.E. Armstrong. A further note on the "running treatment" for anxiety. *Psychotherapy: Theory, Research, and Practice*, 12:385–387, 1975.
204. Naughton, J., J.G. Bruhn and M.T, Lategola. Effects of physical training on physiologic and behavioral characteristics of cardiac patients. *Archives of Physical Medicine and Rehabilitation*, 49:131–137, 1968.
205. Nideffer, R.M. *The Ethics and Practice of Applied Sport Psychology*. Ithaca, NY: Mouvement Publications, 1981.
206. Nideffer, R.M. and C.M. Keckner. A case study of improved athletic performance following the use of relaxation procedures. *Perceptual and Motor Skills*, 30:821–822, 1979.
207. Moble, B.J., C.M. Maresh and M. Ritchey. Comparison of exercisesensations between females and males. In J. Borms, M. Hebbelinick, and A. Venerando (Eds.) *Women and Sport*. S. Karger, Basel, Switzerland, p. 175–179, 1981.
208. Oldridge, N.G. Compliance and exercise in primary and secondary prevention of coronary heart disease: a review. *Preventive Medicine*, 11:56–70, 1982.
209. Oldridge, N.B., A.P. Donner, and C.W. Buck et al. Predictors of dropout from cardiac exercise rehabilitation: Ontario Exercise Heart Collaborative Study. *Am J. Card*, 51, 70–74, 1983.
210. Orwin, A. The running treatment: A preliminary communication on a new use for an old therapy (physical activity) in the agoraphobic syndrome. *British Journal of Psychiatry*, 122:175–179, 1973.
211. Orwin, A. Treatment of a situational phobia—a case for running. *British Journal of Psychiatry*, 125:95–98, 1974.
212. Pandolf, K. Perceived exertion. In R. Terjung *Ex. Sport Sci. Rev.*, Philadelphia, Franklin Institute Press, 2:1983.
213. Patton, J.F., W.P. Morgan and J.A. Vogel. Perceived exertion of absolute work during a military physical training program. *Eur J Appl Physiol*, 36:107–114, 1977.
214. Paxton, S.J., J. Trinder and I. Montgomery. Does aerobic fitness affect sleep? *Psychophysiology*, 20:320–324, 1983.
215. Perkins, K.A., P.M. Dubbert, J.E. Martin, M.E. Faulstich and J.K. Harris. Cardiovascular reactivity to psychological stress in aerobically trained versus untrained mild hypertensives and normotensives. *Health Psychology*, 5:407–421, 1986.
216. Peronnet, F., P. Blier, and G. Brisson et al. Relationship between trait-anxiety and plasma catecholamine concentration at rest and during exercise. *Medicine and Science in Sports and Exercise* (abstract), 14, 173, 1982.
217. Pert, C.B. and D.L. Bowie. Behavioral manipulations of rats causes alterations in opiate receptor occupancy. In E. Usdin, W.E. Bunney and N.S. Kline (Eds.) *Endorphins in Mental Health*. New York: Oxford University Press, p. 93–104, 1979.
218. Peyrin, L., and J.M. Pequignot. Free and conjugated 3-methoxy-4-hydroxyphenyl glycol in human urine: Peripheral origin of the glucuronide. *Psychopharmacology*, 79:16–20, 1983.
219. Pierce, D., I. Kupprat, and D. Harry. Urinary epinephrine and norephinephrine levels in women athletes during training and competition. *Europ J App Physiol.*, 36:1–6, 1976.
220. Pinel, J. and T. Schultz. Effect of antecedant muscle tension levels on motor behavior. *Medicine and Science in Sports*, 10:177–182, 1978.
221. Pollock, M.L. Prescribing exercise for fitness and adherence, In R.K. Dishman (Ed.) *Exercise Adherence: Its Impact on Public Health*. Human Kinetics Publishers, Champaign, IL, 1988.
222. Porter, L.W. and E.E. Lawler. *Managerial attitudes and performance*. Homewood, IL: Dorsey, 1968.
223. Post, R.M. and J.L. Ballenger. *Neurobiology of mood disorders*. Williams and Wilkins, Baltimore, 1984.
224. Post, R.M., J. Kotin, F.K. Goodwin. Psychomotor activity and cerbrospinal fluid amine metabolites in affective illness. *American Journal of Psychiatry*, 130:67–72, 1973.
225. Prosser, G., P. Carson, and R. Phillips. Morale in coronary patients following an exercise program. *Journal of Psychosomatic Research*, 25:587–593, 1981.
226. Purvis, J. and K. Cureton. Ratings of perceived exertion at the anaerobic threshold. *Ergonomics*, 24:295–300, 1981.
227. Rejeski, W.J., D. Morely and H.S. Miller. The Jenkins Activity Survey: Exploring its relationship with compliance to exercise prescription and MET gain within a cardiac rehabilitation setting. *Journal of Cardiac Rehabilitation*, 4:90–94, 1984.

PSYCHOLOGICAL FACTORS AND PROLONGED EXERCISE **351**

228. Riegel, P.S. Athletic records and human performance. *American Scientist*, 69(3):281–291, 1981.
229. Risch, S.C. and D. Pickar. Symposium on endorphins. *Psych. Clin. N. Am.*, 6(3):363–521, 1983.
230. Robbins, J.M. and P. Joseph. Experiencing exercise withdrawl: Possible consequences of therapeutic and mastery running. *Journal of Sport Psychology*, 7:23–39, 1985.
231. Robertson, R.J., R.L. Gillespie, J. McCarthy and K.D. Rose. Perceived exertion and the field independence dimension. *Perceptual and Motor Skills*, 46:495–500, 1978.
232. Robertson, R.J., R.L. Gillespie, J. McCarthy and K.D. Rose. Perceived exertion and stimulus intensity modulation. *Perceptual and Motor Skills*, 45:211–218, 1977.
233. Robins, L.N., J.E. Helzer, M.M. Weissman, H. Orvaschel, E. Gruenberg, J.D. Burke, and D.A. Regier. Lifetime prevalence of specific psychiatric disorders in three sites. *Archives of General Psychiatry*, 41:949–958, 1984.
234. Roskies, E., P. Seraganian, R. Oseasohn, J.A. Hanley, R. Collu, N. Martin and C. Smilga. The montreal Type A Intervention Project: Major Findings. *Health Psychology*, 5:45–69, 1986.
235. Roth, D.L. and D.S. Holmes. Influence of physical fitness on determining the impact of stressful life events on physical and psychological health. *Psychosomatic Medicine*, 47:164–173, 1985.
236. Roviaro, S., D.S. Holmes and R.D. Homsten. Influence of a cardiac rehabilitation program on the cardiovascular, psychological, and social functioning of cardiac patients. *Journal of Behavioral Medicine*, 7:61–81, 1984.
237. Rumball, W.M. and C.E. Coleman. Analysis of running and the prediction of ultimate performance. *Nature*, 228:184, 1970.
238. Russell, P.O., L.H. Epstein and K.T. Erickson. Effects of acute exercise and cigarette smoking on autonomic and neuromuscular responses to a cognitive stressor. *Psychological Reports*, 53:199–206, 1983.
239. Ryan, E.D. and R. Foster. Athletic participation and perceptual augmentation and reduction. *Journal of Personality and Social Psychology*, 6:472–476, 1967.
240. Ryan, E.D. and C.R. Kovacic. Pain tolerance and athletic participation. *Perceptual Motor Skills*, 22:383–390, 1966.
241. Ryder, H.W., H.J. Carr and P. Herget. Future performance in footracing. *Scientific American*, 234:109–119, 1976.
242. Sacks, M.H. and M.L. Sachs. *Psychology of running*. Champaign, IL: Human Kinetics Publishers, (Eds.) 1981.
243. Sallis, J.F., W.L. Haskell, S.P. Fortmann, K.M. Vranizan C.B. Taylor and D.S. Solomon. Psychological predictors of adoption and maintenance of physical activity in a community sample. *Preventive Medicine*, 15:331–341, 1986.
244. Saltin, B. and P. Gollnick. Skeletal muscle adaptability and significance for metabolism and performance. *Handbook of Physiology*, Bethesda, MD: Am Physiol Soc., 555–631, 1987.
245. Scanlan, T.K. and M.W. Passer. Factors related to competitive stress among male youth sport participants. *Med Sci Sports*, 10:103–108, 1978.
246. Scanlan, T.K. and M.W. Passer. Factors influencing the competitive performance expectancies of young female atheletes. *J of Sport Psy*, 1:151–159, 1979.
247. Schwartz, G.E., R.J. Davidson and D. Coleman. Patterning of cognitive and somatic processes in the self-regulation of anxiety: effects of meditation versus exercise. *Psychosomatic Medicine*, 40:321–328, 1978.
248. Schwartz, G.E., D. Weinberger and J.A. Singer. Cardiovascular differentation of happiness, sadness, anger and fear following imagery and exercise. *Journal of Psychosomatic Medicine*, 43:343, 1981.
249. Severtsen, B. and M.A. Bruya. Effects of meditation and aeronic exercise of EEG patterns. *Journal of Neuroscience Nursing*, 18:206–210, 1986.
250. Sforzo, G.A., T.F. Seeger, C.B. Pert, A. Pert and C.O. Dotson. In vivo opioid receptor occupation in the rat brain following exercise. *Medicine and Science in Sports and Exercise*, 18:380–384, 1986.
251. Shapiro, C.M. R. Bortz, D. Mitchell P. Bartel, and P. Jooste. Slow wave sleep: a recovery period after exercise. *Science*, 214: 1253–1254, 1981.
252. Shapiro, S. E.A. Skinner, L.G. Kessler et al. Utilization of health and mental health services. *Archives of General Psychiatry*, 41:971–978, 1984.
253. Shephard, R.J. T. Kavanagh and P. Klavora. Mood state during postcoronary cardiac rehabilitation. *Journal of Cardiopulmonary Rehabilitation*, 5:480–484, 1985.
254. Shulhan, D., H. Sher and J. Furedy. Phasic cardiac reactivity to psychological stress as a function of aerobic fitness level. *Psychophysiology*, 23:562–566, 1986.
255. Siconolfi, S.F., C.E. Garber, G.D. Baptist et al. Hemodynamic effects of mental stress during exercise in coronary artery disease patients. *Medicine and Science in Sports and Exercise* (abstract), 16:140, 1984.

256. Sime, W. A comparison of exercise and meditation in reducing physiological response to stress. *Medicine and Science in Sports and Exercise* (abstract), 9:55, 1977.

257. Sinyor, D., M. Golden, Y. Steinert and P. Seraganian. Experimental manipulation of aerobic fitness and the response to psychological stress: Heart rate and self-report measures. *Psychosomatic Medicine*, 48:324–337, 1986.

258. Sinyor, D.A., Schwartz, S.G., and Peronnet, F. (1983). Aerobic fitness level and reactivity to psychosocial stress: Physiological, biochemical, and subjective measures. *Psychosomatic Medicine*, 45:205–217.

259. Skubic, E., and Hilgendorf, J. (1964). Anticipatory, exercise, and recovery heart rates of girls as affected by four running events. *Journal of Applied Physiology*, 19:853–856.

260. Smutok, M.A., Skrinar, G.S., and Pandolf, K.B., (1980). Exercise intensity: subjective regulation by perceived exertion. *Arch. Phys. Med. Rehab.*, 61:569–574.

261. Solomon, R.L. (1980). The opponent process theory of acquired motivation. *American Psychologist*, 35:691–712.

262. Sonstroem, R.J. (1984). Exercise and self-esteem. In R. Terjung (Ed.), *Exercise and Sport Sciences Reviews*, 12:100–130.

263. Sothmann, M.S., Horn, T.S., Hart, B.A., and Gustafson, A.B. (1987). Comparison of discrete cardiovascular fitness groups on plasma catecholamine and selected behavioral responses to psychological stress. *Psychophysiology*, 24:47–54.

264. Sothmann, M.S., and Ismail, A.H. (1985). Factor analytic derivation of the MHPG/NM ratio: Implications for studying the link between physical fitness and depression. *Biological Psychiatry*, 20:570–583.

265. Sothmann, M.S. and Ismail, A.H. (1984). Relationships between urinary catecholamines, metabolites, particularly MHPG, and selected personality and physical fitness characteristics in normal subjects. *Psychosomatic Medicine*, 46:523–533.

266. Sothmann, M.S., Ismail, A.H., and Chodzko-Zajko, W.J. (1984). The influence of catecholamine activity on hierarchical associations involving physical fitness and personality. *Journal of Clinical Psychology*, 40:1308–1317.

267. Starzec, J.J., Berger, D.F., and Hesse, R. (1983). Effects of stress and exercise on plasma corticosterone, plasma cholesterol, and aortic cholesterol levels in rats. *Psychosomatic Medicine*, 45:219–226.

268. Stephens, T., Jacobs, D.R., and White, C.C. (1985). A descriptive epidemiology of leisuretime physical activity. *Public Health Reports*, 100:147–158.

269. Stern, J.J., Gorman, P.A., and Kaslow, K.L. (1983). The group counseling and exercise therapy study. *Archives of Internal Medicine*, 143:1719–1725.

270. Stern, M. and Cleary, P. (1981). National Exercise and Heart Disease Project: Psychosocial changes observed during a low level exercise program. *Archives of Internal Medicine*, 141:1463–1467.

271. Stern, M.J., and Cleary, P. (1982). The national exercise and heart disease project: long term psychosocial outcome. *Archives of Internal Medicine*, 142:1093–1097.

272. Stone, E.A. (1973). Accumulation and metabolism of norepinephrine in rat hypothalamines after exhaustive stress. *Journal of Neurochemistry*, 21:589–601.

273. Stones, M.J. and Kozma, A. (1984). In response to Hartley and Hartley: Cross-sectional age trends in swimming records; decline is greater at the longer distances. *Experimental Aging Research*, 10:149–150.

274. Strnad, J. (1985). Physics of long-distance running. *American Journal of Physiology*, 53:371–373.

275. Suinn, R. (1972). Behavior rehearsal training for ski racers. *Behavior Therapy*, 3:519.

276. Sweeney, D.R., Leckman, J.F., Maas, J.W., Hattox, S., and Herringer, G.R. (1980). Plasma free and conjugated MHPG in psychiatric patients. *Archives of General Psychiatry*, 37:1100–1103.

277. Sweeney, D.R., Maas, J.W., and Heninger, G.R. (1978). State anxiety, physical activity, and urinary 3-methoxy-4-hydroxyphenethylene glycol excretions. *Archives of General Psychiatry*, 35:1418–1423.

278. Tang, S.W., Stancer, H.C., Takahashi, S., Shephard, R.J., and Warsh, J.J. (1980). Controlled exercise elevates plasma but not urinary MHPG and VMA. *Psychiatry Research*, 4:13–20.

279. Tharp, G.D. and Carson, W.H. (1975). Emotionality changes in rats following chronic exercise. *Medicine and Science in Sports*, 7:123–126.

280. Thaxton, L. (1982). Physiological and psychological effects of short-term exercise addiction on habitual runners. *Journal of Sport Psychology*, 4:73–80.

281. Thompson, C.E. and Wankel, C.M. (1980). The effects of perceived activity choice upon frequency of exercise behavior. *Journal of Applied Social Psychology*, 10:436–444.

282. Thompson, J.K., and Blanton, P. (1987). Energy conservation and exercise dependence: a sympathetic arousal hypothesis. *Medicine and Science in Sports and Exercise*, 19:91–99.

PSYCHOLOGICAL FACTORS AND PROLONGED EXERCISE **353**

283. Torsvall, A., Akerstedt, T., and Lindbeck, G. (1984). Effects of sleep stages and EEG power density of different degrees of exercise in fit subjects. *Electroencephalography and Clinical Neurophysiology*, 57:347–353.
284. Trinder, J., Paxton, S.J., Montgomery, I., and Fraser, G. (1985). Endurance as opposed to power training: Their effect on sleep. *Psychophysiology*, 22:668–673.
285. Trinder, J., Stevenson, J., Paxton, S.J., and Montgomery, I. (1982). Physical fitness, exercise, and REM sleep cycle length. *Psychophysiology*, 19:89–93.
286. Usdin, E., Bunney, W.E., and Kline, N.S. (Eds.) (1979). *Endorphins in mental health research*. Oxford University Press, New York.
287. Vroom, V. (1964). *Work and motivation*. New York: Wiley.
288. Wankel, L.M. (1984). Decision-making and social support strategies for increasing exercise adherence. *Journal of Cardiac Rehabilitation*, 4:124–135.
289. Wardlaw, S.L. and Frantz, A.G. (1980). Effect of swimming stress on brain B-endorphin and ACTH. *Clinical Research*, (abstract), 28:482.
290. Weber, J.C. and Lee, R.A. (1968). Effects of differing prepuberty exercise programs on the emotionality of male albino rats. *Research Quarterly*, 39:748–751.
291. Weinberg, R.S., Bruya, L.D., and Jackson, A.W. (1985). The effects of goal proximity and specificity on endurance performance. *Journal of Sport Psychology*, 7:296–305.
292. Weinberg, R.S., Smith, J., Jackson, A., and Gould, D. (1984). Effect of association, dissocation, and positive self-talk strategies on endurance performance. *Canadian Journal of Applied Sport Sciences*, 9:25–32.
293. Wiese, J., Singh, M. and Yeudall, L. (1983). Occipital and parietal alpha power before, during, and after exercise. *Medicine and Science in Sports and Exercise*, (abstract), 15:117.
294. Wilmore, J.H., Roby, F.B., Stanforth, R.R., et al. (1985). Ratings of perceived exertion, heart rate, and treadmill speed in the prediction of maximal oxygen uptake during submaximal treadmill exercise. *Journal of Cardiopulmonary Rehabilitation*, 5:540–546.
295. Yates, A., Leehey, K., and Shisslak, C. (1983). Running—an analogue of anorexia? *New England Journal of Medicine*, 308:(5), 251–255.
296. Ziegler, S.G., Klinzing, J., and Williamson, K. (1982). The effects of the stress management training programs on cardiorespiratory efficiency. *Journal of Sport Psychology*, 4:280–289.

DISCUSSION

LANDY: Allow me to address a couple of experimental design issues that are pertinent. One is that the sample sizes for the most part in a lot of studies are atrocious. The possibility of detecting a difference between Group A and Group B, or demonstrating covariation between variable A and variable B is vanishingly small. You are looking for modest effects that might account for 10 to 20% of the variance. In your wildest imagination, that's how much variance you are going to have to account for. The question then becomes, "Is a nonsignificant effect trivial?" If you need sample sizes in the range of 100 or 200 or 300, should we be messing around with this anyway, because the effect must be trivial? The answer is, "Yes," we should be messing around with this for two reasons.

First, for the scientist, no systematic variance is trivial. And secondly, for the elite athlete, if all other things were held constant, such as ability, training programs, and environmental conditions, and if the only systematic variation then turned out to be the variation in cognitive constructs in goals that are set, or in perceptions or expectations, that variance is magnified enormously, and it is that variation that will separate first place from last.

BLAIR: I would like to comment on the adherence story that Rod told us about and simply point out that he told it from a clinical perspective, that is, "Who dropped out of exercise programs?" There is another side to the issue, which I would call a public health aspect of adherence. An analogy can be drawn from the smoking literature. If you read the recidivism rate in smoking cessation programs, you find that for years it was around 20% who remained nonsmokers after a year; 80% who had quit smoking became recidivists. That's a very pessimistic view, just as I think our clinical view of exercise is very pessimistic. But, if you take the public health view and realize there are now 50 million ex-smokers out there, some people are quitting and staying quit. And if you look at the joggers and tennis players, a lot of people are starting to exercise and continuing to exercise. I urge us to take a population-based view with a defined population and to monitor the exercise adoption and maintenance within that population. I think that it gives a more optimistic view than focusing just on the clinical studies.

DISHMAN: Based on available technology, I think the estimates of population physical activity probably aren't any more encouraging than those for supervised samples of subjects.

BLAIR: Well, the rates are low, but if you are looking at a starting point, there were 2% active 20 years ago, and it's now increased five-fold. That's not trivial.

DISHMAN: The only problem is that the percentage of the population which is sedentary has not changed. We've still got approximately 40% since the early '70s data that, by best estimate, aren't doing anything. I'd like to see more people trying to do more things.

LANDERS: Much of the literature reviewed is focused on the cognitive model and not so much on the sociocultural. Rod did at least incorporate in his model some of the social and environmental factors. But is seemed more of it was social structures and physical structures in the environment that could be a carrier of the message rather than the influence that stirs to action. If everyone else gets caught up in the fitness boom, people will say, "Well, everyone else is doing it, maybe I can do it, too." I don't think we have really got a good handle on that, but I think we should be aware of it.

8

Training for Performance of Prolonged Exercise

CHRISTINE L. WELLS, PH.D.

RUSSELL R. PATE, PH.D.

INTRODUCTION
I. PRINCIPLES OF TRAINING FOR PROLONGED EXERCISE
   A.   Background
   B.   Physiologic Rationale
       1.   Maximal Oxygen Uptake
       2.   Economy of Motion
       3.   Lactate Threshold
       4.   Fractional Utilization of $\dot{V}O_2$max
       5.   Fuel Supply
   C.   Training Techniques
       1.   Long Slow Distance (LSD)
       2.   Aerobic Interval Training
       3.   Pace/Tempo Training
       4.   Anaerobic Interval Training
       5.   Weight Training
II. CURRENT TRAINING REGIMENS
   A.   Running
       1.   Training Systems
       2.   Current Approaches
   B.   Swimming
       1.   Unique Determinants of Swimming Performance
       2.   Training for Swimming
   C.   Cycling
III. SPECIAL TRAINING PROBLEMS
   A.   Overtraining
   B.   Detraining/Retention of Training
       1.   Detraining
       2.   Retention of Training Effects
   C.   Tapering/Peaking

SUMMARY
BIBLIOGRAPHY
DISCUSSION

INTRODUCTION

"Training" might be defined as systematic and regular participation in exercise for the purpose of enhancing sports performance.
Our current beliefs about appropriate training have evolved over a
very long period and are based largely on the experiences of many
thousands of athletes and coaches. This chapter is intended to provide a review of the scientific literature on training for enhanced
performance in long duration, endurance sports. However, it should
be noted that scientific inquiry has had, at best, a limited impact on
the training practices of successful endurance athletes. To date, sport
scientists have focused much of their efforts on explaining why al-
ready-accepted training practices result in enhanced performance.
Far less frequently have "scientific breakthroughs," arising from the
laboratory, precipitated major changes in accepted training practices.

The circumstance described above constitutes a central premise
upon which this chapter is based. Appropriate training, we believe,
is not purely a scientific endeavor, and it would be fallacious of us
to present it as such. Certainly we believe that scientific studies have
contributed to our understanding of training, and certainly we believe that future studies hold out the hope of helping us solve the
many issues that currently confront endurance athletes. However,
we must recognize and emphasize that, to date, conscientious and
enlightened observations of field-based experiences by coaches and
athletes have had by far the greatest impact on the training practices
of endurance athletes. It is our hope that this somewhat humbling
observation will aid the reader in placing the material in this chapter
in proper perspective. Our primary focus will be on "the scientific
literature." However, we shall endeavor to keep our bearings by
noting the many limitations of the current scientific literature, and
by citing some of the contributions of noteworthy coaches and athletes.

The specific purposes of this chapter are: (1) to review the principles of endurance training and the physiologic bases that underlie
them, (2) to describe currently-accepted approaches to training for
enhanced performance for long distance running, cycling and swimming, and (3) to examine several of the special training problems
that confront endurance athletes.

I. PRINCIPLES OF TRAINING FOR PROLONGED EXERCISE

A. Background

Many physiological responses or reactions occur as a result of acute physical stress. The exercise and medical physiology literature is replete with descriptions of these responses. This literature includes descriptions of respiratory, circulatory, endocrine, nervous, muscular, renal, and thermoregulatory deviations from the baseline, resting condition. These responses can usually be classified as either morphological or biochemical deviations from the resting state. In some cases these physiological responses to exercise have been monitored continuously throughout the period of exercise and until the resting state is once again attained following a period of recovery. But more often, the responses of interest to the investigator(s) have been monitored only at selected time periods during or immediately following the exercise. With the gradual development of improved technology, investigations of various responses to acute exercise have progressed from purely descriptive designs toward examinations of causation and underlying mechanisms. Through such studies we have learned much about the responses in various organisms, systems, organs, and tissues that result from the acute physical stress of exercise.

Unfortunately, we know far less about how acute responses to exercise *change* with the application of training (i.e., chronic exercise). While we know that there is often a general improvement (sometimes remarkable) in physical performance capacity with regularly performed vigorous exercise, we know relatively little about the rate at which these changes occur or about the interrelationships among the changes that develop in various tissues or systems. Much research effort has been directed toward the study of the effects of various forms of chronic exercise on muscle function (mostly strength and endurance), muscle metabolic variables, cardiorespiratory responses to exercise, thermoregulation and endocrine control factors. Through this research, we have learned much about the system-specific, organ-specific and tissue-specific adaptations to training. However, because few of the completed training studies have been truly comprehensive, we lack a clear understanding of the *interrelationships* among the various training adaptations.

This deficiency in the scientific literature is unfortunate because it limits our ability to apply the findings of basic research studies to the athlete who seeks to optimize performance. Perhaps what is needed to overcome this deficiency is a more interdisciplinary approach to the study of training than has been possible in the past.

Our current knowledge and technology should allow for the study of carefully selected questions regarding the relationships among the individual training adaptations identified by previous research. In our opinion, exercise and sport science are at important crossroads. Considerable research effort should now be directed toward study of the organism as an integrated whole, rather than as a set of independent tissues or organ systems. This approach should facilitate development of a closer relationship between basic exercise science and applied sport science.

B. Physiologic Rationale

Prolonged exercise performance is limited by the ability of metabolic processes to provide a continuous supply of adenosine triphosphate (ATP) to the contractile complex of the active muscle fibers. This requires adequate "fueling of the metabolic process" (56), and removal of metabolic end-products. These processes operate in a highly integrated fashion, and both are important in prolonged exercise performance. Centrally, an efficient oxygen transport system, characterized by a well-developed heart and vascular system, seems vital for success (18,44). Peripherally, a high relative proportion of type I (slow twitch, oxidative) muscle fibers, highly active heart-specific lactate dehydrogenase (H-LDH) in skeletal muscles, and high capillary density in muscle for elite-level performance in prolonged exercise appear to be important (42,75,77). The extent to which these factors are "trainable," as opposed to genetically determined, is a topic of considerable current discussion.

Many studies have attempted to identify the physiologic variables that are the most important determinants of endurance performance. Typically, this has been approached by correlating a number of factors with a performance measure and assuming that the variables most highly correlated with that measure are the most important determinants of that performance. For example, there are studies dealing with the relationships of numerous variables to long-distance running performance in children and adults. Sjodin and Svedenhag (77) have applied this approach in their extensive review of the determinants of marathon running performance. They identify and describe variables that are significantly related to performance of endurance running. These include:

1) maximal oxygen uptake ($\dot{V}O_2$max)
2) economy of motion
3) lactate threshold
4) fractional utilization of $\dot{V}O_2$max (% $\dot{V}O_2$max)
5) fuel supply.

Since these variables probably relate to performance of all prolonged exercise activities, we shall use this list as the basis for a review of specific training methods used for prolonged exercise. Following are brief descriptions and discussions of each of these key factors.

1. **Maximal Oxygen Uptake.** Maximal oxygen uptake ($\dot{V}O_2$max), the greatest rate at which oxygen can be consumed during exercise, is a reflection of the individual's maximal rate of aerobic energy expenditure. Substantial evidence indicates that $\dot{V}O_2$max is a key determinant of endurance exercise performance. $\dot{V}O_2$max in elite marathon runners usually exceeds 70 mL $\cdot$ kg^{-1} $\cdot$ min^{-1}, and $\dot{V}O_2$max values are significantly different among groups of elite, good, and slow runners. Correlations between $\dot{V}O_2$max and marathon race pace range between 0.63 and 0.91. Somewhat higher $\dot{V}O_2$max values are found for elite middle-distance runners, who perform at faster race paces than marathon (or ultramarathon) runners. Therefore, while a high maximal oxygen uptake is of considerable importance for endurance running performance, it is probably not as important a factor for marathon performance as it is for shorter duration, faster paced long-distance running, e.g., 5,000- or 10,000-meter distances. When groups of marathon runners who have similar performance times are studied, little correlation between performance and $\dot{V}O_2$max is found. This observation suggests that factors other than $\dot{V}O_2$max must be responsible for performance differences among relatively homogeneous groups of endurance runners.

2. **Economy of Motion.** Economy, defined as the oxygen uptake required to produce a specific rate of power output or speed of movement, may vary considerably among subjects with similar $\dot{V}O_2$max values. Better economy of motion is advantageous in endurance performance because a lower oxygen cost of movement is associated with a lower % $\dot{V}O_2$max at any rate of power output and with a slower rate of utilization of energy stores. Exceptionally good running economy has been observed in some outstanding marathon runners. As with $\dot{V}O_2$max, however, within a subgroup of runners who have similar performance times, running economy and performance are not highly correlated. Although not a consistent finding, both Costill (13) and Pollock (67) have reported significantly lower oxygen costs of running in marathon runners than in runners who specialize in competitive shorter distances. In comparing long with middle distance runners, Sjodin and Svedenhag (77) suggested that the better running economy of the longer distance runners helps them compensate for their lower $\dot{V}O_2$max values. As a result, long and middle distance runners demonstrate similar relationships between running speed and relative exercise intensity (% $\dot{V}O_2$max). In endurance sports, such as cycling and swimming, which involve

novel motor skills, economy may vary more among athletes than is the case for running. If this is the case, economy may be more highly correlated with performance in these activities.

3. **Lactate Threshold.** Terms such as "onset of blood lactate accumulation" (OBLA) and "lactate threshold" have been used to describe the kinetics of lactate accumulation during steady-state submaximal exercise (43). In this chapter, the term lactate threshold (LT) will be used to denote this phenomenon. Lactate threshold may be operationally defined as the speed of movement, e.g., running, swimming or cycling speed, or % $\dot{V}O_2$max at which a specific blood lactate concentration, e.g. 4 mM, is observed, or as the exercise intensity at which lactate first increases above resting concentration of approximately 1.0 mM. Ventilatory measures have been used to determine "ventilatory anaerobic threshold" (V_{Ant}) which, in most subjects, occurs at an exercise intensity similar to that for LT.

Regardless of how it is measured or estimated, there is a close relationship between lactate threshold and endurance performance. Correlations from 0.88 to 0.99 have been reported between LT and running times for races from 3.2 km to half marathon distance (77). Sjodin and Svedenhag (77) reported correlations from 0.94 to 0.98 between LT and marathon speed. Since lactate accumulation in blood and muscle has long been associated with fatigue, it is not surprising that LT correlates highly with performance of prolonged exercise. The exercise intensity at LT reflects the highest exercise intensity that the athlete can sustain for an extended period without accumulating limiting amounts of lactate.

4. **Fractional Utilization of $\dot{V}O_2$max.** Very high correlations ($r = 0.92$ to 0.94) have been reported between % $\dot{V}O_2$max at a specific submaximal treadmill running speed and mean marathon race pace in good and elite marathon runners (77). This close relationship no doubt occurs because % $\dot{V}O_2$max reflects the effects of both $\dot{V}O_2$max and running economy, each of which is independently related, albeit imperfectly, to performance. The lower an athlete's % $\dot{V}O_2$max at any movement speed, the greater the speed will be at the lactate threshold.

Fractional utilization of $\dot{V}O_2$max during distance running is dependent on the distance run (14), ambient temperature and humidity (13), altitude, body fluid losses (14), age or number of years of endurance training (16), and other factors. At marathon running race pace, % $\dot{V}O_2$max has been reported to vary between 86% in top level athletes (13) and 75% to 76% in performers who complete the 42.2 km distance in 2:46 to 3:12 (28,85). The fractional utilization of $\dot{V}O_2$max at marathon race pace is determined by two factors: (1) the percentage of the $\dot{V}O_2$max utilized at lactate threshold, and (2) the percentage of running speed at LT utilized (77). Marathon runners of differing abilities run at different percentages of the running speed at LT. Sjodin and Jacobs (76) reported a significant correlation (0.86) between performance time and percentage of running speed at LT for marathon race pace. It is also well known that LT occurs at a higher % $\dot{V}O_2$max in more highly trained endurance athletes (43).

   5. Fuel Supply. A prolonged period of exercise at a high power output is very costly in terms of total energy expenditure. It has been estimated that the energy expenditure for marathon running ranges between 9,000 to 12,000 kJ and that the rate of energy expenditure is roughly 75 kJ $\cdot$ min^{-1} (77). Muscle glycogen may be utilized more readily than blood glucose or fatty acids and seems to be used preferentially for the first 85 min of prolonged exercise, at which time the muscle glycogen is substantially depleted. Glucose and fatty acids provided to the muscles by the circulation become more important during the latter stages of prolonged exercise. At high exercise intensities, there is a greater reliance on carbohydrate than lipid substrates, but more highly adapted endurance athletes make greater use of fat for energy during submaximal exercise. A major benefit is conservation of muscle and liver glycogen stores (56). The onset of fatigue is closely associated with glycogen depletion in the active motor units (56).

   In summary, physiological requirements for high level performance in prolonged exercise include the following:

1) a high, but not necessarily exceptional, $\dot{V}O_2$max;
2) good economy of motion;
3) a high lactate threshold;
4) the ability to perform at a high % $\dot{V}O_2$max for a prolonged period;
5) ability to utilize fat as a metabolic substrate at a high rate (so as to spare muscle and liver glycogen).

C. Training Techniques

   In planning a training program for enhancement of performance of prolonged exercise, the athlete and coach must seek answers to the following questions:

1. What physiological and psychological demands will be placed on the athlete, and what is the athlete's ability to meet those demands? For example, to meet performance objectives, how much improvement will be required in the athlete's muscular strength, muscular endurance, $\dot{V}O_2$max, lactate threshold, and anaerobic capacity? Are these improvement requirements reasonable for this athlete?

2. What muscles are involved in the movements performed, and exactly how do these muscles contribute to the performance, i.e., as prime movers, synergists, or stabilizers? What forms of contraction are utilized by each active group of muscles, i.e., concentric, eccentric, or static? Are sudden powerful contractions required, or are the movements of a less intense, more sustained quality?
3. What environmental stress will be encountered, e.g., extremes in air or water temperature, relative humidity, wind, rain, or altitude? What will be the fluid replacement demands? What, if anything, should be consumed to maintain substrate supply for energy production?
4. Should the training program capitalize on the athlete's strengths or attempt to counteract or reduce weaknesses?
5. How intensely should the athlete train? What volume of training should be accomplished? When should rest periods be employed? What is the proper amount of training and the proper amount of rest for each athlete? How can injury be avoided? When is the athlete too tired?

Obviously, the coach and athlete are in need of great insight and, perhaps a well-polished crystal ball! The questions listed above provide for a careful analysis of training needs for endurance sport performance. Central to this analysis is adherence to the general principles of "overload" and "specificity." Ultimately, in applying these principles, one must design appropriate, specific training protocols and organize them in an effective manner.

In this section, we briefly describe several popular training techniques. The techniques described are "generic," in that they are used to a greater or lesser extent in most endurance sports. In discussing each training technique, we shall describe, in general terms, the physiologic adaptations we deem likely to result from the technique. Table 8-1 provides a more detailed listing of the physiologic adaptations that may accrue from each technique. However, we emphasize that the scientific literature pertaining to the *unique* effects of specific training procedures on functional capacities in *already trained persons* is very fragmentary. As was noted in the introduction to this chapter, endurance athletes train the way they do primarily because they and their predecessors have found empirically that certain techniques are effective.

Current knowledge of the physiologic basis of endurance training provides some good clues as to why specific procedures seem to be effective for highly trained athletes. Excellent reviews of the physiologic adaptations to endurance training have been presented elsewhere (9,26,48,69,70,71,72). The material in the following paragraphs and the summary provided in Table 8-1 reflects the authors' interpretations, interpolations, and extrapolations, of this scientific literature.

   1. **Long Slow Distance.** In long, slow distance (LSD) training, emphasis is on long distances that are covered at an easy and relaxing pace. LSD is usually recommended once a week, or once every two weeks, to aid in the establishment of a sound "aerobic base." For running the 10-km distance, LSD training in the range of 25 to 30 km is recommended; for the marathon, LSD training of distances up to 32 to 50 km is often utilized. Depending upon the nature of the swim for which the athlete is training, LSD swim training may be 5 to 10 km, often in open water. For cycling, LSD training may involve 130 to 250 km of cycling at a low gear ratio (spinning), depending on the terrain (hills) and environmental (wind) conditions.

   The athlete should practice the fluid replacement techniques planned for competition during LSD training sessions. This not only avoids possible problems associated with heat stress and fatigue, but allows the athlete to experiment with various fluid replacement protocols that may enhance performance. Long slow distance training is obviously done to promote endurance. Its unique physiologic benefits ascribed to LSD training include enhancement of cardiovascular function, i.e., oxygen delivery to the active muscle cells, enhancement of thermoregulatory function (heat acclimatization), enhancement of mitochondrial function and oxidative capacity of skeletal muscles, and enhancement of the body's ability to mobilize fatty acids from adipose tissue and use them as fuel in aerobic metabolism. Also, LSD training probably aids in the development of endurance in supporting musculature.

   The psychological benefits of LSD running may be substantial. Many athletes have cited the "mental toughness" that results, and others note an increased ability to concentrate and relax when fatigued. A major benefit may be development of confidence in one's ability to cover a very long competitive distance.

   The benefits of training that may be specific to LSD training include improvements in anaerobic threshold performance economy, fractional utilization of $\dot{V}O_2$max and fat utilization with corresponding "glycogen sparing." Also, LSD training probably aids in the development of endurance in supporting musculature. Often the regular mileage of daily practice does not sufficiently tax supporting or secondary musculature. First attempts at LSD training often reveal these shortcomings, which can be overcome with futher utilization of this training technique.

   Because LSD training is merely one part of a well-planned training program it is impossible to be absolutely certain about the specific physiological benefits that accrue from it. However, it seems logical to suggest that LSD training provides a "volume load" (as opposed to a "pressure load") (9) on the heart, that stimulates improved myocardial function and increased peripheral conductance via a reduction in vascular resistance to blood flow. The end result would be improved cardiac output and stroke volume with enhanced ability to deliver oxygen and remove metabolic wastes from active tissues. An improved sweating capacity to aid in the dissipation of metabolic heat also accompanies LSD training.

In addition, LSD training creates metabolic demands in muscle that may result in unique training adaptations. Prolonged exercise causes muscle glycogen depletion and results in an increased rate of fat utilization. Exposure to sustained activity in the glycogen-depleted state may result in adaptations that enhance the athlete's ability to metabolize fat at a high rate. Neuromuscular recruitment patterns may also be developed in such a manner as to facilitate maintenance of a high rate of power output despite glycogen depletion in some motor units.

The major disadvantage of LSD training is that intensity is markedly lower than that used during racing. Such training does not stimulate neurological patterns of muscle fiber recruitment needed during a race (12). Athletes who train only at speeds slower than race pace do not train all the muscle fibers used in competition. (This would also be true for those who would train only at short distances at very fast paces).

2. **Aerobic Interval Training.** Aerobic interval training (AIT) has been a basic element in swimming conditioning for many years but is used less frequently by other endurance athletes. This form of training involves repeated short intervals at slightly slower than race pace with very brief rest intervals (5 to 15 s) (12). The brief rest intervals keep the circulatory system working at a high level, but allow the athlete a relief from the muscular strain produced by faster paced training. During the brief rest intervals, there is little recovery of heart rate or oxygen uptake. However, there is little lactate accumulation, because the pace is not fast enough to demand significant anaerobic metabolism.

The benefits of this form of training are probably similar to LSD training, but may involve less muscular strain and may be more mentally stimulating to the athlete. Because the exercise intensity employed with aerobic interval training approaches lactate threshold and race pace, this form of training is probably better than LSD training for improving economy at race pace, lactate threshold, and fractional utilization of $\dot{V}O_2max$. However, because aerobic interval training sessions can be quite prolonged, muscle glycogen depletion and increased fat use can be induced.

3. **Pace/Tempo Training.** Pace or tempo training employs exercise of a sustained nature performed at a pace slightly faster than race pace. This form of training is sometimes referred to as aerobic-anaerobic interval training (12,29). It involves long intervals alternating with periods of slower paced activity or complete rest. Pace training is designed to improve both aerobic and anaerobic metabolic responses to exercise. A major advantage of pace training compared to LSD training is that pace training involves the same pattern of muscle fiber recruitment that occurs in competition. Primary objectives of pace training are to develop a sense of race pace and to expose the various physiologic systems to sustained exercise at that pace (12). Therefore, only enough rest should be given to enable the athlete to hold the desired pace for all the intervals planned. Obviously, the selected pace should match the pace that can realistically be expected in competition. Rest periods should be 30 to 90 s long. In this time, not all lactate is removed, so lactate accumulation ultimately becomes the limiting factor. While there are many potential benefits from this form of training, it is also very stressful. Pace training of this nature probably should not be performed more than two or three times per week.

Pace training probably carries specific benefits for performance economy at race pace and for increasing the lactate threshold. If race pace economy improves, the pace associated with a given % $\dot{V}O_2$max would be increased and, thereby, performance would be enhanced. Improved economy may accrue from the prolonged use of neuromuscular recruitment patterns that are used at race pace. Pace training may enhance lactate threshold by improving the capacity to remove lactate. Also, tolerance for exercise with elevated lactate may be enhanced by increased buffering capacity.

4. **Anaerobic Interval Training.** This common form of interval training is sometimes referred to as "speed training." This training technique is very stressful and must be used sparingly by the endurance athlete. While the stresses involved promote increased speed and power, there is a high risk for muscular injury, due to the high muscle tensions developed. Many believe it has little place in a training program for prolonged performance.

Anaerobic interval training employs relatively short, high intensity (maximal to supramaximal) work bouts. Rest intervals should be about two min in duration. Hill running or cycling is another form of anaerobic interval training. In this case, the pace is not as fast as it would be on flat terrain, but the effect is still to elicit major involvement of anaerobic metabolic processes. Both runners and cyclists have found hill work to be of great value. This form of training should not be utilized until a firm base of aerobic training and muscular fitness has been attained. Speed training is used more frequently in swimming as compared to running or cycling, probably because most swim training occurs in pools with convenient lengths for speed work. Speed work may be a desirable form of preparation for the mass swim starts of most endurance swimming or triathlon events.

For the endurance athlete, two aims of anaerobic interval training are to develop strength and to increase capacity for and tolerance of anaerobic metabolism. As listed in Table 8-1, enhanced anaerobic metabolism is the primary physiologic adaptation to this form of training.

5. **Weight Training and Stretching.** We have just outlined the techniques that constitute the core of successful endurance training programs. However, weight training and stretching are also used regularly by many endurance athletes, and these probably contribute to enhanced performance. Unfortunately, there is little scientific documentation of such a benefit. Both of these procedures may reduce injury risk if applied appropriately to the muscle groups that are most active in the athlete's endurance activity. Maintenance of good flexibility through stretching may enhance performance by reducing muscle soreness and by enhancing economy of movement. High levels of muscular strength probably are not critical to performance of prolonged exercise, but adequate muscular strength and endurance may be helpful in avoiding local fatigue in supporting musculature. Specific weight training and stretching procedures for endurance athletes will not be discussed here.

II. CURRENT TRAINING REGIMENS

A. Running

Experience indicates that optimal training programs for enhancement of long-distance running performance should incorporate most of the training techniques mentioned in the previous section. This section is intended to describe several of the so-called "training systems" that have been developed over the past four decades and to discuss the approaches to training that are now being used by elite long-distance runners.

1. **Training Systems.** During the forty years since World War II, the training practices of elite long distance runners have evolved through several identifiable stages. These stages can be associated with several famous coaches, each of whom has been credited with

TABLE 8-1. *Summary of training techniques for prolonged exercise and presumed benefits*

	Long Slow Distance	Aerobic Interval Training	Pace/Tempo Training	Anaerobic Interval Training
		TRAINING TECHNIQUE		
	I: 65% to 70% $\dot{V}O_2$max (slower than race pace; steady state $\dot{V}O_2$) D: >1 h F: $1 \cdot wk^{-1}$ RPE: 10, 11, 12 (fairly light)	I: 70% to 80% $\dot{V}O_2$max (pace slightly less than race pace or below lactate threshold) D: 5 to 15 min; depends on exercise mode and competitive distances REPS: 5 to 20 F: 3 to $4 \cdot wk^{-1}$ RPE: 13, 14, 15 (somewhat hard)	I: 80% to 95% $\dot{V}O_2$max (pace slightly faster than race pace; slightly *above* lactate threshold) D: 3 to 10 min; depends on exercise mode and competitive distances F: 1 to $2 \cdot wk^{-1}$ RPE: 15, 16, 17 (hard to very hard)	(As adapted for prolonged performances) I: 95% to 120% $\dot{V}O_2$max (pace well above lactate threshold) D: 30 s to 4 min REPS: 5 to 20 F: no more than $1 \cdot wk^{-1}$ RPE: 18, 19, 20 (very, very hard)
		ACUTE RESPONSES		
	Marked reduction in muscle glycogen stores Elevated body temperature (unless cold environment) Decreased body weight due to sweat loss Perceived muscle and joint fatigue Some protein metabolism (5% to 10% of caloric expenditure)	Slight increase in blood lactate (at or below 4 mM) Elevated body temperature Same responses as LSD, but at higher level	Moderately high levels of blood lactate (8 to 15 mM) Respiratory distress (O_2 debt)	Depleted phosphagens Marked elevation in blood lactate (15 to 20 mM) with longer intervals Considerable respiratory distress (O_2 debt)

I: Intensity.
D: Duration.
F: Frequency.
RPE: Rating of Perceived Exertion.
REPS: Repetitions.

TABLE 8-1. (*continued*)

Long Slow Distance	Aerobic Interval Training	Pace/Tempo Training	Anaerobic Interval Training
		PRIMARY BENEFITS	
Elevated free fatty acid (FFA) oxidation; sparing of muscle glycogen stores -increased oxidative enzymes, particularly those associated with FFA catabolism -blood glucose homeostasis improved -increased hormone sensitive lipase activity -greater use of cirulating lipoproteins and intramuscular fat Enhanced utilization of amino acid shuttles (e.g., pyruvate to alanine) Increased capacity of cardiovascular system: increased left ventricular mass, heart volume, stroke volume	Improved $\dot{V}O_2$ kinetics, but little change in $\dot{V}O_2$max Improved economy of performance Improved ability to maintain a high level steady state of $\dot{V}O_2$ Decreased fractional utilization of $\dot{V}O_2$max at specific pace Increased mitochondrial mass Increased activities of oxidative enzymes; particularly those associated with carbohydrate catabolism Improved oxygen transport across membranes -increased myoglobin Possible increase in lactate threshold: enhancement of lactate removal Increased hexokinase: greater use of blood glucose, lesser use of muscle glycogen	Increased lactate threshold -enhanced lactate removal Increased lactate tolerance -enhanced respiratory response -enhanced lactate buffering Improved $\dot{V}O_2$ kinetics: probable increase in $\dot{V}O_2$max -enhanced cardiovascular responses to intense exercise -enhanced mitochondrial responses specific to carbohydrate catabolism and oxygen utilization Neuro-muscular recruitment patterns specific to competition (more fast twitch muscle involvement than in LSD or AIT)	Enhanced power production of fast twitch muscle fibers (with shorter intervals) Increased phosphagen utilization Increased creatine kinase and myokinase activities Increased lactate tolerance (with longer intervals) Increased muscular strength (particularly with hill work) Increase in hexokinase activity

PRIMARY BENEFITS

-increased vagal tone: decreased resting heart rate
-improved venous return: increased stroke volume
-enhanced blood pressure regulation
-increased muscle vascularity
Improved temperature regulation (enhanced heat tolerance—largely the result of circulatory adaptations)
Increased respiratory endurance: improved ability to ventilate lungs for prolonged period
-gradual reduction in cost of breathing
Improved oxygen transport across cell membranes
-increased myoglobin
Increased mitochondrial protein (particularly in slow, oxidative muscle fibers)

Enhanced glycolytic capacity of fast twitch muscles
Enhanced glycogen storage capacity

TABLE 8-1. *(continued)*

Long Slow Distance	Aerobic Interval Training	Pace/Tempo Training	Anaerobic Interval Training
		SECONDARY BENEFITS	
Increased muscle glycogen storage capacity Decreased cardiovascular, metabolic, and respiratory "drift" -improved capacity to maintain cardiac output, blood pressure and muscle blood flow for prolonged periods Increased plasma volume and blood volume -increased plasma renin and antidiuretic hormone Musculo-skeletal adaptations resulting in increased resistance to muscle cell damage during heavy exercise -increased endurance of supporting muscle structures Decreased body fat stores Improved pacing ability	Improved blood flow patterns and enhanced venous return (increased stroke volume) Decreased heart rate at specified pace Improved breathing patterns Improved biomechanics and economy	Enhanced lactate utilization by cardiac and slow twitch muscle tissue Increased mitochondrial material Increased muscular strength	Hypertrophy of fast twitch muscles Increased activities of glycolytic and glycogenolytic enzymes Increased muscle mass Increased speed

developing an impressive number of world-class runners. In addition, and more importantly in the present context, each of these coaches developed and popularized approaches to training that seem, in retrospect, to have had an important impact on our current view of appropriate training. Each of these coach's systems will be discussed briefly.

Franz Stamfl served as advisor to many of the great British middle- and long-distance runners of the 1950s. These included Roger Bannister, the first sub-four minute miler, and Chris Chataway, a world record holder at 5,000 m. The hallmark of Stamfl's system was interval training, which he recommended be employed, in varying forms, five days per week nearly year around (81). Stamfl's training schedules incorporated interval sessions of both the aerobic, anaerobic and pace/tempo interval sessions. By today's standards, Stamfl's advisees ran relatively few miles per week, although they did perform fartlek runs of 60–90 min duration once per week.

Percy Cerutty has been credited with developing the impressive stable of Australian distance runners who dominated international competitions in the late 1950s and early 1960s. Most notable of the group were Herb Elliott and John Landy. Cerutty's athletes performed prodigious weekend training sessions near his beach-side home in Portsea. Included in the program were exhaustive interval runs up sand-hills, extensive weight training sessions and occasional runs of durations up to two h (7). Cerutty's most unique, lasting contribution to our concept of proper training may have been his emphasis on development of strength and power. He recommended that all distance runners spend at least one-third of their training time in non-running activities, weight training in particular. Also, Cerutty's athletes ran 50 miles per week or more, a modest dose by current standards, but more than had been run by their predecessors.

Arthur Lydiard, a New Zealander, was the coach who catalyzed the development of his country's great middle- and long-distance runners of the 1960s. Among his proteges were Peter Snell, a double Olympic gold medalist in 1964, and Murray Halberg, a gold medalist in 1960. Lydiard was one of the first coaches to prescribe marked seasonal variations in training techniques and to design programs that build the athlete to a distinct performance "peak." However, Lydiard is probably best known for his popularization of "marathon training" even for middle-distance runners. His athletes regularly performed training runs of two h duration and frequently ran as many as 100 miles per week (51). The success of Lydiard's athletes across competitive distances ranging from 800 meters to the marathon seemingly convinced the distance running world of the value of high volume training. The "one hundred mile week," once viewed as an absurdity, was converted to a widely accepted training procedure by Lydiard and his athletes.

Bill Bowerman was track coach at the University of Oregon for over 25 years, and during his tenure, he developed a remarkable number of world class distance runners. One of these athletes, Steve Prefontaine, held the American records for every competitive distance between 3,000 and 10,000 meters during the early 1970s. Bowerman's "Oregon system" includes liberal doses of aerobic and pace/tempo intervals, fartlek runs on roads and grass surfaces, near-race pace "tempo runs," and prolonged runs of 90–120 min duration. Perhaps the most creative and lasting contribution of Bowerman's system was his "hard-easy" approach to organization of training sessions (3). This approach involves alternating days of heavy and light training. The technique is based on the concept that desirable physiologic adaptations to training require an adequate recovery period following the application of a demanding training stimulus. Bowerman's hard-easy system has done much to sensitize distance runners and their coaches to the risks of overtraining and the benefits of applying "optimal," as distinct from "maximal," training doses.

2. **Current Approaches.** The training techniques and programs of the current generation of elite long-distance runners vary considerably in accordance with individual needs and preferences. However, these programs, collectively, manifest certain consistencies which constitute the core of our current perception of appropriate training for long-distance runners (12,21). Several of these key factors have been drawn from the training systems described above. Among the central elements in the training programs of currently elite long distance runners (10 km or longer) are the following.

A. *High volume of training.* Weekly training mileages in the range of 80 to 120 miles per week are now commonplace and are generally accepted as essential to elite performance.
B. *Faster than race pace training.* Elite long-distance runners typically employ interval training and/or fartlek running at least once per week (and often two or three times per week).
C. *Prolonged, moderate intensity runs.* Sustained LSD runs of one and one-half to three h duration at considerably slower than race pace are a prominent feature of current training programs. These are typically performed on a weekly basis.
D. *Hard-easy training pattern.* Though employed in various specific formats, the hard-easy approach to organization of

training sessions is now widely accepted by elite endurance athletes.

E. *Seasonal variation and peaking.* Current training programs generally are structured so that the greatest training volume is accomplished during the non-competitive season, and the more intense forms of training are emphasized in the immediate pre-competition period. Marathon runners typically aim for performance peaks once or twice per year.

F. *Strength Training.* Elite distance runners typically engage in weight training, particularly for the upper body musculature. Two to three weight training sessions per week is a common frequency in the non-competitive season; somewhat lower frequencies are usually employed during periods of regular competition.

B. Swimming

1. **Unique Determinants of Swimming Performance.** The "generic" determinants of endurance performance, as discussed above, all relate to performance of prolonged swimming. However, because swimming involves a very novel motor skill, economy is a particularly important factor in this activity. The energy cost of swimming has been studied extensively (49). LePere and Porter (50) and Montpetit et al. (60), have presented linear regression equations (for both male and female swimmers) relating oxygen uptake to swimming velocity. The cost of crawl swimming is significantly higher in men than in women due to the differences in body size (increased drag), body density (bouyancy), and torque about the center of volume (30). A swimmer is rotationally unstable in the prone position because of the torque produced by the bouyant force and body weight. Therefore, the energy expenditure of swimming involves two components: (1) the cost of maintaining a horizontal position (combating the rotational effect), and (2) the cost of translational motion, i.e., overcoming drag. The relative contribution of these two components varies with swimming velocity. Essentially, the cost of overcoming drag increases as speed increases, while the cost of opposing gravity decreases (49). Thus, the cost of fast swimming is directly related to the passive body resistance of the swimmer. Probably the single most important aspect of endurance swimming is economy of motion and efficiency of stroke mechanics. Generally, this means long hours of instruction and coaching in one's early years, with careful attention to detail throughout the competitive years.

Studies of substrate utilization during typical swim training suggest that the primary energy sources are phosphagens and carbohydrates (41,83). Haralambie and Senser (36), however, have shown that lipid oxidation is very important during prolonged swimming. Much more research needs to be done on this topic.

2. Training for Swimming. Most competitive distances in swimming are 200 m or less. Consequently, typical swim team training has focused on developing faster speeds for short distances, and there has been great emphasis on anaerobic metabolism and the use of fast interval training. Excellent work has been done on determining swimming velocity at maximal lactate levels, on estimating proper training paces, and on evaluating the effectiveness of training programs (49). The East Europeans have been particularly active in applying poolside lactate measures to determine training paces and to monitor training progress.

However, while typical swim team training is about 40% to 60% interval work in 25 yd to 50 m pools, endurance swimming is more typically performed in open water. Consequently, a large part of the preparatory training for endurance swimming should be done in open water. Open water swimming can be quite different than pool swimming. The water is colder and rougher, and sighting is required since there are no pool bottom lines to follow. Sighting in relatively calm water requires "peeking" the instant before the face rolls back into the water on the crawl stroke. In particularly rough water, peeking is not sufficient, and some strokes must be done with the head completely above the water. Swimmers accustomed to open water usually sight about every 8 to 10 strokes and develop a bit more body roll than accomplished pool swimmers. An elevated head position, even for an instant, means that the ideal "planing" position is lost (if attained at all). The final outcome is that the kick must be accentuated whenever sighting is required. Swim times in open water are always slower than in pools, and this is, no doubt, at least part of the reason. A higher head and lower legs increases drag, and swimming economy is reduced.

A typical training program for endurance swimming involves long-distance swimming, with the target distance determined by the competition objective. The total swim distance should be accomplished using proper stroke mechanics. Practicing a shortened stroke, or slower than race pace stroke cadence is not likely to improve performance. Interval swim distances and work-rest times are individualized and specific to the training needs of the swimmer, but long intervals are usually emphasized for prolonged swimming performance. Swim training aids, such as pull-bouys to hold the legs up while stroking and styrofoam kick boards to support the upper body while kicking, allow the athlete to concentrate on developing strength in the arms and legs separately.

C. Cycling

Previous research has shown that the physiologic determinants of endurance performance discussed earlier in the chapter are important in cycling (6,46,54,78). Technique is very important in cycling as well as swimming. Developing a smooth and efficient leg stroke at a fast cadence ("spinning") takes considerable practice. Many miles of endurance cycling are performed by endurance cyclists at a high cadence (90 to 120 rpm) in a low gear ratio. This sort of training is analogous to long, slow distance running, although the actual speeds may be quite high. Hill work for strength and shifting practice, as well as long-interval work on flat terrain for development of anaerobic-aerobic power, round out a well-planned cycling training program. Variation, as in running and swimming training programs, is important to prevent boredom. Group training rides are commonly used to sharpen attention, hone skills, and to provide a measure by which to gauge improvement. Basically the same techniques used in running are employed in cycling training: acceleration sprints, intervals, speed play (fartlek), continuous riding at race pace, and continuous slow riding. The distances, intensity levels, duration, and frequency of training must be individualized according to one's competitive goals and distances.

Training programs of highly competitive cyclists tend to manifest the following characteristics (46,78,84):

A. *High Volume of Training.* Elite, male road cyclists train and race 575 to 825 km (350 to 500 miles) per week to prepare for stage racing. Female cyclists average 425 to 500 km (250 to 300 miles) per week.

B. *Faster Than Race Pace Training.* Elite, long-distance cyclists use interval training at least once per week, along with a session of speed training.

C. *Prolonged, Moderate Intensity Rides.* Long rides of four to six h for men and two to four h for women, at considerably slower than race pace, are used by endurance cyclists. These are performed several times per week during the peak of the season.

D. *Hard-Easy Training Pattern.* Rarely do cyclists perform two very intense days of cycling back-to-back, although, long mileage sessions may be used several days in a row.

E. *Seasonal Variation and Peaking.* Weekly mileage is gradually increased during pre-season training, and sessions of intervals, pace training and speed work are incorporated into the training program as the season progresses. Top road cyclists peak several times during the season for major events.

F. *Strength Training*. As with elite distance runners, road cyclists use weight training primarily for upper body musculature during the off-season. During the season, they tend to use only calisthenic exercises for the upper body.

III. SPECIAL TRAINING PROBLEMS

Increased competitiveness in endurance sports has led to numerous changes in the training practices of elite athletes. Among the most noteworthy of these changes are: (1) increased volume of training, and (2) extension of the "training year." It is now commonplace for endurance athletes to maintain high training volumes on virtually a year-around basis. This chronic exposure to demanding training has raised several issues that have significance for athletes and sport scientists alike. This section is dedicated to discussion of three of these issues: overtraining, detraining/retention of training and tapering/peaking.

A. Overtraining

Today's endurance athletes and coaches are confronted by a paradoxical and frustrating situation. As discussed above, it is now widely accepted that very heavy training doses are needed to optimize performance, and, yet, paradoxically, excessive training can lead to a maladaptive state in which performance is impaired. It is frustrating that there are no well-established, objective markers that can be used by coaches, athletes and sports medicine practitioners to identify optimal training doses for individual athletes. However, the sports medicine literature and the experiences of many coaches and athletes do provide some guidance regarding the overtraining issue.

The term "overtraining" has been used to describe a broad range of states observed in endurance athletes. Overtraining sometimes describes participation in more exercise than is needed to optimize performance. This may have no major negative health consequences, but the athlete may become chronically fatigued, and performance may either fail to improve or may decline moderately. This condition has sometimes been called "overwork." The term "overtraining" has also been used to describe a serious and chronic maladaptation to training, in which performance is clearly impaired, and injury or illness is likely to develop. The latter condition is much more overt and has a much more severe impact on performance. This section will deal with this more severe form of overtraining.

Coaches and athletes have long recognized that the severely overtrained condition arises in some athletes and that it is inconsistent with optimal performance. However, it is only recently that sport scientists have begun to examine this problem in a systematic way. As a consequence, most of the available pertinent information is descriptive in nature and has focused on identification of objective markers of the overtrained state.

While no definitive markers of overtraining have yet been identified, the existing sports medicine literature indicates that changes in several physiological, biochemical and psychological factors may be associated with and/or predictive of the overtrained state. Among the physiological factors associated with overtraining are some observed during rest and others that involve responses to acute exercise bouts. Increased morning resting heart rate and T-wave changes in the electrocardiogram have been associated with overtraining (23,87). Also, various metabolic and cardiorespiratory responses to submaximal and maximal exercise may change in systematic ways with overtraining. Among the potentially useful markers are decreased muscular strength, decreased $\dot{V}O_2$max, increased $\dot{V}O_2$ during standard submaximal exercise (i.e., decreased economy), decreased oxygen pulse, increased ratings of perceived exertion, and increased blood lactate responses to submaximal exertion (12,17,40,55,58,73,87).

A substantial number of blood-borne biochemical factors have been suggested as useful markers of overtraining. Serum creatine phosphokinase is often taken as an indicator of skeletal muscle damage, and increased activity of this muscle enzyme in serum may be associated with overtraining (23,63). Recently, much attention has been focused on measures of endocrine and immune function as possible markers of overtraining. It is well documented that the body's response to physical and/or psychological stress involves interactions between the nervous, endocrine and immune systems (66,80,88). Altered functions in these systems may cause some of the symptoms of overtraining (1,2,4,58,68,87). Among the endocrine factors that may be helpful in identifying and predicting development of the overtrained state are responses of catecholamines (12,31,68), endogenous opiates (22,31), ACTH, and cortisol (2,31,68) to submaximal and maximal exercise. Also, the resting levels of plasma testosterone and cortisol (and the ratio between these two) has been used as an index of overall metabolic state (anabolic vs. catabolic activity) (31,34,86). Since the overtrained state is often associated with an increased risk of illness, measures of immune status may be helpful in predicting development of overtraining. Among the potentially helpful markers of immune function are determinations of lymphocyte subpopulations and T lymphocyte function (27,35,37,53,59,74,82).

In the psychological domain, factors such as apathy, lack of appetite, irritability and sleep disturbances have been suggested to be indicators of overtraining (4,58,61). The Profile of Mood States instrument may be a particularly helpful indicator of the overtrained state (57).

The many factors cited above constitute a list of *potentially* useful markers of overtraining. However, it must be emphasized that our knowledge of the biological basis of overtraining is very limited. Much more research of various types is needed. First, the factors that are associated with an existing overtrained state must be clearly identified. Second, experimental and prospective epidemiological studies should be conducted to find factors that are predictive of the overtrained state. In addition, there is a need for clinical studies that will expand our knowledge of appropriate methods for: (1) prevention of overtraining in athletes who show the early signs of its development, and (2) treatment of the condition in those athletes who manifest a full-blown maladaptation to training.

B. Detraining/Retention of Training

Consistency in training is a key feature of successful endurance training programs. Indeed, some of today's elite endurance athletes seem almost compulsive in their adherence to training regimens that may involve as many as 10 to 20 exercise sessions per week. Nonetheless, endurance athletes do, on occasion, experience periods in which training is reduced or ceased altogether. These detraining periods may be voluntary or may result from injury or illness. Whatever the cause of the detraining period, endurance athletes often express great concern about losing the physiologic benefits that had been gained through previous heavy training. Consequently, it is important that the physiologic response to detraining be understood and that methods for retaining a trained state during periods of detraining be developed.

1. Detraining. Our knowledge of the physiologic responses to detraining in highly trained endurance athletes is limited to that gained from a relatively small number of studies. The available evidence indicates that most of the central and peripheral physiologic adaptations to training regress rather rapidly toward pretraining levels with cessation of training (24,25,45,62). $\dot{V}O_2$max has been observed to decrease by 15% to 20% after 12 weeks of detraining in highly trained endurance athletes (19). About half of the decline in $\dot{V}O_2$ occurred in the first two to three weeks of detraining, and this rapid decrease was associated most closely with decreased stroke volume and maximal cardiac output. However, decreased maximal arteriovenous oxygen difference also contributed to the decreased $\dot{V}O_2$max.

It appears likely that the decline in stroke volume is due to a reduction in blood volume and consequent decreases in venous return of blood to the heart and left ventricular end-diastolic diameter (11,20,32). It is not established that cardiac contractility decreases with relatively short periods of detraining.

Detraining results in a regression of many of the adaptations in skeletal muscle that are associated with training. Mitochondrial enzyme activities decrease rapidly with detraining (8,38). However, muscle capillarization may be maintained during a detraining period, particularly in those who are highly trained (19).

The available literature on the physiology of detraining suggests that highly trained persons respond somewhat differently to the absence of the training stimulus than do the moderately trained (8,19,20). The studies of Coyle and colleagues (19,20) have indicated that athletes who had engaged in endurance training for a very prolonged period experience only a partial loss of some training-induced adaptations during three months of detraining. Specifically, $\dot{V}O_2$max, maximal arteriovenous oxygen difference and mitochondrial enzyme activities appear to decrease to levels that remain well above those observed in untrained persons. In contrast, persons participating in short-term training regimens tend to revert to pretrained levels for most pertinent variables. An exception may be muscle capillarization, which may be partially maintained in moderately-trained persons and totally maintained in athletes who trained for a prolonged period.

2. Retention of Training Effects. As noted above, cessation of training results in a marked and rapid loss of many of the physiologic adaptations to training. In an effort to minimize the loss of these adaptations during periods of detraining, many athletes have made use of alternate, secondary modes of exercise training. At first glance, this "cross training" technique appears to be a logical approach to retention of training during periods in which a primary mode of exercise cannot be used. However, the available physiological literature indicates that the benefits of cross training may be quite limited.

There are several reasons to be skeptical about the benefits of cross training. First, "specificity" is one of the most extensively-documented principles of training. As discussed in previous sections of this chapter, many of the physiologic adaptations to training are situated in the specific skeletal muscles that are stressed in the training activity (56). Even some of the so-called "central circulatory" adaptations to training may be very mode-specific. For example, Clausen et al. (10) observed the response to submaximal leg work before and after arm training and found only small changes in several cardiorespiratory and metabolic variables, and Magel et al. (52) found no change in running $\dot{V}O_2$max with 10 weeks of swim training. Thus, the literature on specificity of training seems to argue against the efficacy of cross training as a means of retaining a training effect.

Although cross training has been widely recommended and utilized in recent years as a technique for retention of training adaptations, it has not been studied extensively in this context. Pate and co-workers (64) examined the effects of arm crank training on the retention of training effects originally generated by leg cycling. After a four-week cross training period, responses to leg cycling were no different in the arm training group than in a group that simply detrained. While the results of this study seeem to imply that cross training is useless as a means of retaining training effects, it may be that different results would accrue from studies of very highly trained subjects or from observations of longer periods of cross training/detraining.

At present the scientific literature indicates that the most certain way to retain a training effect is to continue using the primary mode of exercise or one that is very similar in terms of neuromuscular function. It has been demonstrated that training adaptations can be maintained, for at least a few weeks, with training of reduced frequency (but with constant mode, duration and intensity) (5). Thus, when possible, it appears that endurance athletes should attempt to minimize the effects of detraining by continuing to use the primary mode of exercise at reduced frequency. Of course, this recommendation is of no use to the athlete who has been forced into inactivity by an injury that precludes participation in the primary activity. Recently, sports medicine practitioners have developed some techniques for dealing with this problem. An example is "water running." With this procedure, the athlete, wearing a flotation device in a swimming pool, performs the running motion against the resistance provided by the water. The technique has the apparent advantages of avoiding weight-bearing, often problematic for injured runners, while allowing the athlete to exercise with a motion that is rather similar to normal running. While this procedure has not yet been subjected to rigorous scientific study, the potential benefits would seem to warrant such investigation.

C. Tapering/Peaking

"Tapering" of the training regimen has become a widely accepted component of the endurance athlete's preparation for major competitions. Tapering typically involves reduction of the training dose for three to 21 days prior to the competition. Often this reduced training volume is accompanied by ingestion of a high carbohydrate diet and performance of "sharpening" activities, such as short-duration, high-intensity interval training. The goal of tapering the training regimen is to achieve a performance "peak" at the desired time (e.g., major championship competition).

The available scientific literature supports the value of tapering but suggests that many athletes may not taper sufficiently prior to competitions. Costill, who has studied tapering in collegiate swimmers, has reported 3% to 4% improvements in performance with a 15-day taper, during which training yardage was reduced by two-thirds (15). Such a regimen, though apparently quite effective, involves a longer and more marked reduction in training load than is currently used by most endurance athletes. Many athletes fear a loss of training adaptations with tapering protocols that involve more than minor reductions in training dose. The relevant scientific studies indicate that this fear is unwarranted. The work of Costill (15) and other authors (39) shows quite clearly that $\dot{V}O_2max$ and other markers of training status are well maintained for at least two to three weeks with training loads that are markedly reduced.

The available scientific literature indicates that the optimal taper is relatively prolonged and involves a very marked reduction in training load. However, it should be noted that this conclusion is based on very few controlled studies. Clearly there is a need for much more investigation of precompetition tapering techniques. Various levels of reduced training should be studied in athletes of different competitive levels and sport specialties. Broad generalizations about optimal tapering procedures would be premature at the present time.

SUMMARY

We believe that the scientific material presented in this chapter carries important implications for athletes, coaches and sports medicine practitioners. In this final section we shall present several recommendations that should be heeded by those who strive for optimal performance in endurance sports activities.

1. *Base training programs on a careful analysis of the physiological and psychological demands of the specific sport involved.* Training procedures should be designed to enhance the physiological and psychological variables that are critical to performance. Much has been learned about the physiological determinants of endurance performance, and the relevant knowledge should be applied to the selection of training activities and the emphasis given to each activity. Although there is less specific

knowledge available on the psychological determinants of endurance performance, that which is known should be applied. (See Dishman and Landy, this book.)

2. *Assess the physiological and psychological status of the individual athlete and apply training techniques that are consistent with the athlete's needs and limitations.* Each athlete is an individual who has unique traits and needs. While all endurance training programs should meet certain general criteria, the "optimal training regimen" is that which leads to the greatest rate of improved performance for the *individual* athlete. Physiological and psychological testing and medical evaluation can be helpful in identifying the needs of the individual athlete. However, there is no substitute for the athlete "listening to his or her body" and for the coach and medical practitioner maintaining an open line of communication with the athlete.

3. *Avoid overtraining.* In our opinion, many serious endurance athletes train too hard. The old adage that hard training should be followed by rest so that the body can respond is often ignored. Rather, "hard days" are followed by *more* "hard days," rather than "easy days" that allow for recovery.

4. *Be alert to the signs and symptoms of overtraining ("relative energy drain").* The result of excessive training often is a series of overuse injuries, such as stress fractures, illnesses (e.g., colds, sore throats, mononucleosis, Barr-Epstein virus), frequent and recurring minor musculoskeletal injuries, iron-deficiency anemia, or undue and prolonged fatigue, with a corresponding loss of "competitive edge" or desire to compete. Many athletes "burnout" before they achieve their full performance potential.

The incidence of such multidimensional problems as secondary amenorrhea, overtraining syndromes, and overuse injuries in endurance trained athletes may be indicative of an overall "relative energy drain." With the use of this term, we refer to a state of maladaptation caused by a long-term imbalance between energy expenditure and nutritional intake, excessive psychological stress, lack of rest, and possibly other factors. While a somewhat nebulous term that defies exact definition, we believe that "relative energy drain" can nevertheless be monitored. Failure to recognize and reverse such a state can lead to various signs and symptoms that are not only deleterious to performance, but to one's general health.

Clinical features of the obligatory athlete may include anemia, leukopenia, bone marrow hypoplasia, anorexia nervosa, bradycardia, increased blood urea nitrogen, increased morning cortisol level, hypotension, oligomenorrhea or amenorrhea, an absence of normal cyclical variations in reproductive hormones, low sperm count, fatigue, and body fat levels below the normal range. Although not so evident as menstrual dysfunction, reproductive variations are seen in men as well as women athletes. With acute exercise, plasma testosterone levels are elevated in proportion to exercise intensity (47). Basal levels of testosterone, however, are depressed in some athletes.

5. *Avoid excessive weight loss and extreme dietary practices.* The cardinal sign or symptom of long-term relative energy drain seems to be a loss of body weight or a very low level of body fat. Although the safety level or tolerance threshold appears to be a very individual matter, body fat is a variable that a coach or physician can monitor with reasonable accuracy. When an athlete, either male or female, becomes too emaciated, strength and endurance may decline, and general body resiliency to the strain of prolonged athletic training will fail. When that occurs, performance declines, and training must be curtailed.

   All too frequently, the endurance athlete becomes obsessed with body weight and body fat. Many realize that excess weight is costly to performance, and some strive to lower body fat levels below healthful levels. It is becoming commonplace today to hear of young female athletes with eating disorders such as anorexia nervosa and bulimia (79). While there is less documentation of these disorders in men, compulsive training may be an analogous disorder. Yates et al. (89) reported that obligatory runners resemble anorectic patients who have a preoccupation with food and an obsession with lean body mass. Many of these runners adopt very limited or bizarre diets, become vegetarians without sufficient nutritional knowledge, or fast on a regular basis. Their response to a poor performance is usually to eat less and train harder.

6. *Peak for major competitions by markedly reducing training load.* For what may be primarily psychological reasons, many endurance athletes are reluctant to reduce their training loads— even before major competitions. This probably leads many endurance athletes to enter competition in a semi-fatigued state that is inconsistent with optimal performance. While our scientific knowledge of peaking for competition is incomplete, available evidence suggests that training loads should

be reduced drastically to as little as perhaps one-third to one-half of normal during the two to three weeks before a major competition.

BIBLIOGRAPHY

1. Ayers, J.W.T., Y. Komesu, T. Romani, and R. Ansbacker. Anthropomorphic, hormonal, and psychologic correlates of semen quality in endurance-trained male athletes. *Fertil Steril.* 43:917–921, 1985.
2. Barron, J.L., T.D. Noakes, W. Levy, C. Smith, and R.P. Millar. Hypothalmic dysfunction in overtrained athletes. *J Clin Endo Metab.* 60:803–806, 1985.
3. Bowerman, W.J. and W.H. Freeman. *Coaching track and field.* Boston: Houghton Mifflin Co., 1974.
4. Brown, R.L., E.C. Frederick, H.L. Falsetti, E.R. Burke, and A.J. Ryan. Overtraining in athletes: a round table. *Phys Sportsmed.* 11(6):93–110, 1983.
5. Brynteson, P. and W.E. Sinning. The effects of training frequencies on the retention of cardiovascular fitness. *Med Sci Sport.* 4:29–33, 1973.
6. Burke, E.R., E. Cerney, D. Costill, and W. Fink. Characteristics of Skeletal Muscle in Competitive Cyclists. *Med Sci Sport.* 9(2):109–112, 1977.
7. Cerutty, P.W. *Athletics—how to become a champion.* London: Stanley Paul, 1960.
8. Chi, M.M.-Y., C.S. Hintz, E.F. Coyle, W.H. Martin III, et al. Effects of detraining on enzymes of energy metabolism in individual human muscle fibers. *Am J Physiol.* 244:C276–C287, 1983.
9. Clausen, J.P. Effect of physical training on cardiovascular adjustments to exercise in man. *Physiol Reviews.* 57:779–815, 1977.
10. Clausen, J.P., K. Klausen, B. Rasmussen and J. Trap-Jensen. Central and peripheral circulatory changes after training of the arms or legs. *Amer J Physiol.* 225:675–682, 1973.
11. Convertino, V.A., P.J. Brock, L.C. Keil, E.M. Bernauer, et al. Exercise training-induced hypervolemia: role of plasma albumin, renin, and vasopressin. *J Appl Physiol.* 48:655–699, 1980.
12. Costill, D.L. *Inside Running: Basics of Sports Physiology.* Indianapolis: Benchmark Press, Inc., 1986.
13. Costill, D.L. Physiology of marathon running. *J Amer Med Assoc.* 221:1024–1029, 1972.
14. Costill, D.L. and E.L. Fox. Energetics of marathon running. *Med Sci Sports.* 1:81–86, 1969.
15. Costill, D.L., D.S. King, R. Thomas and M. Hargreaves. Effects of reduced training on muscular power in swimmers. *The Physician and Sportsmedicine.* 13(2):94–101, 1985.
16. Costill, D.L. and E. Winrow. Maximal oxygen intake among marathon runners. *Arch Phys Med Rehab.* 51:317–320, 1970.
17. Costill, D.L., W.J. Fink, M. Hargreaves, D.S. King, R. Thomas, and R. Fielding. Metabolic characteristics of skeletal muscle during detraining from competitive swimming. *Med Sci Sports Exerc.* 17:339–343, 1985.
18. Costill, D.L. Metabolic responses during distance running. *J Appl Physiol.* 28:251–255, 1970.
19. Coyle, E.F., W.H. Martin III, D.R. Sinacore, M.J. Joyner, et al. Time course of loss of adaptations after stopping prolonged intense endurance training. *J Appl Physiol.* 57:1857–1864, 1984.
20. Coyle, E.F., M.K. Hemmert, and A.R. Coggan. Effects of detraining on cardiovascular responses to exercise: role of blood volume. *J Appl Physiol.* 60:95–99, 1986.
21. Daniels, J., R. Fitts, and G. Sheehan. *Conditioning for Distance Running.* New York: John Wiley & Sons, 1978.
22. Davis, J.M., D.R. Lamb, G.K.W. Yim and P.V. Maluen. Opioid modulation of feeding behavior following repeated exposure to forced swimming exercise in male rats. *Pharm Biochem Behav.* 23L 709–714, 1985.
23. Dressendorfer, R.H., C.E. Wade, and J.H. Scaff Jr. Increased morning heart rate in runners: a valid sign of overtraining? *The Physician and Sportsmedicine.* 13(8):77–86, 1985.
24. Drinkwater, B.L. and S.M. Horvath. Detraining effects on young women. *Med Sci Sports.* 4:91–95, 1972.
25. Ehsani, A.A., J.M. Hagberg, and R.C. Hickson. Rapid changes in left ventricular dimensions and mass in response to physical conditioning and deconditioning. *Am J Cardiol.* 42:52–56, 1978.
26. Ekblom, B. Effect of physical training on the oxygen transport system in man. *Acta Physiol Scand.* 328 (Suppl.):11–45, 1969.
27. Eskola, J., O. Ruuskanen, E. Soppi, M.K. Viljanen, M. Jarvinen, H. Toivonen, and K. Kouvalainen. Effect of sport stress on lymphocyte transformation and antibody formation.

Clin Exp Immunol. 32:339–345, 1978.

28. Farrell, P.A., J.H. Wilmore, E.G. Coyle, J.E. Billing, and D.L. Costill. Plasma lactate accumulation and distance running performance. Med Sci Sports. 11:338–344, 1979.
29. Fox, E.L., R.L. Bartels, C.E. Billings, R. O'Brien, et al. Frequency and duration of interval training programs and changes in aerobic power. J. Appl Physiol. 38:481–484, 1975.
30. Gagnon, M., and R. Montpetit. Technological development for the measurement of the center of volume in the human body. J Biom. 14:235–241, 1981.
31. Galbo, H. Hormonal and metabolic adaptation to exercise. Thieme-stratton, Inc. New York, 1983.
32. Green, H.J., J.A. Thomson, M.E. Ball, R.L. Hughson, et al. Alterations in blood volume following short-term supramaximal exercise. J Appl Physiol. 56:145–149, 1984.
33. Hagan, R.D., M.G. Smith, and L.R. Gettman. Marathon performance in relation to maximal aerobic power and training indices. Med Sci Sports Exerc. 13:185–189, 1981.
34. Hakkinen, K., A. Pakarinen, A. Mackku and P.V. Komi. Serum hormones during prolonged training for neuromuscular performance. Eur J Appl Physiol. 53:287–293, 1985.
35. Hanson, P.G. and D.K. Flaherty. Immunological responses to training in conditioned runners. Clin Sci. 60:225–228, 1981.
36. Haralambie, G., and L. Senser. Metabolic changes in man during long-distance swimming. Eur J Appl Physiol. 43:115–125, 1980.
37. Hedfors, E., G. Holm, and B. Ohnell. Variations of blood lymphocytes during work studied by cell surface markers, DNA synthesis and cytotoxicity. Clin Exp Immunol. 24:328–335, 1976.
38. Henriksson, J., and J.S. Reitman. Time course of changes in human skeletal muscle succinate dehydrogenase and cytochrome activity and inactivity. Acta Physiol Scand. 99:91–97, 1977.
39. Hickson, R.C. and M.A. Rosenkoetter. Reduced training frequencies and maintenance of increased aerobic power. Med Sci Sports Exerc. 13:13–16, 1981.
40. Houston, M.E., H. Bentzen, and H. Larsen. Interrelationships between skeletal muscle adaptations and performance as studied by detraining and retraining. Acta Physiol Scand. 105:163–170, 1979.
41. Houston, M.E. Metabolic responses to exercise, with special reference to training and competition in swimming. In: Swimming Medicine IV, Eriksson and Furberg, Eds., Baltimore: University Park Press, 1978, pp. 207–232.
42. Ingjer, F. Capillary supply and mitochondrial content of different skeletal muscle fiber types in untrained and endurance-trained men: a histochemical and ultrastructural study. Eur J Appl Physiol. 40:197–209, 1979.
43. Jacobs, I. Blood lactate: Implications for training and sports performance. Sports Med. (New Zealand) 3:10–25, 1986.
44. Keul, J., H.-H. Dickhuth, M. Lehmann, and J. Staiger. The athlete's heart-haemodynamics and structure. Inter J Sports Med. 3:33–43, 1982.
45. Klausen, K., L.B. Andersen, and I. Pelle. Adaptive changes in work capacity, skeletal muscle capillarization and enzyme levels during training and detraining. Acta Physiol Scand. 113:9–16, 1981.
46. Krebs, P.S., S. Zinkgraf, and S.J. Virgilio. Predicting competitive bicycling performance with training and physiological variables. J Sports Med and Physical Fitness. 26(4):323–329, 1986.
47. Lamb, D.R. Androgen and exercise. Med Sci Sports. 7:1–5, 1975.
48. Lamb, D.R. Physiology of Exercise: Responses and Adaptations, 2nd ed. New York: Macmillan Publishing Co., 1984.
49. Lavoie, J.M. and R.R. Montpetit. Applied physiology of swimming. Sports Medicine (New Zealand). 3:165–189, 1986.
50. LePere, C.B. and G.H. Porter. Cardiovascular and metabolic responses of skilled and recreational swimmers during running and swimming. In: Application of Science and Medicine to Sport. A. Taylor, Ed., Springfield, IL.: Charles Thomas, 1975, pp. 234–247.
51. Lydiard, A. and G. Gilmour. Run to the top. Auckland: Minerva, 1962.
52. Magel, J.R., G.F. Foglia, W.D. McArdle, B. Gutin, G.S. Pechar and F.I. Katch. Specificity of swim training on maximum oxygen uptake. J Appl Physiol. 38:151–155, 1975.
53. Makinodan, T., S.J. James, T. Inamizu, and M-P. Chang. Immunologic basis for susceptibility to infection in the aged. Gerontology. 30:279–289, 1984.
54. Malhorta, M.S., S.K. Werma, R.K. Gupta, and G.L. Khanna. Physiological basis for selection of competitive road cyclists. J Sports Med and Phys Fit. 24:49–57, 1984.
55. Maron, M.B., S.M. Horvath, and J.E. Wilkerson. Blood biochemical alterations during recovery from competitive marathon running. Eur J Appl Physiol. 38:231–238, 1977.
56. Matoba, H. and P.D. Gollnick. Response of skeletal muscle to training. Sports Medicine (New Zealand) 1:240–251, 1984.
57. McNair, D.M., M. Lorr, and L.F. Droppleman. Profile of Mood States Manual. San Diego,

CA: Educational and Industrial Testing Service, 1971.

58. Mellerwowicz, H. and D.K. Barron. Overtraining. In: *Encyclopedia of Sports Science and Medicine*, L.A. Larson and D.E. Hermann, eds. New York: McMillan, 1971, pp. 1310–1312.

59. Monjan, A.A. and M.I. Collector. Stress-induced modulation of the immune response. *Science*. 196:307–308, 1977.

60. Montpetit, R.R., J.M. Lavoie, and G. Cazorla. Aerobic energy cost of swimming the front crawl at high velocity in international class and adolescent swimmers. In: *Biomechanics and Medicine in Swimming*, Hollander, Huijing, DeGroot, eds: International Series on Sports Sciences, Vol. 14, Champaign, IL: Human Kinetics Publishers, 1983, pp. 228–234.

61. Morgan, W.P. Selected psychological factors limiting performance: A mental health model. In: D.H. Clarke and H.M. Eckert, eds. *Limits of Human Performance*. American Academy of Physical Education Papers, Vol. 18, 1985, pp. 77–80.

62. Orlander, J., K-H. Kiessling, J. Karlsson, and B. Ekblom. Low intensity training, inactivity and resumed training in sedentary men. *Acta Physiol Scand*. 101:351–362, 1977.

63. Pate, R.R., P. Palmieri, D. Hughes and T. Ratliffe. Serum enzyme response to exercise bouts of varying intensity and duration. In: F. Landry and W. Orban, eds. *Third International Symposium on Biochemistry of Exercise*. Symposia Specialists: Miami, 1978.

64. Pate, R.R., R.D. Hughes, J.V. Chandler and J.L. Ratliffe. Effects of arm training on retention of training effects derived from leg training. *Med Sci Sports*. 10:71–74, 1978.

65. Pate, R.R. and A. Kriska. Physiological basis of the sex difference in cardiorespiratory endurance. *Sports Medicine*. 1:87–98, 1984.

66. Plotnikoff, N.P. and A.J. Murgo. Enkephalins-endorphins: stress and the immune system. *Federation Proc*. 44:89–90, 1985.

67. Pollock, M.L. Submaximal and maximal working capacity of elite distance runners. Part I.: Cardiorespiratory aspects. *Ann N Y Acad Sci*. 301:310–322, 1977.

68. Prokop, L. Adrenals and Sport. *J Sports Med Phys Fitness*. 3:115–121, 1963.

69. Rowell, L.B. Human cardiovascular adjustments to exercise and thermal stress. *Physiol Rev*. 51:75–159, 1974.

70. Saltin, B. Physiological effects of physical conditioning. *Med Sci Sports*. 1:50–56, 1969.

71. Saltin, B., K. Nager, D.L. Costill, E. Stein, J. Jansson, B. Essen, and P.D. Gollnick. The nature of the training response; peripheral and central adaptations to one-legged exercise. *Acta Physiol Scand*. 96:289–305, 1976.

72. Scheuer, J. and C.M. Tipton. Cardiovascular adaptations to physical training. *Ann Rev Physiol*. 39:221–251, 1977.

73. Sherman W.M., L.E. Armstrong, T.M. Murray, F.C. Hagerman, D.L. Costill, R.C. Staron, and J.L. Ivy. Effect of a 42.2 km footrace and subsequent rest or exercise on muscular strength and work capacity. *J Appl Physiol*. 57:1668–1673, 1984.

74. Simon, H.B. The immunology of exercise: A brief review. *JAMA*. 252:2735–2738, 1984.

75. Sjodin, B. Lactate dehydrogenase in human skeletal muscle. *Acta Physiol Scand*. (Suppl. 436), 1976.

76. Sjodin, B. and I. Jacobs. Onset of blood lactate accumulation and marathon running performance. *Int J Sports Med*. 2:23–26, 1981.

77. Sjodin, B. and J. Svedenhag. Applied physiology of marathon running. *Sports Med*. (New Zealand) 2:83–99, 1985.

78. Sjogaard, G., B. Nielsen, F. Mikkelsen, B. Saltin, and E.R. Burke. *Physiology of Bicycling*, Ithaca, NY, Mouvement Publications, 1985.

79. Slavin, J.L. Eating disorders in athletes. *J Phys Educ Rec Dance*. March 1987, pp. 33–36.

80. Solomon, G.F. Psychoneuroendocrinological effects on the immune response. *Ann Rev Microbiol*. 35:155–184, 1981.

81. Stamfl, F. *Franz Stamfl on running*. London: Herbert Jenkins, 1955.

82. Tomasi, T.B., F.B. Trudeau, D. Czerwinski, and S. Erredge. Immune parameters in athletes before and after strenuous exercise. *J Clin Immunol*. 2:173–178, 1982.

83. Troup, J.P. Review: energy systems and training considerations. *J Swimming Res*. 1:13–16, 1984.

84. Van Handel, P. Specificity of Training. *Bike Tech*. 6(3):6–12, 1987.

85. Wells, C.L., L.H. Hecht, and G.S. Krahenbuhl. Physical characteristics and oxygen utilization of male and female marathon runners. *Res Quart Exerc Sport*. 52:281–285, 1981.

86. Wheeler, G.D., S.R. Wall, A.N. Belcastro, and D.C. Cumming. Reduced serum testosterone and prolactin levels in male endurance runners. *JAMA*. 252:514–516, 1984.

87. Wolf, W. A contribution to the question of overtraining. In: *Health and fitness in the modern world*. The Athletic Institute Publishers, 1961, pp. 291–301.

88. Wybran, J. Enkephalins and endorphins as modifiers of the immune system: present and future. *Federation Proc*. 44:92–94, 1985.

89. Yates, A., K. Keehey, and C.M. Shisslak. Running—an analogue of anorexia? *New Engl J Med*. 308:251–255, 1983.

388 *PERSPECTIVES IN EXERCISE*

DISCUSSION

GISOLFI: What percent of $\dot{V}O_2$max do you think most athletes achieve during long, slow distance (LSD) work?

WELLS: It depends a great deal on the athlete. The "recreational" athlete is running around 60% to 70%, well below lactate threshold, so it's an easy pace for them. They are talking while they are running. But, I think it varies considerably. Somewhere around 60% to 75%. It varies with person's ability to run.

TIPTON: But what should it be? Not what people are doing, but what should it be?

WELLS: We don't really know, there are not many good studies. That's the problem.

GOLLNICK: I think you can get that information if you want to. You can monitor heart rate during the training and then do laboratory tests.

PATE: I don't think there is any question that some information is available. My personal preference has always been to resist listing specific kinds of approaches to training and rather try to communicate the general principles. Now, here is LSD training. Should it be at 50% of max, 60% of max, 70% of max? I don't know. What I do believe is that it varies. And what one athlete will call LSD is probably a bit different from what another one would. I don't think we know what it should be, because the answer to that question implies that we have research data to answer the question.

BURKE: I also think that if you were to bring 50 coaches into this room right now you would get 50 different interpretations of what LSD training is. I know cyclists who go out for LSD training and do 35% of their max. They are out there talking and having a good time. They put hours on the bike.

LANDY: LSD contains the words long and slow. You use the words long and slow, so it would seem that somebody should be able to at least describe the range of what is long and the range of what is slow.

DEMPSEY: Should you always be in a steady state? Can you maintain a steady state?

WELLS: Certainly.

DEMPSEY: You should?

WELLS: In long, slow distance, you should.

DEMPSEY: Could you exert a training effect if you always stay in a steady state?

WELLS: Yes.

DEMPSEY: Well, will it enhance max $\dot{V}O_2$?

WELLS: I don't think so, no.

PATE: I think the one reason the prolonged endurance athlete needs to be out there for two or more hours is to force glycogen depletion, i.e., force the system to operate to a greater extent on fat, probably something that is going to be encountered in a competitive situation. I think it's difficult to create that kind of physiologic environment with any other kind of training.

MICHELI: Some coaches talk about the bones and ligaments and tendons and so forth; we shouldn't forget those aspects of training.

WELLS: I think everybody realizes that movement patterns change, muscle recruitment patterns change with fatigue, and that sort of thing. You are not going to go out and run a marathon if you run 30 min every day. You are going to fall apart in an hour.

COYLE: This whole idea of training longer to increase your ability to utilize fat is a mystery to me. For example, if you put in more than 45 to 60 min a day, you probably don't show any additional enhancement of adaptation. So, regarding your selected adaptations for fat oxidation, I am not sure they have been quite well documented. It might be more than cardiovascular. It might be more than mitochondrial oxidation.

PATE: I think we do most of the things we do in training because they evolved out of common practice in the field. I don't believe we have very good answers for why we do many of the things we do in training. I suppose coaches stick with what works, and certain misconceptions then fall by the wayside. Other misconceptions are refuted by research. I don't believe that there exists adequate, experimental, scientific literature which allows us to be very direct in making the linkage between the changes we note in a laboratory and specific training advice.

SUTTON: There is a tremendous need to try to understand training in physiological terms, and I think that's where we are. It may well be that in the final analysis, we can't help the coach. But we certainly can't help anyone if we don't ask questions and provide answers in quantifiable terms. That would be a very major contribution.

GISOLFI: There's accumulating literature now which suggests that with overtraining or when you really overdo it, you sometimes have frank diarrhea, certainly loose stools, with finding of blood in the stools of people who were training at 30 to 40 miles a week and then ran 26 miles in one day.

PATE: Randy Eichner will address the GI bleeding issue. I think that in some areas of training research, the scientific literature is helpful and maybe even adequate. We know rather clearly that with absolute cessation of exercise, there is a reversal of the training adaptation that is fairly rapid and manifested both in skeletal muscle adaptations and in cardiorespiratory adaptations. From the pragmatic perspective of the athlete, the issue really is not so much what happens with detraining but what can be done to offset it, so that the deleterious effect of detraining is minimized. I guess I'm a bit of a skeptic in this area in terms of common practice, which now is leaning towards the cross training concept. I think the literature indicates that the best approach to training is to stay with the primary mode of activity to the extent that is possible. There are studies that show that reduced frequency or dose of activity does lead to a maintenance of a training effect for up to a substantial number of weeks. Cross training literature right now is not so encouraging. That, of course, is not a very helpful observation for the athlete that cannot perform due to injury.

HAGBERG: I thought I heard George Brooks talking about studies of active and inactive muscle builders, particularly in terms of lactate uptake and a couple of other things, that led me to believe that he would disagree with what you just said.

BROOKS: Well, that had to do with the specific point about fuel distribution. Runners ask the question, "Can I do arm training to improve the aerobic capacity of my arms and enhance lactate removal?" The premise is if I have more fit arms, my legs should benefit. I usually say no, because you don't want to raise the activity of the arms for economy reasons. But I am curious about the taper. Why does the taper work?

COYLE: I think the athletes that taper well are the ones that probably didn't need all the aerobic training in the first place and were failing to adapt.

HAGBERG: Swimmers are on the verge of overtraining every day. We had an orthopedic study going on with them, and they all said, "I don't want to do this; I don't want to overtrain." And one of the ex-swimmers who works with them said, "You overtrain in your normal training regimen; all we are going to do is measure you."

I just want to make one other point that I think we skipped over: the exercise training prescription based on lactate. Swimmers do it all the time. Cyclists are now into it, because an Italian cyclist a few years ago was trained by an exercise physiologist who prescribed the training very precisely, say an hour at anaerobic threshold on this day and 75 minutes below anaerobic threshold on that day, etc. And I would like to go on record as saying I don't think we have a lick of evidence to support either of those recommendations. Maybe I've set myself up to be shot down, but that's fine. I don't mind if someone can disprove it, but the coaches are just going wild with this stuff.

PATE: That's the primary reason we chose to overlook that. I don't think much of it either.

9

Injuries and Prolonged Exercise

Lyle J. Micheli, M.D.

INTRODUCTION
   I. TYPES OF OVERUSE INJURIES
  II. RUNNING INJURIES
 III. RISK FACTORS: RUNNING
  IV. ASSESSING RISK FACTORS
   V. SITES OF RUNNING INJURIES
  VI. LOWER LEG OVERUSE INJURIES
 VII. SWIMMING INJURIES
VIII. CYCLING INJURIES
  IX. TRIATHLON INJURIES
SUMMARY
BIBLIOGRAPHY
DISCUSSION

INTRODUCTION

In North America, a number of different exercise techniques or fitness activities have been used or recommended to attain and maintain aerobic fitness. These activities include running, swimming, cycling, rowing, paddling, rope skipping, various types of dance activities and, perhaps, walking (1,11,26,40,51). The common denominator of these activities is, of course, attaining and maintaining, for at lease 30–40 min a level of work that places the heart rate in an appropriate range (49). Recently, certain training programs and competitions have been introduced which combine some of these activities, such as the triathlon, a combination of running, cycling, and swimming (17).

Ideally, individuals participating in one of these "aerobic activities" will enjoy themselves, feel better and, improve their health. Unfortunately, certain individuals will sustain injuries, primarily to the musculoskeletal system, that will render them less healthy and may cause them to discontinue exercise. A small number may actually sustain sudden death in the course of performing aerobic activity (20,51). This chapter will discuss the musculoskeletal injuries occurring with sustained exercise and techniques of injury prevention.

Injury in sustained exercise may result from either macrotrauma or microtrauma. Single impact macrotrauma, such as a blow or a twisting injury may injure bone, muscle, tendon, ligament, or even neurovascular elements. Repetitive microtrauma, i.e. the repeated exposure of tissue to low magnitude force, may eventually result in injury to the same tissues, though often at the microscopic level (30,32).

Occasionally, a combination of the two mechanisms may result in injury, as when a tissue weakened by repetitive microtrauma is suddenly exposed to a single excessive load. While accidental macrotrauma injuries may occur in any sport or work situation, the overuse injuries resulting from repetitive microtrauma are seen much more frequently with sustained exercise.

These overuse injuries are usually characterized by the inflammatory response which accompanies the tissue injury, as with "tendinitis," "bursitis," "fasciitis," or "neuritis." With bone and articular cartilage, however, pain is the usual presentation, with the other characteristics of the inflammatory response—swelling and erythema—less evident.

It is evident that these heterogenous injuries to very different tissues are classed together because of their shared mechanism of injury—repetitive microtrauma. However, microtrauma injuries may result from a combination of extrinsic and intrinsic factors, including the relative rate and intensity of this microtrauma exposure, the fitness of the individual, and environmental factors, such as shoe choice, and running surface (32).

While once thought to be sustained primarily by adults, recent observations have demonstrated large numbers of overuse injuries in children performing sustained exercise (30). It is striking that overuse injuries in children were a rarity before the introduction of organized and competitive sports training for them. In adults, as less and less repetitive activity is occurring in the work place, there is, ironically, an increase in overuse injuries resulting from sports and fitness exercise, particularly at the beginning of an aerobic training program.

I. TYPES OF OVERUSE INJURIES

Every major tissue of the musculoskeletal system is subject to overuse injuries. In the muscle-tendon units, the major overuse injury is tendinitis. However, muscle strains, the result of microtrauma to muscle tissue or supporting tissue, have been observed in muscle biopsies of marathon runners following their run (46). It is important to remember that the inflammatory phase of tendinitis, with heat, swelling, pain, and erythema, is really the body's normal initial healing response to injured tissue, and this response must be respected. Treatment or training techniques that increase pain, swelling, or erythema following injury must be avoided. While it is rarely necessary to totally discontinue the use of the injured extremity, and complete rest may actually delay the healing, a period of relative rest may be required during which the extremity is used, but with a different stress pattern. A runner with an acute Achilles tendonitis who is swimming five miles a day may not be running, but he or she is certainly not resting.

It is important to maintain the strength and flexibility of a muscle-tendon unit while one is recovering from an acute tendinitis. Pain and swelling are good guides to the limits of training; applications of ice packs and gentle compression are often invaluable aids to maintaining conditioning during the recovery phase. Some recent work from Dalhousie University suggests that dynamic eccentric work can safely be done with tendinitis and may actually speed healing (48).

Microinjury to the support structures of joints, the ligaments and tendons, may also result in inflammation to adjacent bursae and be labeled bursitis. A bursa is actually only a pocket or space lined by synovial cells which excrete lubricating fluid. Overuse of adjacent ligaments and tendons may become evident by inflammation of the bursa, but therapy must be directed to restoring the strength and motion of the actual joint, and not to simply eradicating the inflammation in the bursa.

The overuse injury of bone is stress fracture or fatigue fracture. Although most often seen in the long bones of the lower leg it is the great masquerader (9). In any persistent, activity-related extremity pain, whether of foot, hip, knee, or ankle, stress fracture must be suspected. During a seven month period in the sports medicine clinic of Boston's Children's Hospital, a total of 53 stress fractures of the lower extremity were diagnosed, including five hip fractures (31). In ballet dancers, persistent foot pain, often initially diagnosed as tendonitis or metatarsalgia, will often finally be determined to be a stress fracture. This diagnosis can be very difficult to make by physical examination or even by x-ray techniques, and a Te^{99} bone scan may be necessary for final confirmation (43).

In articular cartilage, repetitive microtrauma appears to result in a pattern of injury starting with softening and progressing to shredding and thinning of the articular surface i.e. chondromalacia. The most common articular cartilage overuse injury involves the articular cartilage of the patella (29,44).

The characteristic history of activity-related aching pain in the front of the knee, increased by climbing stairs and, ironically, by prolonged sitting with the knees bent (called the "movie sign"), combined with tenderness on palpation of the patella or its adjacent retinaculum, is usually due to patella-femoral stress syndrome. If training is continued in the face of this parapatellar pain, further injury of the articular cartilage may occur resulting in chondromalacia of the patella (1,6).

II. RUNNING INJURIES

Of the various aerobic exercise activities, distance running has enjoyed a particular increase in popularity. In addition to the easy availability, convenience, and economy of running, certain other factors including the "running fad" have played a part. It is ironic that one of the first published reports on the high rate of overuse injury from running, and its relationship to intensity and duration of training, was, in actuality, a cardiovascular physiology study.

In 1969, Pollock et al. (39) reported a study of adult males involved in a running program in which intensity and duration of training were related to changes in aerobic capacity. This study demonstrated increased aerobic fitness and an increased injury rate with increased intensity and duration of training. Subjects training at 70% $\dot{V}O_2$max for 40 min, four times per week, sustained a 12% rate of injury. Those training at 85% to 90% $\dot{V}O_2$max for 15 min three times per week sustained a 22% injury rate, and those trained at 85% to 90% $\dot{V}O_2$max for 45 min, three times per week, had a 54% rate of injury. These observations suggested that the changes in the duration and intensity of training could be an important factor in the occurrence of overuse injury during a running program.

In running gait, a force in the range of three to five times body weight ascends up the lower extremity at heel strike (4). This force behaves like a sound wave, with a short duration (20–40 milliseconds) and rapid dissipation. In certain individuals, perhaps those with inappropriate training or mechanical or physiologic pre-dispositions, injury to bone, tendon, or articular cartilage may result from this force.

Unfortunately, at the present we know little about the training effect at the tissue level which results from the progressive exposure to these forces. We do know that remodeling and increases in the size and density of bones occur in response to repetitive stress from forces of this magnitude in exercising humans (9). Tipton et al. (50)

similarly demonstrated increases in the size and strength of ligaments of the extremities in running animals when compared to inactive controls.

It is not yet feasible to measure bone strength, ligament strength, or articular cartilage strength in a runner, swimmer, or cyclist, or to assess changes in these as a result of training. While we can measure in muscle-tendon units low velocity or static characteristics, such as strength, flexibility, or power, there is no evidence that changes in these variables as a result of training positively affect performance or the rate of injury (13).

Work by Raden et al. (42,47) on the etiology of osteoarthritis in animals suggested that increased muscular bulk of the extremities decreases the forces on the joints by absorbing a portion of the impacting force applied to the extremity. Increasing the size and bulk of the muscles of the legs with resistive training may thus indirectly decrease the potential for bone and joint injury, but this has yet to be proven with human studies.

III. RISK FACTORS: RUNNING

Most of the information and impressions concerning additional factors which may predispose to injury come from the assessments of athletes who have sustained overuse injuries. From this review has come a checklist of risk factors for overuse injury which has been proven useful for better management and prevention of these injuries (Table 9-1).

While studies of running have been the primary source of risk factor information on overuse injuries of the legs, these factors are also useful for the study of injuries in a variety of other endurance activities, including dance, cross-country skiing, rope skipping, etc. For dance, poor technique must be added as an additional risk factor.

It is noteworthy that the gender of the participant is not on the list of risk factors. While it appears that the female runner may sustain a higher incidence of overuse injuries than similar groups of males by age, this may be primarily a cultural phenomenon, the result of significantly less running by teenage girls (29). In actuality, many of the leg injuries in females appear to be the result of training error. This is especially true for culturally deconditioned women who begin running programs designed for men; this is seen in female military academy entrants.

An additional factor that may be present in certain female athletes who sustain overuse injuries is abnormality of the menstrual

TABLE 9-1. *Risk Factors in Running*

1. Training errors, including abrupt changes in intensity, duration, or frequency of training.
2. Musculotendonous imbalance of strength, flexibility, or bulk.
3. Anatomical malalignment of the lower extremities, including differences in leg lengths, abnormalities or rotation of the hips, position of the kneecap, and bow legs, knock knees, or flat feet.
4. Footwear: improper fit, inadequate impact-absorbing material, excessive stiffness of the sole, and/or insufficient support of hindfoot.
5. Running surface: concrete pavement versus asphalt, versus running track, versus dirt or grass.
6. Associated disease state of the lower extremity, including arthritis, poor circulation, old fracture, or other injury.

cycle. Recent studies have suggested that females engaged in heavy athletic training, particularly aerobic training, may have absent or irregular menstrual cycles (10). Concomitant with this, decreases in femoral and vertebral bone density have been demonstrated in some of these athletes (25). This decrease in bone density may increase the risk of leg or back injury (21).

IV. ASSESSING RISK FACTORS

As noted above, the occurrence of a given overuse injury in an individual may be the result of interactions of a number of risk factors. It is important for the physician to determine, as exactly as possible, which risk factors may have contributed to the occurrence of the overuse injury being assessed. This will aid in managing the injury and may help prevent the occurrence or reoccurrence of the same or similar injuries (32,34).

The task of assessing risk factors is rendered more difficult, because of the lack of normative values for many of these factors, and because of the difficulty of measuring them. As an example, we know little about the range of "safe progression" for training the musculoskeletal system, and we cannot easily measure the training effect at the tissue level. We can contrast this with the training of the cardiovascular system, where the time course of training is better known, and measures of relative fitness level, such as $\dot{V}O_2max$, are rather easily attainable.

While increases in cardiovascular fitness can safely be attained in a matter of months, the time course of musculoskeletal conditioning and strengthening, particularly of the bones, may be much slower. These tissues may take much longer to remodel and strengthen themselves in response to increased physical demands, particularly when underutilized for a number of years. In addition, we cannot easily measure the "fitness level" of bone. It is obviously a much more complex issue than simple bone density or size.

With the musculotendon units, measurements of strength and endurance are now more readily available; this is due largely to the increased popularity of isokinetic dynamometers (13). Yet, there is no clear relationship between these low velocity load response characteristics and the resistance to injury from high velocity forces, such as the footfall of running. Thus, although we know that rapid changes in the rate, intensity, or duration of repetitive microtrauma are an extremely important contributor to injury, we still do not know enough about these factors to recommend a specific exercise prescription for a specific individual.

While it is difficult to quantify exactly the intensity of training, changes in intensity, or the effect of intensity at the tissue level, there are studies suggesting that training errors are the most frequent contributor to overuse running injuries (1,18,22). Our own study of stress fractures in adult runners supported this (32). More recently, Lysholm and Wiklander's (22) study of injuries in runners also found training error to be the most common injury-provoking factor, occurring in 72% of the injuries which they studied.

Perhaps the most useful clinical guideline for a safe rate of training progression comes from experience with running injuries and is called "the ten percent rule." In general, the rate or intensity of running training should not be progressed more rapidly than 10% a week. Therefore, if a person is running 30 min at a session, four times a week, for a total of 120 min, he or she can probably safely increase running time to 132 min (120 ± 10%) the following week, if all other factors remain equal.

Terrain is also a very important factor in training. From both cardiovascular and orthopedic perspectives, running 30 min on a flat surface is very different, from running 30 min up hills (4,35). A coaching recommendation which may help prevent injury is to advise the runner to lean forward when running downhill.

It is important to remember that certain sports, if participated in exclusively, may actually contribute to muscle-tendon imbalance. Running, exclusively, tends to tighten and strengthen low back muscles and fascia, as well as the quadriceps and calf muscles, and results in a relative imbalance with the opposing muscles. If supplemental flexibility exercises are not also done, this muscle-tendon imbalance may predispose one to back, hip, knee, or lower leg injuries (14,19).

Anatomic malalignment can be the risk factor for which it is most difficult to compensate. If a dancer begins to suffer knee pain and injuries because the hips lack sufficient turnout (external rotation) for a technically satisfactory plie, little can be done. Similarly, runners lacking rotation about the hips, particularly internal rotation, may never be able to run without a repetitive pattern of injuries and might be counseled to consider biking or swimming.

On the other hand, some rather dramatic malalignments about the knee, lower leg, or foot may be completely compatible with injury-free participation. Some of the more effective runners we have seen have evident tibia vara and genu varum, and yet run without problems. Similarly, flat or pronated feet are often indicated as a major factor in the occurrence of lower-extremity overuse injury, and yet a number of world class runners and premier dancers have severely pronated feet and function without a problem. In other athletes, however, compensation for these alignments may be necessary to treat or prevent injury. The use of orthotic inserts in the shoes may prove helpful. The use of these devices in the management of knee and lower-leg problems in some athletes has been especially successful (33,35).

Thus, it is usually a combination of factors that result in a given overuse injury in a given athlete. In the study of stress fractures noted previously, training error was the most prevalent risk factor associated with the occurrence of injury, followed closely by muscle-tendon imbalance and anatomic malalignment (31).

It is important to recognize that overuse injury is not seen only in the recreational or less-skilled athlete. A nationally ranked runner who had been training at more than 90 miles a week dropped below 70 miles during a three-week examination period and then immediately resumed his 90 mile pace. A stress fracture of the tibia resulted, somewhat to his embarrassment. Additional risk factors in this injury appeared to be the use of a worn pair of racing flats from the previous season and tight calf muscles.

V. SITES OF RUNNING INJURIES

In addition to this review of the types of injury and associated risk factors, it is beneficial to review the anatomic sites of injury and discuss the injuries most frequently seen at each site.

Low back pain can be a distressing overuse injury, particularly for the runner. As noted previously, running tends to tighten the posterior low back muscles and fascia. The resulting tendency to low back sway, or lordosis, increases the risk for a number of low back conditions, including ruptured disc, facet syndrome, and spondylolysis (14). Supplemental stretching of the low back and hamstrings and strengthening of the abdominal muscles can reverse this tendency and may decrease the risk of low back injury (29).

Overuse injuries about the hip include trochanteric bursitis, iliopsoas tendonitis and, although frequently unsuspected, stress fractures (19). In trochanteric bursitis, tight fascia lata and hamstrings, as well as minor leg length discrepancy (the bursitis usually occurs in the longer leg), are frequently associated risk factors.

The most frequent overuse injury about the knee, as already noted is chondromalacia or patello-femoral stress syndrome (17,19,29). In addition, lateral knee pain can be frequently encountered in runners. This may be unilateral or bilateral and has a high association with the anatomic malalignment of genu valgum and tibia vara. Again, unilateral lateral knee pain may be seen in the long leg of an athlete who has a leg length discrepancy. A number of anatomic structures and conditions have been indicted as the cause of this pain. These include, popliteal tendinitis, impingement of the fascia lata on the lateral femoral condyle, and chondromalacia of the patella. This lateral knee pain appears to be one of the conditions which can be helped by orthotics in the shoes. Again, relative training error is often seen as an associated risk factor in overuse knee pain. Tight hamstrings should also be watched for in these syndromes.

A program of static straight leg raising exercises done with progressive resistance and combined with leg flexibility exercises, has helped to resolve this problem (31). A recent survey of young patients with patello-femoral stress syndrome showed that more than 90% of them were cleared of pain and resumed function with this program. It is interesting to observe that the ability to lift 12 pounds 10 times with a straight leg appears to be a threshold. Patients who reach this will almost always have a satisfactory result if lifting is maintained for six months at these levels. The maximal goal of lifting is generally between 15 and 18 pounds, performed with three sets of 10 repetitions with each leg.

VI. LOWER LEG OVERUSE INJURIES

"Shin splints" is a term used to refer to training related to pain over the front of the lower leg. Pain at this site may actually be due to stress fracture, tendinitis, irritation of the bone covering (the periosteum) at sites of muscle insertion, or increased pressure in the muscle compartments of the lower leg. For this reason, the term "shin splints" is rarely used by the sports medicine practitioner. The specific diagnosis responsible for the pain should be made (6,19).

Pain in this area is usually the result of repetitive impacting of the legs from the running and jumping sports, with distance running, aerobic dance, and rope jumping potentially more damaging. It is important to determine the exact site of pain and tenderness, the chronology of the pain, and any change in its severity.

Tenderness at a specific site over the tibia or fibula, combined with the ability to reproduce the pain at the same site by applying indirect pressure, as by bending the affected bone, usually is suggestive of stress fracture as a cause of the pain (9). This diagnosis may be confirmed by obtaining a Te[99] bone scan (43). Tenderness over specific tendons of the lower leg muscles and exacerbation of the pain by resisting motion performed by a given muscle is suggestive of tendinitis.

Tenderness over the muscle bellies of one of the four muscle compartments of the lower leg immediately after exercise suggests compartment pressure elevation, i.e., compartment syndrome, as a possible cause of "shin splints." This can be tested by obtaining the pressures within the compartment immediately after exercise. Elevation of the compartment pressure by more than 20 mmHg following exercise, or more than 10 mmHg greater than the opposite, uneffected side, is very suggestive of compartment syndrome as a cause of the lower leg pain (19,36).

Recently, Clancy (6), Puddu (41) and others have called attention to tendonosis or aseptic necrosis of tendon tissue as an additional cause of dysfunction and pain in major tendons, including the Achilles tendon. These sites undergo ischemic death, much as can occur in the bone, and are not successfully healed and revascularized by the body. Continued pain, and in some cases, complete tendon rupture may result if significant mechanical compromise has occurred. Clancy (6) has emphasized the importance of a complete exploration of the involved tendon if tendonosis is suspected and surgical exploration required. The important risk factors in these cases appear to be inflexibility of musculo-tendon units and, often, training error that is repetitive in nature. Perhaps the single most important preventative step is daily slow stretching, particularly of the Achilles, and maintenance of the dorsiflexor strength by heel walking or resistive exercises.

One of the most difficult overuse injuries of all, plantar fascitis, occurs in the foot. The plantar fascia is a heavy layer of tissue running from the base of the heel bone, or oscalcis, to the base of the metacarpo-phalangeal joints along the arch of the foot. Progressive tightening of the structure, usually in association with a tight Achilles tendon, appears to be the prime factor in its occurrence. Again, slow stretching of this structure and of the Achilles tendon is probably the best preventor. Well cushioned, stable running shoes are also important, as is slow, progressive training.

VII. SWIMMING INJURIES

Overuse injuries from sustained swimming occur in both the upper and lower extremities. While overuse injuries at these sites can be encountered with any swimming stroke, certain techniques, such as the butterfly and breast stroke, appear to have an increased potential for injury.

In the upper extremity, the shoulder is the primary site of overuse injury. Dubbed "swimmer's shoulder," the usual complaint at presentation is anterior shoulder pain at the initiation of the swimming stroke (5).

The pathomechanics of this condition are debated, with anterior or multiaxial instability of the glenohumeral joint indicted by most observers (3,7,27). Instability and excessive excursion of the humeral head beneath the coracoacromial arch results in injury to the rotator cuff, biceps tendon, or anterior glenoid labrum.

Factors in injury occurrence include excessive distance or duration of training, use of hand paddles in training, and errors in stroking technique, such as using too wide a stroke (8).

Overuse injuries to the knee in swimming occur at the patellofemoral joint or to the medial structures of the knee (12,16,44,52). In one study of swimmers, an extremely high incidence of overuse type of knee pain was discovered in 73% of breast stroke swimmers (44).

In breaststroke swimmers, the site of tissue injury included the patello-femoral joint, medial retinaculum, and medial collateral ligament (52). In pain localized to the patello-femoral joint of swimmers, there appeared to be a higher incidence of injury to medial retinacular plica than other anterior knee disorders.

Preventive techniques currently recommended for overuse knee injuries in swimmers include decreasing the intensity of training, altering the technique of kick, and strengthening the medial structures of the knee.

VIII. CYCLING INJURIES

Reported overuse injuries from cycling include injuries to the low back, to the patello-femoral joint of the knee, and tendinitis or joint impingement about the ankle (15,26,45). Cycling involves a constrained posturing of the body and lower extremity with force application over a defined range. There are, however, variations in frame size, seat height and angle, crank length, the use of toe clips, and internal or external posturing of the foot which can effect the comfort, the mechanical efficiency of cycling, and the occurrence of overuse injury (27,40).

As with other overuse injuries discussed above, the management of patello-femoral pain, in particular with cycling, includes institution of a proper rehabilitative exercise program, altering the intensity of training, and, especially, avoiding hills and heavily-loaded pedaling. In addition, techniques of cycle adjustment may decrease the stress across the patello-femoral joint. Studies of cycling mechanics have suggested that elevating the seat and positioning the foot more posteriorly over the pedal decreases the stress across the knee. Cycling shoes and toe clips, properly adjusted, may also decrease the stress on the patella (15,27).

Other relatively rare overuse injuries have been reported with cycling. These include ulnar neuropathy, caused by poor posturing of the hand along the handle bars, bursitis of the ischeal tuberosities caused from poor positioning of the saddle and ischemic neuropathy of the penis from excessive anterior saddle pressure (11,49,45).

In cycling, of course, acute accidents are a much more serious and prevalent injury than overuse injury. With children in particular, this is the leading cause of sports and exercise injury (45). Simple preventive measures, such as wearing a protective head-gear and safety instruction have not yet been mandated in most states and are an obvious first step in the prevention of these serious injuries.

IX. TRIATHLON INJURIES

Triathlons are growing rapidly in interest as a form of varied endurance training. It has been hypothesized that the very different types of training required for each stage of the activity might well exert a protective effect on the individual and decrease the incidence of overuse injury. While this is an attractive hypothesis, and is supported, to some extent, by studies which have shown more injuries in runners who do not participate in other types of training activities than from those who do, there are inadequate data from triathletes to confirm this phenomenon. Our own study of triathlon injuries shows that the majority of overuse injuries occurs as a result of run training and that triathlon-related injuries and injury rates are similar to those seen in athletes engaged exclusively in run training (17).

SUMMARY

Overuse injuries sustained by the endurance athlete can be as debilitating as the acute injuries of the contact sport athlete, especially if proper care is not taken to attain early diagnosis and proper treatment.

The problem, of course, is distinguishing between a serious overuse injury and the aches, pains, and sore muscles encountered with normal training. A useful guideline for the endurance athlete or coach is that any painful site associated with swelling or loss of motion of an adjacent joint should be evaluated immediately. If the athlete has access to an athletic trainer, the first step may be to seek his or her advice. A certified athletic trainer, while not qualified to make a diagnosis, may help the athlete decide which physician may be best suited to assess and treat the injury. In addition, the athletic trainer may recommend first-aid measures that can help reduce pain and swelling. If the athlete does not have access to an athletic trainer, the team physician or a physician with an interest in athletic injuries should be consulted.

Pain over an anatomic site which is not associated with swelling or loss of motion, but which presents in the same pattern and at the same level or increased levels of discomfort beyond one week, should also receive medical attention.

Too many athletic training and fitness programs have been delayed or even ended by inattention to an overuse injury. Ironically, many of these overuse injuries, and, in particular, tendinitis and stress fractures, may require little more than medication, ice therapy and corrective exercises to reverse their course. Often, a short period of "relative rest" may be sufficient to reverse the stress patterns and tissue injury responsible for the pain and inflammation. Trying to run, swim, or cycle "through the pain" may be an invitation to disaster.

Methods of preventing certain types of these problems are just beginning to be understood. Proper training, with slow progression, is the most important step in preventing the occurrence of overuse injuries, despite the great variety of tissues involved. Since recreational athletes frequently have no coach, physicians must become more knowledgeable in the practical aspects of training and conditioning—particularly of running—in order to safely prescribe exercise for their patients.

BIBLIOGRAPHY

1. Brubaker C.E. and S.L. James. Injuries to runners. *Am J Sports Med.* 2:189–98, 1974.
2. Buxbaum, R. and L.J. Micheli. *Sports for Life.* Boston: Beacon Press, 1979.
3. Cain, P.R., T.A. Mutschler, F. Fu and S.K. Lee. Anterior stability of the glenohumeral joint: A dynamic model. *Am J Sports Med* 15:144–148, 1987.
4. Cavanaugh, P.R. and M.A. Lafortune. Ground reaction forces in distance running. *J Biomech.* 13:397–406, 1980.
5. Ciullo, C.V. Swimmer's shoulder. *Clin Sports Med* 5:115–137, 1986.

6. Clancy, W.G. Runners injuries. Part II: Evaluation and treatment of specific injuries. *Am J Sports Med* 8:287–89, 1980.
7. Cofield, R.H. and W.T. Simonet. The shoulder in sports. *Mayo Clinic Proceedings* 59:157–164, 1984.
8. Councilman, J.E. The role of the coach in training for swimming. *Clin Sports Med* 5:3–7, 1986.
9. Devas, M.B. *Stress Fractures*. Churchill-Livingston, Edinburgh, 1975.
10. Drinkwater, B.L., K. Nilson, C.H. Chestnut, W.J. Bremner, S. Shaninholtz, and M.B. Southworth. Bone mineral content of amenorrheic and eumenorrheic athletes. *N Engl J Med* 311:277–281, 1984.
11. Eckman, P.B., G. Perlstein and P.H. Altrocchi. Ulnar neuropathy in bicycle riders. *Arch Neurol.* 32:130–131, 1975.
12. Fowler, P.J. and W.D. Regan. Swimming injuries of the knee, foot and ankle, elbow, and back. *Clin in Sports Med* 5:139–148, 1986.
13. Gleim, G.W., J.A. Nicholas and J.W. Webb. Isokinetic evaluation following leg injuries. *Phys Sports Med* 6:74–81, 1978.
14. Guten, G. Herniated nucleus pulposus in the runner. *Am J Sports Med* 9:155–159, 1981.
15. Hannaford, D.R., G.T. Moran and H.F. Hlavac. Video analysis and treatment of overuse knee injury in cycling: A limited clinical study. *Clin Podiat Med Surg* 3:671–678, 1986.
16. Heckman, J.D. and C.C. Alkire. Distal patella pole fractures. A proposed common mechanism of injury. *Am J Sports Med* 12:424–428, 1984.
17. Ireland, M.L. and L.J. Micheli. Triathletes: Biographic data, training and injury patterns. *Annals Sport Med* 3:117–120, 1987.
18. Jacobs, J.S. and B.L. Berson. Injuries to runners: A study of entrance in a 10,000 meter race. *Am J Sports Med* 14:151–155, 1986.
19. Jones, D.C. and S.L. James. Overuse injuries of the lower extremity: Shin splints, iliotibial band friction syndrome, and extertional compartment syndromes. *Clin Sports Med* 6:273–290, 1987.
20. Koplan, J.P., D.S. Sistovick and G.M. Goldbaum. The risks of exercise: A public health view of injuries and hazards. *Public Health Rep* 100:189–196, 1985.
21. Lloyd, T., E.R. Triantafyllou, P.S. Houts, J.A. Whiteside, A. Kalenak and P.G. Stumpf. Women athletes with menstrual irregularity have increased musculoskeletal injuries. *Med Sci Sports* 18:374–378, 1986.
22. Lysholm, J., and J. Wiklander. Injuries in Runners. *Amer J Sports Med.* 15:168–171, 1987.
23. Mann R.A. Biomechanics of running. In: R. D'Ambrosia, and D. Drezeds. *Prevention and treatment of running injuries*. Thorfore: Charles B. Slack Inc., 1982, 1–14.
24. Marcus, R., et al. Menstrual function and bone mass in elite women distance runners. *Ann Int Med* 102:158–163, 1985.
25. Mayer, P.J. Helping your patient avoid bicycling injuries. *J Osteoskeletal Med* 2:31–38, 1985.
26. McLeod, W.D., and T.A. Blackburn. Biomechanics of knee rehabilitation with bicycling. *Am J Sports* 8:175–180, 1980.
27. McMaster, W.C. Anterior glenoid labrum damage: A painful lesion in swimmers. *Am J Sports Med* 14:383–387, 1986.
28. Micheli, L.J. Female runners. In D'Ambrosia, R.D., ed. *Prevention and treatment of running injuries*. Thorofore: Charles B. Slack Inc., 1980.
29. Micheli, L.J. Overuse injuries in children's sports: The growth factor. *Ortho Clin North Am* 14:337–60, 1983.
30. Micheli, L.J. Special considerations in children's rehabilitation programs. In: Hunter L.Y., F.J. Funk, Jr., eds. *Rehabilitation of the injured knee*. St. Louis: C.V. Mosby, 1984, 406–413.
31. Micheli, L.J., F.J. Santopietro, et al. Etiological assessment of overuse stress fractures in athletes. *Nova Scotia Medical Bulletin*, 1980, 43–47.
32. Micheli, L.J., F.J. Santopietro and R.S. Sohn. Shoewear and Orthotics. In: Nicholas, J.A., ed. *Lower extremity injuries*. St. Louis: C.V. Mosby, 1985.
33. Monsour, J.M., M.D. Lesh, M.D. Nowak and S.R. Simon. A three dimensional multi-segmental analysis of the energetics of normal and pathological human gait. *J Biomechanics* 15:51–59, 1982.
34. Nicholas, J.A. The value of sports profiling. *Clin Sports Med* 3:3–10, 1984.
35. Nigg, B.M., J. Denoth, B. Ken, S. Luethi, D. Smith, A. Staeoff. Load, sports shoes and playing surfaces. In: Frederick, E.C., ed. *Sports shoes and playing surface*. Champaign: Human Kinetics Publishing, 1984, 1–23.
36. Owen, C.A. Clinical diagnosis of acute compartment syndromes. In: Mubarak, S.J., A.R. Hargens, eds. *Compartment Syndromes and Volkman's Contracture*. Philadelphia: W.B. Saunders, 1981, 98–105.
37. Paffenbarger, R.S., A.L. Wing and R.T. Hyde. Physical activity as an index of heart attack risk in college alumni. *Am J Epidemiology* 108:161–175, 1978.

38. Paffenbarger, R.S., R.T. Hyde, W.L. Wing and C.H. Steinmetz. A natural history of athleticism and cardiovascular health. *J Amer Med Assoc* 252:491–495, 1984.
39. Pollock, M.L., T.K. Cureton, and L. Greninger. Effects of frequency of training on work capacity, cardiovascular function and body composition of adult men. *Med Sci Sports* 1:70–74, 1969.
40. Powell, B. Correction and prevention of bicycle saddle. *Phys J M* 10:62–67, 1982.
41. Puddu, G. Method for reconstruction of the anterior cruciate ligament using the semitendonosus tendon. *Am J Sports Med* 8:402–404, 1980.
42. Radin, E.R. Role of muscles in protecting athletes from injury. *Acta Med Scand Suppl* 711:143–147, 1986.
43. Rosen, P.R., L.J. Micheli and S. Treves. Early scintigraphic diagnosis of bone stress and fractures in athletic adolescents. *Pediatrics* 70:11–15, 1982.
44. Rovere, G.D. and A.W. Nichols. Frequency associated factors, and treatment of breaststroker's knee in competitive swimmers. *Am J Sports Med* 13:99–104, 1985.
45. Selbert, S.M. and D. Alexander. Bicycle related injuries. *Am J Disease of the Child.* 141:140–144, 1987.
46. Siegel, A.J., L. Silverman, W. Evans. Elevated skeletal muscle creatine kinase MB isoenzymes levels in marathon runners. *JAMA* 250:2835–2837, 1983.
47. Simon, S.R., E.R. Radin, I.L. Paul and R.M. Rose. The response of joints to impact loading, *J. Biomechanics* 5:267, 1972.
48. Stanish, W. And S. Curwin. *Tendonitis: Its etiology and treatment.* Lexington: D.C. Heath Company, 1985.
49. The American College of Sports Medicine. *Guidelines for graded exercise testing and exercise prescription.* Philadelphia: Lea and Febiger, 1985.
50. Tipton, C.M., A.C. Vailas and R.D. Matthes. Experimental studies on the influence of physical activity on ligaments, tendons and joints: A brief review. *Acta Med Scand Suppl* 157–158.
51. Van Camp, S.P. Sudden death in the athlete. ASCM Clinical Conference. Keystone, Colorado, 281–288, 1987.
52. Vizsolyi, P., J. Taunton, G. Robertson, et al. Breaststroker's knee: An analysis of epidemiology and biomechanical factors. *Am J Med* 15:63–71, 1987.

DISCUSSION

MICHELI: Our clinical approach with injured athletes is to try to factor out the various host factors, the various environmental factors, to separate acute trauma from overuse injuries, to try to work backwards and figure out why the athlete got injured in the first place. Was it the way they were training? Was it observed muscle-tendon imbalances or the way their body was shaped, (for instance their leg length ratio between the femur and the tibia)? Are they bowlegged, knock-kneed, flat-footed? In the case of running or dancing, we want to know the surface they are working on. Are they in the midst of a growth spurt? This is what we have done, trying to work backwards from injury to causation.

Training seems to be the most important problem. Obviously there is some relationship between the intensity, and duration or progression of training and injury rate, and this seems to be the case with many people.

BROOKS: What do you mean by injury? Is it defined as an occurrence serious enough to stop training?

MICHELI: That's how most injuries are defined in the epidemiology of trauma. But, in many instances an injury is hard to define. A patient comes to you and says he's injured, an athlete goes to the athletic trainer or personal physician and says, "I am injured." In some cases, you can prove it's an injury. You look at a bone scan, and there's a stress fracture. But some of these things are hard to define and hard to diagnose. One of the problems with looking at the injury potential aspect of the musculoskeletal system, and that's my primary emphasis, is that it is hard to noninvasively assess the training effect at the musculoskeletal level. We know that when animals are trained, the bones get stronger, the ligaments get stronger, and the muscle-tendon units get stronger. We don't have a good idea of the time course of those events in humans, and we don't have very good noninvasive ways of measuring them.

RAVEN: With some cases of the tendinitis, could they not be biochemically or physiologically induced?

MICHELI: There may be biochemical components. There is a small group of people, for instance, that feels that patello-femoral, articular cartilage overuse injuries may be a biochemical problem. But most of us feel that it starts as a biomechanical problem and then may become biochemical. Hence, the use of medications, for instance, to try to stabilize the articular cartilage.

BLAIR: I'm reminded of a study in which the researchers looked at dancers exposed to differences in the shock absorbing qualities of floors, and there was really no difference in the injury rates among these dancers.

WEIKER: It's tough for me to accept that, though, because they worked with completely different dance instructors, choreographers, and companies. And no two are the same. If you go to a few different dance companies and watch, they don't dance the same. They will adapt to the type of floor they are working on and the type of dancers they have. So that study meant nothing except that given smart instructors, a variation in dances, and a variation in floors, they all came out at the same end point as far as injury.

BLAIR: Well, I don't think it's fair to say it meant nothing. There were people dancing on different floors. They were monitored prospectively.

WEIKER: But you are making the assumption that dancing is dancing, and it's not. There's a wide variation.

BLAIR: I'm aware of that, but the only data we have suggests that the floor is not important. The other things you suggest may well be important, but we need data.

WEIKER: Consider The American Ballet Theater. When they go on the road and have to dance on different floors, they assume a higher injury rate and take extra dancers. They have the same technique of dancing, the same dancers, and the same choreography. The only change they are aware of is the change in floor surfaces when they go on the road, where they don't have quality floors.

They take along a group of spares because of the expected injury rate.

BLAIR: There's another difference; they're on the road. They perform more; they are more tired.

WEIKER: No, they don't perform any more. They practice at the same rate as they perform.

MICHELI: Obviously the dance technique and so forth is an additional factor in the occurrence of various injuries to dancers. I didn't include aerobic dancing in this chapter, because it typically doesn't fit the definition of prolonged exercise.

Just to change direction for a moment, I'd like to mention an excellent example of an overuse injury in the upper extremities. It is the so called "swimmer's shoulder." Some people say there are many orthopedic problems in swimming and many typical overuse injuries. We are seeing a tremendous amount of shoulder problems in our young swimmers. There is an absolute epidemic in age group swimmers. These kids are doing 9 to 12 thousand yards a day. A nine-year-old kid comes in, and he has sore shoulders, a subluxating shoulder. You examine these kids, and they have a muscle-tendon contracture. The forces involved in overhand swimming are very different from most any other activity. Muscle-tendon imbalance, I think, is a formidable contributor to some of the overuse tissue injuries. And, in particular, these kids develop a relative external rotation contracture. They lose internal rotation and they lose the ability to adduct the arm, suggesting development of a tight posterior capsule. They do get a so-called tendinitis, but I think it's secondary to this contracture. The arm slips out of the joint with an anterior subluxating shoulder, which, in turn, secondarily impinges on the so-called rotator cuff muscle. And then, if you go in there with a big cortisone needle and inject the tendinitis, you've missed the entire etiology of this condition. I think it's as good an example of an overuse injury as is a stress fracture. If it's a stress fracture, you can usually show it by x-ray or bone scan.

WEIKER: I'm concerned about the implication I often hear and read that running can cause spondylolysis. I am unaware of any statistical studies that show that. I do think that running causes dramatic accentuation in the symptomatology of spondylolysis and spindylolisthesis. Work long ago showed that over 95% of spondys occurred between the ages of five and seven, so, maybe, as we are getting younger marathon runners, we might start to see a cause. The runners I see with spondylolysis—and that is a fairly rare occasion—show no evidence of active disease with a bone scan. They have long-standing chronic spondy that has gotten symptomatic because of the hyperlordotic posture. And I wonder if we should criticize running as causing that. At the same time, I think we should point out that, although it has been said that swimmers don't have back problems, I have had to take numerous kids out of butterfly because of recurrent spondylolysis symptoms. The hyperextension of the butterfly stroke is devastating to somebody who is a spondy or has frank spondylolisthesis.

MICHELI: We know that if you don't assume the upright posture, the incidence of spondy is zero. So I think there is a big shift in thinking about spondylolysis, because it is an overuse injury. Maybe there is a congenital predisposition to get it. On the other hand, these kids doing repetitive flexion and extension, such as running, gymnastics, diving, and so forth, have an increased incidence.

WEIKER: I agree with that, but spondy occurs at a younger age than that at which most people get into running.

Let me mention one more thing. We have a lot of people running rural roads. If they don't learn to alternate sides of the road, running on one single side of a dome-shaped road throws everything out of whack. They come up with all sorts of knee and hip problems related to posturing, so we should try to get them to alternate.

Also, I think we need to be more definitive in our position on shin splints. The coach or trainer reading this chapter will be looking for a section on shin splints. I think we need to put in some explanation as to whether we believe it's a periostitis or whatever. But it is a syndrome in the early stages of overuse. We treat it the same as we treat a stress fracture, and we get basically the same results.

RAVEN: Dr. Weiker, you say the treatment of stress fractures is rest, is that correct?

WEIKER: Basically the treatment of stress fractures is avoidance of impact loading. You go to a smooth function, whether it's cycling or swimming without kick-off turns.

RAVEN: But there's a lot of discussion of shin splints suggesting that you should just run through them.

WEIKER: Well, that's why we get to treat a lot of stress fractures.

MICHELI: Shin splints covers about four different pain syndromes of the lower legs, one of which may be a stress fracture. It's a differential diagnosis. It may be compartment syndrome, such as periostitis. But the diagnostic techniques are now available to sort this out very readily. I didn't perceive this chapter to be something for the orthopedist to try to sort out how to make a differential diagnosis of shin splints.

WEIKER: I have just three other points. One is the rule of 10% on progression. I think that's an excellent guideline, and I use it with my patients. In addition, I have adopted another rule for runners specifically called "The Rule of Controllable Variables." Runners can select their shoes, their distance, their speed, the terrain they run on, the surface they run on, and the time of day they run. I don't allow my runners, once I have them under my control, to ever change more than one of those variables in a given two week period. The quickest way to get in trouble is to change shoes, terrain, and speed, during the same period of a training program. It's too much for the body to adjust to. If you take a history of patients presenting with overuse problems, invariably you find that they have changed several of these variables at once.

I think we should also add some other problems, such as the ulnar nerve neuropathy of the wrist and occasional median nerve compartment syndrome seen in cyclists. Whether you believe it is caused by ischemia or direct nerve pressure, the pudendal neuropathy and numbness that also goes with cycling should be discussed. For men, especially, if they haven't at least read about it, pudendal numbness can be very frightening.

BLAIR: I wonder if we should imply that training errors are in fact causing most injuries. It may be more appropriate to suggest that in the clinical management of these patients, making suggestions that training errors may have caused injury is appropriate, clinical management. However, we should not leave the implication that these errors are in fact etiologic factors. Now they may well be, but we have to get that data.

MICHELI: I think many of these injuries may be multifactorial problems—psychological, nutritional, and so forth. But when we give a talk to athletes on how to prevent injuries, we should certainly not omit mention of training errors.

DEMPSEY: You mentioned that you knew a coach who suggested that moderate jogging would be a good injury preventer because it might strengthen connective tissue and ligaments surrounding the knees or ankles. Do you believe that's really true, that jogging really does strengthen? Wouldn't it be better to do specific exercises to strengthen the knees and ankles of runners?

MICHELI: Well, that's a classic debate. Do the velocity of training and the specificity of training have real injury prevention potential? Some people say you should train athletes with weight training and employ Russian plyometric techniques and so forth, and that doing so will strengthen their connective and muscular tissues and enhance their performance without injury. But I think that at some point you have to train the body to tolerate the specific insults of an athletic event. Simply doing squats or other such drills will not do it.

WEIKER: There's a general misconception or misunderstanding regarding the relationship between bone density and bone strength that we should address. I think bone density is important. Osteomalacia and osteoporosis illustrate this importance. On the other side, the architectural structuring of the bone is equally important. Bone density is not the whole answer. Several diseases result in dense bone that is also very fragile bone. What counts is the integrity of the architectural structure, and that's where the impact loading of training comes in. Cybex training may strengthen muscle, but it does not adequately stimulate bone. The bone needs a stimulus in order to restructure. When you change sports, you restructure your skeleton. The bone is taken through urban renewal. It's stripped of its architecture and rebuilt to do its new job.

RAVEN: What do you need to do this? Impact?

WEIKER: Well, impact is certainly important if the athlete is involved in an impact sport. The runner needs impact loading. If kids swim all winter long, like a lot of high school students, doing virtually nothing of impact during the winter, they will have a different bony architecture in the spring than they would have has if they had run all winter.

MICHELI: Radiographic studies of tennis players indicate that the service arm develops dramatic differences in bony architecture and in density. I know of no study that correlates bone density with bone strength.

DEMPSEY: I have measured foot plant pressures in terms of gastric pressure and the effect on what the diaphragm does, and those pressures are absolutely huge. It's important to try to absorb those pressures. What about the importance of muscle mass on the lower limbs?

MICHELI: Animal work has shown that soft tissue bulk may be very closely related with force absorption.

DEMPSEY: Why can't you get thicker, stronger tendons and more muscle mass to absorb the shock if you do specific muscle training for the lower limbs in addition to the running?

BLAIR: This issue is very interesting. We have some very crude data in which we find no association between 1 RM leg press strength and leg injuries among runners and walkers.

WEIKER: I have two comments to add to this discussion. I think we are confusing the protective benefit of muscle strength when the real issue is muscle fatigueability. It's the muscle that rapidly fatigues that lets the athlete down. An athlete's one RM capability has very little to do with muscle fatigueability.

My final comment is that the majority of coaches do not work with elite athletes. The person who becomes elite has already proven that he or she is a different animal from the rest of us mere mortals. If the average high school coach takes what we just talked about and starts applying that to his or her high school athletes, orthopods are going to be swamped with athletic injuries. You just can't train all people the same way.

10

Other Medical Considerations in Prolonged Exercise

Edward R. Eichner, M.D.

I. SPORTS HEMATOLOGY
    A.   The Anemias of Athletes
    B.   Dilutional Pseudoanemia Versus Stress Erythrocytosis
    C.   True Anemias in Athletes
    D.   Iron Deficiency Without Anemia
    E.   Iron Deficiency Anemia
    F.   Footstrike Hemolysis
    G.   Other Types of Intravascular Hemolysis in Athletes
    H.   Blood Doping
    I.   The Acute Phase Response: Blood Markers of Overtraining?
II. PROLONGED EXERCISE AND THE URINARY TRACT
    A.   Exercise-Induced Proteinuria
    B.   Exercise-Induced Hematuria
    C.   Exercise-Induced Acute Renal Failure
III. PROLONGED EXERCISE AND THE GASTROINTESTINAL TRACT
    A.   Gastrointestinal Disturbances in Runners
    B.   Management of Common Gastrointestinal Disturbances
BIBLIOGRAPHY
DISCUSSION

I. SPORTS HEMATOLOGY

Regular aerobic exercise evokes diverse hematologic adaptations that expand the blood while making it more fluid and less likely to clot. In concert, these healthy hematologic adaptations to exercise offer the elite athlete enhanced performance and the everyday exerciser reduced risk of blood clots, heart attack, and stroke.

Prolonged exercise, however, takes a toll on the blood. The acute hematologic changes during prolonged, intense exercise can be opposite to the long-term, healthful adaptations which result from regular exercise. Stress leukocytosis and thrombocytosis are common.

Severe hemoconcentration can occur. Red blood cells can be destroyed. Major abnormalities of blood clotting can appear. Paradoxically, the clotting abnormalities can take either extreme: distance running has caused thrombotic strokes, as well as gastrointestinal hemorrhages. Bleeding during distance running, in fact, can be massive (63) and even fatal (89). Sports hematology, then, comprises the beneficial and the detrimental changes in the blood during exercise.

A.   The Anemias of Athletes

In the athletic world, one of the best-known examples of a change in the blood is sports anemia. The term "sports anemia" is an imprecise misnomer. It is imprecise when applied to the true anemias of individual athletes; it is a misnomer when applied to the false anemia common to many endurance athletes. The term "sports anemia," then, should be dropped. Instead, specific diagnostic terms should be used for true anemias in athletes; the term "dilutional pseudoanemia" could be used for the false anemia of endurance athleticism.

The most common cause of a low hemoglobin concentration in an endurance athlete is a dilutional pseudoanemia. Teleologically, it is an overcompensation for the acute hemoconcentrations of repeated bouts of vigorous exercise. As such, it is one of the earliest bodily adaptations to exercise and a cardinal component of aerobic fitness. It enhances athletic performance by increasing the cardiac stroke volume and increasing the sweat output (22,78).

The inciting mechanism for dilutional pseudoanemia is the acute hemoconcentration of exercise. For example, upon running 1.5 miles, the hematocrit increases 5% to 12%, with the increase proportional to running speed (45). Such exercise drives plasma water into the tissues. To compensate for this acute hypovolemia, the body holds onto salt and water by releasing renin, aldosterone, and vasopressin and increases plasma oncotic pressure by making more albumin. This expands the baseline plasma volume.

The plasma volume expands quickly in response to daily exercise and shrinks quickly when exercise ceases. Vigorous cycling two hours a day for one week increases the plasma volume about 400 mL without changing the red-cell mass. This rapid exercise-induced increase in plasma volume recedes to normal in one week or less if the exercise is stopped (14).

The increase in plasma volume with aerobic training is correlated with the fitness achieved. For example, when four subjects trained at 70% to 80% of maximal oxygen uptake one hour a day for 10 days, their gains in plasma volume closely paralleled their gains in maximal aerobic power (59).

The exercise-induced expansion of plasma volume dilutes the hemoglobin and creates a pseudoanemia. The degree of dilutional anemia is correlated with the amount of regular exercise. As a rough guideline, plasma volume increases 5% with a moderate jogging program, 15% in a 20-day road race, and 20% with the regimen of an elite distance runner (22).

The regular exerciser, then, tends to have a high plasma volume and a low hematocrit. But the red-cell mass is generally normal. In contrast, the elite athlete often has an increased red-cell mass. In 1974–1975, studies of 12 elite runners in London, 40 competitive runners in California, and one young man who ran across the United States (3,000 miles in 70 days) each found an 18% increase in red-cell mass (6,7,20). The mechanism is uncertain but presumably involves intermittent tissue hypoxia that stimulates the release of erythropoietin.

The elite aerobic athlete, with a high red-cell mass, nonetheless tends to have a low hematocrit, because his gain in plasma volume outstrips his gain in red-cell mass. He has more blood, but it has a low viscosity. Teleologically, this physiological adaptation should increase oxygen delivery and may enhance maximal athletic performance. It should increase oxygen delivery because, by the Fick equation, the large increase in stroke volume overcompensates for the small decrease in hemoglobin concentration. In other words, the rise in cardiac output overrides the fall in oxygen-carrying capacity per unit of blood, so oxygen delivery increases.

B. Dilutional Pseudoanemia versus Stress Erythrocytosis

The healthful blood changes of dilutional pseudoanemia are the reverse of the blood abnormalities of stress erythrocytosis. In dilutional pseudoanemia, the blood has a low viscosity; in stress erythrocytosis, the blood has a high viscosity. These sharp differences in blood rheology have vital clinical implications.

The viscosity of the blood varies with the hematocrit, the deformability of the red cells, and the concentrations of plasma proteins, especially large, asymmetrical proteins like fibrinogen. In general, the higher the hematocrit, the higher the viscosity, the greater the chance of stasis and thrombosis, and the greater the risk of heart attack or stroke (23).

Stress erythrocytosis has been defined as an elevated hematocrit (over 52%) in a patient whose red-cell mass is normal. The hematocrit is high because the plasma volume is low. Why the plasma volume is low is uncertain; possibilities include excessive catecholamines from stress or smoking, diuresis from alcohol or other drugs, or, in some patients, physiological adjustments to hypertension.

The typical patient with stress erythrocytosis is a hard-driving, obese, middle-aged man under stress at work or at home. Many such men smoke; some abuse alcohol; some have hypertension; few exercise regularly. Men with stress erythrocytosis are at increased risk of heart attack and stroke. Whether the high hematocrit, per se, increases this risk is debated, but some experts advocate phlebotomy to keep the hematocrit under 45% in patients with stress erythrocytosis (23).

Besides increasing blood viscosity, a high hematocrit predisposes to thrombosis by increasing the so-called turbulent mixing effect. That is, when blood flows through an artery, the red cells tend to flow in the center of the stream, where they rotate and collide with one another to create turbulence that drives platelets against the vessel wall. The higher the hematocrit, the more forcefully the platelets are driven against the arterial wall. In various laboratory models, when blood is pumped through arteries denuded of en dothelium, the higher the hematocrit, the greater the platelet adhesion and thrombus formation (1,91).

The high hematocrit in stress erythrocytosis, therefore, may increase the risk of thrombosis for two reasons: it increases blood viscosity, and it increases the adhesion of platelets to arterial walls. Men with stress erythrocytosis may be prone to thrombosis for a third reason: lack of exercise.

Lack of exercise increases the risk of thrombosis, because it decreases fibrinolysis (24). Exercise releases from blood vessels the body's endogenous fibrinolysin, tissue plasminogen activator (TPA). TPA travels through the blood, binds to plasminogen in the clot, and converts plasminogen to plasmin, which dissolves the clot. Obesity, a marker of inactivity, is linked with decreased fibrinolysis and increased thromboembolism. Conversely, exercise has an antithrombotic role.

Inactivity—six hours in a car or 40 hours watching television— enhances coagulability and decreases fibrinolysis, but exercise augments fibrinolysis (24). Moderate conditioning programs increase fibrinolysis, either at rest or after stimulation by venous occlusion. Fibrinolysis also increases appreciably after bouts of exercise ranging from five minutes of cycling to running a marathon. Augmented fibrinolysis can last up to 90 minutes after as little as five minutes of strenuous exercise (24).

A 1987 study suggested that physical conditioning also enhances the fibrinolytic response to maximal exercise (35). Sixty nonobese, nonsmoking, healthy men, with a mean age of 35, had blood sampled before and after maximum exercise on a treadmill via the Bruce protocol. Twenty were marathoners, 20, joggers, and 20, sedentary. Marathoners had the greatest increase in fibrinolytic activity with exercise: 76% versus 63% for joggers and 55% for sedentary men (35).

Whether strenuous exercise activates platelets is controversial, but recent studies (25,53) suggest it does not, and a 1986 randomized trial in middle-aged, overweight Finnish men showed that 12 weeks of jogging can decrease baseline platelet aggregability (69).

Regular exercise, then, is anti-thrombotic. It decreases blood viscosity, lowers the hematocrit, retards platelet adherence, and enhances fibrinolysis. These anti-thrombotic actions of exercise complement its better-known actions—lowering body fat, blood cholesterol, and blood pressure—to ward off heart attack and stroke. Dilutional pseudoanemia is the healthy mirror image of stress erythrocytosis (Table 10-1).

During prolonged, exhaustive exercise in hot weather, however, the blood of the athlete can begin to resemble that of the patient with stress erythrocytosis. This potentially hazardous transformation will be discussed under the section entitled Blood Doping.

C. True Anemias in Athletes

A hemoglobin under 13 $g \cdot dL^{-1}$ in a male athlete or under 11 $g \cdot dL^{-1}$ in a female athlete usually denotes a true anemia rather than dilutional pseudoanemia. However, an individual athlete can be anemic despite a hemoglobin level within the normal range for the general population. Hence, the only practical way to detect true anemia early is to know the individual's normal hemoglobin level. For example, if an athlete normally has a hemoglobin of 16 $g \cdot dL^{-1}$ despite heavy aerobic training, he is probably anemic at 15 $g \cdot dL^{-1}$ and definitely anemic at 14 $g \cdot dL^{-1}$, although one must always consider state of hydration and laboratory variability when evaluating such subtle differences.

TABLE 10-1. *Dilutional pseudoanemia versus stress erythrocytosis*

Feature	Dilutional Pseudoanemia	Stress Erythrocytosis
Hematocrit	Low	High
Red-cell mass	Normal (or high)	High-normal
Plasma volume	Increased	Decreased
Body fat	Decreased	Increased
Blood Pressure	Normal	Increased (often)
Smoking	No	Yes (usually)
Exercise	High	Low
Risk of Thrombosis	Low	High

If the hemoglobin level suggests a true anemia, the physician should take into account the mean corpuscular volume (MCV) and the peripheral blood smear, because the two most common causes of true anemia in athletes—iron deficiency and footstrike hemolysis—are characterized by red cells that are too small and too large, respectively. For example, if the hemoglobin is 11 $g \cdot dL^{-1}$ and the MCV is 85 fL or below, iron deficiency anemia is probably present; if the MCV is 95 fL or above, footstrike hemolysis is probably the culprit (22,26). Of course, certain runners can have both problems simultaneously. Iron deficiency anemia can range from mild to severe, but footstrike hemolysis is always mild.

D. Iron Deficiency without Anemia

The notion that iron deficiency without anemia impairs athletic performance is a myth founded on misinterpretation of research and nourished by placebo responses. Actually, it has never been shown that humans with marginal iron stores but no anemia have any symptoms or athletic limitations.

It is true that even very mild iron deficiency anemia impairs maximal performance. For example, when Guatemalan agricultural laborers performed Harvard step tests, there was a performance difference according to whether the hemoglobin concentrations were just over or just under 15 $g \cdot dL^{-1}$ (16). And when nine female college athletes with mild iron deficiency anemia (mean hemoglobin 12.2 $g \cdot dL^{-1}$) underwent maximal exercise tests before and after two weeks of iron therapy, there was significantly less lactate generated after iron treatment, even though the mean hemoglobin had risen to only 12.7 $g \cdot dL^{-1}$ (76).

It is not true, however, that iron deficiency without anemia impairs maximal performance. This myth arose because animal research was misinterpreted. Rodents deprived of iron from birth developed severe iron deficiency anemia (16). Then the anemia was obviated by transfusing them. However, their running was subpar because their muscles were still iron deficient (16). This model obviously studied the effects of iron deficiency severe enough to cause anemia, not marginal iron deficiency without anemia.

The above model was misinterpreted, however, and soon famous runners with marginal plasma ferritin concentrations but no anemia were having placebo responses to iron therapy. A myth was born: iron-deficiency without anemia impairs maximal performance.

The relevant question is: Does an athlete who is beginning to run out of iron stores, but who still has a normal hemoglobin concentration, have impaired maximal performance because of iron-deficient muscles? The answer is no. The best proof that the answer is no comes from a recent experiment in which iron deficiency anemia was induced by venesection of nine healthy men. During a period of five weeks, they were bled an average of 3.5 L. For the next four weeks, they were severely iron deficient (mean serum ferritin $7 \ ug \cdot L^{-1}$) and mildly anemic (mean hemoglobin $11 \ g \cdot 1 \ dL^{-1}$). At week nine, they were transfused to a normal hemoglobin. At this point, their mean maximal aerobic power (about $4.5 \ L \cdot min^{-1}$) and running endurance (about 50 min) were unchanged from baseline (13).

Iron deficiency without anemia, then, did not curb performance. Moreover, it did not decrease the maximal activities of muscle enzymes. In these subjects, quadriceps biopsies showed no effect of four weeks of severe iron deficiency on cytochrome C oxidase and various enzymes in the glycolytic pathway and the citric acid cycle (26).

The myth should die. Iron deficiency curtails athleticism only when anemia is present.

E. Iron Deficiency Anemia

The most common cause of true anemia in athletes is iron deficiency. The diagnostic triad for iron deficiency anemia is: subnormal hemoglobin concentration, microcytosis, and subnormal serum ferritin concentration (under $12 \ ug \cdot L^{-1}$). The red-cell distribution width (RDW), which quantifies the variation in red-cell size, rises early in iron deficiency anemia, because the newborn red cells are ever smaller. Most electronic counters print the RDW with the complete blood count, so a rise in the RDW may help detect early iron deficiency anemia in athletes (23).

Does prolonged exercise increase the need for iron beyond that supplied by a normal diet? Probably not, although this area is controversial, because some studies have stressed iron loss in urine or sweat, and others have found occult blood in the stool after marathons.

Recent studies illustrate the controversy over iron deficiency in distance runners. In an Israeli study of 21 competitive distance runners, bone marrow iron stores were generally reduced or absent, but hemoglobin and serum ferritin values were generally normal or low-normal (31). It was speculated that such athletes might store iron preferentially in the liver, i.e., that footstrike hemolysis might produce hemoglobin-haptoglobin complexes that are removed by hepatocytes (31). Iron in hepatocytes, unlike iron in reticuloendothelial cells, may not raise the serum ferritin. In contrast, another group found normal red cell survival and no footstrike hemolysis in six female marathoners and speculated that iron deficiency in such athletes reflects inadequate dietary iron (81).

My perusal of the literature and our ongoing research suggest that most endurance athletes do not lose meaningful amounts of iron in the urine, sweat, or stool. Little iron is lost in the urine, because intravascular hemolysis is rarely severe enough to exhaust haptoglobin. Marathons can exhaust haptoglobin, but it usually begins to rebound the next day. And high-mileage training often lowers but rarely totally depletes haptoglobin.

Although some studies emphasize iron loss in the sweat, one meticulous study suggests such loss is trivial. When 11 healthy men were studied in a sauna, mean iron content of cell-free sweat was only 22.5 ug$\cdot$L^{-1} (8). At such a concentration, one would have to sweat 50 L a day to lose even 1 mg of iron! To be fair, however, one must note that the composition of sweat in a sauna can be different from that during exercise and that earlier studies have found higher values for sweat iron content than that emphasized here.

Some athletes may, however, lose iron via gastrointestinal (GI) bleeding during races. One study cited the case of a 28-year-old man who bled to death from hemorrhagic gastritis after jogging (89). A report from Greece noted major upper GI bleeding in three distance racers aged 16, 18, and 22 years (63). Each had hematemesis just after a race. All three had clues to mild, preexisting iron deficiency anemia; one had hemorrhagic gastritis by endoscopy (63). A recent Yale report concluded that GI blood loss in competitive runners is now established (36). This report involved four women who developed iron deficiency anemia from repeated GI bleeding during distance running. Two were collegiate athletes, 20 and 22 years old, vegetarians, with guaiac-positive stools but no GI symptoms and negative colonoscopies. After graduation, they stopped competitive running and had no further guaiac-positive stools or anemia. The other two, 33 and 37 years old, had negative colonoscopies but abdominal cramps and bloody diarrhea while running. One tended to bleed during heavy training or marathon racing, sometimes when also taking aspirin (36).

To be sure, then, some persons bleed from the gut during endurance racing. I have seen a few such patients in my practice. The possible mechanisms are debated. Exercise-induced intestinal ischemia is often invoked, as is mechanical trauma, for example, the so-called cecal slap syndrome (66). I doubt such mechanisms are important causes of GI bleeding. Many individuals with exercise-induced bleeding have histories that suggest gastritis, peptic ulcers, or irritable bowel syndrome. They probably bleed from gastritis or colitis evoked by the stress of racing and/or aspirin therapy. However, relative gut ischemia is still favored by some to explain running-related bouts of bloody diarrhea and crampy abdominal pain that can even mimic appendicitis (11).

How serious a problem is GI bleeding during marathons? Five studies from 1983–1986 tested a total of 283 marathoners for occult blood loss (47,56,57,67,83). The positivity rate ranged from 0% to 11% before and from 13% to 30% after the race. Those who had guaiac-positive stools after the race did not bleed much or for long (Table 10-2).

In one study, the runners who bled were younger and faster than those who did not, as if bleeding correlated with exertion (57). In another, bleeding did not correlate with age, sex, or running time (56). That most subjects had quaiac-negative stools before the race despite heavy training suggests that occult blood loss correlates with racing, not training. Granted, many may have tapered training before the race. If occult GI blood loss indeed occurs only during racing, it cannot be a major drain of iron for most athletes.

Our research suggests that GI blood loss is not a major problem for elite runners. We are following the 14 distance runners on the Oklahoma State University track team through a competitive season. None had anemia or a subnormal serum ferritin concentration at baseline. Each is tested for occult blood loss in the stool twice a week and after races. So far, most have had few quaiac-positive stools.

More research is needed to clarify how often prolonged exercise causes significant GI bleeding. Studies of endurance swimmers or cyclists would be of interest.

Iron deficiency could be prevented in many athletes, especially female athletes, by emphasis on diet. Basically, meat iron is easy to absorb, but grain iron is difficult. To increase iron supply, one could: eat more lean red meat or dark meat of chicken; drink orange juice instead of tea or coffee with meals (vitamin C increases, but tannates in tea decrease, iron absorption from grain); cook in cast iron pots and skillets; and eat poultry or seafood with beans or peas (the animal protein increases the absorption of the iron in the vegetables).

The final proof of iron deficiency anemia is the return of the hemoglobin concentration to normal with iron therapy. If the physician is unsure whether he is dealing with dilutional pseudoanemia or early iron deficiency anemia, he should treat the athlete with iron (ferrous sulfate, 325 mg three times a day) for 1 to 2 months. If the hemoglobin concentration does not rise, the iron should be stopped. Injudicious, long-term use of iron supplements should be avoided, especially in men, because they can contribute to iron overload in

TABLE 10-2. *Occult GI bleeding before and after marathons (references 47,56,57,67,83)*

Year	Place	n	No. Pos. Before	No. Pos. After (%)
1983	England	39	0	3 (13)
1984	Yale	32	1	6 (19)
1984	Mayo Clinic	24*	0	7 (29)
1986	Norway	63	5	8 (13)
1986	Walter Reed	125#	14	37 (30)

*Some were 10,000-meter races.
#Biased sample: 17% had bloody diarrhea after races.

the 5% to 10% of the population that is heterozygous for the gene for primary hemochromatosis.

In summary, prolonged exercise probably does not increase the need for iron beyond that supplied by a normal diet. The causes of iron deficiency anemia in athletes are generally the same as in non-athletes: in women, too little iron in the diet to match physiological iron losses; in men, occult bleeding from GI lesions. Athleticism, per se, rarely causes iron deficiency anemia.

F. Footstrike Hemolysis

Footstrike hemolysis was discovered in German soldiers in 1881 and explored in American cross-country runners in the 1940s. In the 1960s it was shown that padded shoes prevented hemolysis. One might assume, then, with modern running shoes, that footstrike hemolysis is no longer a problem.

Indeed, footstrike hemolysis is not a problem for most athletes. For distance runners, however, it can make a small contribution to anemia, and more importantly, it can limit the increase in red-cell mass needed for world-class performance. And evidence suggests that America's best distance runners suffer from footstrike hemolysis.

The best evidence comes from the two-year profile of nine elite American distance runners training for the 1984 Olympic Games (54). Although only two had low hemoglobin concentrations (13.4 and 14.1 $g \cdot dL^{-1}$, respectively), seven had hematologic clues to footstrike hemolysis: reticulocytosis and/or low haptoglobin concentrations. And the two with the lowest hemoglobin concentrations—a steeplechaser and a marathoner—also had the lowest serum haptoglobin concentrations (54). Olympic distance training seems to cause footstrike hemolysis.

Our research has shown that the diagnostic triad for footstrike hemolysis is: mild reticulocytosis, subnormal haptoglobin concentration, and mild macrocytosis. Footstrike hemolysis destroys preferentially older (smaller) red cells, and the compensatory reticulo-cytosis reflects younger (larger) red cells, so the mean cell volume (MCV) rises to produce the so-called runner's macrocytosis (26).

Footstrike hemolysis is especially likely to occur in heavy persons who run in thin shoes on hard roads with stomping gaits. The degree of hemolysis waxes and wanes with the amount of running, but generally remains mild. It usually increases during a marathon, when the plasma haptoglobin can be exhausted, with resultant hemoglobinuria and, thereby, loss of a small amount of iron in the urine. Switching to better-cushioned shoes does not always abolish hemolysis at high weekly mileage, but footstrike hemolysis can be mitigated by attention to weight, gait, shoes, and terrain (26).

G.   Other Types of Intravascular Hemolysis in Athletes

Our research has shown that prolonged, exhausting exercise causes intravascular hemolysis from other than the footstrike. For example, we have shown that swimmers develop intravascular hemolysis during distance races (3). We studied the University of Oklahoma swimming team and a group of community masters swimmers. Almost 20% of the swimmers had low haptoglobin concentrations at baseline, and in races ranging from one mile to 10,000 meters, 16 of 17 swimmers had reductions in haptoglobin. The degree of reduction correlated with distance and effort. The winner of the 10,000-meter race had the greatest fall in serum haptoglobin concentration; it was equivalent to the hemolysis of 5 to 10 mL of blood (78).

The mechanism for intravascular hemolysis in swimmers is unknown. It may relate to turbulence and osmotic forces in the microcirculation of working muscles. Our recent discovery in racing triathletes, however, introduces a novel possibility for hemolysis in endurance athletes: the formation of spiculated red cells, or echinocytes (40).

We studied 25 male triathletes immediately before and after a 1986 race (1/2-mile swim, 18-mile bike ride, 5-mile run). The race evoked considerable stress leukocytosis and thrombocytosis and a moderate rise in muscle enzymes. All serum proteins rose in concert with hemoconcentration, except for haptoglobin, which fell modestly, reflecting mild intravascular hemolysis. Most athletes had the expected hemoconcentrational rise in hemoglobin concentration, but the three who lost the most weight (4% to 5% of body weight) had slight, paradoxical falls in hemoglobin concentration, suggesting possible hemolysis. Unexpectedly, we found up to 10% echinocytes in the peripheral blood smears of some triathletes after the race. The number of echinocytes formed correlated with postrace acidosis.

We continue to investigate, in vivo and in vitro, the implications of athletes' echinocytes. They form quickly during anaerobic running and disappear quickly when exercise ceases. Similar echinocytes have been seen in racehorses, deep-sea divers, and mountain climbers, suggesting a common denominator of tissue hypoxia. How athleticism causes echinocytes remains unknown, but they appear stiffer than normal red cells. Hence, they may impair blood rheology, curtail maximal performance, and contribute to anemia in athletes (40).

H. Blood Doping

Blood fascinates man. Mentioned more than 500 times in the Bible, blood still has mystical allure. Just as gladiators of yesterday drank the blood of foes to gain courage, Olympians of today infuse the blood of friends to gain endurance. It must be stressed that blood doping is widely regarded as unethical and has been declared illegal by the United States Olympic Committee.

Blood doping—also called blood boosting, blood packing, or induced erythrocythemia—is the transfusion of blood to improve oxygen delivery and, thereby, endurance. Typically, autologous blood is used. The athlete donates one liter of blood. The red cells are frozen for 8–12 weeks while the athlete retrains from the deconditioning effect of donating blood and returns his hemoglobin concentration to normal. Then, in the week before the competition, the red cells are infused, diluted to a hematocrit of 50%. This increases the athlete's hemoglobin concentration 5% to 15% over baseline.

Blood doping, although unethical and illegal, may nonetheless be the racer's edge. Finnish Olympic distance runners have been accused of doing it. Today's top Italian marathoners are suspected of doing it. And at the 1984 Los Angeles Summer Games, seven United States cyclists, including four medalists (one a gold medalist), did it, receiving whole blood from relatives and friends (28).

But does it really work? In theory, it should. As reviewed above, a cardinal adaptation to prolonged exercise is expansion of the blood volume. Top endurance athletes have more blood, but it has a low viscosity. If one could further augment the red cell mass, one could further increase maximal aerobic power. Blood doping, it is argued, could do this, provided viscosity were kept within reasonable bounds by keeping the final hematocrit below 50%.

In the laboratory, blood doping does work. In a benchmark double-blind, sham-controlled, crossover study, 11 elite male track athletes underwent treadmill testing before and after phlebotomy with reinfusion of 900 mL of autologous, freeze-preserved red cells (9). The blood doping increased the mean hemoglobin concentration 8%, maximal oxygen consumption 5%, and running time to exhaustion 35%. In a corroborating 24-week, double-blind, placebo-controlled, crossover study, 12 experienced male distance runners who received 920 mL of blood had a mean 7% increase in hemoglobin concentration and a mean 45-second improvement in a 5-mile treadmill run, compared with when they received 920 mL saline (94).

Blood doping seems also to work in the field. In a double-blind, placebo-controlled, crossover 1987 study of six highly trained distance runners, 400 mL of autologous red cells improved race times (5). All six men ran faster after receiving the blood, and the mean 10-km race time dropped 69 seconds, or about 3%.

Another double-blind, placebo-controlled study was of six soldiers in whom blood doping increased the mean maximal oxygen consumption 11% (72). However, a 43-year-old platoon sergeant—the oldest person known to have been blood-doped—had no increment in maximal oxygen consumption (73). Surprisingly, when this 1987 study was analyzed with three prior blood-doping studies, individual increases in hemoglobin concentration did not correlate with increases in maximal oxygen consumption. The authors concluded that moderately fit (as opposed to poorly fit or supremely fit) persons benefit the most from blood doping, but the authors' rationale is unconvincing. They also found that blood doping provided a small thermoregulatory benefit during exercise in the heat (72).

Other recent blood-doping research suggests that more is better. When four elite runners got 1.5 L of autologous blood over two weeks, there was a 4% increase in maximal oxygen consumption after one liter and a 7% increase after 1.5 L. There were no adverse cardiovascular responses to exercise despite a peak mean hemoglobin of $17.6 \text{ g} \cdot \text{dL}^{-1}$ (80).

Theoretically, the routine use of blood doping, especially in hot environments, could be harmful. In the late stages of a hot-weather marathon, hemoconcentration can be severe. If, from blood doping, the athlete starts the race with a hematocrit of 50%, he can end the race with a hematocrit approaching 60%. At the end, he has developed stress erythrocytosis: low plasma volume, high hematocrit, increased blood viscosity, and, potentially, increased adhesion of platelets to arterial walls. Theoretically, he now risks a stroke.

In fact, thrombotic strokes have occurred (although not in blood-doped runners) during distance runs and marathons (50,64), and recent laboratory research in lambs has shown that blood doping, by increasing blood viscosity, decreases cerebral blood flow. That is, raising the hematocrit from 30% to 55% cuts cerebral blood flow in half (55).

In summary, blood doping works, but is unethical, illegal, and dangerous.

I. The Acute Phase Response: Blood Markers of Overtraining?

The acute phase response is a purposeful, generalized, host-defense biological response to infection or injury that has evolved in vertebrates over the past 800 million years. The response comprises fever, leukocytosis, muscle wasting, fall in serum iron and zinc, rise in serum copper and in erythrocyte sedimentation rate (ESR), and activation of lymphocytes and leukocytes (21).

Prolonged or strenuous exercise can evoke the acute phase response. Several studies show that: prolonged exercise can cause sustained, albeit mild, fever; a marathon evokes leukocytosis, thrombocytosis, and elevations in acute phase proteins such as C-reactive protein; a 20-day, 320-mile road race decreases serum iron and zinc but increases serum copper and causes muscle wasting; and strenuous exercise seems to activate lymphocytes and leukocytes (29,74,87).

A 1987 study looked at markers of the acute response during and after a 160-kilometer triathlon (87). The mean time taken to complete the event by the 18 subjects was 10.6 h. The mean white cell count and plasma lactoferrin concentration were significantly increased immediately after the race, while the plasma iron concentration was significantly decreased. In addition, there was evidence of muscle injury; plasma ferritin tended to rise during the race; and C-reactive protein rose sharply the day after the race. The authors attributed these triathlon-induced changes to the acute phase response initiated by muscle injury (87).

Indeed, the acute phase response is governed by interleukin-1 released by activated monocytes (21), and the monocytes responsible for the acute phase response in endurance athletes are probably those shown infiltrating damaged muscles (32).

In fact, it has been shown directly that strenuous exercise can release interleukin-1 and cause the acute phase response (10). Plasma obtained before and after 14 subjects cycled vigorously for one hour was injected into rats. The plasma taken after (but not before) exercise elevated the rats' body temperatures and lowered their plasma iron and zinc concentrations. Blood monocytes seemed to be the source of the small peptide (consistent with interleukin-1) that evoked this biological response to strenuous exercise (10).

In summary, prolonged exercise can damage the body. The ideal level of training, then, should probably be just below that which evokes the acute phase response. In fact, the syndrome of staleness or overtraining in athletes, may in part, be a day-to-day, or "chronic," acute phase response. A battery of blood markers of the acute phase response might be a practical way to monitor elite athletes training for competition, but much more research is needed to support this hypothesis (Table 10-3).

II. PROLONGED EXERCISE AND THE URINARY TRACT

Strenuous exercise has long been linked with renal abnormalities. In 1713, the Italian physician Bernardino Ramazzini, father of occupational medicine, devoted a chapter of his classic book, *Diseases of Workers*, to runners (4). In it, he said that runners sometimes pass bloody urine, and quoted Celsus, the first-century Roman writer, who advised against running if the kidneys are already affected.

Of course, Ramazzini might have seen myoglobinuria, not hemoglobinuria, but myoglobinuria was not postulated until 1910 and not tied to acute renal failure until the study of crush injuries during the Battle of Britain (48). Exercise-induced proteinuria was documented earlier, in 1878, in healthy soldiers after strenuous marches (21), and march hemoglobinuria was described in 1881 (22).

The benchmark concept of "athletic pseudonephritis" was born in 1956, when Gardner (43) showed that the urine of college football players could contain protein, red cells, and red cell casts. These abnormalities mimicked acute glomerulonephritis but were correlated with the degree of exertion and disappeared with rest. They were benign renal abnormalities caused by exercise-induced renal vasoconstriction.

During exercise, blood is shunted from the splanchnic and renal circulations to the working muscles. Renal blood flow, inversely related to intensity of exercise, can reach a nadir of 20% of baseline (12,65). Renal autoregulation increases the filtration fraction (the ratio of glomerular filtration rate to renal blood flow), but glomerular filtration rate falls, and both creatinine clearance and urine flow can fall 30%. The sluggish flow of blood in the glomerulus enhances diffusion of protein into the tubules. In addition, urinary sodium

TABLE 10-3. *The acute phase response to prolonged exercise*

Fever and muscle wasting
Leukocytosis and thrombocytosis
Activation of leukocytes and lymphocytes
Fall in serum iron and zinc
Rise in serum copper
Rise in ESR and certain serum proteins

excretion falls while potassium excretion rises. These changes are mediated by exercise-induced increases in plasma renin, aldosterone, and antidiuretic hormone, as well as by renal hemodynamic factors.

The renal changes of exercise, even prolonged, exhausting exercise, are generally transient and benign. Prolonged exercise can thus cause pseudonephritis. It can also cause real nephritis—acute renal failure, and exercise-induced renal failure can kill (30).

A. Exercise-Induced Proteinuria

Proteinuria is almost invariable during strenuous or prolonged exercise. Documented in rowers in 1907 and in marathoners in 1910, proteinuria (along with hematuria and cylinduria) occurs in a wide variety of sports: running, swimming, rowing, cycling, skiing, boxing, lacrosse, football, baseball, and others (12,33,43,65).

Postexercise proteinuria has been best characterized by Poortmans (65) and Castenfors (12). The amount of protein in the urine correlates with intensity more than with duration of exercise and can vary from the normal physiologic range (30 to 100 $ug \cdot min^{-1}$) to as high as 5 $mg \cdot min^{-1}$. The maximal rate of protein excretion usually occurs during the first 20 to 30 min after stopping exercise. Runners, for unknown reasons, excrete more protein than cyclists, rowers, or swimmers.

At rest, only proteins with a molecular weight of 160,000 daltons or less are found in the urine. Plasma proteins constitute one-third of basal urinary protein; the rest being uromucoid (a proximal tubular protein) and small glycopeptides from extrarenal tissues (65).

Prolonged exercise—a marathon, for example—can increase 50-fold or more the urinary excretion of a wide variety of high molecular-weight plasma proteins. Albumin is the main postmarathon urinary protein, but substantial amounts of alpha-1- and alpha-2-glycoproteins, transferrin, and IgG and IgA immune globulins are found, along with lesser amounts of haptoglobin and many other plasma proteins (65). Brief, strenuous exercise also increases the urinary excretion of low-molecular-weight proteins such as lysozyme and beta-2-microglobulin (65).

Three major variables in protein excretion are glomerular permeability, tubular reabsorption, and disposal of the absorbed proteins. Tubular reabsorption is vital for conservation of the low-molecular-weight proteins, which pass readily through the normal glomerulus even at rest. With moderate exertion, the predominant urinary protein is the so-called glomerular type, albumin and other large molecules, suggesting enhanced glomerular permeability (65).

Exactly how exercise enhances glomerular permeability is unknown, but the renal vasoconstriction, with its sluggish glomerular blood flow and increased filtration fraction, seems to drive diffusion of macromolecules, and the glomerular membrane may be more porous because of exercise-induced fever, a rise in plasma renin and kallikrein, and a fall in the glomerular electrostatic barrier (12,65).

With severe exertion, the clearance of low-molecular-weight proteins rise sharply. For example, during brief, maximal exercise, the clearance of albumin rises 30-fold, but the clearance of beta-2-microglobulin rises 160-fold (65). This suggests that peak exertion swamps the tubules with more low-molecular-weight protein than they can resorb. In other words, proteinuria of moderate exercise is mainly glomerular, but that of maximal exercise is both glomerular and tubular (65).

Exercise-induced proteinuria is transient and benign. After exercise ceases, urinary protein excretion declines rapidly with a half-time of just under one hour (65). When tested, the urine is generally protein-free within one to two days after a marathon (3,17). Even during a challenging 20-day, 320-mile road race, proteinuria was inconspicuous in basal overnight urine collections (93).

B.   Exercise-Induced Hematuria

The hematuria story parallels the proteinuria story but generates more intensity, because hematuria, unlike proteinuria, evokes emotional responses in patients and diagnostic urges in doctors. That is, bloody urine makes patients and physicians nervous.

Prolonged exercise commonly causes microscopic hematuria. Marathons cause microscopic hematuria which disappears in one to two days, in about 20% of runners (3,79). More sensitive counting methods show that distance running increases the number of urinary red cells in 90% of runners (33). Microscopic hematuria may occur equally in men and women (3), but gross hematuria, much rarer than microscopic hematuria, seems more common in men (2,41).

The mechanism of exercise-induced hematuria is less understood than that of exercise-induced proteinuria. Even the site of bleeding is debated. The focus has moved back and forth from the kidney to the lower urinary tract (46). Probably, different mechanisms and idiosyncracies during exercise can cause bleeding either from the kidney, the bladder, or the posterior urethra.

Despite recent disclaimers (46,79), the glomerulus seems to be the most common source for microscopic hematuria in the runner. The morphology of urinary red cells by phase microscopy reflects their source (51). Normal red cells come from the lower urinary tract; dismorphic (echinocytic) red cells and red cell casts come from the glomerulus. In a phase-microscopy study of the urine of 48 distance runners, 44 had increased urinary red-cell counts after running (38). In all 44, the red cells were dysmorphic (and 10 had red cell casts), indicating a glomerular source.

On the other hand, some athletes bleed from the lower urinary tract. Some men, especially after long runs in hot weather, void bloody urine, sometimes with small clots, often with suprapubic discomfort or burning pain in the glans penis or perineum (2,41). Of 18 such patients in whom no upper tract lesion was found, eight had bladder contusions on cystoscopy, presumably from the posterior wall of the empty bladder banging into the trigone (2).

Likewise, male cyclists have reported painless gross hematuria after bumpy rides, presumably because of trauma to the perineum (62,71). And exercise occasionally unmasks bladder pathology: a young woman and man with gross hematuria while running were found to have, respectively, a bladder stone and a papillary carcinoma (92), and I have seen a runner who had gross hematuria from bladder angioma.

In general, microscopic hematuria after prolonged exercise is transient and benign. It needs no investigation. Gross hematuria from bladder contusions can be prevented by better hydration and not voiding before running. Bicycle-seat hematuria can be prevented by lowering the nose of the saddle, using a special seat cover, and rising off the saddle for railroad tracks and other bumps.

Experts seem to agree that microscopic hematuria that persists two to three days after prolonged exercise merits investigation. Good diagnostic schemes are available (4,30,32).

C. Exercise-Induced Acute Renal Failure

Exercise-induced acute renal failure is rare but can be fatal. It is, in fact, the cause of the exercise deaths in sickle cell trait (30). How does it happen? Who gets it? How can it be prevented or treated? The sickle-trait story serves as an example.

The pattern of exercise death in sickle cell trait is severe exertional rhabdomyolysis (sometimes with heat stress), acute renal failure, acidosis, hyperkalemia, and death in 20 to 48 h. Not all cases have been fatal; some persons have had two episodes. A football player collapsed on the first day of practice two years in a row; the second time, he died. A cross-country runner was hospitalized after collapsing in two races a year apart; he survived (87).

In the exercise deaths associated with sickle cell trait, heat and poor fitness seem to play roles, especially in military recruits who collapse on the first day of basic training. Altitude, viral illnesses, and extreme exercise may also be involved especially in fit athletes who collapse. Other possible contributing factors, such as alcohol, drugs, hypokalemia, or muscle enzyme deficiencies, have not been found (30).

Is this cataclysmic illness unique to sickle cell trait? Not at all. It is the syndrome of acute exertional rhabdomyolysis and myoglobinuria (with or without heat stroke), known since 1910 and reported in depth in military populations in 1967 (19,61,77,92). Serial studies, beginning with "squat-jump" myoglobinuria in 1960 and continuing through the 1970s, outlined the scope of this illness in recruits (44,70). The rate and severity of clinical cases varied markedly by platoon and by individual fitness and could be reduced by conditioning and by paying attention to hydration, heat, and rate and type of exercise (30).

In civilian life, severe exertional rhabdomyolysis, often with acute renal failure, has been described as a result of football, basketball, wrestling, ice-skating, karate, conga drumming, mechanical-bull riding, mountain climbing, and marathon running (58). Tae Kwon Do is also a risk: when a young man broke 2,035 boards in four hours to raise money for charity, he developed acute renal failure eight hours later, but survived after four hemodialyses (58).

Despite the many case reports, athleticism, even prolonged exhausting competition, rarely causes acute renal failure. However, during prolonged exercise, myoglobinemia is common. In recent studies, myoglobinemia, sometimes with myoglobinuria, was found in 25 of 44 ultramarathoners and in all of 24 triathlon finishers (75,88).

Myoglobin, however, like hemoglobin, is not especially toxic to the kidney unless accompanied by major heat stress and dehydration, and/or shock and acidosis (48). So, even grueling endurance events, such as the Comrades Marathon (56.3 miles) rarely cause acute renal failure—only 10 known cases among about 20,000 runners (0.05%) in nine years. Four of the 10 required dialysis, but all 10 survived and seemed generally to recover normal renal function.

Perusal of individual cases of exercise-induced acute renal failure reveals clearcut predisposing factors in most cases. These factors include pre-race viral infection, crash dieting, vomiting, or diarrhea, along with heroic but foolhardy attempts to continue running despite heat exhaustion, muscle pain, dark urine, vomiting, diarrhea, and even confusion (48,52,82).

Is sickle cell trait a risk factor for exertional rhabdomyolysis? Probably not. This area is controversial, but there is no compelling evidence that either the risk or severity of exertional rhabdomyolysis is increased in persons with sickle trait (38). One might speculate that the kidney in sickle cell trait, with subtle abnormalities in the medulla, might excrete poorly the massive load of myoglobin, creatinine, uric acid, and potassium from severe rhabdomyolysis. Indeed, the proximate cause of death seems often to be a hyperkalemic cardiac arrhythmia (30). But the uniquely fulminant form of acute renal failure from exertional rhabdomyolysis threatens any patient, and often requires fast rehydration, Kayexelate for hyperkalemia, and early dialysis to save a life (48).

What should physicians tell athletes with sickle cell trait? Sickle trait is no barrier to outstanding athletic performance. Athletes with the trait should take the same precautions as any other athletes. They should not charge into vigorous exercise without careful training. They must avoid dehydration and overheating. They should not exercise strenuously when they have diarrhea or a viral infection (certain viruses cause or augment exercise-induced rhabdomyolysis). If they collapse or get sick during physical activity, they should see a doctor (30).

The medical advice given to runners of the London Marathon, i.e., tips on training, diet, fluids, clothing, and racing, is invaluable (90). Major heat stress can potentially trigger severe exertional rhabdomyolysis and acute renal failure in any athlete. Proper training and common sense during competition can prevent acute renal failure.

III. PROLONGED EXERCISE AND THE GASTROINTESTINAL TRACT

Research on exercise and the GI tract is sparse. I have reviewed athleticism and GI bleeding. Most of the remaining literature is on distressing, but rarely disabling, disturbances of GI function in distance runners and triathletes.

A. Gastrointestinal Disturbances in Runners

Many runners experience occasional, mild-to-moderate abdominal cramping, bloating, and frequent loose bowel movements, sometimes watery, sometimes mixed with a little blood. These symptoms, termed "runner trots," tend to be exacerbated during a rapid increase in running mileage or a stressful race.

The original "runner's trots" report was of two men (39). One, 31 years old, had crampy periumbilical pain and diarrhea that prevented his training buildup for a marathon. His GI workup was negative, and his symptoms subsided when he tapered his running. After a more gradual buildup, he completed his first marathon without symptoms.

The second man, 24 years old, had running-induced cramping and watery diarrhea for one year. During a buildup for a marathon, he developed bloody diarrhea. GI workup, including barium studies and sigmoidoscopy, was negative, and his symptoms gradually abated despite strenuous training. Over the next two years, he had rare cramping and bloody diarrhea during stressful marathons (39).

A survey of 57 members of a community running club gives an idea of the frequency of GI complaints in dedicated runners (84). Respondents comprised men and women whose mean age was 38 years and who ran an average of 40 miles a week. Two-thirds were recreational runners; one-third were racers. Thirty percent had the occasional or frequent urge to defecate during a run. Twenty-five percent had toublesome abdominal cramps or diarrhea during or after races. Ten percent had heartburn, and 6% had severe nausea or retching associated with racing. GI symptoms, then, are common in recreational and competitive runners (84).

Many marathoners also have GI symptoms, predominantly from the lower tract. A survey of 707 marathoners showed that one-third had bowel movements or diarrhea immediately after running, and almost 20% had to interrupt races to defecate (49). Lower GI disturbances were more frequent in women than in men and in younger than older runners.

Most triathletes also have GI symptoms during exercise. In a New Zealand survey, four out of five Enduro athletes had at least an occasional GI symptom: the urge to defecate (54%), belching (36%), indigestion (30%), chest pain (26%), nausea (21%), diarrhea (20%), regurgitation (17%), heartburn (11%), or vomiting (6%) (95). Only four percent regarded their symptoms as severe and limiting.

One might think that the heartburn, regurgitation, belching, and chest pain in triathletes is from esophageal dysfunction. When six asymptomatic young athletes ran moderately for two hours on a treadmill, however, esophageal contraction remained normal, and lower esophageal sphincter pressure increased, thus decreasing the chance of regurgitation (96). No subject developed GI symptoms. The mechanism of the increase in sphincter pressure during exercise is unknown, but may be related to rises in plasma motilin, gastrin, or catecholamines (96).

Thus, moderate exercise in asymptomatic athletes causes no esophageal dysfunction. Of course, it is possible that certain athletes may be susceptible to esophageal spasm and chest pain with prolonged, strenuous exercise. Research on symtomatic athletes is needed.

In fact, we need more research on exercise and GI physiology in general. Little is known about exercise and the gut. We know that light exercise speeds gastric emptying, but strenuous exercise slows it. The literature on exercise and gastric acid secretion is contradictory (37,85). Consensus suggests that in normal subjects, light exercise has little effect, whereas vigorous exercise decreases meal-stimulated secretion, but not basal secretion. In patients with duodenal ulcers, however, one study has shown that exercise increases the secretion of acid (37,85).

There is scant scientific support for the notion that exercise promotes regular bowel function. That is, while light exercise speeds gastric emptying, it seems not to affect small bowel transit, and there is no proof that it speeds colonic transit. Still, anecdotal experience and pilot studies suggest that running somehow increases the frequency of defecation (85), and a 1986 study of 17 college students suggested that six weeks of aerobic running accelerated bowel transit (15).

How, then, does exercise cause diarrhea and increased defecation? To test the hypothesis that running stimulates gut motility through hormonal mechanisms, the effects of a 30-km run on plasma concentrations of GI regulatory peptides were studied in seven male marathon runners (86). Concentrations of insulin, enteroglucagon, neurotensin, and gastric inhibitory polypeptide did not increase during the run. In contrast, running did increase plasma concentrations of gastrin, motilin, somatostatin, pancreatic glucagon, pancreatic polypeptide, and vasoactive intestinal peptide. Plasma catecholamines also increased. In a control study at rest in a sauna, there were no changes in any GI regulatory peptides (86).

Running thus increases plasma levels of certain GI regulatory peptides. Whether the increases are from increased release or decreased clearance is unknown. The exercise-induced increase in motilin level is theoretically sufficient to stimulate gastric emptying and colonic motility. But more research is needed to determine if these hormonal changes indeed alter GI function.

There are other nonhormonal mechanisms that probably affect GI function in the runner. These include possible intestinal ischemia from splanchnic vasoconstriction during running, the upright posture and gravity, jiggling of the colon, and dietary fiber (85,86).

A novel mechanical cause of "runners' trots" has been proposed. A 36-year-old man had for three years the urge to defecate every 30 minutes during 10-mile training runs and competitive marathons. He had less frequent bowel movements while running on soft surfaces and no increase in frequency while cycling. Routine GI workup, including sigmoidoscopy, was negative, and his whole gut transit time was only slightly shortened (from 47.3 to 44.5 h) by a 32-km run. The mystery was solved when ultrasonography showed grossly enlarged psoas muscles that compressed the colon during hip flexion. It was proposed that, during running, his psoas muscles massaged his colon to empty it (18). This putative mechanism for "runner's trots," while innovative, seems fanciful.

Cecal volvulus may be a "different twist" for the serious runner. A 42-year-old man who ran marathons had acute abdominal pain from cecal volvulus that required resection (68). A 60-year-old man, a world-class marathon runner, had sudden hypogastric pain from a cecal volvulus which was reversed during a barium enema. He later had colonic resection because of recurrent crampy pain. His cecum was very mobile and tethered on a thin mesentery (68).

That these men ran, however, may have been a red herring. It was not stated whether pain in either man began during running. A thin runner with a thin visceral mesentery may, as the authors claim, be predisposed to cecal volvulus, but this report may be an artifact of case finding.

B. Management of Common Gastrointestinal Disturbances

Some relief of exercise-induced GI symptoms can be achieved by not eating for three to six hours beforehand. If there is any suggestion of lactose intolerance, one can also try a lactose-free diet.

On the run, drinks containing concentrated amounts of carbohydrate (e.g., >10% sugar) can slow gastric emptying and cause belching, nausea, and cramping. For hydration during short races (45 min or less), cool water is as good as anything. For long races, especially ultramarathons, glucose-electrolyte sports drinks may be best, because they do not slow gastric emptying and, late in the race, they provide needed energy and may ward off hyponatremia (42,60).

To curb race-induced diarrhea, one can eat a low-residue diet for one to two days beforehand and stimulate peristalsis and defecation before the race by coffee or light exercise. Antidiarrheal drugs (diphenoxylate/atropine or loperamide) have been used successfully (18) but are not recommended for long-term use.

For heartburn, antacids before competition may help. For refractory cases, and for the rare athlete with hematemesis after races, prophylactic treatment with histamine H2 receptor antagonists (cimetidine or ranitidine) can be considered, but such an athlete ought to be under the care of a physician.

Athletes who have exercise-induced GI bleeding should avoid aspirin for at least four days before a race; 1987 research corroborates that aspirin can cause occult GI bleeding (38).

BIBLIOGRAPHY

1. Aarts, P.A.A.M., P.A. Bolhui, K.S. Sakariassen, R.M. Heethaar, and J.J. Sixma. Red blood cell size is important for adherance of blood platelets to artery subendothelium. *Blood.* 62:214–217, 1983.

2. Blacklock, N.J. Bladder trauma in the long-distance runner: "10,000 metres haematuria." *Br J Urology*. 49:129–132, 1977.
3. Boileau, M., E. Fuchs, J.M. Barry, and C.V. Hodges. Stress hematuria: athletic pseudo-nephritis in marathoners. *Urology*. 15:471–474, 1980.
4. Brieger, G.H. The diseases of runners: a view from the eighteenth century. *Pharos* 43 (Fall): 29–32, 1980.
5. Brien, A.J., and Simon, T.L.: The effects of red blood cell infusion on 10-km race time. *JAMA* 257:1761–1765, 1987.
6. Brotherhood, J., B. Brozovic, and L.G.C. Pugh. Haematological status of middle- and long-distance runners. *Clin Sci Mol Med*. 48:139–145, 1975.
7. Bruce, R.A., F. Kusumi, B.H. Culcer, and J. Butler. Cardiac limitation to maximal oxygen transport and changes in components after jogging across the U.S. *J Appl Physiol*. 39:958–964, 1975.
8. Brune, M., B. Magnusson, H. Persson, and L. Halberg. Iron losses in sweat. *Am J Clin Nutr*. 43:438–443, 1986.
9. Buick, F.J., N. Gledhill, A.B. Froese, L. Spriet, and E.C. Meyers. Effect of induced ery-throcythemia on aerobic work capacity. *J Appl Physiol*. 48:636–642, 1980.
10. Cannon, J.G. and M.J. Kluger. Endogenous pyrogen activity in human plasma after ex-ercise. *Science*. 220:617–619, 1983.
11. Cantwell, J.D.: Gastrointestinal disorders in runners. *JAMA*. 246:1404–1405, 1981.
12. Castenfors, J. Renal function during prolonged exercise. *Ann NY Acad Sci*. 301:151–159, 1977.
13. Celsing, S., E. Blomstrand, Werner, P. Pihlstedt, and B. Ekblom. Effects of iron deficiency on endurance and muscle enzyme activity in man. *Med Sci Sports Exer*. 18:156–161, 1986.
14. Convertino, V.A., P.J. Brock, L.C. Keil, E.M. Bernauer, and J.E. Greenleaf. Exercise train-ing-induced hypervolemia: role of plasma albumin, renin, and vasopressin. *J Appl Physiol*. 48:665–669, 1980.
15. Cordian, L., R.W. Latin, J.J. Behnke. The effects of an aerobic running program on bowel transit time. *J Sports Med*. 26:101–104, 1986.
16. Dallman, P.R. Manifestations of iron deficiency. *Semin. in Haematol*. 19:19–30, 1982.
17. Dancaster, C.P., S. J. Whereat. Renal function in marathon runners. *S Afr Med J*. 45:547–551, 1971.
18. Dawson, D.J., A.N. Khan, and D.R. Shreeve. Psoas muscle hypertrophy: mechanical cause for "jogger's trots?" *Br. Med J*. 391:787–788, 1985.
19. Demos, M.A., E.L. Gitin, and L.J. Kagen. Exercise myoglobinemia and acute exertional rhabdomyolysis. *Arch Intern Med*. 134:669–673, 1974.
20. Dill, D.B., K. Braithwaite, W.C. Adams, and E.M. Bernauer. Blood volume of middle-dis-tance runners: effect of 2,300-m altitude and comparison with non-athletes. *Med Sci Sports*. 6:1–7, 1974.
21. Dinarello, C.A. Interleukin-1 and the pathogenesis of the acute-phase response. *N Engl J Med*. 311:1413–1418, 1984.
22. Eichner, E.R. The anemias of athletes. *Phys Sportsmed*. 14:122–130, 1986.
23. Eichner, E.R. Stress erythrocytosis versus runner's anemia: mirror images? *IM—Int Med for Spec*. 8:109–120, 1987.
24. Eichner, E.R. Coagulability and rheology: hematologic benefits from exercise, fish, and as-pirin. Implications for athletes and nonathletes. *Phys Sportsmed*. 14:102–110, 1986.
25. Eichner, E.R. Platelet, carotids, and coronaries. *Am J Med*. 77:513–523, 1984.
26. Eichner, E.R. Runner's macrocytosis: a clue to footstrike hemolysis. Runner's anemia as a benefit versus runner's hemolysis as a detriment. *Am J Med*. 78:321–325, 1985.
27. Eichner, E.R. Common anemias: Update on diagnosis and therapy. *IM—Int Med for Spec*. 8:183–189, 1987.
28. Eichner, E.R. Blood doping: results and consequences from the laboratory and the field. *Phys Sports Med*. 15:121–129, 1987.
29. Eichner, E.R. The marathon: is more less? *Phys Sports Med*. 14:183–187, 1986.
30. Eichner, E.R. Sickle cell trait, exercise, and altitude. *Phys Sports Med*. 144–157, 1986.
31. Eliraz A., R. Wishnitzer, A. Berrebi, N. Hurwitz, E. Vorst. Decreased cellularity and he-mosiderin of the bone marrow in healthy and overtrained competitive distance runners. *Phys Sportsmed*. 14:86–100, 1986.
32. Evans, W.J. Exercise-induced skeletal muscle damage. *Phys Sports Med*. 15:89–100, 1987.
33. Fassett, R. Exercise hematuria. *Austr Fam Phys*. 13:518–519, 1984.
34. Fassett, R.G., J.E. Owen, J. Fairley, D.F. Birch, and K.F. Fairley. Urinary red-cell mor-phology during exercise. *Br Med J*. 285:1455–1457, 1982.
35. Ferguson, E.W., L.L. Bernier, G.R. Banta, J. Yu-Yahiro, and E.B. Schoomaker. Effects of exercise and conditioning on clotting and fibrinolytic activity in men. *J Appl Physiol*. 62:1416–1431, 1987.

36. Fisher, R.L., L.F. McMahon, Jr., M.J. Ryan, D. Larson, and M. Brand. Gastrointestinal bleeeding in competitive runners. *Dig Dis Sciences*. 31:1226–1228, 1986.
37. Fisher, R.L. Exercising the gut—therapy or complications? *Am J Gastroenterol*. 81:299–300, 1986.
38. Fleming, J.L., D.A. Ahlquist, D.B. McGill, A.R. Zinsmeister, R.D. Ellefson, S. Schwartz. Influence of aspirin and ethanol on fecal blood levels as determined by using the HemoQuant assay. *Mayo Clin Proc*. 62:159–163, 1987.
39. Fogoros, R.N. "Runner's Trots." Gastrointestinal disturbancs in runners. *JAMA* 243:1743–1744, 1980.
40. Frame, D.B., K.K. Eichner, G.B. Selby, and E.R. Eichner. Spiculated red cells (echinocytes) and hemolysis in triathletes (Abstract). Presented at Amer Coll Sports Med., May 28, 1987.
41. Fred, H.L. and E.A. Natelson. Grossly bloody urine of runners. *South Med J*. 70:1394–1396, 1977.
42. Frizzell, R.T., G.H. Lang, D.C. Lowance and R. Lathan. Hyponatremia and marathon running. *JAMA* 255:772–774, 1986.
43. Gardner, K.D. "Athleticc psuedonephritis"—alteration of urine sediment by athletic competition. *JAMA* 161:1616–1617, 1956.
44. Gitin, E.L. and M.A. Demos. Acute exertional rhabdomyolysis: a syndrome of increasing importance to the military physician. *Milit Med*. 139:33–36, 1974.
45. Godesen, R.H. Hemoconcentration is associated with superior aerobic performance (abstract). *Med Sci Sports Exerc*. 18:S59, 1986.
46. Goldszer, R.C. and A.J. Siegel. Renal abnormalities during exercise. In: *Sports Medicine*, R.H. Strauss (Ed.). Philadelphia: W.B. Saunders Company, 1984, pp. 130–139.
47. Halvorsen, F.A., J. Lyng, and S. Ritland. Gastrointestinal bleeding in marathon runners. *Scand J Gastroenterol*. 21:493–497, 1986.
48. Honda, N. and K. Kurokawa. Neghrology forum: Acute renal failure and rhabdomyolysis. *Kidney Internat*. 23:888–898, 1983.
49. Keeffe, E.B., D.K. Lowe, J.R. Goss, R. Wayne. Gastrointestinal symptoms of marathon runners. *West J Med*. 141:481–484, 1984..
50. Kelly, W.F. and J. Roussak. Stroke while jogging. *Br J Sports Med*. 14:229–230, 1980.
51. Kincaid-Smith, P. Hematuria and exercise-related hematuria. *Br Med J*. 285:1595–1596, 1982.
52. MacSearraigh, E.T.M., J.C. Kallmeyer, and H.B. Schiff. Acute renal failure in marathon runners. *Nephron* 24:236–240, 1979.
53. Mant, M.J., C.T. Kappagoda, J. Quinian. Lack of effect of exercise on platelet activation and platelet reactivity. *J Appl Physiol*. 57:1333–1338, 1984.
54. Martin, D.E., D.H. Vroon, D.F. May, and S.P. Pilbeam. Physiological changes in elite male distance runners training for the Olympic Games. *Phys Sports Med*. 14:152–167, 1986.
55. Massik, J., Y. Tang, M.L. Hudak, R.C. Koehler, R.J. Traystman, and M.D. Jones, Jr. Effect of hematocrit on cerebral blood flow with induced polycythemia. *J Appl Physiol*. 62:1090–1096, 1987.
56. McCabe, M.E., D.A. Peura, S.C. Kadakia, Z. Bocek, and L.F. Johnson. Gastrointestinal blood loss associated with running a marathon. *Dig Dis Sciences* 31:1229–1232, 1986.
57. McMahon, L.F., Jr., M.J. Ryan, D. Larson, and R.L. Fisher. Occult gastrointestinal blood loss in marathon runners. *Ann Intern Med*. 100:846–847, 1984.
58. Morton, A.R. and S. Walder. Myogobinuric renal failure after prolonged sponsored activity. *Br Med J*. 291:1767, 1985.
59. Nadel, E.R. Physiological adaptations to aerobic training. *Am Scien*. 73:334–343, 1985.
60. Noakes, T.D., N. Goodwin, B.L. Rayner, T. Branken, R.K.N. Taylor: Water intoxication: A possible complication during endurance exercise. *Med Sci Sports Exer*. 17:370–375, 1985.
61. Olerud, J.E., L.D. Homer, and H.W. Carroll. Incidence of acute exertional rhabdomyolysis: serum myoglobin and enzyme levels as indicators of muscle injury. *Arch Intern Med*. 136:692–697, 1976.
62. Palmer, H.A. More on Huffy-bike hematuria (Letter). *N Engl J Med*. 316:632, 1987.
63. Papaioannides, D., C.H. Giotis, N. Karagiannis, and C. Voudouris. Acute upper gastrointestinal hemorrhage in long-distance runners (letter). *Ann Intern Med*. 101:719, 1984.
64. Phillips, J., B. Horner, T.O. Doorley and J. Toland. Cerebrovascular accident in a 14-year-old marathon runner. *Br Med J*. 286:351–352, 1983.
65. Poortmans, J.R. Postexercise proteinuria in humans: facts and mechanisms. *JAMA* 253:236–240, 1985.
66. Porter, A.M.W. Marathon running and the caecal slap syndrome. *Br J Sports Med*. 16:178, 1982.
67. Porter, A.M.W. Do some marathon runners bleed into the gut? *Br Med J*. 287:1427, 1983.
68. Pruett, T.L., M.E. Wilkins, and W.G. Gamble. Cecal volvulus: a different twist for the serious runner (Letter). *N Engl J Med*. 312:1262–1263, 1985.
69. Rauramaa, R., J.T. Salonen, K. Sppanen, et al. Inhibition of platelet aggregability by mod-

OTHER MEDICAL CONSIDERATIONS **439**

erate-intensity physical exercise: a randomized clinical trial in overweight men. *Circulation.* 74:939–944, 1986.

70. Ritter, W.S., M.J. Stone, and J.T. Willerson. Reduction in exertional myoglobinemia after physical conditioning. *Arch Intern Med.* 139:644–647, 1979.
71. Salcedo, J.R. Huffy-bike hematuria (Letter). *N Engl J Med.* 315:768, 1986.
72. Sawka, M.N., R.C. Dennis, R.R. Gonzalez, et al. Influence of polycythemia on blood volume and thermoregulation during exercise-heat stress. *J Appl Physiol.* 62:912–918, 1987.
73. Sawka, M.N., A.J. Young, S.R. Muza, R.R. Gonzalez, and K.B. Pandolf. Erythrocyte reinfusion and maximal aerobic power. An examination of modifying factors. *JAMA* 257:1496–1499, 1987.
74. Schaefer, R.M., K. Kokot, A. Heidland, and R. Plass. Jogger's leukocytes (letter). *N Engl J Med.* 316:223–224, 1987.
75. Schiff, H.B., E.T.M. MacSearraigh, and J.C. Kallmeyer. Myoglobinuria, rhabdomyolysis and marathon running. *Quart J Med.* 47:463–472, 1978.
76. Schoene, R.B., P. Escourrou, H.T. Robertson, K.L. Nilson, J.R. Parsons, and N.J. Smith. Iron repletion decreases maximal exercise lactate concentrations in female athletes with minimal iron-deficiency anemia. *J. Lab Clin Med.* 102:306–312, 1983.
77. Schrier, R.W., H.S. Henderson, C.C. Tisher and R.L. Tannen. Nephropathy associated with heat stress and exercise. *Ann Intern Med.* 67:356–376, 1967.
78. Selby, G.B. and E.R. Eichner. Endurance swimming, Intravascular hemolysis, anemia, iron depletion. New perspective on athlete's anemia. *Am J Med.* 81:791–794, 1986.
79. Siegel, A.J., C.H. Hennekens, H.S. Solomon, and B.V. Boeckel. Exercise-related hematuria: findings in a group of marathon runners. *JAMA* 241:391–392, 1979.
80. Spriet, L.L., N. Gledhill, A.B. Froese, and D.L. Wilkes. Effect of graded erythrocythemia on cardiovascular and metabolic responses to exercise. *J. Appl Physiol.* 61:1942–1948, 1986.
81. Steenkamp, I., C. Fuller, J. Graves, T.D. Noakes, P. Jacobs. Marathon running fails to influence RBC survival rates in iron-replete women. *Phys Sportsmed.* 14:89–95, 1986.
82. Stewart, P.J. and G.A. Posen. Case report: acute renal failure following a marathon. *Phys Sports Med.* 8:61–64, 1980.
83. Stewart, J.G., D.A. Ahlquist, D.B. McGill, D.M. Ilstrup, S. Schwartz and R.A. Owen. Gastrointestinal blood loss and anemia in runners. *Ann Intern Med.* 100:843–845, 1984.
84. Sullivan, S.N. The gastrointestinal symptoms of running (letter). *N Engl J Med.* 304:915, 1981.
85. Sullivan, S.N. The effect of running on the gastrointestinal tract. *J Clin Gastroenterol.* 6:461–465, 1984.
86. Sullivan, S.N., M.C. Champion, N.D. Chritofides, T.E. Adrian, and S.R. Bloom. Gastrointestinal regulatory peptide responses in long-distance runners. *Phys Sportsmed.* 12:77–82, 1984.
87. Taylor, C., G. Rogers, C. Goodman, et. al. Hematologic, iron-related, and acute-phase protein responses to sustained strenuous exercise. *J Appl Physiol.* 62:464–469, 1987.
88. Thomas, B.D., Jr. and C.P. Motley. Myoglobinemia and endurance exercise: a study of 25 participants in a triathlon competition. *Am J Sports Med.* 12:113–119, 1984.
89. Thompson, P.D., E.J. Funk, R.A. Carleton, and W.Q. Sturner. Incidence of death during jogging in Rhode Island from 1975 through 1980. *JAMA* 247:2535–2538, 1982.
90. Tunstall-Pedoe, D.S. Medical support for marathons in the United Kingdom: the London Marathon. In: *Sports Medicine for the Mature Athlete.* J.R. Sutton and R.M. Brock (eds.). Indianapolis: Benchmark Press, 1986, pp. 181–192.
92. Vertel, R.M. and J.P. Knochel. Acute renal failure due to heat injury: an analysis of ten cases associated with a high incidence of myoglobinuria. *Am J Med.* 43:435–451, 1967.
93. Wade, C.E., R.H. Dressendorfer, J.C. O'Brien, and J.R. Claybaugh. Overnight basal urinary findings during a 500 km race over 20 days. *J Sports Med.* 22:371–376, 1982.
94. Williams, M.H., S. Wesseldine, T. Somma, and R. Schuster. The effect of induced erythrocythemia upon 5-mile treadmill run time. *Med Sci Sports Exer.* 13:169–175, 1981.
95. Worobetz, L.J. and D.F. Gerrard. Gastrointestinal symptoms during exercise in Enduro athletes: prevalence and speculations on the etiology. *N.Z. Med J.* 98:644–646, 1985.
96. Worobetz, L.J. and D.F. Gerrard. Effect of moderate exercise on esophageal function in asymptomatic athletes. *Am J Gastroenterol.* 81:1048–1051, 1986.

DISCUSSION

BROOKS: I'm a little concerned about anemia and iron deficiency and the interpretation of the literature. How would you summarize these studies?

EICHNER: Some investigators had taken weanling rodents and made them iron deficient by never feeding them any iron. It made them severely iron deficient with anemia. They drove their hemoglobins down to 5 or 6. Both their red cell mass and their muscles were very iron deficient. Then they transfused them up to normal, ran them immediately on the treadmilll, and of course, they had poor performance. They had been anemic all their lives—terribly anemic. So then, some athletes and coaches concluded that iron deficiency can cause weak muscles without anemia, forgetting that the animals had terrible anemia.

PATE: I'm not sure that we ought to latch onto that as the definitive study.

EICHNER: Well, the relevant question is, does an athlete who is beginning to run out of iron have iron deficient muscles? The trouble that we face as clinicians is that we treat individuals, not populations. If an athlete comes in with a hemoglobin of 14 and is not running well, I may try iron if I'm not sure. But the key thing is that after two months, if it's still 14, that means he didn't have iron deficiency. The gold standard is whether hemoglobin goes up with iron treatment.

STRAUSS: Your blood doping section says that it helps performance to have a much higher hematocrit. So how do you resolve the apparent paradox between that statement and your previous suggestion that the relatively low hematocrit—around 40 to 42—found in elite marathoners may be ideal?

EICHNER: Well, here's how I resolve it. What the runner wants is the highest red cell mass. To win the gold medal, you have to expand your red cell mass and your plasma volume. The problem is when you're running, you're decreasing the red cell mass every day a little bit by foot strike hemolysis. So you're losing 5 mL of red cells every day in your training. At the last minute, you infuse more red cell mass, but not enough to really make the blood too thick. You've artifically given him what he was striving for anyway and what he would have had if he hadn't been having foot strike hemolysis. Blood doping works.

RAVEN: It's a real concern to me that we're now generalizing that the optimum hematocrit is 42 to deliver the most oxygen to the tissue.

EICHNER: I think most hemotologists would have trouble accepting 42, or any given number, as an ideal hematocrit.

RAVEN: I feel we have a problem here because we're accepting sports anemia as being normal. I don't think it is.

PATE: My concern is with the optimistic interpretation of the dilutional pseudoanemia as being a normal part of the adaptive process. I agree with just about everything you've said about the potential benefits of the end results of the adaptive process. Blood doping studies pretty clearly indicate that an athlete can have the best of both worlds. Expand the plasma volume and also take red cells up; then performance is, in fact, enhanced.

11

Exercise, Health, and Longevity

Steven N. Blair, P.E.D.

INTRODUCTION
  I. EPIDEMIOLOGY OF PHYSICAL ACTIVITY
    A. Assessment of Physical Activity
      1. Seven-day Physical Activity Recall
      2. Mail Surveys
      3. Physiologic Markers of Inactivity
  II. PARTICIPATION IN PHYSICAL ACTIVITY
    A. Present Status
      1. Federal Surveys
      2. Other National Surveys
      3. Change in Physical Activity
  III. PROLONGED PHYSICAL ACTIVITY AND HEALTH
    A. Physical Fitness
      1. Functional Capacity
      2. Chronic Fatigue
    B. Cardiovascular Disease
      1. Mechanisms of Protection
      2. Vigorous versus Moderate Activity
    C. Cancer
    D. Diabetes
    E. Other Health Habits
  IV. TREATMENT AND REHABILITATION
    A. Cardiovascular Disease
    B. Pulmonary Rehabilitation
  V. RISKS OF EXERCISE AND PHYSICAL ACTIVITY
    A. Cardiovascular Deaths
      1. Cardiac Rehabilitation
      2. Leisure Time Physical Activity
    B. Musculoskeletal Problems
  VI. PROLONGED PHYSICAL ACTIVITY AND LONGEVITY
    A. Studies in Athletes
    B. College Alumni
  VII. RECOMMENDATIONS
  VIII. PUBLIC HEALTH APPROACH TO PHYSICAL ACTIVITY AND EXERCISE
    A. Targeted Interventions

    B.   Physical Activity at the Worksite
        1. Program Implementation
SUMMARY
BIBLIOGRAPHY
DISCUSSION

INTRODUCTION

Fortunately for many of us, it has become respectable, and perhaps even fashionable, to study exercise (64). Research in exercise science has focused on basic mechanisms, such as body temperature regulation, metabolic adaptation to acute and chronic exercise stress, and the specific relationships between components of the training program and changes in physical fitness. Ultimately, the underlying goal and practical utility for much of this research has been to understand better the relationship between exercise and health. Another important stimulus for research has been the desire to enhance peak athletic performance.

The public's interest in exercise is due to a great extent to its presumed health benefits. It is difficult, if not impossible, to determine whether scientific interest in exercise contributed to public interest or vice-versa. Nonetheless, it is clear that both scientific and lay interest in exercise has grown considerably in recent years, and that health issues are intimately related to this trend. This paper considers the hazards and benefits of exercise, physical activity, and physical fitness in relation to health, primarily from an epidemiological perspective.

Epidemiologic studies of chronic disease frequently require consideration of lifestyle factors and health habits which are well known and commonly referred to in everyday social discourse. In order to bring precision to studies of chronic disease and lifestyle, it is necessary to carefully and specifically define terms and concepts in order to develop accurate and valid measurement of the items of interest. Definitions of several key items are presented below. Several of the definitions are taken from Caspersen et al. (26).

> Physical activity—"any bodily movement produced by skeletal muscles that results in energy expenditure" (26).
> Exercise—"physical activity that is planned, structured, repetitive, and purposeful in the sense that improvement or maintenance of one or more components of physical fitness is an objective" (26). Additional objectives of exercise may include elevation of mood and recreation.
> Prolonged exercise or physical activity—refers to the degree to which a person engages in regular exercise or physical activity;

the time frame is weeks, months or years, rather than hours.

Physical fitness—"a set of attributes that people have or achieve that relates to the ability to perform physical activity" (26).

Health related physical fitness—physical fitness components that are associated with some aspect of health; components include: cardiorespiratory endurance, muscular endurance, muscular strength, body composition, and flexibility (8).

Health—"physical, mental, and social well-being, not merely the absence of disease or infirmity" (117).

Longevity—length of life, although quality of life is an important additional consideration.

As defined here, physical activity is a generic term, with exercise as a component. Other useful subsets of physical activity, such as occupational or leisure time physical activity, are also discussed in this paper. Discussions of physical fitness in this report will primarily address health related physical fitness. Unless otherwise noted, these two terms will be used synonymously.

The definition of repeated and prolonged exercise or physical activity in this chapter differs from other chapters in this book. Most of the other chapters deal with the effect of prolonged bouts of exercise in a single session. The thrust of this discussion is health and physical activity; since there is little health benefit to be gained from a single bout of exercise, repeated sessions or regularity in physical activity is of interest. In general, the dose of physical activity can be considered as the total energy expended (above resting levels) over time. The spectrum of physical activity considered here varies widely, from a totally sedentary existence to one including very high energy expenditures.

The World Health Organization definition of health quoted above is a general guideline which helps focus attention on the spectrum of health, from complete absence (death) to the highest levels of functional capability. Health, as defined here, is difficult to measure and quantify, and it is frequently necessary to adopt other definitions to conduct appropriate studies. For example, cardiovascular disease is a major cause of morbidity and mortality and is a frequent outcome variable in research studies on health. The major form of cardiovascular disease, atherosclerosis, exists on a spectrum from completely clear arteries to total occlusion. For practical reasons, however, atherosclerosis is usually defined as significantly present or absent, based on clinical criteria or postmortem analysis. Therefore, although the concept of optimal health is useful for conceptualizing issues, frequent departures into specific clinical diagnoses are required to perform analyses.

I. EPIDEMIOLOGY OF PHYSICAL ACTIVITY

This section contains a review of methods of assessment for exercise and physical activity, including some still-unresolved issues. Current levels of physical activity and recent changes in physical activity in North America are discussed.

A. Assessment of Physical Activity

Physical activity assessment methods have been reviewed in several recent papers (66,69,112,116). LaPorte et al. note that more than 30 different methods have been used to assess physical activity (66). They describe major categories of methods, including: calorimetry, job classification, survey procedures, physiological markers, behavioral observations, mechanical or electronic monitors, and dietary measures. A complicating factor is that physical activity is a very complex behavior, and different aspects of activity may be important in different studies. In studies on coronary heart disease, total energy expenditure or cardiovascular stimulation may be important; in other studies, activities related to muscular strength and endurance or weight bearing may be of primary interest.

The various review papers generally agree that questionnaire methods of physical activity assessment are most feasible for population-based studies of physical activity and health (66). The existing methods have problems, such as limited data on reliability and validity; impracticability due to excessive time, respondent burden, equipment, and expense of data acquisition; or reactive effects of the procedure (66). Authorities agree that much more work is needed to develop and validate survey and other procedures which are personally and socially acceptable and which provide adequate detail to completely characterize physical activity (66,69,112,116). Major issues that need to be addressed include indentification of a suitable validation standard against which new techniques can be compared, time frame of assessment (past week, past month, or estimate of usual activity?), categorization of vigorous physical activity, assessment methods for muscular conditioning activities, development of appropriate indices, and the value of exercise intensity adjustments. Although there are numerous measurement difficulties, several studies show regular physical activity to be strongly and positively related to a lower incidence of coronary heart disease (86). Because of attenuation of correlations, these findings, based in part on some studies that use less than optimal assessment methods, suggest that the true relationship between physical activity and health may be even stronger than reported in current studies (66).

1. **Seven-day Physical Activity Recall.** The seven-day physical activity recall was developed for use in a community health survey (92). This recall was designed to provide estimates of total daily energy expenditure; occupational, leisure time and other activities are included. The physical activity recall is interviewer-administered, and the procedure asks the participant to recall activities over the preceding seven days. Most Americans spend the majority of their waking hours in light activities (<three METs (MET = work metabolic rate/resting metabolic rate, one MET = approximately 4.2 $kJ \cdot kg^{-1} \cdot h^{-1}$ (1 $kcal \cdot kg^{-1} \cdot h^{-1}$)). The recall ignores light activities and asks participants to recall time spent in moderate (3.0 − 5.0 METs), hard (5.1 − 6.9 METs), and very hard (≥7.0 METs) activities. Hours of sleep are also ascertained, then hours of light activity are obtained by subtraction (light hours = 24 − sleep − moderate, hard, and very hard activities). For most individuals, only a few hours per week are spent in moderate, hard, and very hard activities, and it is typically not difficult to identify and recall these activities. The outcome measures are estimates of kJ (kcal) $\cdot kg^{-1} \cdot day^{-1}$ in total physical activity and for the individual activity components (6,10). The physical activity recall has been validated in community surveys, worksite health promotion programs, and experimental studies (10,105).

2. **Mail Surveys.** In some population studies, there is no direct contact with participants because funds for survey centers are inadequate or subjects are geographically dispersed. Mail surveys for data collection are feasible alternatives in these projects. Perhaps the best known of this type of research on physical activity and health is Paffenbarger's longitudinal survey of Harvard alumni (78,79,81). Reports from this study show a strong inverse relationship between baseline questionnaire assessments of physical activity and subsequent mortality. Kohl et al. (62) show evidence of the validity of physical activity assessment by a mail questionnaire. Patients from a preventive medicine clinic were surveyed by mail for health habits and health status (9). Several questions on physical activity and exercise habits were included. A sub-set (n = 375) of the total surveyed population was examined in the clinic within 60 days before or after the return of questionnaires. Physical activity and exercise questions from the mail survey were compared to maximal treadmill exercise test performance. Multiple regression analyses were done, with treadmill time as the dependent variable and age and physical activity questions as independent variables. A multiple correlation coefficient of 0.65 was found for the model, which included age; a simple index of walking, running, and jogging participation; and frequency of sweating. This relatively high correlation suggests that

mail surveys of endurance type of physical activity are feasible and have validity.

3. **Physiologic Markers of Inactivity.** Kannel et al. (58) report that persons who were overweight (>120% of ideal weight), had resting tachycardia (≥85 beats · min), and low vital capacity (<3.0 L in men, <2.0 L in women) were at greatly increased risk for cardiovascular problems. Framingham study participants who had the sedentary traits listed above had five times the coronary heart disease mortality (after adjustment for other risk factors), when compared to those persons who had none of the three traits. In another population, these sedentary traits were associated with maximal exercise performance on a treadmill test (multiple correlations of $R = 0.45$ to $R = 0.62$ in various age and sex groups). These analyses have been extended in large groups of men (n = 15,501) and women (n = 3,937) (61). Regression models, with treadmill performance as the dependent variable, and age, sedentary traits, and a simple exercise index show very high associations ($R = 0.75$ in women and $R = 0.79$ in men) (61). These analyses suggest that using physiological markers of sedentary living might sharpen estimates of physical activity.

II. PARTICIPATION IN PHYSICAL ACTIVITY

Many observers of the American scene have the impression that regular participation in exercise is common. From commercials on television to joggers on the streets and the sales of exercise videotapes, the image is one of a physically active society; but are these impressions valid? What is the scientific evidence suggesting high levels of exercise by Americans, and can a significant change in exercise habits over the past 15 to 20 years be documented? These and related questions are discussed in this section.

A. Present Status

Current physical activity participation in North America has been assessed in several surveys. As reviewed earlier, it is extremely difficult to obtain valid estimates of physical activity in large populations, and these limitations must be kept in mind (66). The studies reviewed here all used survey methodology, with self-report of physical activity and exercise participation. The shortcomings of these procedures have been recently discussed (31,100), but the data are the best available.

1. **Federal Surveys.** The U.S. National Center for Health Statistics collected information on physical activity in 1985 as a part of the National Health Interview Survey (NHIS) (77). Participants in

NHIS are a representative sample of noninstitutionalized adults (aged 18 and older) in the United States. They were asked a series of questions about specific participation in several physical activities during the previous two weeks (77). Caspersen et al. (25) recently re-scored the NHIS data to estimate the percentage of adults who meet the U.S. Surgeon General's 1990 objectives (83) on exercise. One of these objectives states: "By 1990, the proportion of adults 18–65 years old participating regularly in vigorous physical exercise should be greater than 60%." Their analysis of the NHIS data shows that only 8.1% of men and 7.0% of women currently achieve the objective. Regular, but less intensive, activity was done by 36.2% of the men and 31.5% of the women indicating that a total of 44.3% of the men and 38.5% of the women engage in at least a minimal amount of regular physical activity.

The U.S. Centers for Disease Control recently reported on the prevalence of a sedentary lifestyle in selected states (28). Data were analyzed from the Behavioral Risk Factor Surveillance System (BRFSS). BRFSS is a telephone survey administered to representative samples of residents in states participating in BRFSS (22 states in 1985). Sedentary lifestyle in the BRFSS analyses was defined as persons who reported no physical activity or activity less than three times per week and/or less than 20 minutes per occasion. In 1985, 25,221 adults in the 22 states participated in the survey. Overall, 55% of the survey participants were classified as sedentary. Sedentariness was more common in women than in men, and rates increased with age. Residents of southeastern states were most sedentary, and the southwest/mountain region had the lowest rates of sedentary living. This study agrees with others in concluding that there are large numbers of adults in the United States who are sedentary.

Other national surveys give somewhat more optimistic estimates of physical activity participation (104). The 1981 Canada Fitness Survey is probably the most extensive survey of a nation's physical activity status, in that a large sample was surveyed, and a detailed physical activity questionnaire was used (103). A representative sample of more than 17,000 adults was queried about their leisure time physical activity over the previous year. Extensive detail was obtained on type of activity and frequency and duration of participation. The authors estimate that approximately 25% of adult Canadians are sufficiently active to benefit their cardiovascular health. Conversely, approximately 58% of Canadians were quite sedentary.

2. Other U.S. National Surveys. Brooks (20,21) has recently published results from nonfederal surveys on physical activity participation in United States adults. In one large, representative sam-

ple of more than 15,000 adults, she reports that over 18.6% participate in vigorous activity 60 days or more per year (20). This analysis
also shows that nearly 50% did not participate in any vigorous activity during the previous year. In another study in which participants kept time diaries, Brooks reports that only 14% expended more
than 1,600 kcals · week^{-1} in leisure time physical activity; and only
10% meet the 1990 objective ·for vigorous activity (21).

Virtually all studies, including smaller (but representative) samples of communities (41,92), as well as national surveys indicate a
decline in physical activity with age (although this could be a cohort
effect), less activity in the lower socioeconomic strata, and generally
higher levels of activity in men (104). It appears that no more than
20%, and possibly less than 10%, of adult North Americans get optimal amounts of physical activity. Furthermore, from 40% to 50%
of adults are almost totally sedentary. These findings suggest that
much more change is needed before we can declare that North
Americans are highly physically active.

    3. Change in Physical Activity. Physical activity participation
may be relatively low in adults, but Stephens suggests that there
have been increases in the prevalence of physical activity over the
past ten years (102). Figure 11-1 shows the percentage of the adult
United States population classified as vigorously active (≥12.6 kJ (3
kcal) · kg^{-1} · day^{-1}) in three national surveys conducted in 1978, 1982
and 1985 (29,77,82). Within the limitations of differing instruments,

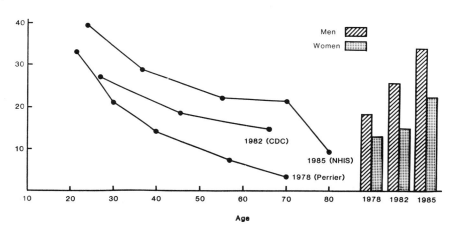

FIGURE 11-1. *Percentage of U.S. adult population who are vigorously active, 1978–85
(>12.6 kJ (3 kcal)·kg^{-1}·day^{-1} of leisure-time activity) (102). Reprinted by permission of the
American Alliance for Health, Physical Education, Recreation, and Dance, 1900 Association
Drive, Reston, Virginia 22091.*

the data suggest significant increases in vigorous physical activity in all age groups.

Figure 11-2 (also from Stephens (102)) shows the percentage of the United States adult population categorized as sedentary. Data are from four United States national surveys conducted by the National Center for Health Statistics between 1971 and 1985 (73,75,93). All four surveys focused on nationally representative samples and used similar physical activity assessment methods. The definition of sedentary was that the person did essentially no leisure time physical activity. Overall, there is a decline in the prevalence of sedentariness from approximately 40% in the early 1970s to about 27% in 1985. In general, the overall pattern holds for the various age and sex groups. These data show a similar percentage of persons classified as performing no activity in 1985, as reported by the BRFSS.

Unfortunately, ambiguous definitions of physical activity and different measurement techniques make it difficult to quantify any change in physical activity habits. Furthermore, the national studies on which we can base estimates of participation are repeated cross-sectional samples. No representative United States cohort has been

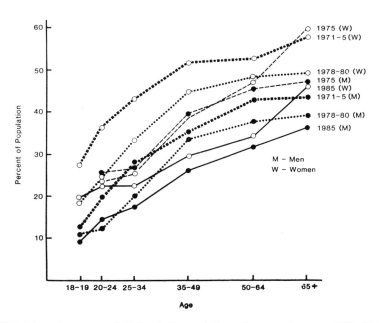

FIGURE 11-2. *Percentage of U.S. adult population who are sedentary, 1971–85 (102). Reprinted by permission of the American Alliance for Health, Physical Education, Recreation, and Dance, 1900 Association Drive, Reston, Virginia 22091.*

followed to more precisely estimate change in exercise and physical activity. Striking increases in vigorous exercise participation have been reported in select and nonrepresentative cohorts (15). It is unclear how these data might relate to the population as a whole.

III. PROLONGED PHYSICAL ACTIVITY AND HEALTH

Regular participation in physical activity is a common sense health habit that has been advocated by physicians, essayists, and philosophers for hundreds of years. Scientific documentation of the health value of physical activity is relatively recent. In this section, studies on exercise or physical activity and health are reviewed and summarized.

A. Physical Fitness

Numerous exercise studies over the past 20 years clearly confirm a causal contribution of physical activity to physical fitness. Controlled exercise training studies permit the description and quantification of a dose-response relationship between exercise and fitness (2). Some might question why physical fitness is included as a health item. First, physical fitness is related to several other health variables. These include actual diagnosed medical conditions, as well as clinical variables, such as low glucose tolerance or high blood pressure, which are themselves related to a disease endpoint. The second reason for listing physical fitness as a health variable is that it specifically determines functional capacity or the type and amount of physical work that can be performed. Functional capacity is, in turn, considered a health variable and is also related to other health conditions.

1. **Functional Capacity.** The concept of functional disability is well established in medical and social research. It typically refers to an inability to perform, or to perform easily, common tasks of daily living and is related to quality of life. Examples include the ability to feed, groom, and dress oneself; walk upstairs; walk a given distance; and carry or move specific objects (33). The definition of functional disability described here is useful in identifying individuals with various levels of disability and for public health and social welfare planning purposes. The prevalence of functional disability in the United States is relatively low in the total population, but higher at older ages. The number of disabled individuals does, however, produce a societal burden and the impact will increase with the aging of the population.

In this chapter, emphasis also is placed on functional capability, rather than functional disability. These two terms describe different segments of a spectrum of function, and any particular categorization of this continuum is arbitrary. A basic premise of this chapter is that physical fitness is a very important determinant of functional disability and functional capability. Some of the basic causes of disability are disease processes or trauma (arthritis, multiple sclerosis, or accidents) but even in these cases, an improvement in some aspects of physical fitness (muscular strength and endurance or flexibility) can lessen the impact of the disabling condition. In other instances, and this is more likely in the elderly, the disability may be primarily due to a very low level of some physical fitness component. For example, persons who have been extremely sedentary for decades may have so little muscular strength that they cannot carry bags of groceries, move pieces of furniture, or lift themselves out of the bath or a soft chair.

On the functional capability side of the spectrum, peak rate of sustained energy expenditure is determined by the maximal aerobic power. People in our society are seldom required to exert themselves at maximal levels, unless they choose to do so in sports or other voluntary activities. The highest rate of energy expenditure routinely demanded for most persons is well within the maximal aerobic power of the average middle-aged individual (9–11 METs). The average rate of energy expenditure that the typical sedentary, middle-aged individual can sustain over the waking hours may be 20% to 30% of maximal aerobic power. More active and fit persons can utilize a higher percentage of maximal aerobic power for extended periods. Thus, the sedentary man or woman has a low maximal aerobic power and can utilize a relatively low percentage of it without developing chronic fatigue or exhaustion. This individual is limited to a less active lifestyle, owing to a relatively low energy expending capability, which means that he or she becomes fatigued more easily, cannot enjoy as much active leisure time as more fit individuals, and may be unable to perform some occupational and household tasks. For most people, the reduced functional capacity that accompanies low physical fitness is an inconvenience and perhaps reduces the quality of life. For the elderly, however, the consequences may be more serious. Shephard (95) postulates that a $\dot{V}O_2max$ of 15–16 mL $\cdot$ kg^{-1} $\cdot$ min^{-1} is required for independent living. At lower aerobic power levels, individuals cannot care for themselves and may have to be institutionalized. This loss of independence and subsequent economic burden have serious societal ramifications. As the United States population ages, these problems will become more severe and make maintaining functional capability and reducing functional disability important goals.

Maximal aerobic power (estimated from maximal treadmill exercise tests) was determined for more than 4,400 male patients of the Cooper Clinic. These men were classified as sedentary or active, based on responses to a medical history questionnaire. At every age, active men were considerably more physically fit, with maximal METs 1.5–2.5 higher than sedentary men. There was about a 20 year difference in capacity between sedentary and active men; that is, an active 60 year old was as physically fit as a sedentary 40 year old man. Such data indicate that sedentary persons will reach the fitness threshold for independent living much sooner than active individuals. These data probably represent an optimistic view of functional capability in elderly men, since men with low capacities are less likely to come for a preventative medical examination.

Examples of the magnitude of the functional disability problem in the elderly are presented in Table 11-1. These data are derived from three epidemiological studies on aging, sponsored by the National Institute on Aging (33). The samples surveyed are representative of the communities from which they are drawn. The table makes clear that the prevalence of functional disability is substantial beyond age 80, at least for these routine activities. Rates are higher in the older groups and are generally higher in women than in men. Rates differ considerably across the three studies: differences are probably due to demographically and geographically different populations from which the survey samples were drawn. Hopefully, increased exercise habits throughout life with the concomitant higher levels of physical fitness may help reduce the burden of disability in the elderly (see Table 11-1).

2. Chronic Fatigue. Chronic fatigue may result from low levels of physical fitness. Persons with very low maximal aerobic power

TABLE 11-1. *Physical function and restriction of activity in three elderly white populations (National Institute on Aging (33)).*

Restriction of Activity	East Boston				New Haven				Rural Iowa			
	Age				Age				Age			
	80–84		>85		80–84		>85		80–84		>85	
	M	F	M	F	M	F	M	F	M	F	M	F
Walk across room	12*	23	22	38	8	9	10	31	10	15	17	22
Move from bed to chair	4	14	11	22	1	9	5	14	8	9	8	9
Climb stairs	15	31	29	50	12	12	10	30	12	17	16	26
Do heavy housework	57	70	74	89	31	54	53	68	43	56	68	69
Use the toilet	3	12	12	19	2	5	1	8	6	8	7	10

* Percent of individuals needing assistance to perform the activity. M = males; F = females.

may not be able to easily provide the energy expenditure necessary for required activities; they may be able to meet day-to-day demands but become exhausted if additional exertion is needed for emergencies or unexpected activities.

The first U.S. National Health and Nutrition Survey was conducted by the National Center for Health Statistics during 1971–1974 (74). This survey focused on a representative sample of non-institutionalized United States adults aged 25–74 years. More than 4,000 men and women responded to a question on whether or not they suffered from chronic fatigue. Persons who reported that they felt tired or worn out "quite a bit of the time," "most of the time," or "all the time" were classified as experiencing frequent fatigue (30). Using this definition of fatigue, 14.3% of the men and 20.4% of the women suffered from frequent fatigue. Individuals who were physically inactive were twice as likely to report frequent fatigue as the active respondents. High body weight was associated with fatigue in women but not in men. Psychological conditions such as anxiety, depression, and stress were also related to fatigue. A multivariate logistic analysis indicated that physical inactivity remained a significant predictor of fatigue after age, sex, body weight, and psychological factors.

Kohl et al. (63) compared histories of chronic fatigue to maximal treadmill test time in 285 men and 97 women with at least two visits to the Cooper Clinic. Baseline prevalence of chronic fatigue was 9.5% in men and 29.9% in women. These rates are lower in men and higher in women when compared to those reported by Chen (30). This may be due to differences in the populations, methods of ascertaining chronic fatigue, or both. Subjects who significantly improved their treadmill test performance at the second visit were less likely to report chronic fatigue at the follow-up visit. Multivariate analyses suggested that cardiorespiratory fitness is a determinant of chronic fatigue.

The two studies mentioned here confirm that chronic fatigue is prevalent in United States adults. Furthermore, clinical experience indicates that many visits to physicians include vague, non-specific complaints of tiredness. Lack of physical fitness may be an important cause of fatigue in our society.

B. Cardiovascular Disease

Modern scientific studies on physical activity and cardiovascular disease began in the 1950s (70). Since then, several dozen studies have been reported. These studies have been reviewed many times, but a recent review by Powell et al. (86) extends our understanding of the issue. Powell and colleagues carefully evaluated each study on the quality of the measurement of physical activity, the clarity of the diagnoses of disease, and the appropriateness of the epidemiologic methods. Table 11-2 is reproduced from their chapter and shows a summary of 16 cohort studies on physical activity and coronary heart disease. In all, Powell et al. reviewed 43 studies and concluded that the direct association between sedentary living and coronary artery disease is consistent across studies (in particular the better studies), follows an appropriate temporal sequence, shows a graded response, and is coherent with existing knowledge. A relative risk of 2.0 for fatal coronary artery disease seems plausible for sedentary, compared to active individuals. This risk ratio is similar to that for other major coronary artery disease risk factors, such as hypertension, cigarette smoking, and hyperlipidemia.

1. **Mechanisms of Protection.** If regular physical activity protects against fatal coronary heart disease, what are the mechanisms? A heart attack is essentially a disparity between myocardial oxygen supply and demand, although dysrhythmic causes of cardiac events are also a problem. Haskell (53) discussed mechanisms by which physical activity may affect both the supply and demand sides of the equation. In order to affect myocardial oxygen supply, either the atherosclerotic process must be prevented or retarded, or the coronary blood flow must increase via increased capillarization or by an increase in arterial diameter. There is little evidence in humans that physical activity increases capillarization or arterial diameter. It seems more likely that the atherosclerotic process might be retarded by regular physical activity.

Physical activity appears to have a favorable impact on the major risk factors. Habitual physical activity and a high level of physical fitness protect against and help correct physician-diagnosed hypertension (9,81). Experimental trials of exercise training appear to reduce blood pressure in mild hypertensives (37). Exercise also has a favorable affect on plasma lipoproteins (52). Regular exercise (approximately equivalent to 16 km of walking/running per week) probably decreases low density lipoprotein-cholesterol and increases high density lipoprotein-cholesterol (HDL-C), especially HDL_2, which is the specific lipoprotein that appears to lower risk of atherosclerosis. The association between physical activity and cigarette smoking is complex and is confounded by demographic factors, such as educational level, but occupational physical activity is positively associated with smoking rates, whereas exercise (especially vigorous exercise) is associated with lower smoking rates (11).

Thus, the favorable impact of physical activity on risk factors may well prevent or reduce the rate of progression of coronary artery disease and enhance myocardial oxygen supply.

Physical activity may also be beneficial in decreasing myocardial oxygen demand. This may result from a decrease in circulating cate-cholamines and from a reduction in heart rate and blood pressure at rest and during moderate exercise (37,53). Aerobic exercise also enhances the intrinsic muscular function of the myocardium which may make the heart better able to withstand damages from myocardial infarction.

2. **Vigorous versus Moderate Activity.** One major issue still unresolved is whether protection comes only from vigorous exercise or whether more moderate activity is sufficient. The data of Morris et al. (71) suggest that vigorous activity is required. Other studies support the concept that total energy expenditure is the important factor (80). Furthermore, it may not be necessary to participate in extreme amounts of physical activity to get some benefit. Individuals with moderate physical activity participation have a substantially lower risk of cardiovascular disease than persons who are totally sedentary (67,80).

C. Cancer

Investigators recently began to examine cancer risk in sedentary and active groups. Several studies on physical activity and colon and rectal cancer are available. Garabrant et al. (46) studied 2,950 cases of males with colon cancer in a population based registry in Los Angeles. Occupational physical activity for these men was rated as sedentary, moderate, or high. Examples include: sedentary—accountants, social workers, and bus drivers; moderate—machinists, sales clerks, and entertainers; and high—gardeners and mail carriers. Persons in sedentary jobs had a colon cancer risk 1.6 times higher than men in the high job activity category. The risk gradient across occupational categories was seen along each socioeconomic stratum and in different racial and ethnic groups. No relation was seen for rectal cancer and occupational physical activity.

A 19-year follow-up study of 1.1 million Swedish men reports results similar to the Los Angeles study (48). Men in sedentary jobs had a 1.3-fold increased risk for colon cancer, compared to their more active peers. The greatest risk for sedentary men in the Swedish study was for cancers of the transverse colon (RR = 1.6). Rectal cancer risk was not elevated in sedentary men. Dietary habits and leisure time physical activity were considered, and the authors concluded that these factors did not confound the results.

Vena et al. (109) report increased colon cancer risk in 430,000 men in Washington state who had sedentary jobs (coded from "usual occupation" as listed on the death certificate). Proportionate mortality ratios for the most sedentary men were approximately 120 for

Study location	Outcome (1)	High-activity group	Low-activity group
1. Chicago Western Electric employees	CHD	leisure, sport participant	non-participant
2. Harvard Alumni	MI,SD	>2000 kcal/wk in leisure activity	<2000 kcal/wk
	SD	>2000 kcal/wk in leisure activity	<2000 kcal/wk
	fatal MI	>2000 kcal/wk in leisure activity	<2000 kcal/wk
	nonfatal MI	>2000 kcal/wk in leisure activity	<2000 kcal/wk
Harvard Alumni	CHD death	>2000 kcal/wk leisure activity	500–1999 kcal/wk < 500 kcal/wk
3. British Civil Servants	CHD Total	Vigorous exercise (VE) in sports (>5 min at ≥1.5 kcal/min)	no VE in sports or around the house
	CHD Nonfatal	VE sports	no VE
	CHD Fatal	VE sports	no VE
	A	VE sports	no VE
	CHD Total	VE around the house (≥30 min digging, moving heavy objects)	no VE in sports or around the house
	CHD Nonfatal	VE house	VE house
	CHD Fatal	VE house	VE house
Framingham, Male residents	CHD death	Physical Activity Index scores of 38–83	Scores 34–37 Scores 30–33 Scores 24–29
4. Framingham, Male residents	CHD death	Multiple regression on physical activity index	
Framingham, Female residents	CHD death	Multiple regression on physical activity index	
5. Puerto Rico, rural residents	CHD	Multiple regression on Framingham physical activity index	
Puerto Rico, urban residents	CHD	Multiple regression on Framingham physical activity index	
6. Honolulu Heart Program, Japanese	CHD	Multiple regression on Framingham physical activity index	
7. Los Angeles firemen and policemen	MI,SD	Above median cardiovascular fitness	Below median cardiovascular fitness
8. Gothenberg, Sweden, residents	MI,SD	Multiple regression on fitness level	

Relative Risk	Score (2)	Adjustments (3)	Evaluation (4) act	CHD	epi
2.0 (1.3–3.0)	**	none	S	G	U
1.6 (p < .001)	**	A			
1.2 (p = .594)	0	A			
2.0 (p = .001)	**	A	G	U	S
1.5 (p = .002)	*	A			
1.3 (p = .002)	**	A,BP,SM			
1.6 (p = .002)					
2.2 (p < .05)	**	A			
2.0 (p < .001)	**	A			
2.6 (p < .05)	**	A			
2.5 (p < .05)	**	A	G	S	G
2.2 (NA)	?	A			
1.7 (NA)	?	A			
1.3 (NA)	?	A			
1.2 (NA)		A			
1.6 (NA)	*				
1.9 (NA)					
Inverse (p < .05)	**	A,BP,CH,SM,Gl,LVH	G	G	G
(p > .05)	0	A,BP,CH,SM,Gl,LVH			
Inverse (p < .05)	**	A,BP,CH,SM, heart rate			
			G	S	S
Inverse (p < .05)	**	A,BP,CH,SM, heart rate			
Inverse (p < .05)	**	none	G	S	S
2.4 (1.1–5.9)	**	A,BP,CH,SM,O	S	G	G
Inverse (p < .05)	**	A,BP,CH,SM, abnormal EKG	S	S	U

TABLE 11-2. *(continued)*

Study location	Outcome (1)	High-activity group	Low-activity group
9. Gothenberg, Sweden, residents	MI	Multiple regression on leisure time physical activity index	
10. Gothenberg, Sweden, residents	MI	Multiple regression on leisure time physical activity	
11. Gothenberg, Sweden, female residents	MI, CHD death A EKG changes	Multiple regression on occupational activity	
	MI, CHD death A EKG changes	Multiple regression on leisure activity	
12. New York, health insurance subscribers	CHD, CHF, conduction defects	Work, 11–28 points on 28 point scale Leisure, 2–10 points on 10 point scale Work and leisure, 13 more active categ.	1–10 points 0–1 points 3 least active categories
	A	Work, 19–28 points Leisure, 6–10 points Work and leisure, 7 most active categories	1–18 points 0–5 points 9 least active categories
13. San Francisco Federal employees	CHD CHD	Work, moderate and heavy Leisure, regular activities	Sedentary and light Occasional or no activities
14. San Francisco federal employees	CHD	Multiple regression on total daily calories from work and leisure	
15. Oslo, Norway, residents	CHD death CHD death	Work activity, great Leisure activity, intermediate	Intermediate Moderate Sedentary Moderate Sedentary
16a. North Karelia Finland, Male residents	MI CHD death	High work activity High work activity	Low work activity Low work activity
	MI CHD death	High leisure activity High leisure activity	Low leisure activity Low leisure activity
	MI	High work and high leisure activity	High/low or low/high Low/low

Relative Risk	Score (2)	Adjustments (3)	Evaluation (4) act	CHD	epi
(p > .05)	0	A,BP,EKG changes	U	S	U
(p > .05)	0	A,BP,CH,SM	U	S	U
(p > .05)	0	A,BP,CH,SM,O,SES, Educ, TG			
(p > .05)	0				
(p > .05)	0		S	G	G
(p > .05)	0	A,BP,CH,SM,O,SES, Educ, TG			
(p > .05)	0				
(p > .05)	0				
1.6 (1.2–2.1)	**	A			
1.5 (1.1–2.0)	**	A			
1.7 (1.3–2.2)	**	A	S	G	S
0.7 (0.5–1.0)(5)	0	A			
0.8 (0.5–1.1)(5)	0	A			
0.7 (0.5–1.0)(5)	0	A			
0.9 (0.6–1.4)	0	A	U	S	S
1.5 (1.1–2.1)	**	A	S	S	S
1.2 (p = 0.23)	0	A,BP,CH,SM	G	S	S
1.1 (NA)					
1.4 (NA)	*	none			
2.1 (NA)			U	S	S
1.3 (NA)	*	none			
2.5 (NA)					
1.5 (1.2–2.0)(5)	**	A,BP,CH,SM,O			
1.6 (1.1–2.3)(5)	**	A,BP,CH,SM,O			
1.2 (0.9–1.5)(5)	0	A,BP,CH,SM,O			
1.4 (1.0–2.1)(5)	0	A,BP,CH,SM,O	S	S	G
1.3 (1.0–1.7)	***	A			
2.5 (1.8–3.7)					

TABLE 11-2. *(continued)*

Study location	Outcome (1)	High-activity group	Low-activity group
16b. North Karelia, Finland, Female residents	MI MI	High work activity High leisure activity	Low work activity Low leisure activity
	MI	High work and high leisure activity	High/low or low/high Low/low

(1) A = angina, CHD = coronary heart disease, CVD = cardiovascular disease, CHD includes A, MI, and SD; CHD death includes fatal MI and SD.
(2) ** = RR of ≥ 1.5 and p < .05, * = 1.0 < RR < 1.5 and p < .05, trend adds *
(3) A = age. BP = blood pressure, CH = cholesterol, SM = smoking, O = obesity,
(4) G = Good, S = Satisfactory, U = Unsatisfactory.
(5) 90% confidence intervals.
Reproduced, with permission, from the Annual Review of Public Health, vol. 8.

the different study decades. Corresponding figures were approximately 90 for the most active men. The risk of dying from rectal or prostate cancer was approximately the same in the sedentary and active men in this study. Twenty-five thousand deaths in women from 1974–1979 were also studied (109). The women with more active jobs had lower risk of dying from colon and breast cancer, and rectal cancer rates were similar across job classifications.

Vena et al. (110) also report on colon and rectal cancer risk in men by lifetime occupational physical activity categories in a case control study in Buffalo, NY. Men who spent 20 or more years in sedentary or light work were about twice as likely to die from colon cancer as men who spent *no* years in sedentary or light work. Once again, rectal cancer risk was not associated with occupational physical activity.

Lower prevalence of breast cancer and cancers of the reproductive system was reported in former college athletes, as compared to non-athletes (44). More than 5,000 living alumnae from eight colleges and two universities who graduated from 1925 to 1981 were surveyed to ascertain if they had ever been diagnosed with cancer. Non-athletes had a 1.86 relative risk for breast cancer and a 2.62 risk for reproductive system cancer, compared to former athletes. Caution is needed in interpreting these data because current activity was not associated with cancer risk.

The studies reviewed above suggest lower risk for some cancers in more physically active individuals. These results are encouraging, but much more work is needed before firm conclusions can be drawn. The current studies all use relatively crude assessments of physical

Relative Risk	Score (2)	Adjustments (3)	Evaluation (4)		
			act	CHD	epi
2.4 (1.5–3.7)(5)	**	A,BP,CH,SM,O			
1.5 (0.9–2.5)(5)	0	A,BP,CH,SM,O	S	S	G
1.8 (0.9–3.5)					
	***	A			
4.0 (2.1–7.8)					

CHF = congestive heart failure, MI = myocardial infarction, SD = sudden death.

to every value in the series.
Gl = glucose intolerance or diabetes.

activity; and in the occupational activity studies, no adjustments were possible for leisure-time activity. Other potential confounders such as diet, smoking status, body composition, exposure to carcinogens in the environment, and other lifestyle factors need further consideration and careful analyses.

A possible mechanism has been mentioned for the lower colon cancer rates in active individuals. It is possible that vigorous activity causes different bowel habits. Reduced bowel transit time could mean that carcinogens would spend less time in contact with bowel mucosa (32). Preliminary data show different bowel habits between runners (n = 23) and lower extremity amputees (n = 10) (unpublished data—LaPorte, R.E. and Blair, S.N.). Thirteen (56%) of the runners and three (30%) of the amputees reported two or more bowel movements per day. Amputees were much more likely to report three days without a bowel movement (20% versus 4%). These data are not adjusted for total caloric intake or dietary composition.

D. Diabetes

According to the U.S. National Center for Health Statistics (NCHS), there are 5.8 million known diabetics among the civilian non-institutionalized population of the United States (76). The NCHS data do not allow separation of diabetics into Type I and Type II diabetics, but, in the general population, most cases are Type II. Diabetes causes significant disability, with about half of all diabetics reporting some activity limitation (this rate is about three times higher than for the non-diabetic population).

Exercise has long been considered as one aspect of treatment for diabetics (5,118), although the value of exercise in metabolic control in Type I diabetics is not established (59). Type I diabetics obviously need to carefully regulate their physical activity and to balance it with insulin administration (5). Regulation of insulin administration, exercise, and diet in Type I diabetics is a complex problem requiring medical supervision. This subject will not be discussed further here.

Regular physical activity is advocated for Type II diabetes in order to maintain physical fitness and help control coronary heart disease risk factors (59). Type II diabetes is probably a more serious public health problem than Type I, and prevention and treatment of Type II is probably more related to physical activity.

One of the primary characteristics of Type II diabetes is peripheral insulin resistance. Several reviews on physical activity and diabetes conclude that regular exercise increases peripheral insulin sensitivity (5,55,59,107). Holloszy et al. (55) suggest that the decline in insulin sensitivity with age may be prevented by regular vigorous physical activity. Others are more cautious about the long-term impact of exercise on glucose control (118). Richter and Galbo (91) suggest that diet and weight loss for the overweight may be more beneficial than exercise in regulating blood glucose for Type II diabetics.

Leisure time physical activity is inversely associated with glucose intolerance, after control for confounding variables, including body composition (4,27). Frisch et al. (43) report a lower prevalence of diabetes in women who were athletes in college compared to their nonathletic classmates. The age-adjusted relative risk for diabetes was 2.24 for the non-athletes. To my knowledge, this is the first report in which baseline physical activity was associated with later risk of developing diabetes. Other similar studies are urgently needed to determine if a less equivocal measure of regular physical activity is associated with a reduced risk of subsequent diabetes.

E. Other Health Habits

It is intuitively appealing to assume that exercise may be associated with other health habits. If all we have to do is to get people to exercise, and their other health habits automatically improve, intervention efforts would be simplified. The epidemiologist is concerned about the issue, because problems of confounding and difficulties in dissentangling the independent impact of health habits complicate studies of the causes of disease. There are essentially no well-controlled experimental studies which bear on the issue; however, observational and clinical studies do provide some amount of information.

A recent review of the relationship between physical activity and other health behavior examined approximately 40 studies (11). These studies were obtained by a MEDLINE search and from known articles. Articles were excluded from review if they had an uncertain definition of physical activity or other health behaviors, or an incomplete description of the demographic characteristics of the study group. In addition to reviewing existing articles, data from the Center for Disease Control Behavioral Risk Factor Survey and the NCHS National Survey of Personal Health Practices and Consequences were analyzed. Several problems complicated the review: 1) There were no consistent definitions of exercise and physical activity in the various papers; 2) Assessments of exercise and physical activity were typically crude and imprecise, leading to misclassification; and 3) Several other health behaviors, such as habitual diet or stress management practices also are difficult to assess.

The following summary points were developed from the review:

1. Even when significant correlations are found between physical activity and other health habits, the strength of the associations is relatively low, although lack of precision in measuring physical activity and the other health habits undoubtedly is a major factor in the low correlations.
2. High levels of physical activity are associated with lower body weight.
3. Habitually active persons have a generally higher caloric intake.
4. Occupational physical activity is positively associated with cigarette smoking, while leisure time activity is inversely related to smoking. These results are likely to be confounded by socioeconomic factors.
5. Physically active persons may be more likely to practice certain preventive health behaviors, such as obtaining medical check-ups and maintaining their immunizations, getting regular sleep, and eating a good breakfast.

In general, physical activity appears to exert relatively little influence on other health behaviors. This finding is perhaps not surprising, since it is clear that human behavior is complex and is poorly understood. It is recommended that additional studies with improved assessment techniques and designs be planned to further examine the interrelationships among health behaviors. Well-controlled experimental trials, especially in children and youth, would be especially helpful in determining the value of exercise in preventing the adoption of deleterious health habits.

IV. TREATMENT AND REHABILITATION

This chapter has so far emphasized the role of prolonged physical activity in the prevention of disease and disability. Exercise intervention also has a role in the treatment of some diseases. A brief review of some of the key studies follows.

A. Cardiovascular Disease

Cardiac rehabilitation programs became popular in the United States during the 1960s. Prior to that time a person with a myocardial infarction was prescribed several weeks or a few months of bed rest. This treatment further deconditioned the patient and therefore increased his or her disability and lengthened the rehabilitation process. The early experience with cardiac rehabilitation, including exercise, generally led to enthusiastic impressions about its effectiveness. Regular exercise typically enhances feelings of general well-being (7), and this response may even be more pronounced (and maybe even more important) in cardiac patients. The psychological effects of a heart attack are well documented (23), and exercise rehabilitation may make patients feel better because "they are doing something about their disease." The increased physical fitness which follows exercise intervention is an important result of a rehabilitation program. Many cardiac patients had been sedentary before their myocardial infarction and, consequently had a low initial physical fitness, exacerbated by hospital rest. In some cases, rehabilitation after the cardiac event produced higher fitness than the patient had experienced in many years. The improved functional capacity in these cases is associated with a feeling of accomplishment and improved psychological health.

Exercise training improves functional capacity in cardiac patients more than in healthy subjects. Several well-controlled recent studies clearly document the specific changes in myocardial function. Increases in maximal oxygen uptake in selected studies range from 9% to 100% (39,45,72,97,111). Other changes documented in these studies include a decrease in resting and submaximal exercise heart rate and blood pressure, increased ejection fraction, increased maximal systolic blood pressure, decreased rate pressure product at standardized exercise level, and some evidence of improved myocardial perfusion. Exercise training probably does not improve the exercise ECG (72). Overall ventricular function appears to improve with exercise training, functional capacity is increased, and the anginal threshold is increased (50). Thus, exercise is an important part of the treatment of coronary heart disease.

Early enthusiasm for cardiac rehabilitation and the improved functional capacity of patients led to the hypothesis that rehabilitation might reduce reinfarction and death rates in cardiac patients. There have been several randomized clinical trials to test this hypothesis (24,57,89,94,115). The first of these studies was conducted in Goteborg, Sweden by Wilhelmsen et al. (115). They randomly assigned 315 post-myocardial infarction patients to exercise and control groups and followed both groups for four years. There were 28 deaths in the training group and 35 in the control group, but the difference was not statistically significant. The other exercise training studies report similar results. The training group generally had lower rates of reinfarction or death, but the results are not statistically significant (24,89,94). One exception was the study by Kallio et al. (57), which showed a reduction in sudden deaths in the intervention group. The studies reviewed here used random assignment to study groups. All of these studies had a major flaw, however. Studies such as these are very time and labor intensive, and, consequently, quite expensive. Primarily because of these constraints, the studies had inadequate sample size, inadequate follow-up time, or both. They thus lacked the statistical power to detect a clinically significant difference between groups. In an effort to address this problem, Shephard (97) pooled the results of three studies, yielding a total study population of 1,318. He reanalyzed the pooled study findings with a life-table analysis approach and concluded that exercise training provided significant protection against fatal reinfarction, that the greatest benefit occurs during the first two years after the initial event, and that exercise training reduced the death rate by 35% during the first year and 25% during the fourth year.

B. Pulmonary Rehabilitation

Rehabilitation programs for chronic obstructive pulmonary disease patients are not as widespread as cardiac rehabilitation programs, but pulmonary rehabilitation is becoming more common. The American College of Sports Medicine added behavioral objectives on exercise testing and prescription to the third edition of *Guidelines for Exercise Testing and Prescription* (1). Many cardiac rehabilitation programs now accept pulmonary disease patients, and research and clinical activities in pulmonary rehabilitation will continue to expand.

At this point, the data base on pulmonary rehabilitation is relatively sparse. There is general agreement that pulmonary disease patients benefit from exercise training by improving their overall physical fitness and strengthening their respiratory muscles (54). Increases in $\dot{V}O_2$max and muscular strength and endurance in these patients improves their functional capability and enables them to accomplish more easily the routine tasks of daily living. Exercise training probably does not directly impact the pulmonary disease process and is not likely to alter death rates in pulmonary disease patients. Improved function and quality of life is important, however, and comprehensive rehabilitation efforts appear to be cost effective (38).

V. RISKS OF EXERCISE AND PHYSICAL ACTIVITY

There are numerous benefits to prolonged physical activity, as reviewed in previous sections of this chapter. As with every health intervention, exercise training also has some risks. If responsible public health recommendations are to be made, careful consideration must be given to these risks and thought given to risk/benefit analyses. Some individuals have expressed concern about sudden death due to vigorous exercise. There may be as many as 20 million joggers in the United States (77); and if they are at increased risk, we need to know about it. Casual observation and anecdotal accounts do not support the hypothesis that there are very large numbers of sudden deaths due to vigorous exercise. For one thing, sudden death in a jogger is headline news in most communities; this would not likely be the case if it were a common event. Sudden death rates have actually declined over the past two decades (65), the time period during which an increase in exercise participation is thought to have occurred. If exercise were a cause of sudden death, one would expect death rates in the population to increase rather than decrease (unless they increased during bouts of exercise, but decreased elsewhere). Studies on physical activity or exercise and death and on musculoskeletal problems are reviewed in the following sections.

A. Cardiovascular Deaths

1. Cardiac Rehabilitation. It is reasonable to assume that the greatest risk of an untoward cardiovascular event during exercise would be in patients with disease. Haskell (51) surveyed 30 cardiac rehabilitation programs in North America. These programs were in operation during the period 1960–1976, and they held exercise classes in 103 locations. There were 1,629,634 hours of exercise participation represented in the survey. Fourteen fatal and forty-seven nonfatal complications were reported, which results in a complication for every 26,715 hours of exercise. Approximately one half of the fatal events occurred in programs that were among the first cardiac rehabilitation programs, but these groups accounted for less than 10% of the total participation hours. The fatality rates became much lower (one death per 212,182 hours of participation) in later years. Presumably, experience gained in the early years enabled program directors to make modifications that resulted in lower risk for participants. Haskell's study shows that death during exercise is quite rare, even in cardiac patients. A study of complications during cardiac rehabilitation was reported in 1986 by Van Camp and Peterson (108). They surveyed 167 rehabilitation programs in which 51,303 patients exercised 2,351,916 hours during 1980–1984. In this more recent study, complication rates were much lower (cardiac arrest rate was onefourth as great, and fatality rate was one seventh as great) than the overall results reported by Haskell (51). The fatality rate reported by Van Camp and Peterson was less than one third that reported by Haskell for the more recent programs.

2. **Leisure Time Physical Activity.** Cardiovascular complications during leisure time physical activity have been documented in several populations. Gibbons et al. (49) reported on cardiovascular events during 65 months of follow-up in 2,935 exercisers at the Aerobics Activity Center. Exercise participation was monitored by a computerized exercise log system. Participants recorded 374,798 hours of exercise, including 2,726,272 km of running and walking. There were no deaths and two nonfatal cardiovascular complications reported during the 65 month follow-up. Complication rates were 3/ 100,000 hours of exercise for men, and 2/100,000 hours of exercise for women.

Thompson et al. (106) monitored the incidence of death during jogging in Rhode Island for the years 1975–1980. A random digit telephone survey was used to estimate jogging rates. Twelve jogging related deaths occurred during the study. There was one death per year for every 7,620 joggers, or one death per 396,000 hours of jogging. The authors conclude that there is a significantly increased risk of death while jogging, but that the absolute risk of death during jogging is low. It is also clear that most (approximately 90%) exercise-related deaths are due to advanced coronary heart disease and that the death was probably imminent, in any event (88).

The Rhode Island study indicates an increased risk of dying during exercise, as compared to more sedentary activities (106). A study on primary cardiac arrest (PCA) was done in Seattle in order to estimate the absolute and relative risk of death during exercise in men who were sedentary and men who were physically active (99). The investigators interviewed the wives of 133 men who had PCA. Men who were sedentary (<20 minutes of exercise per week in high intensity activity) were 56 times more likely to have PCA during exercise than during the other 23 hours of the day. Men who exercised >139 minutes per week were only five times more likely to have PCA during an exercise session, as compared to non-exercise time. Thus, these data confirm an increased risk during exercise, but that risk is much greater with infrequent exercisers. Furthermore, when overall risk (exercise and sedentary activities) for PCA was considered, the frequent (>20 minutes per week of high intensity activity) exercisers had only 40% of the risk of PCA, as compared to the more sedentary men. There appears to be a transient increase in risk of PCA during exercise, but there is the clear benefit of a low PCA risk in regular exercisers during non-exercise time.

B. Musculoskeletal Problems

There is much concern expressed in the lay press and medical literature regarding the prevalence of orthopedic injuries resulting from exercise participation. A great deal of publicity about injuries in aerobic dance participants resulted from two 1985 studies (42,90). Both studies reported an approximate 75% injury rate for aerobic dance instructors, and Richie et al. (90) reported a 43% injury rate for students. In my opinion, these studies have overstated the problem of injuries in aerobic dance. The first issue regards the definition of injury. Francis et al. (42) provide no specific definition. Richie et al. (90) asked about whether or not the dancer had ever been injured, so their data indicate a lifetime incidence. They defined injury as "any condition causing significant pain and/or limiting participation" (time of limited participation unspecified in the paper). When the "limiting participation" definition was used, 126 out of 1,233 students (10%) and 15 of 58 instructors (26%) were injured. In this study, the students had been participating in aerobic dance for 6.1 months and the instructors 30.5 months. When this difference in participation time is considered, the annual injury rates are 20% per year for students and 10% per year for instructors; these rates are not significantly different from one another. The statement that there is a 10% per year injury rate for instructors is not as dramatic as the assertion that 75% of aerobic dance instructors become injured, but the lower rate is a more accurate indication of the problem.

Garrick et al. (47) published the results of a longitudinal study of aerobic dance injuries. They followed 351 students and 60 instructors in six dance exercise facilities for 16 weeks. Three hundred twenty-seven medical complaints were reported during 29,924 hours of activity. Only 84 of these injuries resulted in any disability ($2.8 \cdot 1,000$ person hours^{-1} of participation), and just 2.1% of the injuries required medical attention. The authors have concluded that aerobic dance has a "minimal risk of injury."

There are major methodological flaws in most of the studies on exercise injuries (84). Failure to provide a clear and specific definition of injury has been alluded to. Another major problem is that many studies are case series in which the number of injuries is tabulated. These studies ignore the population of exercisers from which the injuries arise. In order to calculate a meaningful injury rate, the number of injuries, the number of participants, and the length of time of participation in the population at risk are needed. Another problem is the lack of a control or comparison group. For example, not all injuries in runners are due to running; some may result from routine daily activities.

Several factors have been proposed as possible risk factors for running injuries (84). The case series studies frequently mention structural abnormalities, training errors, body build, age, sex, and lack of flexibility as factors related to injuries. The lack of data on the population from which the cases arise makes these conclusions suspect. It is not enough to state that injuries are caused by too rapid an increase in running distance simply on the basis that some injured runners report increasing the amount of running. One also has to know what proportion of non-injured runners also increased their distance. Our recent review suggests that the risk of running injury is related to distance run per week, and past injury probably makes one more susceptible to future injury (84). Age, sex, body build, running experience, intensity of training, and stretching habits have been examined as risk factors for injury, but present data are insufficient to confirm these as causes.

We studied exercise injuries in three populations (12). The purpose was to estimate injury rates and to search for possible risk factors for exercise injuries. The first study was a retrospective survey of running practices and orthopedic injuries in members of the Aerobics Activity Center in Dallas. Participants were 438 men and women who had recorded at least 16 km of running for at least one week during a three month period. These runners had been running for 6.7 years and averaged about 40 km per week. Runners who reported an injury which caused them to stop running for at least seven days were classified as injured. Twenty-four percent reported an injury during the previous 12 months. Distance run per week was positively associated with risk of injury. Factors not related to injury risk were: age, gender, time and place of running, frequency of stretching, and running speed.

We also examined orthopedic injury rates in a longitudinal study of Cooper Clinic patients. Participants were 2,826 men who had two clinic visits and completed a mail survey. Injury definition for this analysis was that the person had a physician diagnosed orthopedic problem. The participants were classified as runners or non-runners based on their responses to questions on exercise habits on a medical history questionnaire. Injury rates were calculated for specific sites: knee, foot, hip, back, shoulder, and elbow. We initially expected that injury rates for the shoulder and elbow would be the same for runners and non-runners, but that the groups would differ on injury rates in the legs. In fact, only knee injuries differed between groups, with the runners reporting a higher incidence. Overall injury rates in both groups were low, with site specific rates less than 2% per year.

The third study involved approximately 1,000 men and women participating in worksite health promotion programs. Participants were classified into four exercise groups (a) walk/jog/run or other exercise; (b) racket sports or other vigorous sports (e.g., swimming, or cycling); (c) combination of activities (walk/jog/run *and* other exercise); and (d) sedentary. Exercise group assignments were based on responses to exercise questions on a lifestyle survey. Injuries were defined as an affirmative response to the question, "During the past 12 months, have you sustained any bone, muscle, or joint injuries?" Persons who answered "no" to the injury question at baseline, but "yes" at follow-up, were classified as injury incident cases. The annual injury incidence for all exercisers was 44%, and the corresponding rate for the sedentary persons was 32%. Thus, the net injury rate that can presumably be attributed to the exercise program was 12% per year; this may be an overestimate, however, because exercise and non-exercise injuries cannot be separated in the exercisers.

In summary, there is little good information presently available on estimates of injury rates in populations and even less data on risk factors for exercise injuries. There is a great need for improved studies on these issues. Exercise scientists and public health educators need to be able to tell the public what the risks of injury are if they decide to start an exercise program. Furthermore, knowledge of exercise injury risk factors is necessary in order to develop preventive strategies.

VI. PROLONGED PHYSICAL ACTIVITY AND LONGEVITY

A. Studies in Athletes

The athlete is a picture of health, and superbly trained bodies performing at peak functional capability provide an image of invincibility. Athletes do, in fact, appear to live longer, when compared to the general population. Stephens et al. (101) reviewed 17 studies in which the mortality rates of former athletes were compared to population controls. In 16 of the studies, athletes tended to have increased longevity or lower mortality rates. Stephens et al. questioned these results, since most of the former athletes attended a university and thus had a favored socioeconomic status; also, they felt that more appropriate control groups were needed. When university classmates were used as controls, thereby eliminating socioeconomic differences, the athlete versus control comparisons were not consistent. Depending on the study, athletes had higher, lower, or the same mortality rates as their classmates (101). Most of the studies were unable to control for other potential confounding factors, such as differences in body build and in health habits such as smoking, diet, and exercise. These latter issues may be important, although we find that former athletes and non-athletes are similar in middle age on many health-related and clinical variables (22). The former athletes were somewhat more physically fit and were more likely to smoke, but other variables were similar between the two groups. Both groups were equally likely to start an exercise program after the baseline clinic visit, and changes in health variables were the same in athletes and non-athletes.

In summary, there is no conclusive evidence that former athletes enjoy any particular health benefit when compared to non-athletes. In fact, it seems likely that it is the current physical activity, rather than past activity, that may offer some protection (80).

B. College Alumni

Paffenbarger et al. (78) followed 16,936 Harvard alumni for cause specific and all cause mortality for up to 16 years. Men who entered Harvard College from 1916 to 1950 were the study participants. College data on physical examinations and sports participation were available, as were data on health habits and health status, obtained by mail surveys in 1962 and 1966. Official death certificates were obtained on men who died between 1962 and 1978. Several questions on the mail surveys dealt with current physical activity patterns. Data from these questions were used to estimate total energy expenditure in leisure time physical activity.

Previous work by Paffenbarger et al. reported a lower death rate from total cardiovascular disease, respiratory disease, cancer, unnatural causes, and all cause mortality in the physically active alumni. In the 1986 paper, they extended these analyses to estimates of longevity. The more physically active men (8,400 kJ (>2,000 kcal) of leisure time physical activity/week) gained slightly more than two years of life to age 80, when compared to sedentary men (<2,100 kJ (<500 kcal/week)) (see Table 11-3). This is reduced to 1.25 years when the group is split at 8,400 kJ · week^{-1}. The absolute difference between groups is greater at the younger ages, but the relative gain is greatest in the older men. The percent of men in each age group surviving to age 80 is also shown by activity classification in Table 11-3. The authors calculated that if one gets the 8,400 kJ in three hours per week, the gain in longevity per hour of exercise is 1.95 hours for 40 year old men, and 2.47 hours for 70 year old men. This research on Harvard alumni is the most definitive estimate of the extent to which an active lifestyle extends life. Dr. Paffenbarger further stated that these added years of life are not prolonging several months of disability at the end of life, but, rather, extend the time of useful, productive life in earlier years (personal communication). (See Table 11-3.)

VII. RECOMMENDATIONS

The research reviewed here supports the value of prolonged physical activity as an important health habit. There are numerous physical and psychological benefits to be gained from a physically active way of life, and risk/benefit considerations suggest an overall net benefit from regular activity. Furthermore, the prevalence of sedentary living habits in the United States is quite high. These factors lead to a consideration of the total burden of sedentary living relative to the health of the population. The epidemiologic term is "population attributable risk" (PAR), which is how much disease or other problems can be attributed to a particular factor or set of factors. This concept (PAR) must be distinguished from clinical or in-

TABLE 11-3. *Physical activity and longevity in college alumni (adapted from Paffenbarger et al, N. Engl. J. Med., 1986).*

Age at entry	Additional Years of Life		Percent Surviving to Age 80		
	>8400* vs. <2100	>8400* vs. <8400	>8400	vs.	<8400
35–39	2.51+	1.50	68.2		57.8
40–44	2.34	1.39	68.5		58.2
45–49	2.10	1.10	69.0		59.2
50–54	2.11	1.20	69.9		59.8
55–59	2.02	1.13	71.1		61.0
60–64	1.75	0.93	73.0		63.4
65–69	1.35	0.67	76.4		67.6
70–74	0.72	0.44	82.4		74.6
75–79	0.42	0.30	91.8		85.0
35–79	2.15	1.25	69.7		59.8

*Kilojoules expended · week^{-1} in walking, climbing stairs, and playing sports.
+All values adjusted for blood pressure, smoking, change in weight since college, and age of parental death.

dividual attributable risk estimates. A simple example will help clarify this point. Cigarette smoking is conclusively established as a major threat to health and longevity, and anyone who smokes can probably do more for their health by stopping than any other action they may take. Let's consider a population in which smoking prevalence is quite low, say 2%. Stopping smoking is important for that 2%; but even if all smokers quit, population disease and death rates would change only slightly. Assume that the same population has a very low prevalence (<10%) of regular seat belt use while in a motor vehicle. Although not wearing a seat belt represents a lower absolute risk than cigarette smoking for an individual, getting the 90% of non-seat belt users to buckle up will probably have a greater impact on population death rates than getting the 2% to quit smoking. PAR for sedentary living is important, given the substantial risk of inactivity (approximately a doubling of risk for coronary artery disease) (86) and the high prevalence of inactivity (25,28). The PAR for sedentary living relative to all cause mortality in Harvard Alumni is 16.1% (78). Corresponding figures for other variables are: hypertension, 6.4%; cigarette smoking, 22.5%; low weight gain, 10.3%; and early parental death, 4.8%. White (113) estimates that there would be nearly 300,000 fewer cardiovascular disease deaths annually in the United States if inactivity were eliminated. Earlier, the review of physical activity and other health habits showed a few relatively weak relationships. Nonetheless, White estimates that if those relationships are causal, there would be 6.5 million fewer smokers if all sedentary persons became active (113). This would result in 2,900 fewer lung cancer cases. Since vigorous exercisers are slightly more likely to wear seat belts, White estimates that there would be over 8 million more seat belt users if everyone became active. These estimates are highly speculative, and precisely defining the PAR for sedentary habits is risky. The overall thrust of these estimates, however, certainly supports the value of public health efforts to promote increased exercise by the United States population. It is reasonable to expect that such a change would have a major health benefit. As we learn more about relationships between physical activity, other health habits, and chronic disease, the PAR concept may become increasingly more useful and important in public health efforts regarding disease prevention.

VIII. PUBLIC HEALTH APPROACH TO PHYSICAL ACTIVITY AND EXERCISE

Efforts by the U.S. federal government to promote health and prevent disease began to crystallize in the late 1970s (13). In 1980, the U.S. Public Health Service published *Promoting Health/Preventing Disease: Objectives for the Nation*. This report contains 226 discrete objectives in 15 broad areas that are generally referred to as the 1990 Objectives. One of the areas is physical fitness and exercise, and there are 11 specific objectives in this area (83). A discussion of the objectives is beyond the scope of this chapter, but they pertain to surveillance of appropriate physical activity habits, awareness of benefits of physical activity, worksite programs, and further documentation of health benefits. Government activities to help achieve the 1990 Objectives have increased in recent years. Several major United States conferences on various aspects of physical activity and health have been held by the Centers for Disease Control; National Institute of Mental Health; National Heart, Lung, and Blood Institute, and the National Center for Health Statistics (13). More external research initiatives are being supported by the National Institutes of Health; and within the U.S. Public Health Service, the Behavioral Epidemiology Branch at the Centers for Disease Control has its major focus on physical activity and health. The Public Health Service continues to monitor and refine the 1990 Objectives on physical fitness and exercise (26,28,85), and it is clear that the federal government will continue to support efforts in this area. Several of the 1990 Objectives may be achieved, but others probably will not (85). Plans for modification and refinement of the objectives are under way, and given the high prevalence of sedentary living habits, increased efforts to promote physical activity to all segments of the population are needed (26,28).

A. Targeted Interventions

Although there apparently has been an increase in physical activity participation in recent years (102), much remains to be done. It is clear that some sub-groups in the population, notably women, older individuals, persons in the lower socioeconomic strata, and minorities, have been less inclined to adopt regular, vigorous exercise as a way of life (26,28,92,104). Specific plans and activities designed to appeal to these groups are needed.

Another important factor in the public health promotion of exercise is the intensity issue. Many of the promotional campaigns and specific exercise intervention programs have emphasized vigorous activity. The typical advertising image is one of a relatively young professional person participating in vigorous sports or 10K races. The older individual who has been sedentary for decades and is somewhat overweight cannot imagine donning a leotard for a vigorous aerobic dance class, running a 10K race, or competing in the Ironman Triathlon. Exercise scientists have probably helped promote this vigorous activity image with our focus on target heart rates, scientific approaches to exercise prescription, recommending exercise ECG stress tests (at least in the United States), and placing other barriers (real or imaginary) to exercise adoption before the public. Existing research indicates that significant health benefits result from moderate physical activity (67,78,80). While we should continue to give attention to exercise prescription formulae and promote vigorous sports and activities, additional strategies must be developed. A sound behavioral approach to exercise adoption appears to promote moderate changes in habits. For example, a message to the large group of sedentary persons might be "watch a little less television, and try to do 20–30 minutes of walking each day." Alternative messages could be "try a bit of gardening," "join in a folk dance club," "always take the stairs, not an escalator or elevator." There would be significant public health benefit if one half of the most sedentary individuals would begin moderate exercise, such as a few minutes of walking each day.

There have been a few attempts to promote physical activity in the community. The early community intervention studies in California (68) and in Finland (87) did not give a major emphasis to physical activity and did not report improvements in physical activity participation. The second generation of community studies appears to place more emphasis on a reduction in sedentary living habits (35,40). In keeping with the PAR concept described above, there is some limited evidence of success from community intervention (3), but more definitive conclusions must await data from the major community trials now under way.

B. Physical Activity at the Worksite

Exercise and physical fitness programs at the worksite have become quite popular in recent years (56). Since a majority of adults in our population go to work outside the home each day, it is logical to locate health promotion programs at the worksite. The primary reason for promoting exercise at the worksite has been to improve the health of employees. The expectation has been that improved health would result in reduced absenteeism and reduced medical care costs. Several key issues are related to achieving these and other objectives: 1) Can worksite exercise programs be implemented?; 2) Will a large percentage of workers change their exercise habits, and can changes be maintained?; 3) Can workers outside the professional and white collar ranks be helped to change their exercise habits?; 4) Will exercise habit changes in workers lead to improved health status?; and 5) Will changes in exercise and physical fitness (if achieved) result in economic benefit to the company?

1. **Program Implementation.** It is clear that it is possible to implement exercise and physical fitness programs at the worksite (56,60). Successful programs have been established in large and small companies and in a wide variety of industries. Company-wide program impact studies are rare, but a recent report on the Johnson and Johnson "Live for Life" program provides encouraging results (16).

The "Live for Life" program follows a community health model; that is, intervention is directed at the entire workforce and organization, rather than to small groups of volunteers (for further explanation of this model see references (14,114). Evaluation for "Live for Life" extended over two years in a quasi-experimental design with four treatment (n = 2,600 employees) and three control (n = 1,700 employees) companies (16). Striking changes in population physical activity were seen in the treatment companies. Employees in treatment companies increased daily energy expenditure in vigorous (>5.0 METs) activity by 104% from baseline to the two year evaluation. The corresponding change in comparison company employees was 33%. At baseline, 992 treatment company employees were classified as getting less than an optimal amount of exercise (roughly equivalent to three times/week for 30 minutes or more each time, at 50% $\dot{V}O_2max$). By the end of two years, 20% of the initially sedentary women and 30% of the initially sedentary men were regularly exercising at or above the optimal level. These changes in self-reported physical activity and exercise habits were corroborated by objective measures of physical fitness. Population increases in estimated $\dot{V}O_2max$ were 8.4% at year one and 10.5% at year two in treatment company employees; corresponding figures for the comparison group were 1.5% and 4.7%. These results indicate that it is possible to make significant changes in exercise and physical fitness in a large population of workers. Furthermore, the changes persist for a relatively extended time. In fact, changes in nearly all exercise and physical fitness variables were greater at year two than for year one.

Population changes of the magnitude described above probably indicate changes throughout the workforce. This was confirmed by extensive multivariate modeling analyses using various socio-demographic groups as independent variables (16). Results indicate that increases in exercise and physical fitness occurred in young and old, married and single, men and women, clerical and management, white and minority, and various educational sub-groups. These results are highly encouraging, in that they support the hypothesis that a carefully planned and implemented program can be beneficial to the total workforce.

Worksite exercise programs also have a beneficial impact on other health and clinical status variables. Workers exposed to a health promotion program are likely to improve coronary heart disease risk factor status and feelings of general well-being, depression, health attitudes, and health knowledge (7,16).

Do the changes enumerated above have any economic benefit to the company? Shephard et al. (34,96,98) show decreases in absenteeism, turnover, and medical care costs in insurance company employees participating in a worksite exercise program. Employees in a large metropolitan school district had a net reduction in absenteeism of 1.25 days per employee per year (17). Reduction in absenteeism was inversely associated with improvement in physical fitness in these employees.

Economic analyses of the "Live for Life" program show an important reduction in hospitalization costs for employees from "Live for Life" companies (18). More than 10,000 Johnson & Johnson employees were followed for five years. Average annual hospitalization cost increases were $43 and $42 for two "Live for Life" groups and $76 for Johnson and Johnson employees not exposed to "Live for Life." These results cannot be solely attributed to exercise and physical fitness changes in employees, since "Live for Life" is a broadly based program with multiple interventions. However, clinically important improvements in exercise and physical fitness did occur in "Live for Life" (16). The school district study (17) also shows a link between physical fitness and the economic variable fo absenteeism, so perhaps it is reasonable to assume that the "Live for Life" economic results are at least partly due to exercise.

Current scientific evidence supports the success of worksite exercise programs (96). These efforts should be part of a broader health promotion program, but exercise is one of the key program elements (14,60). Evidence is growing that worksite programs can be effective in reaching large numbers of employees, that changes can occur throughout the workforce, that beneficial health changes accompany increases in exercise and physical fitness, and that there is economic benefit for the company (17,19,96,98). Other major systems and institutions can make an important contribution to public health promotion of exercise. The roles of schools, primary care physicians, and churches need to be studied and, if feasible, used in population based exercise promotion.

SUMMARY

Evidence reviewed here strongly supports the beneficial impact of prolonged exercise and physical activity on various measures of disability, functional capability, morbidity, and mortality. Although potential problems of exercise, such as risk of orthopedic injuries, need continued study, evidence at present supports a favorable risk/benefit ratio for regular physical activity. Despite an improvement in recent years, most North Americans are still relatively sedentary; and large scale public health intervention efforts are needed to further encourage regular exercise. Worksite exercise programs are showing some success and are a logical place for continued emphasis and study.

ACKNOWLEDGEMENTS

I thank Drs. Roy Shephard and Carl Caspersen for many helpful comments, Kathryn Albrecht for preparing the manuscript, Jennifer Nelson for proofreading, and Dr. Ron Mulder for research assistance.

BIBLIOGRAPHY

1. American College of Sports Medicine. *Guidelines for Exercise Testing and Prescription*, 3rd ed. Philadelphia, PA: Lea and Febiger, 1986, p. 179.
2. American College of Sports Medicine. Position stand on the recommended quantity and quality of exercise for developing and maintaining fitness in healthy adults. *Med Sci Sports Exercise.* 10:vii-x, 1978.
3. Anderson, G., and S. Malmgren. Changes in self-reported experienced health and psychosomatic symptoms in voluntary participants in a 1-year extensive newspaper exercise campaign. *Scand J Soc Med.* 14:141–146, 1986.
4. Annuzzi, G., O. Vaccaro, S. Caprio, et al. Association between low habitual physical activity and impaired glucose tolerance. *Clin Physiol.* 5:63–70, 1985.
5. Björntorp, P. and M. Krotkiewski. Exercise treatment in diabetes mellitus. *Acta Med Scand.* 217:3–7, 1985.
6. Blair, S.N. How to assess exercise habits and physical fitness. In: *Behavioral Health: A Handbook of Health Enhancement and Disease Prevention*, J.D. Matarazzo, S.M. Weiss, J.A. Herd, N.E. Miller, and S.M. Weiss (Eds.). New York: John Wiley and Sons, 1984, pp. 424–447.
7. Blair, S.N., T.R. Collingwood, R. Reynolds, et al. Health promotion for educators: impact on health behaviors, satisfaction, and general well-being. *Am J Public Health.* 74: 147–149, 1984.
8. Blair, S.N., H.B. Falls, and R.R. Pate. A new physical fitness test. *Physician Sportsmed.* 11:87–95, 1983.
9. Blair, S.N., N.N. Goodyear, L.W. Gibbons, and K.H. Cooper. Physical fitness and incidence of hypertension in healthy normotensive men and women. *J Am Med Assn.* 252:487–490, 1984.
10. Blair, S.N., W.L. Haskell, P. Ho, et al. Assessment of habitual physical activity by a seven-day recall in a community survey and controlled experiments. *Am J Epidemiol.* 122:794–804, 1985.
11. Blair, S.N., D.R. Jacobs, Jr., and K.E. Powell. Relationships between exercise or physical activity and other health behaviors. *Public Health Rep.* 100:172–180, 1985.
12. Blair, S.N., H.W. Kohl, and N.N. Goodyear. Rates and risks for running and exercise injuries: studies in three populations. *Res Q Exercise Sport* 1987. 58:221–228, 1987.
13. Blair, S.N., H.W. Kohl, and K.E. Powell. Physical activity, physical fitness, exercise, and the public's health. In: *The Cutting Edge in Physical Education and Exercise Science Research*, M.J. Safrit and H.M. Eckert (Eds.). Champaign, IL: Human Kinetics, 1987, pp. 53–69.
14. Blair, S.N. and B.S. Mitchell. Cost effectiveness of worksite health promotion programs. In: *Cardiac Rehabilitation and Clinical Exercise Programs: Theory and Practice*, N.O. Oldridge, D.H. Schmidt, and C. Foster (Eds.). Ithaca, NY: Mouvement Publications, 1988, pp. 283–297.
15. Blair, S.N., R.T. Mulder, H.W. Kohl. Reaction to "Secular trends in adult physical activity: fitness boom or bust?" *Res Q Exercise Sport.* 58:106–110, 1987.
16. Blair, S.N., P.V. Piserchia, C.S. Wilbur, and J.H. Crowder. A public health intervention

model for worksite health promotion: impact on exercise and physical fitness in a health promotion plan after 24 months. *J Am Med Assn.* 255:921–926, 1986.

17. Blair, S.N., M. Smith, T.R. Collingwood, R. Reynolds, M.C. Prentice, and C.L. Sterling. Health promotion for educators: impact on absenteeism. *Prev Med.* 15:166–175, 1986.
18. Bly, J.L., R.C. Jones, and J.E. Richardson. Impact of worksite health promotion on health care costs and utilization: evaluation of Johnson & Johnson's Live for Life Program. *J Am Med Assn.* 256:3235–3240, 1986.
19. Bowne, D.W., M.L. Russell, J.L. Morgan, S.A. Optenberg, and A.E. Clarke. Reduced disability and health care costs in an industrial fitness program. *J Occup Med.* 26:809–816, 1984.
20. Brooks, C.M. Adult participation in physical activities requiring moderate to high levels of energy expenditure. *Physician Sportsmed.* 15:118–132 (April), 1987.
21. Brooks, C.M. Leisure time physical activity assessment of American adults through an analysis of time diaries collected in 1981. *Am J Public Health.* 77:455–46 , 1987.
22. Burkhalter, H.E., S.N. Blair, N.N. Goodyear, M.W. Taylor, and D.L. Johnsen. Treadmill performance of former athletes vs. non-athletes in middle-age. *Med Sci Sports Exercise.* 16:124 (abstract), 1984.
23. Cantwell, J.D. Cardiac rehabilitation in the mid-1980s. *Physician Sportsmed.* 14:89–96, April, 1986.
24. Carson, P., R. Phillips, M. Lloyd, et al. Exercise after myocardial infarction: a controlled trial. *J Royal Coll Physicians London.* 16:147–151, 1982.
25. Caspersen, C.J., G.M. Christenson, and R.A. Pollard. Status of the 1990 physical fitness and exercise objectives—evidence from NHIS 1985. *Public Health Rep.* 101:587–592, 1986.
26. Caspersen, C.J., K.E. Powell, and G.M. Christenson. Physical activity, exercise, and physical fitness: definitions and distinctions for health-related research. *Public Health Rep.* 100:126–131.
27. Cederholm, J. and L. Wibell. Glucose tolerance and physical activity in a health survey of middle-aged subjects. *Acta Med Scand.* 217:373–378, 1985.
28. Centers for Disease Control. Sex-, age-, and region-specific prevalence of sedentary lifestyle in selected states in 1985—The Behavioral Risk Factor Surveillance System. *Morbidity Mortality Weekly Rep.* 36:195–198, 203–204, 1987.
29. Centers for Disease Control. Behavioral risk factor surveillance, 1981–1983. CDC surveillance summaries. *Morbidity Mortality Weekly Rep.* 33:1SS-4SS, 1984.
30. Chen, M.K. The epidemiology of self-perceived fatigue among adults. *Prev Med.* 15:74–81, 1986.
31 Converse, P.E., and M.W. Traugott. Assessing the accuracy of polls and surveys. *Science* 234:1094–1098, 1986.
32. Cordain, L., R.W. Latin, and J.J. Behnke. The effects of an aerobic running program on bowel transit time. *J Sports Med Physical Fitness.* 26:101–104, 1986.
33. Cornoni-Huntley, J., D.B. Brock, A.M. Ostfeld, J.O. Taylor, and R.B. Wallace, (Eds.). *Established populations for epidemiologic studies of the elderly: resource data book.* National Institute on Aging, Public Health Service, NIH Pub. No. 86–2443, 1986, p. 428.
34. Cox, M., R.J. Shephard, and P. Corey. Influence of an employee fitness program upon fitness, productivity and absenteeism. *Ergonomics.* 24:795–806, 1981.
35. Crow, R., H. Blackburn, D. Jacobs, et al. Population strategies to enhance physical activity. *Acta Med Scand.* Suppl 711:93–112, 1986.
36. Department of Health and Human Services. *Promoting Health/Preventing Disease: Objectives for the Nation.* Washington, D.C.: U.S. Government Printing Office, 1980.
37. Duncan, J.J., J.E. Farr, S.J. Upton, R.D. Hagan, M.E. Oglesby, and S.N. Blair. The effects of aerobic exercise on plasma catecholamines and blood pressure in patients with mild essential hypertension. *J Am Med Assn.* 254:2609–2613, 1985.
38. Dunham, J.L., J.E. Hodgkin, J. Nichol, III, and G.C. Burton. Cost effectiveness of pulmonary rehabilitation programs. In: *Pulmonary Rehabilitation: Guidelines to Success,* J.E. Hodgkin, I.G. Zorn, and G.L. Connors (Eds.). Stoneham, MA, 1984, pp. 389–402.
39. Ehsani, A.A., D.R. Biello, J. Schultz, B.E. Sobel, and J.O. Holloszy. Improvement of left ventricular contractile function by exercise training in patients with coronary artery disease. *Circulation* 74:350–358, 1986.
40. Farquhar, J.W., S.P. Fortmann, N. Maccoby et al. The Stanford Five City Project: design and methods. *Am J Epidemiol.* 122:323–334, 1985.
41. Folsom, A.R., C.J. Caspersen, H.L. Taylor, et al. Leisure time physical activity and its relationship to coronary risk factors in a population-based sample: the Minnesota Heart Survey. *Am J Epidemiol.* 121:570–579, 1985.
42. Francis, L.L., P.R. Francis, and K. Welshons-Smith. Aerobic dance injuries: a survey of instructors. *Physician Sportsmed.* 13:105–111, February, 1985.
43. Frisch, R.E., G. Wyshak, T.E. Albright, N.L. Albright, and I. Schiff. Lower prevalence of

diabetes in female former college athletes compared with non-athletes. *Diabetes.* 35:1101–1105, 1986.

44. Frisch, R.E., G. Wyshak, N.L. Albright, et al. Lower prevalence of breast cancer and cancers of the reproductive system among former college athletes compared to non–athletes. *Br J Cancer.* 52:885–891, 1985.

45. Froelicher, V., D. Jensen, F. Genter, et al. A randomized trial of exercise training in patients with coronary heart disease. *J Am Med Assn.* 252:1291–1297, 1984.

46. Garabrant, D.H., J.M. Peters, T.M. Mack, and L. Bernstein. Job activity and colon cancer risk. *Am J Epidemiol.* 119:1005–1014, 1984.

47. Garrick, J.G., D.M. Gillien, and P. Whiteside. The epidemiology of aerobic dance injuries. *Am J Sports Med.* 14:67–72, 1986.

48. Gerhardsson, M., S.E. Norell, H. Kiviranta, N.L. Pedersen, and A. Ahlbom. Sedentary jobs and colon cancer. *Am J Epidemiol.* 123:775–780, 1986.

49. Gibbons, L.W., K.H. Cooper, B.M. Meyer, et al. The acute cardiac risk of strenuous exercise. *J Am Med Assn.* 224:1799–1801, 1980.

50. Hammond, H.K. Exercise for coronary heart disease patients: is it worth the effort? *J Cardiopulmonary Rehabil.* 5:531–539, 1985.

51. Haskell, W.L. Cardiovascular complications during exercise training of cardiac patients. *Circulation.* 47:920–924, 1978.

52. Haskell, W.L. Exercise-induced changes in plasma lipids and lipoproteins. *Prev Med.* 13:23–36, 1984.

53. Haskell, W.L. Mechanisms by which physical activity may enhance the clinical status of cardiac patients. In: *Heart Disease and Rehabilitation,* M.L. Pollock and D.H. Schmidt (Eds.). Boston: Houghton Mifflin, 1979, pp. 276–296.

54. Hodgkin, J.E., B.V. Branscomb, J.D. Anholm, and L.S. Gray. Benefits, limitations, and the future of pulmonary rehabilitation. In: *Pulmonary Rehabilitation: Guidelines to Success,* J.E. Hodgkin, I.G. Zorn, and G.L. Connors (Eds.). Stoneham, MA, 1984, pp. 403–414.

55. Holloszy, J.O., J. Schultz, J. Kusnierkiewicz, J.M. Hagberg, and A.A. Eshani. Effects of exercise on glucose tolerance and insulin resistance. *Acta Med Scand., Suppl.* 711:55–65, 1986.

56. Iverson, D.C., J.E. Fielding, R.S. Crow, and G.M. Christenson. The promotion of physical activity in the United States population: the status of programs in medical, worksite, community, and school settings. *Public Health Rep.* 100:212–224, 1985.

57. Kallio, V., H. Hamalainen, J. Hakkila, and O.J. Luurila. Reduction in sudden deaths by a multifactorial intervention programmed after acute myocardial infarction. *Lancet.* 2:1091–1094, 1979.

58. Kannel, W.B., P. Wilson, and S.N. Blair. Epidemiological assessment of the role of physical activity and fitness in development of cardiovascular disease. *Am Heart J.* 109:876–885, 1985.

59. Kemmer, F.W. and M. Berger. Exercise and diabetes mellitus: physical activity as a part of daily life and its role in the treatment of diabetic patients. *Int J Sports Med.* 4:77–88, 1983.

60. Knadler, G.F., T. Rogers, B.S. Mitchell, and S.N. Blair. *Physical Fitness Programs in the Workplace.* WBGH Worksite Wellness Series, R.A. Behrens (Ed.). Washington, D.C.: Washington Business Group on Health, 1986, pp. 1–50.

61. Kohl, H., S. Blair, W. Kannel, N. Goodyear, and P. Wilson. Sedentary traits as objective markers for physical fitness. *Am J Epidemiol,* (abstract). (In press.)

62. Kohl, H.W., S.N. Blair, and R.S. Paffenbarger. Validity of self report exercise habit responses in a mail survey. *Med Sci Sports Exercise.* 18:Supplement S30 (abstract), 1986.

63. Kohl, H.W., D.L. Moorefield, and S.N. Blair. Is cardiorespiratory fitness associated with general chronic fatigue in apparently healthy men and women? *Med Sci Sports Exercise.* 19:Supplement S6 (abstract), 1987.

64. Koplan, J.P., and K.E. Powell. Physicians and the Olympics. *J Am Med Assn.* 252:529–530, 1984.

65. Kuller, L.H., J.A. Perper, W.S. Dai, G. Rutan, and N. Traven. Sudden death and the decline in coronary heart disease mortality. *J Chron Dis.* 39:1001–1019, 1986.

66. LaPorte, R.E., H.J. Montoye, and C.J. Caspersen. Assessment of physical activity in epidemiologic research: problems and prospects. *Public Health Rep.* 100:131–146, 1985.

67. Lie, H., R. Mundal, and J. Ericksen. Coronary risk factors and incidence of coronary death in relation to physical fitness. Seven-year follow-up study of middle-aged and elderly men. *Eur Heart J.* 6:147–157, 1985.

68. Meyer, A.J., J.D. Nash, A.L. McAlister, et al. Skills training in a cardiovascular health education campaign. *J Consult Clin Psychol.* 48:129–142, 1980.

69. Montoye, H.J. and H.L. Taylor. Measurement of physical activity in population studies: a review. *Hum Biol.* 56:195–216, 1984.

70. Morris, J.N., J.A. Heady, P.A.B. Raffle, C.G. Roberts, and J.W. Parks. Coronary heart disease and physical activity of work. *Lancet.* 265:1053–1057, 1111–1120, 1953.
71. Morris, J.N., R. Pollard, M.G. Everitt, et al. Vigorous exercise in leisure time: protection against coronary heart disease. *Lancet.* 2:1207–1210, 1980.
72. Myers, J., S. Ahnve, V. Froelicher, et al. A randomized trial of the effects of 1 year of exercise training on computer-measured ST segment displacement in patients with coronary artery disease. *J Am Coll Cardiol.* 4:1094–1102, 1984.
73. National Center for Health Statistics, Exercise and participation in sports among persons 20 years of age and over: United States, 1975. Advance Data from *Vital and Health Statistics.* No. 19, DHEW Pub. No. (PHS) 78–1250. Public Health Service, Hyattsville, MD, March 15, 1978.
74. National Center for Health Statistics. Plan and operation of the Health and Nutrition Examination Survey. *Vital and Health Statistics,* Series 1, No. 10a. DHEW Pub. No. (PHS) 79–1310. Public Health Service, Hyattsville, MD, 1973.
75. National Center for Health Statistics. Plan and operation of the Second National Health and Nutrition Examination Survey. *Vital and Health Statistics,* Series 10, No. 15. DHHS Pub. No. (PHS) 81–1317. Public Health Service, Hyattsville, MD, 1981.
76. National Center for Health Statistics, T.F. Drury and A.L. Powell. Prevalence, impact, and demography of known diabetes in the United States. Advance Data from *Vital and Health Statistics.* No. 114. DHHS Pub. No. (PHS) 86–1250. Public Health Service, Hyattsville, MD, February 12, 1986.
77. National Center for Health Statistics, O.T. Thornberry, R.W. Wilson, and P. Golden. Health promotion and disease prevention provisional data from the National Health Interview Survey, United States, January-June 1985. Advance Data from *Vital and Health Statistics.* No. 119, DHHS Pub. No. (PHS) 86–1250. Public Health Service, Hyattsville, MD, May 14, 1986.
78. Paffenbarger, R.S., Jr., R.T. Hyde, A.L. Wing, and C.C. Hsieh. Physical Activity, all-cause mortality, and longevity of college alumni. *N Engl J Med.* 314:605–613, 1986.
79. Paffenbarger, R.S., Jr., R.T. Hyde, A.L. Wing, and C.C. Hsieh. Physical activity and longevity of college alumni. *N Engl J Med.* 315:400–401 (letter), 1986.
80. Paffenbarger, R.S., Jr., R.T. Hyde, A.L. Wing, and C.H. Steinmetz. A natural history of athleticism and cardiovascular health. *J Am Med Assn.* 252:491–495, 1984.
81. Paffenbarger, R.S., A.L. Wing, R.T. Hyde, et al. Physical activity and incidence of hypertension in college alumni. *J Am Epidemiol.* 117:245–257, 1983.
82. Perrier. *The Perrier Study: Fitness in America.* New York: Perrier Great Waters of France, Inc., 1979.
83. Powell, K.E., G.M. Christenson, and M.W. Kreuter. Objectives for the nation: assessing the role physical education must play. *J Physical Educ.* 55:18–29, 1984.
84. Powell, K.E., H.W. Kohl, C.J. Caspersen, and S.N. Blair. An epidemiological perspective on the causes of running injuries. *Physician Sportsmed.* 14:100–114, June 1986.
85. Powell, K.E., K.G. Spain, G.M. Christenson, and M.P. Mollenkamp. The status of the 1990 objectives for physical fitness and exercise. *Public Health Rep.* 101:15–21, 1986.
86. Powell, K.E., P.D. Thompson, C.J. Caspersen, and J.S. Kendrick. Physical activity and the incidence of coronary heart disease. *Ann Rev Public Health,* 8:253–257, 1987.
87. Puska, P., J.T. Salonen, A. Nissinen, et al. Change in risk factors for coronary heart disease during 10 years of a community intervention programme: North Karelia Project. *Br Med J.* 287:1840–1844, 1983.
88. Ragosta, M., J. Crabtree, W.Q. Sturner and P.D. Thompson. Death during recreational exercise in the state of Rhode Island. *Med Sci Sports Exercise.* 16:339–342, 1984.
89. Rechnitzer, P.A., D.A. Cunningham, G.M. Andrew, et al. Relation of exercise to the recurrence rate of myocardial infarction in men. *Am J Cardiol.* 51:65–69, 1983.
90. Richie, D.H., Jr., S.F. Kelso, and P.A. Belluci. Aerobic dance injuries: a retrospective study of instructors and participants. *Physician Sportsmed.* 13:130–140, February 1985.
91. Richter, E.A. and H. Galbo. Diabetes, insulin and exercise. *Sports Med.* 3:275–288, 1986.
92. Sallis, J.F., W.L. Haskell, P.D. Wood, et al. Physical activity assessment methodology in the Five-City Project. *Am J Epidemiol.* 121:91–106, 1985.
93. Schoenborn, C.A. Health habits of U.S. Adults, 1985: the "Alameda 7" revisited. *Pub Health Rep.* 101:571–580, 1986.
94. Shaw, L.W. Effects of a prescribed supervised exercise program on mortality and cardiovascular morbidity in patients after a myocardial infarction. *Am J Cardiol.* 48:39–46, 1981.
95. Shephard, R.J. Exercise and Aging. In: *Exercise and Sport Sciences Reviews,* R.S. Hutton (Ed.). Philadelphia, PA: Franklin Institute Press, 1979, pp. 1–57.
96. Shephard, R.J. The impact of exercise upon medical costs. *Sports Med.* 2:133–143. 1985.
97. Shephard, R.J. The value of exercise in ischemic heart disease: a cumulative analysis. *J Cardiac Rehabil.* 3:294–298, 1983.

EXERCISE, HEALTH, AND LONGEVITY   **483**

98. Shephard, R.J., P. Corey, P. Renzland, and M. Cox. The influence of an employee fitness and lifestyle modification program upon medical care costs. *Can J Pub Health*. 73:259–263, 1982.
99. Siscovick, D.S., N.S. Weiss, R.H. Fletcher, et al. The incidence of primary cardiac arrest during vigorous exercise. *N Engl J Med*. 311:874–877, 1984.
100. Slater, C.H., L.W. Green, S.W. Vernon, and V.M. Keith. Problems in estimating the prevalence of physical activity from national surveys. *Prev Med*. 16:107–118, 1987.
101. Stephens, K.E., W.D. Van Huss, H.W. Olson, and H.J. Montoye. The longevity, morbidity, and physical fitness of former athletes—an update. In: *Exercise and Health*, H.M. Eckert and H.J. Montoye (Eds.). Champaign, IL: Human Kinetics, 1984, pp. 101–119.
102. Stephens, T. Secular trends in physical activity: fitness boom or bust? *Res Q Exercise Sport*. 58:94–105, 1987.
103. Stephens, T., C.L. Craig, and B.F. Ferris. Adult physical activity in Canada: findings from the Canada Fitness Survey I. *Can J Public Health*. 77:285–290, 1986.
104. Stephens, T., D.R. Jacobs, Jr., and C.C. White. A descriptive epidemiology of leisure-time physical activity. *Public Health Rep*. 100:147–157, 1985.
105. Taylor, C.B., T. Coffey, K. Berra, R. Iaffaldano, K. Casey, and W.L. Haskell. Seven-day activity and self-report compared to a direct measure of physical activity. *Am J Epidemiol*. 120:818–824, 1984.
106. Thompson, P.D., E.J. Funk, R.A. Carleton, et al. Incidence of death during jogging in Rhode Island from 1975 through 1980. *J Am Med Assn*. 247:2535–2538, 1982.
107. Trovati, M., Q.Carta, F. Cavalot, et al. Influence of physical training on blood glucose control, glucose tolerance, insulin secretion, and insulin action in non-insulin-dependent diabetic patients. *Diabetes Care*. 7:416–420, 1984.
108. Van Camp, S.P. and R.A. Peterson. Cardiovascular complications of outpatient cardiac rehabilitation programs. *J Am Med Assn*. 256:1160–1163, 1986.
109. Vena, J.E., S. Graham, M. Zielezney, J. Brasure, and M.K. Swanson. Occupational exercise and risk of cancer. *Am J Clin Nutr*. 45:318–327, 1987.
110. Vena, J.E., S. Graham, M. Zielezney, M.K. Swanson, R.E. Barnes, and J. Nolan. Lifetime occupational exercise and colon cancer. *Am J Epidemiol* 122:357–365, 1985.
111. Verani, M.S., G.H. Hartung, J. Hoepfel-Harris, D.E. Welton, C.M. Pratt, and R.R. Miller. Effects of exercise training on left ventricular performance and myocardial perfusion in patients with coronary disease. *Am J Cardiol*. 47:797–803, 1981.
112. Washburn, R.A. and H.J. Montoye. The assessment of physical activity by questionnaire. *Am J Epidemiol*. 123:563–576, 1986.
113. White, C.C. The carnage of sloth: what if everybody ran? Presented at the American College of Sports Medicine Annual Meeting. Nashville, TN, May 29, 1985.
114. Wilbur, C.S. The Johnson & Johnson program. *Prev Med*. 12:672–681, 1983.
115. Wilhelmsen, L., H. Sanne, D. Elmfeldt, G. Grimby, G. Tibblin, and H. Wedel. A controlled trial of physical training after myocardial infarction: effects on risk factors, non fatal reinfarction, and death. *Prev Med*. 4:491–508, 1975.
116. Wilson, P.W.F., R.S. Paffenbarger, Jr., J.N. Morris, and R.M. Havlik. Assessment methods for physical activity and physical fitness in population studies: report of a NHLBI workshop. *Am Heart J*. 111:1177–1192, 1986.
117. World Health Organization. Text of the constitution of the World Health Organization. Official records WHO. 2:100, 1948.
118. Zinman, B. and M. Vranic. Diabetes and exercise. *Med Clin North Am*. 69:145–157, 1985.

DISCUSSION

BLAIR: Let me very briefly review some of our data on about 2,000 runners and 700 nonrunners, who had at least two clinic visits and completed a follow-up with a mail-back questionnaire. I think this study illustrates some basic epidemiological applications. The subjects are the kind of typical middle-aged adults we see at the Cooper Clinic. The runners, as you would expect, are much more physically fit than the nonrunners. We assessed injury rate for 1,000 person years of follow-up in runners and nonrunners. Now, at the end of this analysis, I thought that we would see very much different injury rates to the lower extremity and perhaps in the back in the subjects who were running. The runners were, on the average, doing about 12 miles a week of jogging or running, 3–4 times a week, 3–4 miles at a time. Running injury in this context refers to bone/muscle/joint injuries. What I mean by injury here is that these people told us on a mail-back questionnaire that they had physician-diagnosed orthopedic problems. I expected, as I said, that the runners would have much higher rates of these physician-diagnosed injuries for the lower extremities and perhaps the back, and not different for the upper extremities. In fact, for virtually every site we examined, the rates are not statistically different.

SHEPHARD: Isn't there a risk there that a doctor would say to you that you are not to participate in running because you have back problems?

BLAIR: That's true. However, this group reported no history of orthopedic problems before they were enrolled in the study.

SUTTON: Isn't it conceivable that the subjects who are runners may also be golfers or tennis players, as well, and that their injuries could come from activities other than running?

BLAIR: That's conceivable, but they tend not to engage in multiple activities. A runner tends to be a runner, and a tennis player tends to be a tennis player. That's not absolute, but there isn't as much cross-over in activities as I thought there would be.

I should point out that in each case the absolute injury rate is higher in the runners, but it is not significantly so. Only for the knee was the rate significantly higher for runners than nonrunners. Now, this I submit, is a very crude beginning point in our own work to look at the issue of sports-related injuries in adult men and women. Isn't it a little surprising that we didn't see relatively more injuries here in the runners than we did?

CANTWELL: It's the same thing we see all the time in our field; there's a natural process of selection. We see that nonrunners choose to be nonrunners. How many of them, at a younger age, found out that, when they tried to do things, they developed pain and problems and then elected not to be runners? The natural process of selection gives you two totally different populaces to look at.

BLAIR: Well, this group had not reported orthopedic problems at baseline. I think the argument that the nonrunners are people who tried running and became injured and then dropped out of running is not the reason.

CANTWELL: But there is natural selection in all sports.

BLAIR: I wouldn't disagree with that. All I'm saying is these nonrunners denied having orthopedic problems. Now, I wouldn't presume to say that there are no differences between runners and nonrunners, in this population or any other. However, I challenge you to find differences. They are not as obvious as you might think. You might think diets are different. You might think that there are some other health habits that are different. We looked at this extensively, not only in this population but in others, and it's surprising how hard it is to find differences. I'm not claiming that there are none.

I view this as a very crude study. But I am struck by the fact that these rates are pretty low. It's less than 1% per year in a defined population followed over a period of time. It is also important to have some kind of comparison group. There are 70 million nonintentional orthopedic injuries a year in the United States, according to the National Center for Health Statistics. They are not all in athletes.

Allow me to touch just briefly on another topic. Carl Casperson published a recent review in which he looked at all the better studies from around the world and showed a risk ratio of about 2:1 looking at inactive compared to active individuals in terms of risk of dying of coronary heart disease. That's a very powerful risk ratio. It's on the same order as cholesterol, hypertension, cigarette smoking, and the like. Past work has shown, of course, that exercise is a powerful risk factor for coronary heart disease and for total mortality. The other point that I want to bring into this is what the epidemiologist calls "attributable risk," the population attributable risk. How much of the disease and disability in the population can possibly be attributed to sedentary living? You not only have to know the relative risk of sedentary living to make the calculation, you have to know the prevalence of that condition in the population. It's a massive public health problem, and I don't think we as exercise professionals have addressed it well.

SHEPHARD: But I guess you are going to really look at three things. You are going to have to look at the prevalence in the community, the risk of it, and the ability to change it.

BLAIR: Exactly. None of these things are easy, and we are not going to eliminate any of these detrimental problems overnight.

CASPERSON: Epidemiologists face obvious methodological problems in collecting and interpreting data. In assessing physical activity, for example, the problem is that if you are not moving, we suspect you are dead. We don't have much ability to measure how active you actually are. If we look at the percentage of studies reporting inverse associations, *significant* inverse associations, between physical activity and coronary heart disease, we see that when we have an "unsatisfactory" assessment of a person's physical activity, you can find a relationship half the time. If you have a "satisfactory" measure, 76% of the time you see a relationship, and if you have a "good" measure, the relationship exists 88% of the time. That means the methods are really critical. We know that as scientists, but we haven't really thought about it a lot in epidemiology with respect to this particular issue. Overall, 68% of the studies we reviewed showed an inverse association that was significant. We saw that as the methods improved, so did our ability to detect the association.

Here's another example. From the Peachtree Road Race data, which is not a perfect study, we felt a runner would be likely to get an injury about every two years. But runners face other hazards. Runners do get hit by thrown objects. Runners can get bitten by dogs. Fortunately, it takes a bit longer to get bitten by a dog. It takes quite a while longer to get hit by a car. And it takes an average runner about 539 years to have a collision with a bicycle. Also, what can primary care physicians say to their patients about physical activity? How can this advice be integrated into the community at large? How can schools be better utilized?

MICHELI: I read somewhere once that most studies on running seem to show a decrease in body fat, an impact on obesity. Is that becoming increasingly obvious to epidemiologists?

BLAIR: Well, I think epidemiologic studies do in fact show that active people tend to weigh less and have lower body mass index, etc., and that's something that we worry about as we look at other disease end points, such as hypertension and perhaps certain cancers. We need to be sure we are not looking at an indirect effect. Whether the national exercise movement is in some way affecting national data on obesity, I guess the data at this point would suggest no.

PATE: Since the focus of this conference has been on endurance athletes, I'm wondering what if anything the epidemiologic literature indicates about the health prospects of the "radical fringe", that small segment in the population that chronically does a lot of exercise.

BLAIR: Well, the exercise injury would be one aspect to that. But if you're thinking more in terms of chronic disease, I'm not aware that anyone has a large enough population to be able to segment it out to that extent.

CANTWELL: Is it relevant to look at the morbidity of former athletes and those formerly involved in prolonged exercise?

BLAIR: Well I have reviewed some of that work in the paper, and as Roy Shephard has pointed out, some of those studies are really ancient, going back to the 19th century. I guess at this point, the data suggest that it doesn't really matter whether you are a former athlete or not. It's the current physical activity that's the important thing. We have looked at former athleticism in terms of whether or not former athletes who come to the Cooper Clinic for their first visit seem to be much different than those who are not former athletes. Their weight, their height, their cholesterol, their blood pressure, and their activity patterns really are pretty much the same in the two groups. In other words, being former athletes did not give them a better profile. As those people get to the clinic, get the exams, get the counseling, go out and do whatever they do, and then come back for another examination, the former athletes are no more likely to make changes in exercise, smoking, or losing weight.

Index

Abusive exercise, 301
Achilles tendon reflex, 303
Acid-base regulation, 85, 93, 96, 110, 114
Acute phase response, 428-429
Acute renal failure, 430, 432-434
Adipose tissue, 223
ADP (Adenosine diphosphate), 2, 14
Aerobic base, 365
Aerobic fitness, 340, 393, 396, 414
Aerobic interval training, 366-367
Aerobics activity center, 469
Aging, 76, 86, 111-112
Alanine, 223
Aldosterone, 257
Alpha brain wave activity, 303
Alpha receptor responsiveness, 65, 71
Alveolar oxygenation, 106
Amino acid carbon skeletons, 223
AMP, Adenosine monophosphate, 12
Anaerobic, energy, 9; glycolysis, 103;
    interval training, 367; metabolism, 366
Anaerobiosis, 19
Analytic issue, 339
Anatomical shunt, 83
Anatomic malalignment, 399-400
Anger, 300
Anorexia nervosa, 300
Antidepressant properties, 307
Anxiety, 303, 314; disorders, 306; neurotics,
    306; response, 306
Apathy, 380
Applied cognitive intervention, 342
Applied sport science, 360
Arousal responses, 299
Arterial, alanine, 223; oxygenation, 78, 82,
    104
Asceticism, 300
Aseptic necrosis, 402
Asymptomatic, 303
Atherosclerosis, 445
Athlete's neurosis, 301
Athletic competition, 254
Athletic pseudonephritis, 429-430
ATP (Adenosine triphosphate), 2, 14;
    aerobic, 12; anaerobic, 12; energy source,
    10, 14; concentration, 3; defined, 2; loss
    of, 10; production, 15, 31, 41; turnover,
    7-9, 17
Autonomic nervous system, 303
Averse stimuli, 302

B-hydroxybutyrate, 248
Balance theory, 330
Baseline life stress response, 305
Basic exercise science, 360
Behavioral barriers, 286

Behavior modification techniques, 324
Behaviorist theory, 330
Beta-endorphin, 296-297
Beta-lipotropin immunoeractivity, 329
Beverage effects, 263
Bicycle ergometry, 326
Biobehavioral models, 293, 331
Biochemical, deviations, 359; hypotheses,
    309; markers, 299
Biofeedback, 303, 320
Biological characteristics, 310
Bipolar depressions, 309
Blood-borne, biochemical factors, 379; fats,
    224; glucose, 225
Blood, doping, 426-428; epinephrine, 236;
    free fatty acids, 248; glucose, 227, 238;
    glycerol concentration, 250; insulin
    concentration, 224; lipids, 317; packing,
    426-428
Blunted lipolysis, 264
Body water, 253
Body water content, compensatory reflexes,
    138-142; effects of loss, 136-138, 145; shifts
    during exercise, 134-136, 143
Brain neurotransmitter changes, 298
Branching characteristics, 244
Bronchodilation, 100
Bulimia, 301
Bursitis, trochanteric 394-395, 401

C-glucose, 264
Caffeine, 251
Calcium gluconate, 257
Caloric adequacy, 215; consumption, 218
Cancer, 457, 462-463
Carbohydrate-delivery agent, 215
Carbohydrate, feedings, 264; ingestion, 269;
    metabolism, 225; oxidation, 223, 246, 248,
    251-252; source, 249; treatment, 268
Carbohydrates, 376
Cardiac arrhythmias, 243; rehabilitation, 308
Cardiac output, maintenance during
    exercise, 134, 136, 138
Cardiovascular, drift, 44-57, 71, 73; function
    markers, 260; function, 254
Catecholamine, 248
Cecal slap syndrome, 422
Central cardiovascular fatigue, 60
Central circulatory adaptations, 381
Central nervous system fatigue, 265
Central systemic control, 313
Cerebral, circulation, 307; hypoxia, 124;
    neurotransmitter metabolism, 96;
    vasoconstriction, 122
Chloride, 257

Chondromalacia, 395-396, 401
Chronic, behavioral response, 288; exercise, 304; fatigue, 452-453; training stress, 341
Circulating insulin, 248
Circulating renin activity, 257
Circulatory system, 366
Classical-low carbohydrate diet, 241
Cognitive-behavior modification, 305
Cognitive mechanisms, 341
Comfort-sensory system, 313
Compartment syndrome, 402
Complex carbohydrates, 218; diets, 235
Concentrically exercised muscle, 236
Concentric contractions, 364
Consensus elite status, 288
Consumption, preexercise meal, 252
Contact power athletes, 312
Contractions, muscle, 364
Control-mixed diet, 241
Convection, 253
Core temperature, 256
Coronary, angiography, 64; artery disease, 43-44
Cortisol, 257; response to exercise, 170-174, 196
Cross training technique, 381
Cumulative metabolic acidosis, 78
Cutaneous, blood flow, 45-46, 53; vascular capacity, 255; vasodilation, 45, 60, 132, 138
Cycling, 377

Dehydration, 244, 257
De novo synthesis, 223
Depression, 298, 306, 314
Detraining, 380
Diabetes, 463-464
Diastolic fatigue, 72; pressure, 47-48
Diet analysis, 220
Dietary carbohydrate, 229; consumption, 232; intake, 231
Dietary patterns, 220
Dietary practices, 218
Dietary protein content, 218
Dietary protein deficiency, 223
Dietary treatments, 241
Dilutional pseudoanemia, 416-419, 423
Distracting anxiety ruminations, 303
Diuresis, 23
Dopamine, 298, 307
Dyspnea, 97, 100, 113, 115

Early repletion, glycogen stores, 231
Eccentric contractions, 364
Eccentric exercise, 236
Economy of motion, 361
Ectotherm, 125
Efficacy of goals, 337
Ego-strength, 294
Electrocardiogram, 379
Electroencephalograms, 303
Electrolyte, distributions, 256; hormonal response, 192-194; replacement, 260; response to exercise, 191-192; supplements, 260
Electrolytes, 253

Electromyograms, 303
Elevated blood insulin, 264
Elevated insulin concentration, 246
Elevation, 257
Elite athletes, 219
Embden-Meyerhof pathways, 10, 12-13, 15
Emotional, behavior, 301; responses, 301
Emptying rates, 262
Endocrine, pathways, 299; response, 156
Endogenous, carbohydrate oxidation, 268; opiates, 379; pyrogenic effect, 311; triglyceride, 223
Endorphins, 297, 307; effects of exercise, 187-188; effects of training on, 189-191
Endotherms, 125
Endurance athlete, 216
Endurance performance, cycling, 243
Energy expenditure consumption, 215
Enhanced glycogen breakdown, 246
Enkephalins, 187-188, 307
Environment, muscle glycogen breakdown, 227
Enzyme protein, 222
Epidemiologic studies, 323
Epinephrine concentration, 224
Ergogenic effect, 250
Esophageal disfunction, 435
Euglycemia, 37
Evaporation, 253
Exercise, capacity, 215, 248; clinicians, 326; compliance, 324; defined, 444; dependence, 301; diffusion capacity, 108; hyperpnea, 77-80; motivation, 301; pathophysiology, 111; physiologists, 218; prescription, 320; rehabilitation, 309, 466-467; stress, 297; therapy, 339
Exertional, rhabdomyolysis, 432-433; strain indicators, 326
Exhaustive, exercise, 239; interval runs, 373
Exogenous glucose, 264-265
Expectancy theory, 331
Extravascular fluid, 82, 85, 100, 110
Extraverted, 311

Facet syndrome, 400
Fasting treatments, 248
Fasting, 252
Fast-twitch fibers, 223
Fatigue factor, 283
Fatigue, 365
Fat, metabolism, 224; oxidation, 224
Fatty acid, concentration, 251; degradation, 251; oxidation, 224
Fatty acids, 251
Femoral bone density, 398
Fiber types, ATP concentrations in, 2; blood flow to, 26; circumferential, 62; in human skeletal muscle, 2, 11; muscle, 5, 14; of animals, 2-3, 5, 38; of man, 5; oxidative, 5, 25-26; recruitment of, 23
Fibrinalysis, 418
Fluid replacement, 253; techniques, 365
Fluid replenishment, 253, 257; regimens, 259
Fluids, hormonal response, 192-194; response to exercise, 191-192

Footstrike hemalysis, 420-421, 424-425
Fractional utilization, 362
Free fatty acids, 248
Fructose, 230, 249; carbohydrate, 22-23;
function liver, 41-42; oxidation, 268
Fuel, catabolism, 126; depots, 221;
homeostasis, 195; oxidation, 225; supply,
363
Fusimotor feedback, 303

Galactose, 4
Gas exchange surface morphology, 108
Gastric emptying, 261-262
Gastrointestinal, bleeding, 422-423, 434-437;
distress, 269
Generic, contractions, 364; determinants of
performance, 375
Genu varum, 400-401
Glomecular permeability, 430
Gluconeogenesis, 223, 228, 264
Glucose, clamp technique, 166-167;
oxidation, 268; paradox, 40-41; polymer
trial, 251; syrup ingestion, 238
Glycerol, 248; ingestion, 250
Glycolytic pathway, 22
Goal setting, theory, 330-331; mechanisms,
336
Gonadatrophic hormonal response,
androgen levels, 185-186; estradiol levels,
184-185; function, 179-189; progesterone
levels, 184-185
Group, outpatient, 337; psychotherapy, 309
Growth hormone, metabolic actions, 174-
179, 189; response to exercise, 177-178
Guar gum (dietary fiber), 235

Haemoptysis, 100
Haldane Effect, 95
Hard-easy training pattern, 374, 377
Heat, dissipation, 253; stress, 365
Hedonic neutrality, 301
Hemaptysis, 64, 66
Hematuria, 431-432
Hemoblobinuria, 429
Heterogenity, 26
Hexose, 230
High glucagon, 232
High intensity exercise, 225
High liver glycogen stores, 229
High volume training, 374, 377
Hill work, 377
Homeostasis, 261; blood pressure, 113, 140
Homeotherm, 125
Hormonal response, 156, 161; effect of
metabolic change, 157; hydration, 193-194;
importance to glucose homeostasis, 162-
170; rate of endogenous opiates, 188-189;
to heat stress, 193-194; to prolonged
exercise, 194-197
Hormone, concentrations, 259
Hormone-sensitive lipase, 225
Hostile environments, 319
Humoral input, 78, 101, 109
Hydrolysis, 9
Hyperarousal, 310

Hyperinflation, 112
Hyperkalemic cardiac arrhythmia, 434
Hyperpnea, 86, 102, 121
Hypersensitive, 251
Hyperthermia, 45, 67; as consequence of
heat/exercise, 134, 138
Hypertonic sugar solution, 259
Hyperventilatory, compensation, 78; drift,
113
Hypervolemia, 191
Hypnotically hallucinated exercise, 317
Hypnotic suggestion, 303
Hypocapnia, arterial, 78, 94-95, 101
Hypocapnic-induced vasoconstriction, 96
Hypoglycemia, 7, 31, 145, 228; prevention,
156-169, 195-197; prolonged exercise, 159
Hyponatremia, 260
Hypothalamic amenorrhea, 184-185, 198
Hypotonic beverage, 258
Hypovalemia, 136-137, 140
Hypoxemia, 95, 106, 110, 112

Iceberg profile, 289
Idiosyncratic differences, 326
Immune responses, 293
Incongruous motivational profile, 292
Induced erythrocythemia, 426
Ingested fructose, 268
Inhibitory opponent process, 301
Initial muscle glycogen concentrations, 239
Insulin receptors, 158-159, 161
Insulin sensitivity, 247
Intensity of exercise, 226
Intensity prescriptions, 324
Interindividual, 292
Interstitial spaces, 254
Intestinal, absorption, 261; ischemia, 422-
423, 436
Intracellular, concentrations, 257;
dehydration, 38, 55; spaces, 254
Intraindividual, 292
Intramuscular triglyceride stores, 224
Intravascular hemolysis, 422, 425-426
Intrinsic personality, 310
Introversion, 300, 311
Iron deficiency anemia, 420-424
Iron status, 218
Irritability, 380
Ischemic death, 402
Isokinetic bicycle, 267
Isokinetic dynamometers, 399
Isotonic drink, 258; saline, 258

Jenkins Activity Survey, 330

Labile mood shifts, 290
Lack of appetite, 380
Lactate threshold, 227, 362
Lactic acidosis, 109
Left ventricular end-diastolic diameter, 381
Leu-enkephalin, 297, 314
Life stressors, 305
Limbic structures, 299
Lipid, mobilization, 224; oxidation, 264;
stores, 225

Lipolysis, 224
Lipoprotein lipase activity, 224
Liver glycogen synthesis, oral ingestion, 230
Local fatigue, 368
Locomotor muscle, fatigue, 106, 115; oxidative capacity, 109; perfusion, 114
London Marathon, 434
Longevity, 445, 472-474
Long, slow distance (LSD) training, 365
Lordosis, 400
Low back sway, 400
Lower respiratory exchange ratio, 237, 248
Low insulin, 232
Lung, morphology, 108; recoil, 111
Lymphatic drainage capacity, 110

Macrotrauma, 394
Magnesium, 257
Magnetic resonance, 298
Maladaptation to training, 380
Maladaptive state, 378
Maltodextrins, 247, 268
Manual labor, 254
Marathon training, 373
Maximal, oxygen uptake, 361; training doses, 374
Mechano-receptor-type feedback, 78, 80, 102
Meditation, 303, 342
Medium-chain triglycerides, 251
Mental stress tolerance, 294
Meta-analytic strategies, 340
Metabolic, acidosis, 82, 97, 101, 109; capacity, 109; end-products, 360
Metabolism, 307; monoamines, 298
Microtrauma, 394, 399
Minimal protein intake, 223
Mitochondria, ATP site, 9; damage, 65, 72; enzymes, 30; oxidation, 17, 19; protein, 18, 19; volume density, 108
Mitochondrial content, 224
Mode of exercise, 226
Monoamine, 298
Monoamine systems, 297
Mood disturbance, 289
Morphological, 359
Motivation, 288, 330
Motivational responses, 301
Motivation mechanisms, 330
Movement velocity, 216
Muscle, biopsies, 237; biopsy technique, 18; capillaries, 224; damage, 236; energy use in, 126; enzyme, 379; fiber recruitment, 366; hypertrophy, 222; metabolic variables, 359
Muscle glycogen, 222, 225; depletion, 366; limiting factor, 227; normal levels, 231; oxidation, 268; predepletion concentration, 232; stores, 231; synthesis, 231, 233; utilization, 226
Muscle-tendon imbalance, 400
Muscular contraction, 222
Musculoskeletal conditioning, measure of, 398-400
Myocardial, dysfunction, 59-60, 66, 72-73; fatigue, 60; function, 366; infarction, 43,

60, 66; preejection period, 296; transmural anterior, 44, 73
Myofibrils, 72
Myoglobinemia, 433
Myoglobinuria, 429
Myophosphorylase, 23

Need theory, 330
Nephritis, 430, 432-434
Neural, factors, 238; pathway, 299
Neurobiological mechanisms, 296, 341; processes, 306; response, 299
Neurobiology, 298
Neuroendocrine, responses, 295; stress, 299
Neuroleptic, 311
Neurological relaxation response, 304
Neuromuscular, function, 382; recruitment patterns, 366; tension, 320
Neurophysiological patterns, 304
Neuroticism, 314
Neurotransmitters, 307
Nibbling patterns, 216
Norepinephrine, 307
Nuivariate model, 313

Optimal constant rate, 244
Optimal curve, 286
Optimal metabolic strain, 326
Optimal training doses, 374
Oral glucose, 230
Oregon system, 374
Organ-specific, 359
Orthopedic risks, 323
Osteoarthritis, etiology, 397
Overtraining, 378
Overuse injuries, anatomic sites, 400-402; cycling, 403-404; running, 396-397; swimming, 403; risk factors, 397-400; triathlon, 404; types, 394-396
Overwork, 378
Oxidative capacity, 224
Oxidative energy supply, 224
Oxidation of carbohydrate, 225

Pace/tempo training, 367
Pancreatic insulin release, 264
Panic disorder, 306
Patello-femoral stress syndrome, 395-396, 401
Pathological adaptations, 341
Pathological barriers, 286
Perceived, discomfort, 342; environmental stress, 294; exertion, 342
Perceptual conflict, 295
Performance, enhancement, 363; peak, 373, 383
Peripheral, conductance, 366; insulin resistance, 464
Personal adaptability, 294
Personality, 343; research, 311; traits, 300
Phlebotomy, 418
Phobias, 306
Phosphagens, 375
Physical activity, 444; assessment, 446-448; participation status of Americans, 448-452
Physical fitness, 445, 452-455

Physiological, approaches, 303; mediators, 314; reactivity, 295; responses, 342; variables, 338
Physiologic variables, determinants, 360
Pituitary hormones, 296
Planing position, 376
Plantar fascitis, 402
Plantaris, 103-104
Plasma cortisol concentration, 258
Plasma glucose, levels during prolonged exercise, 159-162, 166
Plasma magnesium concentrations, 257
Plasma norepinephrine, 298
Plasma volume, 254
Plasma volume losses, 254, 259
Pleural pressure, 102
Polymerization, 4
Positron emission tomography, 298
Postexercise glycogen synthesis, 234
Postexhaustion disposal, 230
Postmyocardial infarction patients, 321, 335
Postprandial blood glucose, 235
Potassium concentrations, 257
Potential exercise pathology, 334
Power output, 342
Precompetition, hydration, 258; meal, 215
Predepletion muscle glycogen concentration, 240
Preexercise, fructose feeding, 250; meal, 245; water feeding, 258
Preferred exertion, 342
Prehydrated condition, 258
Preoptic anterior hypothalamus, 131-132
Pressure load, heart, 366
Primary, mode of exercise, 382; phase, 301; substrates, 221
Progressive, dehydration, 254; relaxation, 303
Prolactin, 296
Prolonged, exercise, 300, 444-445; fasting, 248
Prolonged moderate intensity runs, 374, 377
Protein, degradation, 222; oxidation, 222; precursors, 223; synthesis, 222
Proteinuria, 430-431
Psychological, hardiness, 294; investigation, 340; states, 311; traits, 311
Psychometric depression, 308
Psychometric test, self-motivation, 290
Psychopathology, 301
Psychophysical responses, 312
Psychophysiological reactivity, 296
Psychosocial stress, 295
Psychosomatic disorders, 293
Pulmonary, gas exchange, 80, 82, 93, 112, 114; rehabilitation, 467-468; vasodilation, 94

Quadrupeds, 107

Radical behaviorism, 330
Range restriction, 340
Rapid eye movement (REM) sleep, 310
Reactive depression, 292
Reactivity to mental stressors, 341

Relative humidity, 253
Relaxation response, 310
Reliability, 340
Reproductive function, 181-191, 197
Respiratory, alkalosis, 97; drift, 71; exchange ratio, 238
Respiratory muscle force development, 106-107
Restricted prescription, 323
Runner's trots, 434-437
Running addiction, 301

Saline, feedings, 258; ingestion, 257; solution, 257
Sarcoplasmic reticulum, 251
Seasonal variation/peaking, 375, 377
Secondary phase, 301
Sedentary counterpart, 216
Self-motivation, 294
Self-perception, 343
Self-regulation, 327
Self-selected power output, 315
Self-selection, 305
Serotonergic, 311
Serotonin, 298, 307
Severe hyponatremia, 260
Sharpening activities, 383
Shin splints, 401-402
Shock-avoidance task, 296
Sickle cell trait, 432-434
Simple carbohydrate, 235
Slave process, 301
Sleep disturbances, 380
Slow-twitch fibers, 223
Social mechanisms, 341
Somatic alternatives, 303
Somatic symptoms, 305
Sound stressors, 295
Specific endurance, 283
Specificity, 364, 381
Speed training, 367
Spinal fluid changes, 298
Spinning, 377
Splanchnic, circulation, 52; glucose, 230
Spondylolysis, 400
Sports anemia, 416
Sports nutritionists, 218
Standard mental stressor, 295
Strength training, 375, 378
Stress, adaptations, 299; coping, 294; erythrocytosis, 417-419, 427; fracture, 395, 399, 401-402; hormone profiles, 300; hormones, 317; modalities, 299
Stress-induced gastric lesions, 299
Stretching, 368
Sucrose feedings, 267
Suppression, 300
Sweating capacity, 366; response, 255
Swimming, 375
Sympathetic nervous system, 299
System-specific, 359
Systolic fatigue, 72; pressure, 47

Tachypneic, hyperventilation, 98, 103, 113, 115; response, 101, 104, 110, 120-121

INDEX **493**

Tapering exercise regimen, 241
Tempo runs, 374
Tendinitis, 394-395; iliopsoas, 401
Tension reduction, 303
Thermal balance, 47, 49, 130
Thermoregulation, 260
Thermoregulatory deviations, 359
Thrombosis, 74; risk, 418
Thrombotic stroke, 427
Tibia vara, 400-401
Tissue-specific adaptations, 359
Training, effects retention, 381; motivation, 288; practices, 378; progression, safe rates, 399-400; systems, 368; techniques, 364, 373; variables, 338; yardage, 383; year, 378
Tranquilizing medication, 342
Trans-diaphragmatic pressure, 105
Transvascular hydrostatic pressure, 82
Triathletes, 218
Tricyclic antidepressants, 310
Triglycerides, 223
Trochanteric bursitis, 401
Tubular reabsorption, 430

Ultraendurance runs, 310
Ultramarathon, 361

Unipolar depression, 308

Valence-expectancy theory, 333
Valences, 331
Vasoconstriction, 49, 52; dermal, 47; regional muscular, 47
Vasopressin, 257
Vastus lateralis, 240
Venous return, 381
Ventilation/perfusion ratio, 49-50
Ventilatory, acclimatization, 113; chemosensitivity, 109; drift, 86, 97, 101, 110; minute volume, 312; response, 86-92, 98, 109; threshold, 327
Ventricular filling pressure, 255
Vertebral bone density, 398
Volitional performance, 108
Volume load, 366
Voluntary dehydration, 257

Water feedings, 258
Water running, 382
Weight training, 368
Wet muscle weight, 257
Worksite fitness facilities, 320
World endurance records, 283